Textbook of
Orthodontics

W0193344

Textbook of
Orthodontics

K Vijayalakshmi MDS (Ortho)
Former Professor and Head
Department of Orthodontics and
Dentofacial Orthopedics, and

Principal
Best Dental Science College
Madurai, Tamil Nadu

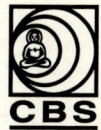

CBS Publishers & Distributors Pvt Ltd

New Delhi • Bengaluru • Chennai • Kochi • Kolkata • Mumbai
Bhopal • Bhubaneswar • Hyderabad • Jharkhand • Nagpur • Patna • Pune • Uttarakhand • Dhaka (Bangladesh)

Disclaimer

Science and technology are constantly changing fields. New research and experience broaden the scope of information and knowledge. The author has tried her best in giving information available to her while preparing the material for this book. Although all efforts have been made to ensure optimum accuracy of the material, yet it is quite possible some errors might have been left uncorrected. The publisher, the printer and the author will not be held responsible for any inadvertent errors, omissions or inaccuracies.

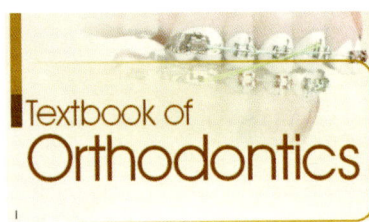

ISBN: 978-93-87964-06-8

Copyright © Author and Publisher

First Edition   2020

All rights reserved. No part of this book may be reproduced or transmitted in any form or by any means, electronic or mechanical, including photocopying, recording, or any information storage and retrieval system without permission, in writing, from the author and the publisher.

Published by Satish Kumar Jain and Produced by Varun Jain for
CBS Publishers & Distributors Pvt Ltd
4819/XI Prahlad Street, 24 Ansari Road, Daryaganj, New Delhi 110 002, India.
Ph: 23289259, 23266861, 23266867   Fax: 011-23243014   Website: www.cbspd.com
                                                                                e-mail: delhi@cbspd.com; cbspubs@airtelmail.in.
Corporate Office: 204 FIE, Industrial Area, Patparganj, Delhi 110 092, India
Ph: 4934 4934   Fax: 4934 4935   e-mail: publishing@cbspd.com; publicity@cbspd.com

Branches

- **Bengaluru:** Seema House 2975, 17th Cross, K.R. Road, Banasankari 2nd Stage, Bengaluru 560 070, Karnataka
  Ph: +91-80-26771678/79   Fax: +91-80-26771680   e-mail: bangalore@cbspd.com
- **Chennai:** 7, Subbaraya Street, Shenoy Nagar, Chennai 600 030, Tamil Nadu
  Ph: +91-44-26260666, 26208620   Fax: +91-44-42032115   e-mail: chennai@cbspd.com
- **Kochi:** 42/1325, 1326, Power House Road, Opp KSEB Power House, Eranakulam 682 018, Kochi, Kerala
  Ph: +91-484-4059061-65   Fax: +91-484-4059065   e-mail: kochi@cbspd.com
- **Kolkata:** No. 6/B, Ground Floor, Rameswar Shaw Road, Kolkata-700014 (West Bengal), India
  Ph: +91-33-2289-1126, 2289-1127, 2289-1128   e-mail: kolkata@cbspd.com
- **Mumbai:** 83-C, Dr E Moses Road, Worli, Mumbai-400018, Maharashtra
  Ph: +91-22-24902340/41   Fax: +91-22-24902342   e-mail: mumbai@cbspd.com

Representatives

Bhopal	0-8319310552	**Bhubaneswar**	0-9911037372	**Hyderabad**	0-9885175004
Jharkhand	0-9811541605	**Nagpur**	0-9421945513	**Patna**	0-9334159340
Pune	0-9623451994	**Uttarakhand**	0-9716462459	**Dhaka (Bangladesh)**	01912-003485

Printed at   HT Media Ltd., Greater Noida, UP, India

to
My parents,
husband
and
children

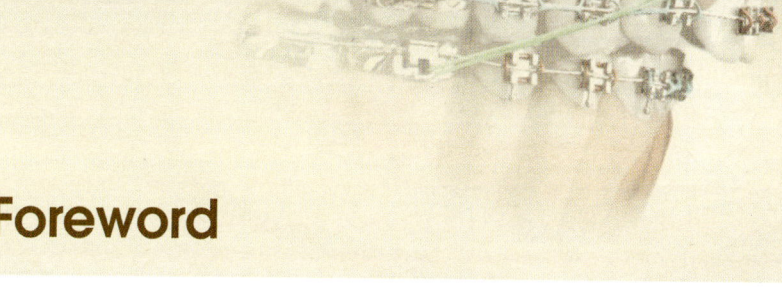

Foreword

I am happy to write foreword and deeply delighted to understand that this beautifully coordinated team effort of all the contributors brings in the new millennium with a fine opus that will provide both the students and clinicians with the very latest and best information in orthodontics.

This extremely comprehensive text can serve as fundamental information with latest technology, current concepts for undergraduate, postgraduate students and other practitioners. It is a veritable gold mine of information.

It is my hope that this book will demystify the nature of orthodontics and enliven the reader's interest. I congratulate the author and all the contributors for the success of this book.

Prof KR Arumugam
Chairman, Ultra Trust
Best Dental Science College
Madurai, Tamil Nadu

Preface

This book is the culmination of the elaborative work done over several years. Compiling and producing the orthodontic subjects in a book form has taken nearly two years. I wish to acknowledge the help and utmost care provided by the contributors.

I sincerely hope that the book fills the lacuna that enliven wide array of knowledge to undergraduate level of education and to certain extent to the postgraduate students and practitioners as a quick reference guide.

This book covers the entire area including current knowledge and subjects like nanotechnology, implants, magnets, laser, invisalign, photography and computers in orthodontics, molar distalizer and all kinds of appliances including fixed functional appliances. A special mention about the chapter of radiography in orthodontics gives better knowledge.

In the following chapters, the reader can be benefited in both theoretical and practical methods for diagnosis and treatment. This book takes a sequential approach to diagnosis and treatment planning with emphasis on esthetic objectives combined with occlusion as well as functional esthetics.

This book emphasizes non-surgical orthodontic treatment and includes important factors in differentiating extraction from non-extraction treatment.

To institute realistic goals and effective mechanotherapy, the clinician requires clear and unequivocal answers to situations they routinely face: Can orthopedic effects to be obtained in the maxilla and mandible? Can arches be stable if expanded? Can lower incisors be flared and what is their optimal position? What is the role of molar distalization in Class II correction? Chief aim of this book is to describe in a scientific context, treatment goals, strategies and sequence which must be defined before appliance therapy.

One essential area addressed in this book is the management of adult cases. As awareness is increasing among adults seeking orthodontic treatment; hence orthodontic practitioner must have a good understanding of the best ways to treat the adult patient.

The long awaited paradigm shift in orthodontics arrived with the introduction of the invisalign system. In this book, enough information have included, what is required to understand.

Orthodontic movements that are considered difficult to accomplish with traditional methods can be achieved with minimal patient cooperation by using mini-screw implants.

I have included 30 chapters covering orthodontic materials, instruments and study model preparation with more than 700 clinical photographs, flowcharts and tables.

I hope this book will give useful information to all readers.

K Vijayalakshmi

Contributors

Arun Jai Kumar MDS, PhD
Senior Lecturer in Prosthodontics
Rajah Muthaiah Dental College and Hospital
Annamalai University, Cuddalore
Tamil Nadu

Pradeep Kumar MDS, MBBS
Oral and Maxillofacial Surgeon
Chidambaram, Cuddalore
Tamil Nadu

N Madhulika Arun Jai Kumar MDS
Sr lecturer in Oral Medicine and Radiology
Adhiparasakthi Dental College and Hospital
Melmaruvathur, Kanchipuram
Tamil Nadu

KS Premkumar MDS
Vice-Principal
Professor in Orthodontics and
Dentofacial Orthopedics
Best Dental Science College
Madurai, Tamil Nadu

Contents

Foreword by KR Arumugam .... *vii*

Preface .... *ix*

Contributors .... *x*

1. Introduction to Orthodontics 1

2. Classification of Malocclusion 4

3. Epidemiology of Malocclusion 22

4. General Principles of Growth and Development 28

5. Development of Dentition and Occlusion 57

6. Functions of Stomatognathic System 68

7. Genetics in Orthodontics 73

8. Etiology of Malocclusion 86

9. Diagnosis and Diagnostic Aids 95

    9.1. Case History and Clinical Examination 95

    9.2. Cephalometric Analysis 108

    9.3. Study Model and Model Analysis 121

    9.4. Skeletal Maturity Indicators 129

10. Biomechanics 141

    10.1. Mechanics of Tooth Movement 141

    10.2. Biology of Tooth Movement 146

    10.3. Anchorage 158

11. Preventive Orthodontics 165

12. Interceptive Orthodontics 173

13. Surgical Orthodontics 180

14. Abnormal Pressure Habits and their Management 204

15. Appliances 223

  15.1. Removable Orthodontic Appliances 223

  15.2. Expansion Appliance 245

  15.3. Removable Functional Appliances 257

  15.4. Fixed Appliances 276

  15.5. Fixed Functional Appliances 296

  15.6. Orthopedic Appliances 299

16. Methods of Gaining the Space 307

17. Treatment Plan 317

  17.1 Management of Class I Malocclusion 317

  17.2. Management of Class II Malocclusion 319

  17.3. Management of Class III Malocclusion 327

18. Early Orthodontic Treatment for Preadolescent Children 332

19. Cleft lip and Palate 353

20. Implants in Orthodontics 371

21. Laser in Orthodontics 375

22. Nanotechnology 383

23. Magnets 386

24. Radiography in Orthodontics 394

25. Retention and Relapse 407

26. Invisalign 419

27. Lab Procedures in Orthodontics 421

  27.1. Study Model Preparation 421

  27.2. Welding and Soldering 425

  27.3. Orthodontic Instruments and Orthodontic Material 430

28. Photography in Orthodontics 435

29. Computers in Orthodontics 456

30. Adult Orthodontics 466

Index *473*

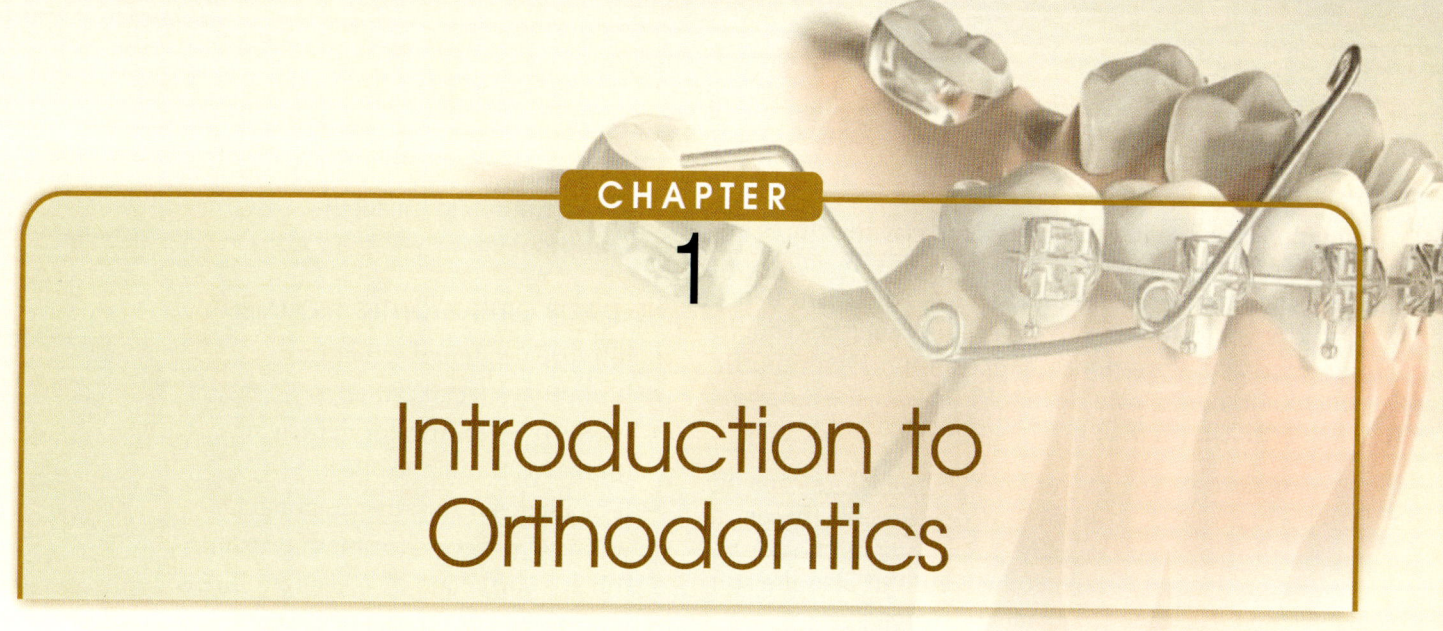

Introduction to Orthodontics

Chapter Outline

- Introduction
- Definitions
- Benefits of orthodontic treatment

- Unfavorable sequelae of malocclusion
- Need for orthodontic treatment
- Branches of orthodontics

INTRODUCTION

Orthodontics is the branch of dentistry concerned with the growth of the face, development of occlusion and the prevention and correction of occlusal anomalies/abnormalities.

The term orthodontics comes from Greek; *Ortho* means right or correct and *Odontos* means tooth. The term orthodontics was first coined by LeFoulon of France in 1839. **Edward Hartley Angle** (1855-1930) is rightly regarded as the **father of modern orthodontics**. The term "malocclusion" was first coined by Guilford. Prior to 1900s, the speciality of orthodontics was referred as "regulation of teeth". The term orthodontics has been used up to 1970s and currently designated as "orthodontics and dentofacial orthopedics". **Carabelli** in the 19th century was probably the first to describe abnormal relationship of the upper and lower dental arches in a systemic way. The terms edge-to-edge bite and overbite are actually derived from "Carabelli" system of classification.

Occlusion: When the teeth in the mandibular arch come into contact with those in the maxillary arch in any functional relation are said to be in occlusion (Wheeler).

Malocclusion: It is a condition in which there is deflection from the normal relation of the teeth to other teeth in the same arch and/or to the teeth in the opposing arch **(Gardiner, White and Leighton).**

Malrelationship: It refers to any deviation from normal relationship of mandible to maxilla in centric occlusion.

DEFINITIONS

Noyes (1911): "The study of the relation of the teeth to the development of the face and the correction of arrested and perverted development".

BSSO (British Society for the Study of Orthodontics) (1922): "The study of growth and development of the jaws and face particularly, and the body generally as influencing the position of the teeth; the study of action and reaction of internal and external influences on the development and prevention and correction of arrested and perverted development".

The American Board of Orthodontics (ABO) and the American Association of Orthodontist (AAO): Orthodontics is that specific area of dental practice that has as its responsibility, the study and supervision of the growth and development of the dentition and its related anatomical structures from birth to dental maturity, including all preventive and corrective procedures of dental irregularities requiring the repositioning of teeth by functional or mechanical means to establish normal occlusion and pleasing facial contour.

Aims

Jackson has summarized the aims of orthodontic treatment that are popularly known as **Jackson's triad** (Fig. 1.1).

They are:

Functional efficiency: Dentocraniofacial structures are involved in a number of functions like mastication, swallowing, respiration and speech. Any disturbance in the normal relationship of various structures should be analyzed for smooth functioning. Orthodontic treatment should increase the efficiency of the functions such as mastication and phonation.

Structural balance: By removing the factors causing disturbances of equilibrium of various forces, a structural balance can be achieved. Orthodontic treatment not only corrects the teeth but also the soft tissue and associated skeletal structures.

Esthetic harmony: Many malocclusions lead to poor esthetics and thus affect the person's psychological status. Orthodontic treatment should enhance the overall appeal of the individual and self-confidence of the person.

BENEFITS OF ORTHODONTIC TREATMENT

- It improves self-confidence.
- Easy to maintain the oral hygiene after proper aligning.
- The space closure after orthodontic treatment obviates the need for prosthetic work.
- It improves stomatognathic system

UNFAVORABLE SEQUELAE OF MALOCCLUSION

- It gives poor facial appearance.
- The patient cannot maintain oral hygiene.
- Poor oral hygiene leads to risk of periodontal diseases.
- Accumulation of food in crowded teeth leads to dental caries.
- Abnormalities of function.
- The patient faces psychosocial problems with malocclusion.

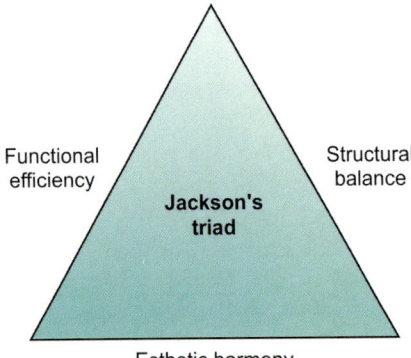

Fig. 1.1: Jackson's triad

- The most proclined anterior teeth are vulnerable for risk of trauma to the teeth.
- TMJ problem.

NEED FOR ORTHODONTIC TREATMENT

- It improves dental esthetics.
- It improves facial esthetics.
- It improves masticatory efficiency.
- It relieves traumatic bite.
- It facilitates restorative treatment.
- It improves access for tooth brushing.
- It helps correction of speech problems.
- It improves respiration in sleep apnea syndrome.

BRANCHES OF ORTHODONTICS

- Preventive orthodontics.
- Interceptive orthodontics.
- Corrective orthodontics.
- Surgical orthodontics.

Certain procedures undertaken may be common to both preventive and interceptive orthodontics. The preventive orthodontic procedures are carried out before the manifestation of a malocclusion, but the interceptive procedures are to intercept a malocclusion that has been developed already.

Preventive Orthodontics

It may be defined as the action taken to preserve "the integrity of what appears to be normal occlusion at a specific time". These actions are generally undertaken during primary dentition period. Some of the preventive procedures are as follows:

- Restoration of carious lesions of deciduous dentition that might change the arch length.
- Monitoring of eruption and shedding time table of tooth.
- Early recognition and elimination of oral habits that might interfere with the normal development of the teeth and jaws.
- Removal of retained deciduous teeth.
- Maintenance of space following premature loss of deciduous teeth to allow proper eruption of their successors.

Interceptive Orthodontics

It involves the procedures used to recognize and eliminate or reduce the severity of the potential developing irregularities and malpositions in the developing dentofacial complex. These actions are undertaken during mixed dentition period especially growth phase. Following are the interceptive procedures:

- Serial extraction.
- Correction of developing anterior crossbite.
- Control of abnormal pressure habits.
- Elimination of bony or soft tissue barrier that prevents the teeth eruption.
- Removal of supernumerary and ankylosed teeth.

Corrective Orthodontics

It recognizes the existence of malocclusion and deals with procedures utilizing mechanical appliances to reduce or correct the malocclusion and to eliminate the possible sequelae of malocclusion.

Surgical Orthodontics

It deals with minor surgical orthodontic procedures as an adjunct to orthodontic therapy and major procedures such as orthognathic surgery.

BIBLIOGRAPHY

1. Graber TM, Vanarsdall RL, et al. Orthodontics, current principles and techniques. Diagnosis and Treatment Planning in Orthodontics. Mosby, 2000.
2. Graber TM. Orthodontics: Principles and Practice. WB Saunders, 1998.

Classification of Malocclusion

Chapter Outline

- Introduction
- Methods of classification of malocclusion
- Angle's classification
- Dewey's modification for Angle's classification
- Lischer's classification
- Andrew's six keys
- Ballard's classification
- Bennett's classification

- Incisor classification
- Skeletal malocclusion
- Canine classification
- Simon's classification
- Katz's classification
- Etiologic classification
- Ackerman and Proffit classification
- Peck and Peck classification

INTRODUCTION

Edward Hartley Angle (1855–1930) started the first school of orthodontia in 1900 named as "The Angle School of Orthodontia" at St Louis. He organized the first orthodontic society and called it as "The Society of Orthodontists". In 1935, the society adopted the name it bears today, "The American Association of Orthodontist (AAO). They also established the magazine, a quarterly titled "The American Orthodontist" which turned today as "The American Journal of Orthodontics and Dentofacial Orthopedics". He promoted orthodontics as a speciality rather than part of dentistry. He contributed various appliances as shown in Fig. 2.1 and Box 2.1.

A classification system, according to **Moyers**, is grouping of clinical cases of similar appearance for ease in handling and discussion. Classification involves the grouping together of various malocclusions into simpler or smaller groups depending upon the similarities and differences. Before classifying malocclusion, standards should be set up to define a normal occlusion.

According to Strang, classification of malocclusion is a process to analysing the cases of malocclusion for the purpose of segregating them into a small number of groups, which are characterized by certain specific and fundamental variations from the normal occlusion of teeth. These variations, in turn, become influential and deciding factor in determining the correct plan of treatment.

Need for Classification (Box 2.2)

Classification is the morphological description of the dental, skeletal and soft tissue deviations from the norm. Morphological deviations from the norm can be compiled into a problem list which is essential for treatment planning.

METHODS OF CLASSIFICATION OF MALOCCLUSION (Table 2.1)

It can be broadly divided into following types.

- Quantitative and qualitative types of malocclusion (Box 2.3)

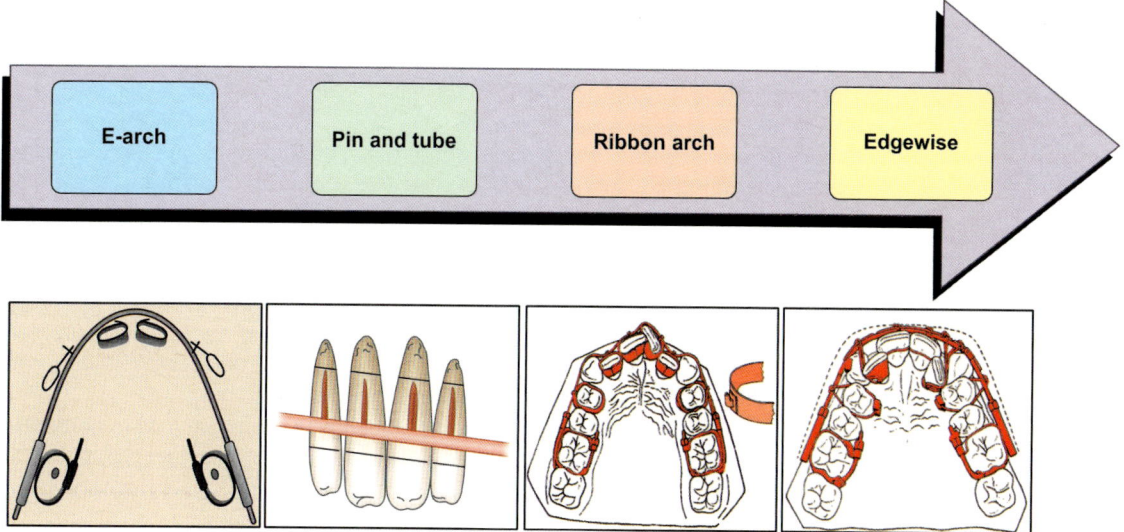

Fig. 2.1: Edward Hartley Angle's various fixed appliances

Box 2.1 Angle's contribution

- Textbook of Irregularities of the Teeth (1st ed) 1887
- Classification of malocclusion   1900
- E-arch appliance   1901
- Pin and tube appliance   1910
- Ribbon arch appliance   1910
- Edgewise appliance   1925

Box 2.2 Need for classification

- Grouping of orthodontic problems
- Location of problems to be treated
- Diagnosis and treatment problem
- Comparison of different types of malocclusion
- For self-communication
- Documentation of problems
- It is used for epidemiological studies
- Assessment of treatment effects of orthodontic appliance

- Intra-arch, interarch problem and skeletal malocclusion (Box 2.4)
- Another way to classify malocclusion: Dental, skeletal and skeletodental.
- The malocclusion can also be classified based on the deviations in different planes of space.
  a. *Malposition in sagittal plane:* These are the conditions due to abnormal relation of teeth or jaws in AP plane of space. They are:
    1. Normal occlusion: Both upper and lower arches are normally related in centric occlusion.
    2. Prenormal occlusion: Lower arch is forward to the normal position in centric occlusion.
    3. Post-normal occlusion: The lower arch is in a distal position to normal in centric occlusion.
  b. *Malposition in vertical plane:* They include normal bite, deep bite and open bite.

Box 2.3 Qualitative and quantitative types of malocclusion

Qualitative methods

- Angle's classification
- Modification of Angle's classification
- Simon's classification
- Bennett's classification
- Skeletal classification
- WHO/FDI classification
- Etiological classification
- Incisor classification
- Canine classification
- Ballard's classification
- Katz classification
- Ackerman-Proffit classification

Quantitative methods

- The PAR index
- The IOTN index by Shaw
- Massler and Frankel
- Malalignment index by Van Kurt and Pennel

Table 2.1: Summary of qualitative methods of recording malocclusion

Angle (1899)	Classification of molar relationship devised as a prescription for treatment
Stallard (1932)	The general dental status, including some malocclusion symptoms, was recorded. No definition of the various symptoms was specified.
McCall (1944)	*Malocclusion symptoms recorded include:* Molar relationship, posterior crossbite, anterior crowding, rotated incisors, excessive over bite, open bite, labial or lingual version, tooth displacements, constriction of arches. No definition of these symptoms was applied. Symptoms were recovered in all-or-none manner.
Sclare (1945)	Specific malocclusion symptoms were recorded which include Angle's classification of molar relationship, arch constriction with incisor crowding, arch constriction without incisor crowding, superior protrusion with incisor crowding, labial prominence of canines, lingually placed incisors, rotated incisors, crossbite, open bite and closed bite. No definition of these symptoms was applied. Symptoms were recovered in all-or-none manner.
Fish (1960)	Dental age was used for grouping patients. Three planes of space were considered. • *Anteroposterior relationship:* Angle's classification, anterior crossbite, overjet (mm), negative overjet (mm). • *Transverse relationship:* Posterior crossbite (manually teeth biting buccally or lingually). • *Vertical relationship:* Open bite (mm), overbite (mm). Additional measurements include labiolingual spread (Draker, 1960), spacing, therapeutic extractions, postnatal defects, congenital defects, mutilation, congenital absence, supernumerary teeth.
Bjork, Krebs and Solow (1964)	Objective registration of malocclusion symptoms based on detailed definitions. Data obtained could be analyzed by computers. Three parts: • *Anomalies in the definition:* Tooth anomalies, abnormal eruption, malalignment of individual teeth. • *Occlusal anomalies:* Deviations in the positional relationship between the upper and lower dental arches in the sagittal, vertical and transverse planes. • *Deviation in space conditions:* Spacing or crowding.
Ackerman and Proffit (1973)	Five-step procedures of assessing malocclusion (no definite criteria for assessment were given). • *Alignment:* Ideal, crowding, spacing, mutilated • *Profile:* Mandibular prominence, mandibular recession, lip profile relative to nose and chin (convex, straight, concave). • *Crossbite:* Relationship of the dental arches in the sagittal plane, as indicated by buccolingual relationship of posterior teeth. • *Angle classification:* Relationship of the dental arches in the sagittal plane. • *Bite depth:* Relationship of dental arches in the vertical plane, as indicated by the presence or absence of anterior open bite, anterior deep bite, posterior open bite and posterior collapse bite.
WHO/FDI (1979)	Five major groups of items were recorded (with well-defined recording criteria): • Gross anomalies • *Dentition:* Absent teeth, supernumerary, malformed incisors, ectopic eruption. • *Space conditions:* Diastema, crowding, spacing. • *Occlusion* – Incisal segment: Maxillary overjet, mandibular overjet, crossbite, overbite, open bite, midline shift – Lateral segment: Anteroposterior relation, open bite, posterior crossbite. • Orthodontic treatment need judged subjectively. Not necessary, doubtful, necessary, urgent
Kinaan and Bruke (1981)	Five features of occlusion measured: • Overjet (mm) • Overbite (mm) • Posterior crossbite (number of teeth in crossbite, unilateral or bilateral). • Buccal segment crowding or spacing (mm). • Incisal segment alignment (classified as acceptable, crowded, spaced, displaced or rotated following defined criteria).

Box 2.4 Another type of classification–problems in intra- and inter-arch

Intra-arch problems (Individual or groups of teeth)	Interarch problems

1. Sagittal problems
    Labioversion
    Linguoversion
    Mesioversion
    Distoversion
	1. Sagittal
	    Class II malocclusion
	    Class III malocclusion
	2. Transverse
	    Crossbite

2. Vertical problems
    Supraversion
    Infraversion
	Scissor bite
	3. Vertical
	    Deep bite

3. Rotated teeth 4. Transposition of teeth	Open bite

c. *Malposition in transverse plane:* They include normal, narrow and wide. It contributes to development of crossbites.

Importance of First Permanent Molars

- First molars are the first permanent tooth to erupt into the oral cavity.
- Upper first permanent molar is the key of occlusion.
- It takes up maximum occlusal load.
- It is the tooth of choice for anchorage.

- Loss of permanent molars may cause marked drifting of other teeth into the space.
- The mesiobuccal cusp is in line with mesiobuccal root and transmits the force to the zygomatic buttress. This is also called as key ridge.

ANGLE'S CLASSIFICATION

In 1899, **Edward Hartley Angle** published the first classification of malocclusion. The classifications are based on the relationship of the mesiobuccal cusp of the maxillary first molar and the buccal groove of the mandibular first molar. He used Roman numerical I, II and III to designate the main classes whereas Arabic numerical 1, 2 denote the divisions of the Class II malocclusion.

Angle's classification was based on the mesiodistal relation of the teeth, dental arches and jaws. Angle's assumption when formulating this classification was that the maxillary first permanent molar is always in the correct position and the variability comes from the mandible. Thus, he fixed 1st permanent molar as a key point and based on lower 1st molar deviation in relation to the upper first permanent molar, he classified the malocclusion. Angle described three classes of malocclusion designated by the Roman numeral I, II, and III, based on the occlusal relationships of the first molars (Figs 2.2 and 2.3).

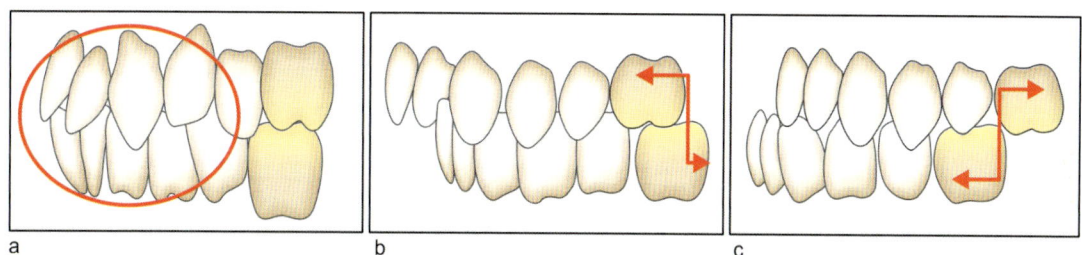

Fig. 2.2: (a) Class I malocclusion; (b) Class II malocclusion; (c) Class III malocclusion

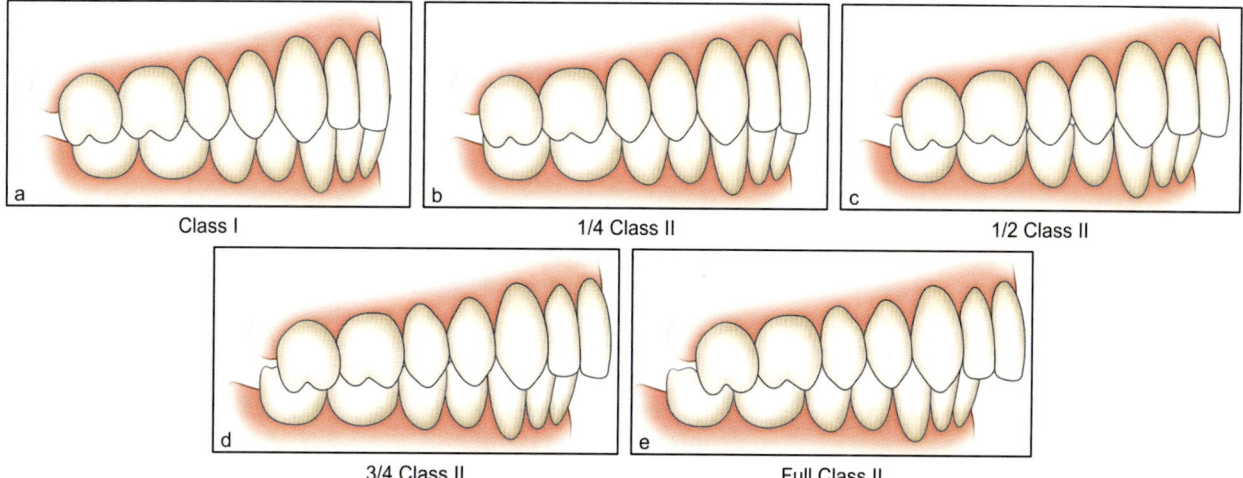

Class I   1/4 Class II   1/2 Class II

3/4 Class II   Full Class II

Fig. 2.3: Variation of molar relationship in class II malocclusion

Though many classifications emerged in course of time, Angle's system of classification is the most widely and globally accepted and used because of its simplicity in application.

Disadvantages

- Severity of malocclusion cannot be described.
- Does not consider vertical/transverse relation.
- Individual tooth malrelation is not considered.
- Does not differentiate skeletal/dental malrelation.
- If the first molar is missing, this classification cannot be applied.
- It cannot be applied to deciduous dentition.
- Did not explain about:
  - Soft tissue
  - Saddle angle
  - Cranial base rotation/gonial angle
  - TMJ associated problems

Angle's Class I Malocclusion (Box 2.5)

The mesiobuccal cusp of the maxillary first permanent molar occludes with the mesiobuccal groove of the mandibular first molar. For all sagittal malocclusion, a variation of 5° or 5 mm is acceptable because of distance between the two buccal cusps of the maxillary first molar is equal to 5 mm. So a 5-mm shift is must to shift the occlusion from normal to a Class II or Class III.

Clinical Features of Bimaxillary Protrusion

Extraoral features

- Decreased nasolabial angle due to proclined maxillary anterior
- Shallow mentolabial sulcus due to proclined mandibular anterior
- Incompetent lips
- Convex profile

Box 2.5   Angle's Class I malocclusion

Extraoral features	Intraoral features
• Mesiocephalic	• Class I molar and Class I canine
• Mesoprosopic facial form	• Good interdental digitations
• Mesomorphic type of patient	• Crowding, spacing, rotation, midline diastema and bimaxillary protrusion
• Straight or orthognathic profile	• Open bite
• Competant lips	
• Normal nasolabial angle	

Intraoral feature: Bimaxillary protrusion is most categorized under Class I, where the patient exhibits a normal Class I molar and canine relationship. It is characterized by forward placement of both upper and lower anteriors in relation to the facial profile.

Angle's Class II Malocclusion (Box 2.6)

In Angle's Class II malocclusion, the distobuccal cusp of upper first permanent molars occluding in the mesiobuccal groove of the lower first permanent molar.

- If upper and lower first molars are seen edge to edge, this is also called Angle's Class II only (Fig. 2.3).
- Class II is subdivided into division 1 and division 2 based on the inclination of the maxillary incisors.
- When a Class II molar relation exists on one side and a Class I relation on the other side, it is referred to as Class II subdivision.

Classification of Class II Malocclusion

Based on incisors relationship: Angle Class II is divided into:

- Angle's Class II division 1 malocclusion (Table 2.2)
- Angle's Class II division 2 malocclusion

Based on abnormal skeletal relationship

- Skeletal Class II division 1
- Skeletal Class II division 2

It may be caused due to any one of the following features:

- Maxillary prognathism
- Mandibular retrognathism
- Maxillary prognathism and mandibular retrognathism

Based on severity of incisor relationship: *Von der Linden:* He classified Angle Class II division 2 malocclusion into following three types based on the severity of incisor relationship.

- *Type-A:* Maxillary central and lateral incisors are retroclined. Degree of retroclination is less severe in nature.
- *Type-B:* Maxillary lateral incisors are overlapping the retroclined maxillary central incisors (Fig. 2.6).
- *Type-C:* Maxillary central and lateral incisors are retroclined and are overlapped by the maxillary canines.

Definition of competency of the lips: Both the lips are approximated without any strain when all the muscles of mastication are in relaxed condition and the teeth are in centric occlusion.

Box 2.6 Angle's Class II malocclusion

Extraoral features (Fig. 2.4)

- Ectomorphic patient (tall and thin built)
- Dolichocephalic
- Leptoprosopic facial form
- Convex profile
- Posterior divergent
- Decreased nasolabial angle
- Curled and everted lower lip
- Flaccid and loose upper lip

Intraoral features (Fig. 2.5)

- Class II molar and canine
- 'V' arch palate and constricted arch
- Oral volume is restricted
- Increased overjet and proclination of upper incisors
- Exaggerated curve of Spee
- Supraeruption of lower anterior
- Flattening of lower arch
- It may be associated with abnormal pressure habit like tongue thrusting and abnormal swallowing habit. Clinically dental open bite is noticed in some cases, there is spacing of upper anterior and lower crowding in some other cases, there is proclination of upper incisors and crowding

- Deep mentolabial sulcus
- Hyperactive mentalis muscle
- Cl II buccinator mechanism

Table 2.2: Differences between Class II division 1 and Class II division 2

Features	Class II div 1	Class II div 2 (Fig. 2.6)
Profile	Convex	Straight
Facial form	Leptoprosopic	Euryprosopic
Lips	Upper—hypotonic, short and flaccid	Upper/lower—normal
	Lower—hypertonic, everted	Competent lips
	Incompetent lips	
Mentolabial sulcus	Deep	Normal
Lower anterior facial height	Increased	Decreased or normal
Mentalis muscle	Hyperactive	Normal
Palate	Deep	Normal
Arch form	"V" shaped—constricted	"U" shaped—square in arch form
Overjet	Increased due to upper proclination	Decreased as the upper central incisors are lingually inclined. The mandibular labial gingival tissue is often traumatized (Table 2.3)
Overbite	Deep bite or open bite	Closed bite
	Classification of deep bite	
	• Mild	
	• Moderate	
	• Severe	
Incisor crown root angulation	Normal	Axes of crown and root are bent and are referred to as Collum angle
Path of closure	Normal	Backward path of closure due to retroclined upper central incisors
Interocclusal clearance	Normal	Increased
Buccinator mechanism	Class II buccinator	Patient exhibit normal perioral muscle activity

Table 2.3: Akerly classification of traumatic overbite

Akerly-1	The lower incisors occlude with the palatal mucosa causing mucosal trauma away from the palatal gingival margin
Akerly-2	The lower incisors occlude with and traumatize the palatal gingival margins of the upper incisors
Akerly-3	Traumatic occlusion leads to stripping of the lower labial and the upper palatal gingivae
Akerly-4	The incisors sheer past each other causing wear on the palatal aspects of the upper incisors and sometimes the labial aspect of the lower incisors. This may be associated with loss of posterior dental support and/or a parafunctional habit

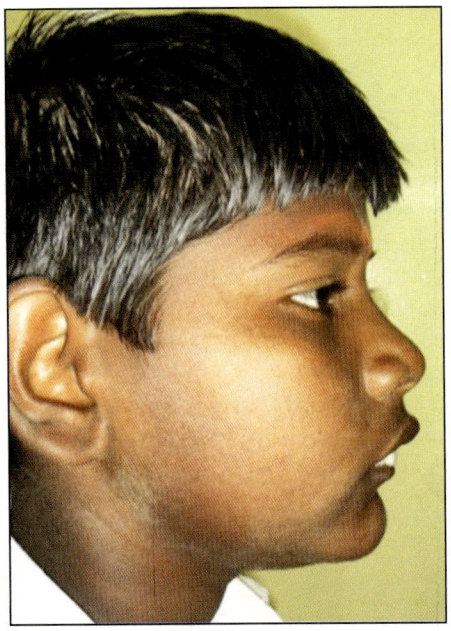

Fig. 2.4: Extraoral picture in Angle Class II

Oral Seal

There are three types of oral seal, namely anterior oral seal, middle oral seal and posterior oral seal.

Anterior oral seal: There is competency of lips and the tip of the tongue lies palatal to the cingulum of incisors.

Middle oral seal: There is contact between the dorsum of the tongue and the vault of the palate.

Posterior oral seal: There is contact between root of the tongue and the soft palate.

When anterior oral seal is broken, the incompetency of the lips is developed and the tongue no longer lies palatal to the cingulum of the incisors but it lies in between the upper and lower incisors.

Variations of Class II Division 2 Incisor Relations

1. Central incisors in lingual inclination with lateral incisors in labial inclination

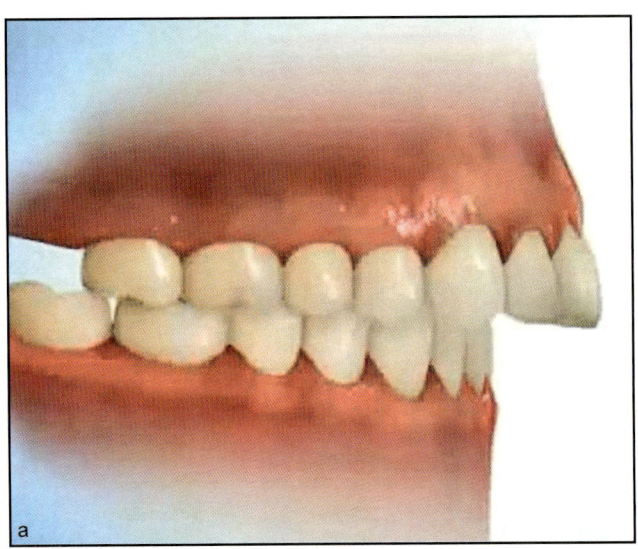

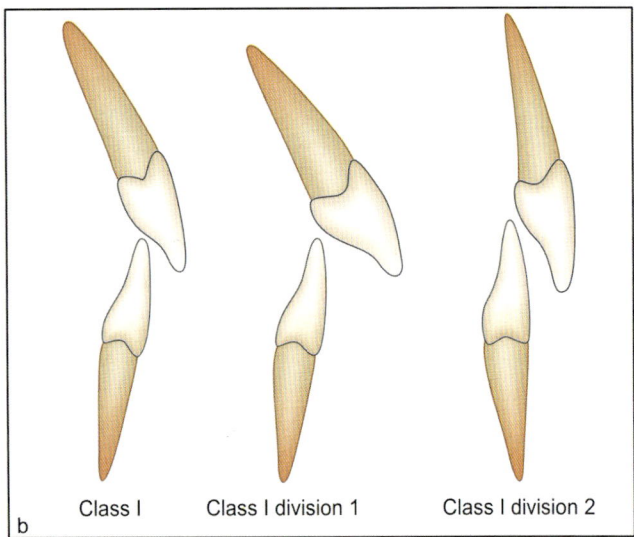

Fig.2.5: Intraoral picture in Angle Class II

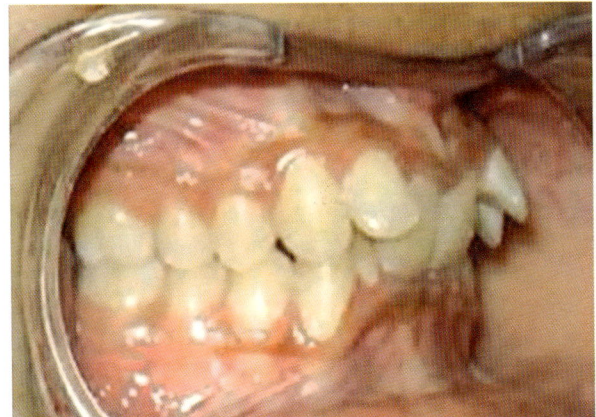

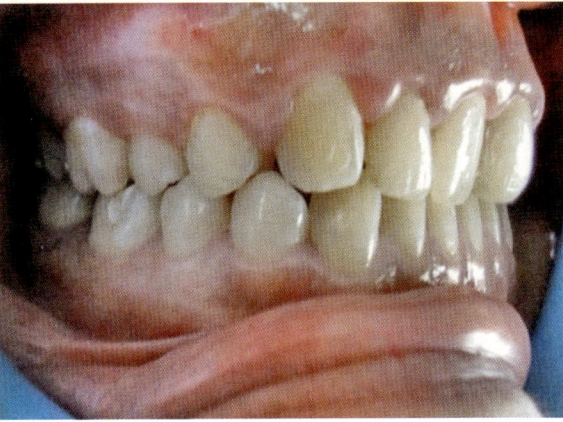

Fig. 2.6: Angle's Class II division 2 malocclusion

2. Central and lateral incisors in lingual inclination with canines labial inclination
3. Centrals, laterals and canines in lingual inclination.

Deck biss: This is a condition in which there is bilateral Class I molar relation, but the incisors are in a pattern resembling division 2 of Class II category.

Angle's Class III Malocclusion

Angle Class III is classified into following two types (Table 2.4):
* Pseudo Class III malocclusion (Fig. 2.7)
* True Class III malocclusion (Fig. 2.8)

    The condition in which Class III molar relationship present only on one side with normal relation on the other side is called Class III subdivision (Fig. 2.9).

* It is again classified into two types:
    – Dental Class III
    – Skeletal Class III

Modification of Class III

Class III molar relation with:
* *Type-1:* Edge-to-edge incisor relationship
* *Type-2:* Mandibular incisor crowding
* *Type-3:* Incisors in crossbite

Tweed in 1966 classified Class III malocclusion: It is genetically determined. The etiology may be due to:
* Normal maxilla but prognathic mandible
* Retrognathic maxilla and normal mandible
* Retrognathic maxilla and prognathic mandible
* Combination of the above

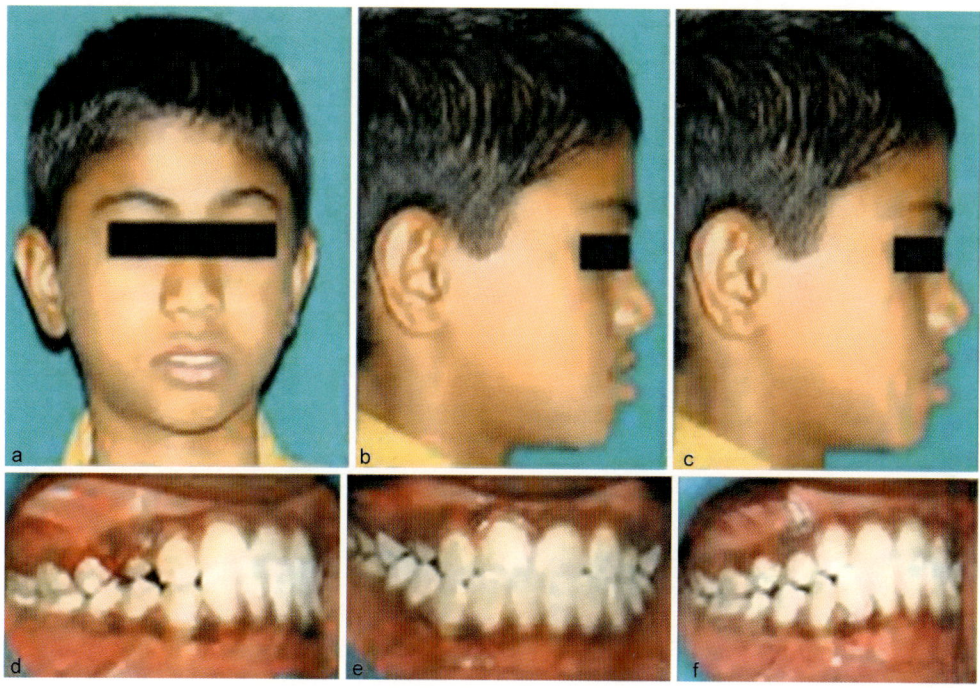

Fig. 2.7: Pseudo Class III malocclusion

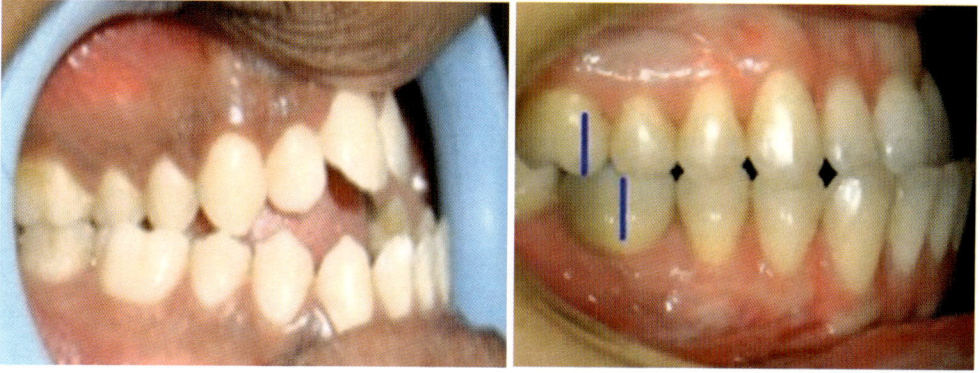

Fig. 2.8: True Class III malocclusion—intraoral picture

Table 2.4: Differences between true and pseudo Class III malocclusion

S.no.	True Class III malocclusion	Pseudo Class III malocclusion
1	Concave profile	Straight or concave profile—acquired or habitual
2	Premature contacts are absent	Premature contacts are present
3	There is forward path of closure	Deviated path closure
4	Increased gonial angle	Normal gonial angle
5	Mandible cannot be further retruded beyond edge-to-edge position	Mandible can be further retruded
6	Retroclined lower incisors	Proclined lower incisor
7	Treatment by orthopedic appliance or by orthognathic surgery after growth is completed	Elimination of premature contacts by leveling the labial surface of lower anterior and palatal surface of upper incisors

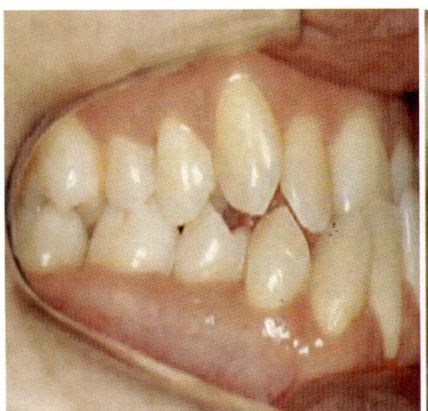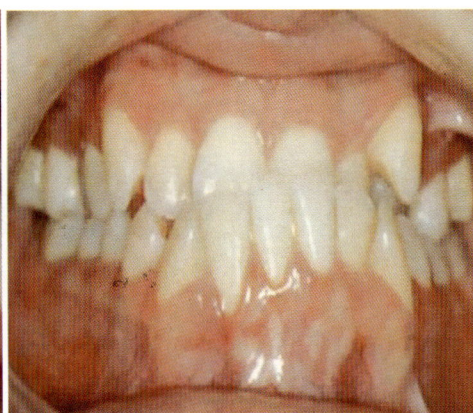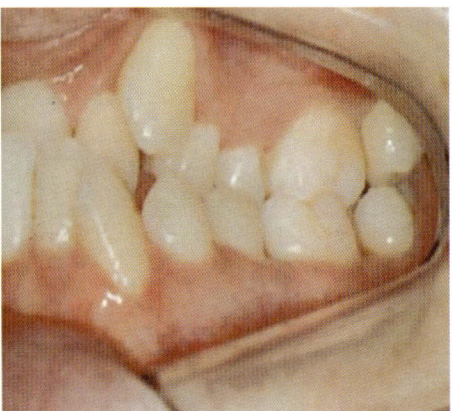

Fig. 2.9: Class III subdivision

Pseudo Class III (Fig. 2.7)

During physiological rest position, the jaws are in normal position. When they come into occlusal contact, the mandible glides anteriorly to the Class III. This is also called postural or habitual Class III malocclusion.

In premature loss of deciduous molars, the child always uses anterior teeth for mastication; thus, the mandible will glide anterioly during function. The presence of any occlusal premature contacts may deflect the mandible forward (Table 2.4).

Variations of Angle's Classes

Although not described originally by Angle in his system, these variations are important for diagnosis and treatment planning of the patients.

Super Class I: This indicates a malocclusion in which there is tendency for Class III relationship but the molar relationship cannot be described as Class I either. However, it may be considered as shift of mandibular first molar mesially by less than half cusp width variation.

Pseudo Class I: Another modification was presented by Jan De Baets and Martin Chiarini in 1995 as Pseudo Class I; a newly defined type of malocclusion. It is an apparent Class I molar and canine relationship with following features that has developed too mesially because of a combination of factors like:

1. Mesial rotation of the upper first permanent molar which may be due to the mesial shift of tooth during loss of leeway space.
2. Lower incisors crowding
3. Lack of space for the lower canines to erupt.
4. Mature pseudo-Class I also have over erupted lower second molar and anterior deep bite.
5. The Class I intercuspation in fact masks a mild dental Class II.

Class IV: It is seen when there is Class III on one side and Class II on the other side. This condition is very rare and seen in gross facial asymmetries. It was not described by Angle in his original classification, but mention in the literature.

Half-cusp relationship: Angle described the variation as full cusp change in the molar relation. However, many cases are seen which have less than full cusp or half cusp variation in molar relation. It may occur due to many factors:

1. Abnormal loss of leeway space
2. Proximal caries
3. Lack of growth
4. Abnormal development due to habits

Half-cusp Class II: Here, the relation of lower first molar with upper first permanent molar is more than one-half cusp distal to that of normal relation. It may be due to either maxillary arch forward or mandibular arch backward or loss of leeway space.

Half-cusp Class III: Here, the relation of lower first molar with upper first permanent molar is more than one-half cusp mesial to normal relation. It may be due to either maxillary arch backward or mandibular arch forward or loss of leeway space in lower arch.

Advantages of Angle's System

1. It is very simple to learn.
2. It is easy to use and reproduce.
3. It is easy for communication with other clinicians.
4. It can be easily used during research to categorize the study subjects.
5. It is not confusing, as it considers only molar relation in sagittal directon only.

Drawbacks of Angle's Classification

1. He did not consider malocclusion in the transverse and vertical planes.
2. Angle considered maxillary first permanent molars as fixed points in the skull which is not true.
3. It gives only a dental relationship rather than skeletal relationship.
4. It does not consider the soft tissues of the face.
5. It does not consider the effect of growth, growth patterns and time factors.
6. It cannot be applied, if any of the first permanent molars is extracted or missing.
7. It cannot be applied to the deciduous dentition.
8. It does not highlight the etiology of the malocclusion.
9. Individual teeth malposition are not considered.
10. It did not consider the partial cuspal variation.

DEWEY'S MODIFICATION FOR ANGLE'S CLASSIFICATION

Martin Dewey (1881–1933)—an ardent champion of non-extraction.

Dewey modified the Angle's classification with his modification in Class I and Class III (Flowchart 2.1 and Table 2.5).

Flowchart 2.1: Dewey's modification for Angle's classification

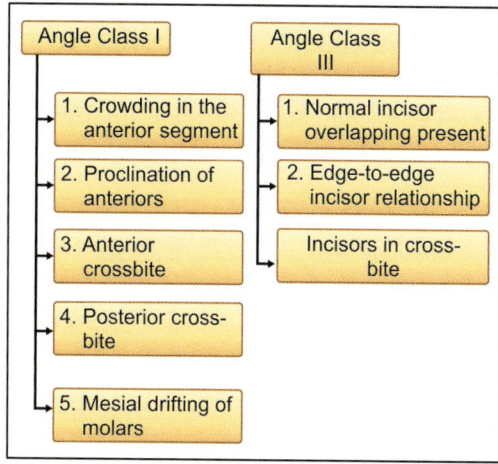

Table 2.5: Class I and Class III modification of Dewey

Class I modification of Dewey

Type-1 Class I malocclusion with crowded anterior

Type-2 Class I malocclusion with protrusive maxillary incisors

Type-3 Class I malocclusion with anterior crossbite

Type-4 Class I malocclusion with posterior crossbite

Type-5 Permanent molar has drifted mesially due to early extraction of second deciduous molar or second premolar

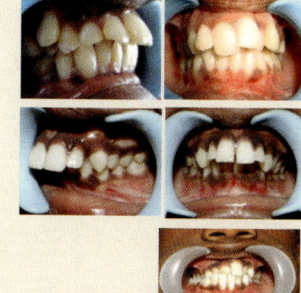
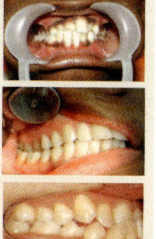
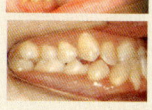
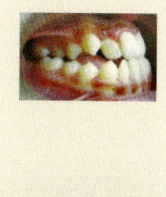

Class III modification of Dewey

Type-1 The upper and lower dental arches when viewed separately are in normal alignment. But when the arches are made to occlude the patient shows edge-to-edge incisor alignment

Type-2 The mandibular incisors are crowded and are in lingual relation to the maxillary incisors

Type-3 The maxillary incisors are crowded and are in crossbite in relation to the mandibular anterior

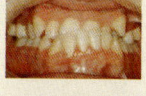
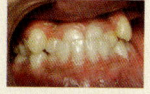

LISCHER'S CLASSIFICATION

Lischer added the suffix "version" to a word to indicate the deviation from normal position. Lischer replaced the terms Class I, II, III Angle's classification of malocclusion, with the terms neutrocclusion, distocclusion and mesiocclusion, respectively. In addition, he described other possible malpositions of a tooth or group of teeth as listed in Flowchart 2.2 and Figs 2.10 and 2.11a to c.

ANDREW'S SIX KEYS (1970) (Fig. 2.12 and Table 2.6)

Andrew extended Angle's classification:

- Correct molar relationship.
- Correct crown angulations.
- Correct crown inclination, i.e. Class I incisor relationship.
- No rotation present.
- Teeth in tight contact with no spacing.
- Occlusal plane/curve of Spee should be flat, i.e. it should not be deeper than 1.5 mm.

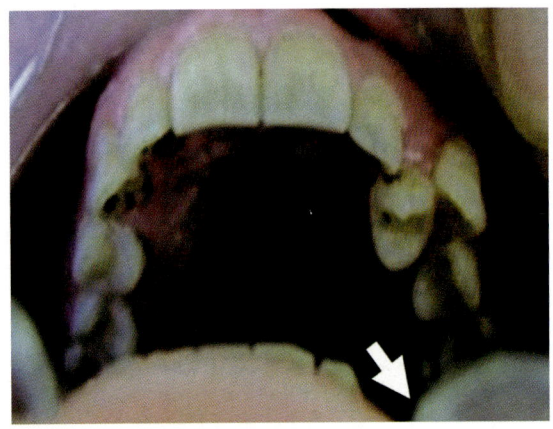

Fig. 2.10: Transposition

BALLARD'S CLASSIFICATION

Ballard's classification is based on skeletal relationship on the jaws which includes three classes (Flowchart 2.3).

Flowchart 2.2: Lischer's nomenclature for individual tooth malpositioned

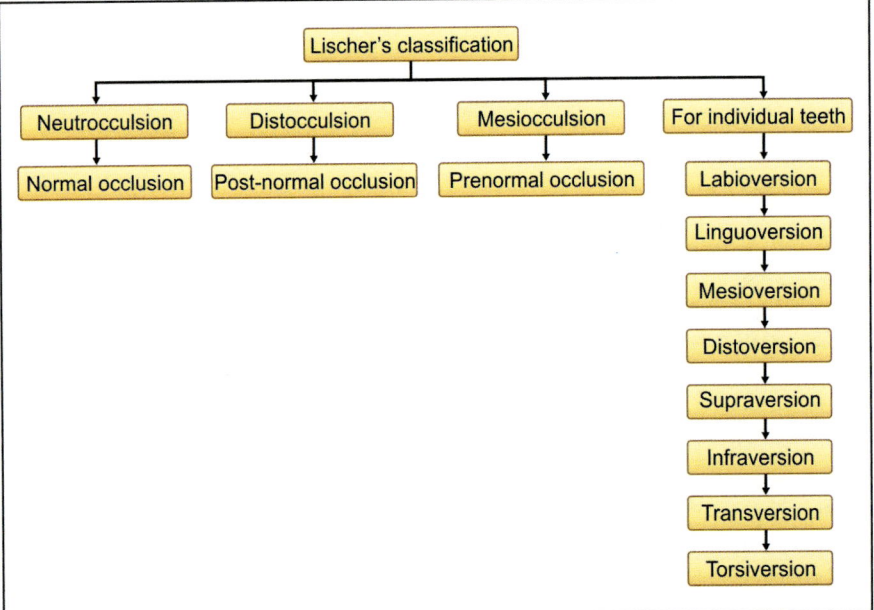

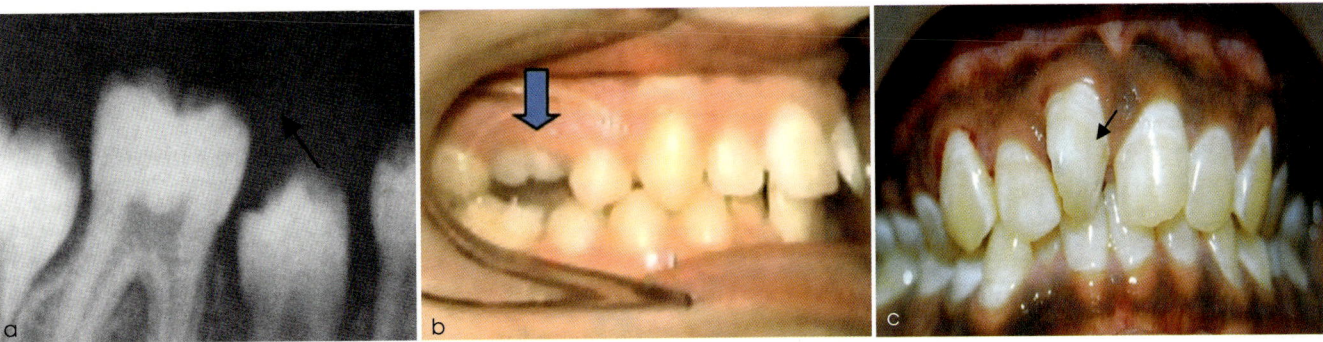

Fig. 2.11: (a) Supraversion; (b) Infraversion; (c) Mesioversion

Table 2.6: Andrew's six keys

Key-1: *Molar relationship.* The distal surface of the distal marginal ridge of the upper first permanent molar occludes with the mesial surface of the mesial marginal ridge of the lower second molar. The mesiobuccal cusp of the upper first permanent molar falls within the groove between the mesial and middle cusps of the lower first permanent molar.

Key-2: *Crown angulation or mesiodistal tip.* The gingival portion of the long axis of each tooth crown is distal to the occlusal portion of that axis. The degree of tip varies with each tooth type.

Key-3: *Crown inclination or labiolingual/buccolingual torque.* For the upper incisors, the occlusal portion of the crowns' labial surface is labial to the gingival portion. In all other crowns, the occlusal portion of the labial or buccal surface is lingual to the gingival portion.

Key-4: *Rotations.* There should be an absence of any tooth rotations within the dental arches.

Key-5: *Spacing.* There should be an absence of any spacing within the dental arches.

Key-6: *Occlusal plane.* The occlusal plane should be flat.

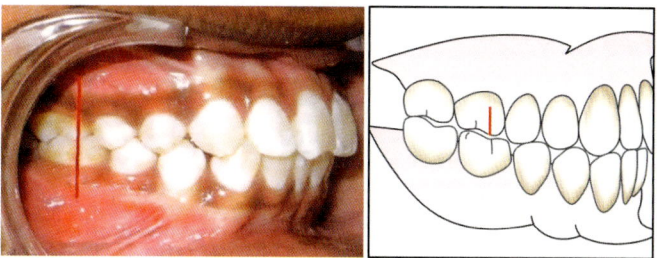

Key-1: Molar relationship

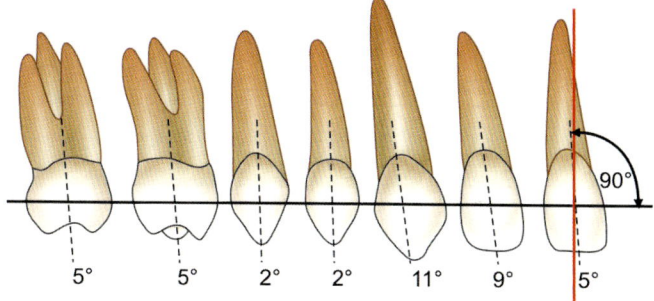

Key-2: Crown angulation

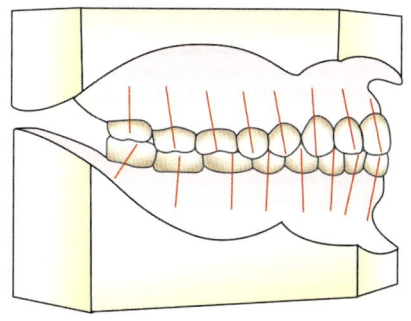

Key-3: Crown inclination

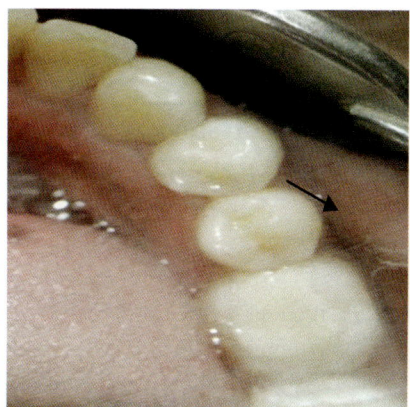

Key-4: Rotation

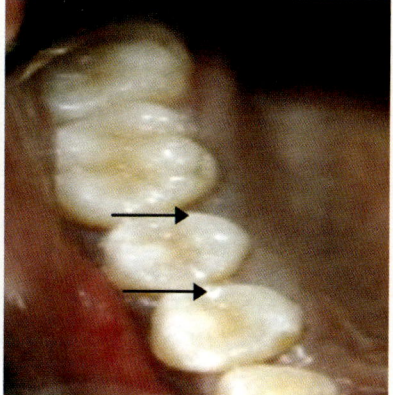

Key-5: Spacing

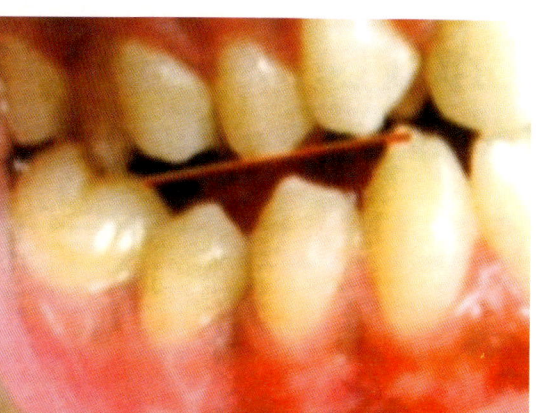

Key-6: Occlusal plane

Fig. 2.12: Andrew's six keys

Flowchart 2.3: Ballard's classification

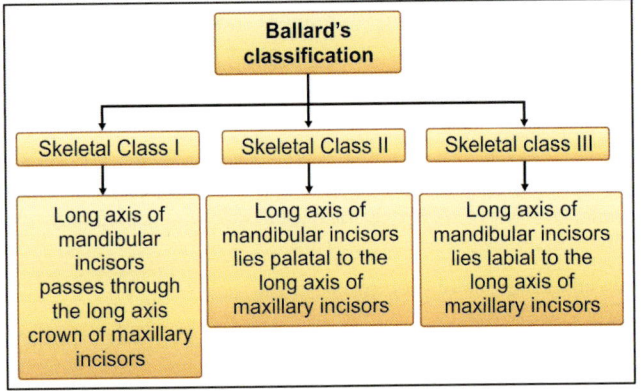

BENNETT'S CLASSIFICATION OF MALOCCLUSION

Sir Norman Bennett's classification is based on its etiology as shown in Flowchart 2.4.

Flowchart 2.4: Bennett's classification

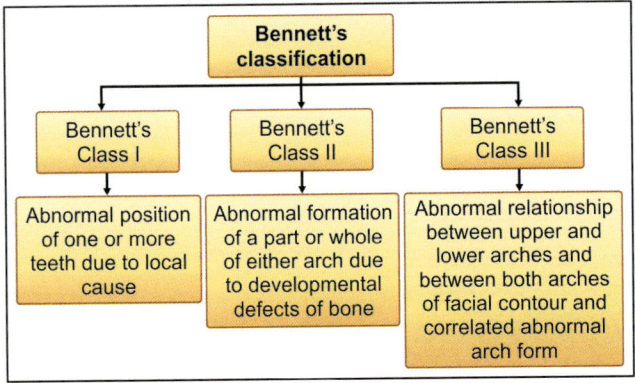

BRITISH STANDARD INSTITUTE CLASSIFICATION (INCISOR CLASSIFICATION)

This is based upon incisor relationship and is the most widely used descriptive classification. The incisor relationship does not always match the buccal segment relationship. In clinical practice, the incisor classification is usually found to be more useful than Angle's classification. The categories defined by British standard are as as given in Flowchart 2.5.

Flowchart 2.5: Incisor classification

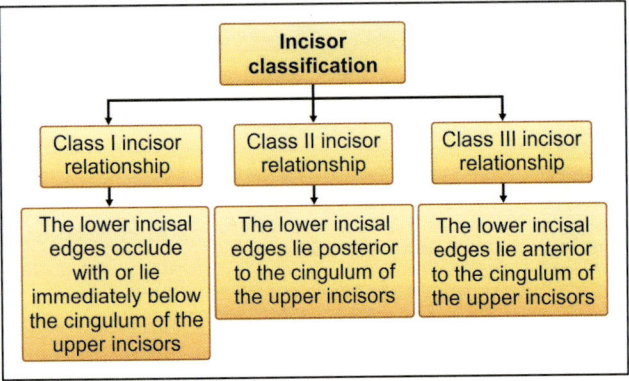

SKELETAL MALOCCLUSION

Skeletal malocclusion can occur in sagittal, vertical and transverse planes. It can be caused by defects in size, position or relationship between the upper and lower jaws. Sagittal plane malocclusion can occur in one or both the jaws or as various combinations (Flowchart 2.6).

Flowchart 2.6: Skeletal malocclusion

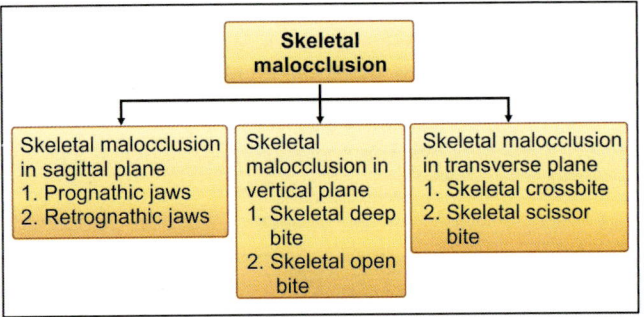

CANINE CLASSIFICATION (Fig. 2.13)

Class I: The mesial slope of upper canine coincides with the distal slope of lower canine.

Class II: The mesial slope of upper canine is ahead of the distal slope of lower canine.

Class III: The mesial slope of the upper canine lies behind the distal slope of the lower canine.

SIMON'S CLASSIFICATION

It was first described by Paul Simon, German Orthodontist in 1926 in which the teeth are related to the Frankfort, midsagittal and orbital planes. One of the best classification efforts has been made by Simon using the gnathostatic approach and orienting the dentition to anthropometric landmarks in an attempt to better show the actual relationship of the dentition in the face. Simon took the suggestion made by Bennett in 1912 that the malocclusion be categorized in three planes.

Reliability of Simon Norms

- No true bilateral symmetry in the human head.
- The orbital plane of Simon was found to pass through the canine in 81% and missed the canine in 19% of cases.
- The raphe or median sagittal plane to be symmetric in 43%, slight deviations (1–2 mm) were found in 37% while 10% showed marked asymmetry.

In Simon's classification system, the dental arches are related to three anthropologic planes (Fig. 2.14):

a. Frankfort horizontal plane or eye-ear plane.
b. Orbital plane.
c. Raphe median plane or mid-sagittal plane.

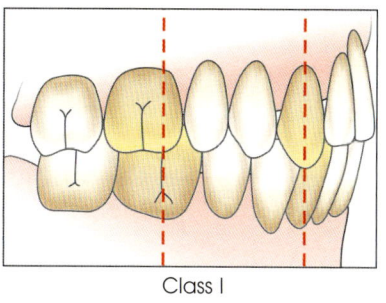 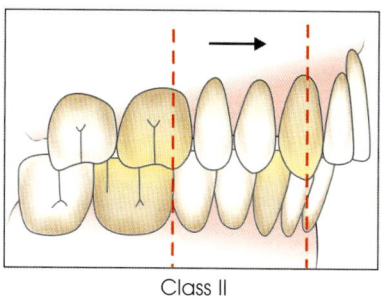

Class I   Class II   Class III

Fig. 2.13: Canine classification

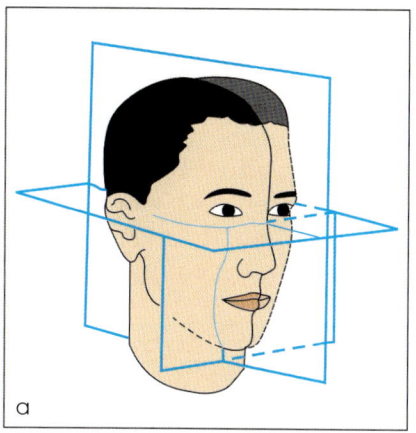

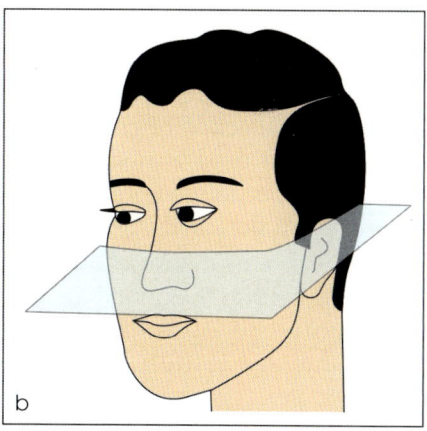 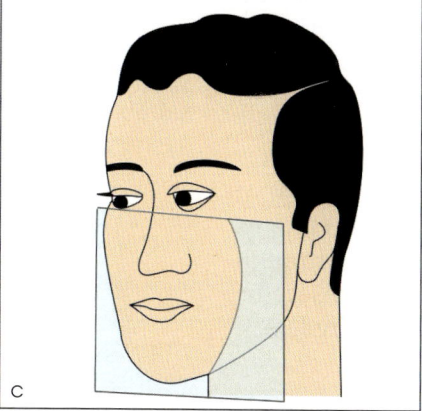 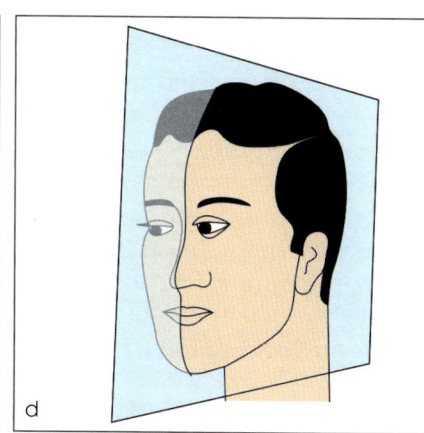

Fig. 2.14: (a) Description of Simon classification in three anthropologic planes; (b) Frankfort horizontal plane; (c) Orbital plane; (d) Sagittal plane

Frankfort horizontal plane: It is determined by the skin landmarks of the eye and ear points and runs parallel to SeN plane.
- Helps to detect deviations in the vertical plane.
- Dental arch closer to the plane is called attraction and farther away is called abstraction.

Orbital plane:
- Helps to detect deviations in the transverse plane.
- Dental arch more anteriorly placed is called protraction and posteriorly placed dental arch is called retraction.

The law of the canine: In normal arch relationship, according to Simon, the orbital plane passes through the distal axial aspect of the canine. This is known as 'the law of the canine'.

Mid-sagittal plane: This plane is formed by points approximately 1.5 cm apart on the median raphe of the palate. This plane passes at right angle to FHP.
- Helps to detect deviations in the sagittal plane.
- Dental arch closer to mid-sagittal plane is called contraction and farther away is called distraction.

KATZ'S CLASSIFICATION

It is a modified form of Angle's classification suggested in 1994 by Katz.

Class I: The most anterior upper premolar fits into the embrasure created by the distal contact of the most anterior lower premolar. With this relationship, the canines also relate correctly in Class I. Here the molar relation is not considered.

Class II: When one upper premolar correctly opposes two lower premolars, the molars are full Angle's Class II position.

Class III: When two upper premolars oppose one lower premolar, the molars are full Angle's Class III position.

Advantages of Katz's Classification

1. It can be applied to the conditions whether all premolars are present or some premolar has been extracted for orthodontic treatment. So, it can be perfectly applied in normal, pretreatment, as well as treated cases.
2. It is useful when the teeth are extracted in only one arch also.
3. It can also be applied in deciduous and mixed dentition, which is an advantage over Angle's classification. Here, the central axis of first primary molar should pass through the embrasure between both lower deciduous molars. The central axis of upper second primary molar is less accurate than first molars. The central axis of upper second primary molar is less accurate than first molars because of the leeway space. In cases, if upper first deciduous molar is prematurely lost, a line drawn through central axis of the edentulous space should bisect the embrasure between two lower deciduous molars.

Quantifying the Classification

Angle's classification lacks a numerical quantification of the degree of Class II or Class III.

Katz's classification designates ideal cusp embrasure occlusion as zero (0). A plus sign (+) is given to Class II direction and a minus sign (–) to Class III tendency.

A study done by Sinh and Rinchuse in 1998 found Katz's classification having the highest reliability. The British Standard Incisor classification system was next highest, and Angle's classification system was the least reliable.

ETIOLOGIC CLASSIFICATION

It is classified based on etiology of malocclusion.
- Osseous
- Muscular
- Dental

Osseous: It includes problems in abnormal growth, size, shape or proportion of any of the bones of the craniofacial complex. For example, Class III due to mandibular hypertrophy and Class II may be due to mandibular deficiency.

Muscular: It includes problems due to malfunction of the dentofacial musculature. They are:
1. Abnormal muscular contraction
2. Sucking habits
3. Abnormal patterns of mandibular closure.
4. Lip posture

Dental: It includes
1. Malposition of teeth
2. Abnormal number of teeth
3. Abnormal size of teeth
4. Abnormal shape or texture of teeth.

ACKERMAN AND PROFFIT CLASSIFICATION

It is a classification scheme for malocclusion in which five characteristics and their interrelationships are assessed. It is a synthesis of two schemes, the Angle's classification and the Venn diagram, both of which were proposed late in the nineteenth century. Venn proposed set theory which deals with collection of groups in this system. Ackerman and Proffit used a modified Venn diagram. In this scheme, a set is defined on the basis of morphologic deviations from the ideal.

Common to all dentitions is the degree of alignment and symmetry of the teeth within the dental arches. It is represented as Universe (group-1). Many malocclusions affect facial aesthetics and it is represented as a major set (group-2) within the Universe. Lateral (transverse), anteroposterior (sagittal) and vertical deviations and their interrelationship (groups 3 to 9) are represented by 3 interlocking subjects within the profile set (Fig. 2.15).

Experience has confirmed that a minimum of 5 characteristics must be considered in a complete diagnostic evaluation. The approach overcomes the major weakness of the Angle system.
- It incorporates an evaluation of crowding and asymmetry within the dental arches and includes an evaluation of incisor protrusion.
- It recognizes the relationship between protrusion and crowding.
- It includes the transverse and vertical as well as the anteroposterior planes of space.

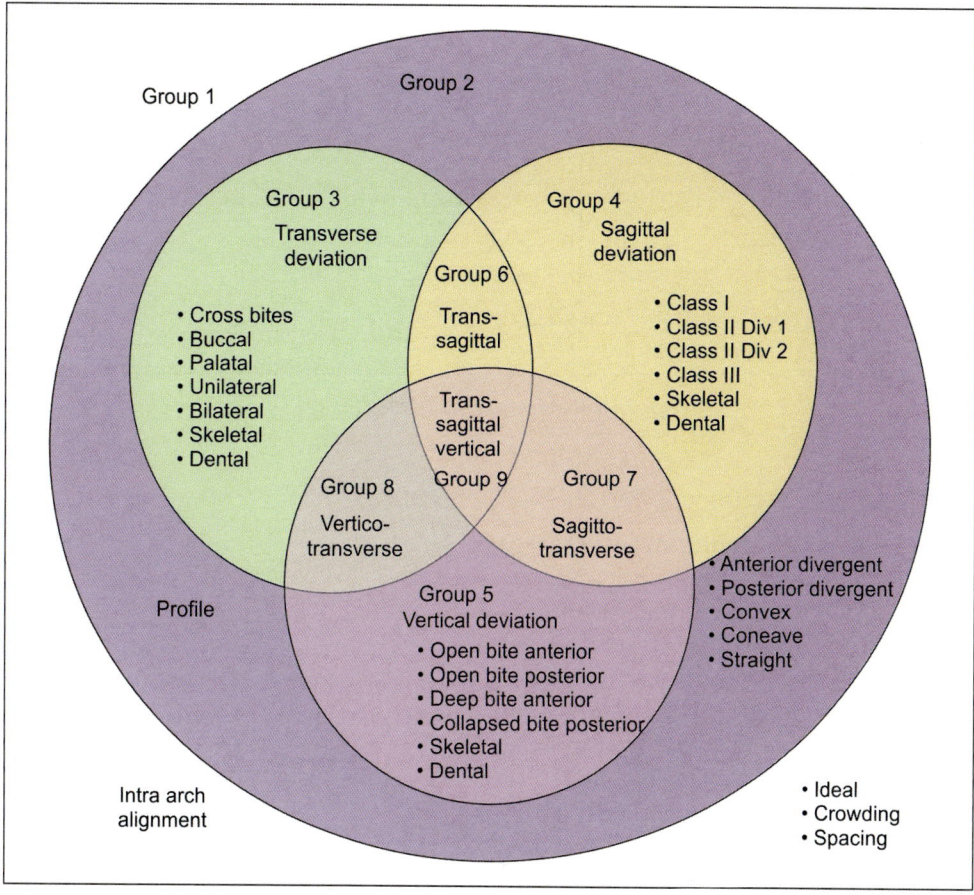

Fig. 2.15: Ackerman and Proffit classification

- It incorporates information about the skeletal jaw proportion at the appropriate point.

The occlusal relationship, dentition and skeletal jaw relationship information are derived from clinical examination, panoramic intraoral radiograph and clinical, photographic or cephalometric evaluation of dental and facial proportions.

Salient Features

- It considers malocclusion in all three dimensions. Transverse and vertical discrepancies are considered in addition to anteroposterior malrelation.
- It takes into consideration the arch length problems that result in crowding, arch asymmetry can be evaluated.
- Incisor protrusion is taken into consideration.
- It is not only classified malocclusion but also diagnoses the malocclusion.

Merits

- It explains the complexities of malocclusion.
- All three-dimensional problems are included.
- Differentiation between skeletal and dental problems is made.
- Profile of the patient is given.

- Arch length problems are evaluated.
- It helps in complete diagnosis and treatment planning.
- It can be used for rating scales for the severity of malocclusion and hence the treatment plan.

Severity Ratings of AP System

The values are assigned to the conditions and the total score is taken which helps to find out the severity of the condition.
- 0 = Ideal, no deviation
- 1 = Slight deviation from the normal, not enough to warrant treatment for this alone.
- 2 = Slight to moderate deviation
- 3 = Moderate deviation from ideal, enough alone to justify treatment
- 4 = Moderate to severe deviation from ideal, definitely needs treatment.
- 5 = Severe deviation to such an extent that the patient is handicapped.

Demerits

- Etiological considerations are not included.
- It is based on static occlusion only.

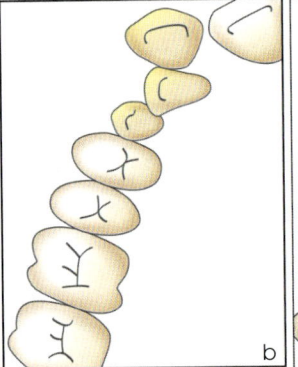 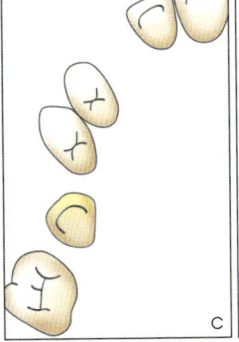 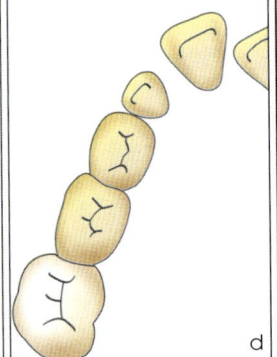 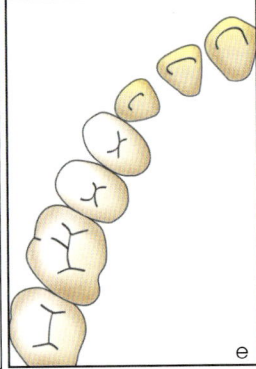

Fig. 2.16: Peck and Peck classification

Pitch, Roll and Yaw in Systematic Description

Pitch: It is the characteristic showing an excessive upward/downward rotation of the dentition around the transverse plane, relative to the lips and cheeks. It shows incisal exposure and the bite depth, i.e. normal bite/open bite/deep bite. Pitch of the jaws and teeth relative to the soft tissue is evaluated by studying the relation with the intercommissure line. Pitch of the jaws and teeth relative to the facial skeleton can be seen with cephalograms where pitch is revealed as the orientation of the palatal, occlusal and mandibular planes relative to the true horizontal plane.

Roll: It is described as rotation of teeth or jaws around the sagittal plane on one or the other side. It depicts the asymmetric inclination/skewing of the incisal plane and the occlusal plane. It is evaluated in relation to the soft tissue using the intercommissure line, while in relation to facial skeleton, the interocular line is used.

Yaw: It is the rotation of the jaws or the dentition to one side or the other around the vertical axis. It produces a skeletal or dental midline discrepancy which is defined as yaw. It also produces different molar relations on both sides.

PECK AND PECK CLASSIFICATION (Fig. 2.16)

- *Canine—1st premolar:* It is due to genetic—polygenic, multifactorial inheritance.
- *Canine—lateral incisor:* It is due to adventitious—early trauma, possible genetic role
- *Canine to 1st molar site:* Adventitious—early loss of 1st molar, canine drift.
- *Lateral incisor–central incisor:* Adventitious—early loss of 1st molar, canine drift
- *Canine to central incisor:* Adventitious—main reason is trauma.

BIBLIOGRAPHY

1. Contemporary Orthodontics, William R. Proffit (5th edition).
2. Graber Tm Orthodontics: Principles and Practice, 3rd Ed. WB Sounders. 1988.
3. Introduction to Orthodontics, Laura Mitchell (3rd edition).
4. James L. Ackerman, William R. Proffit. The characteristic of malocclusion; a modern approach to classification and diagnosis. Am J Ortho 1969;56(5):443–454.

PREVIOUS YEAR'S UNIVERSITY QUESTIONS

Essay

1. Classify malocclusion and explain in detail about Angle's classification.
2. Classify malocclusion and explain in detail about Ackermann and Proffit classification.
3. Describe the intraoral and extraoral features of Class II malocclusion.
4. What are the different methods of classification of malocclusion and write about the drawback of Angle's classification.
5. What are the differences between True and false Class III malocclusion.
6. Write about Venn diagram and explain Ackerman-Proffit classification.

Short Questions

1. Simon's classification
2. Modification of Angle's classification
3. Bimaxillary protrusion
4. Incisor classification

MCQs

1. *Who modified Angle's classification?*
   a. Dewey
   b. Lischer
   c. Both 1 and 2
   d. None of the above   **(Ans: c)**

2. *Who classified malocclusion in all 3 planes of space?*
   a. Angle
   b. Andrew
   c. Simon
   d. Ackerman and Proffit   **(Ans: c)**

3. *Malocclusion in vertical plane includes:*
   a. Open bite
   b. Deep bite
   c. Crossbite
   d. Both a and b   **(Ans: d)**

4. *Malocclusion in vertical plane includes:*
   a. Scissor bite
   b. Deep bite
   c. Crossbite
   d. Both a and c   **(Ans: d)**

5. *In which year did Angle introduce his classification of malocclusion:*
   a. 1898
   b. 1989
   c. 1789
   d. 1689   **(Ans: a)**

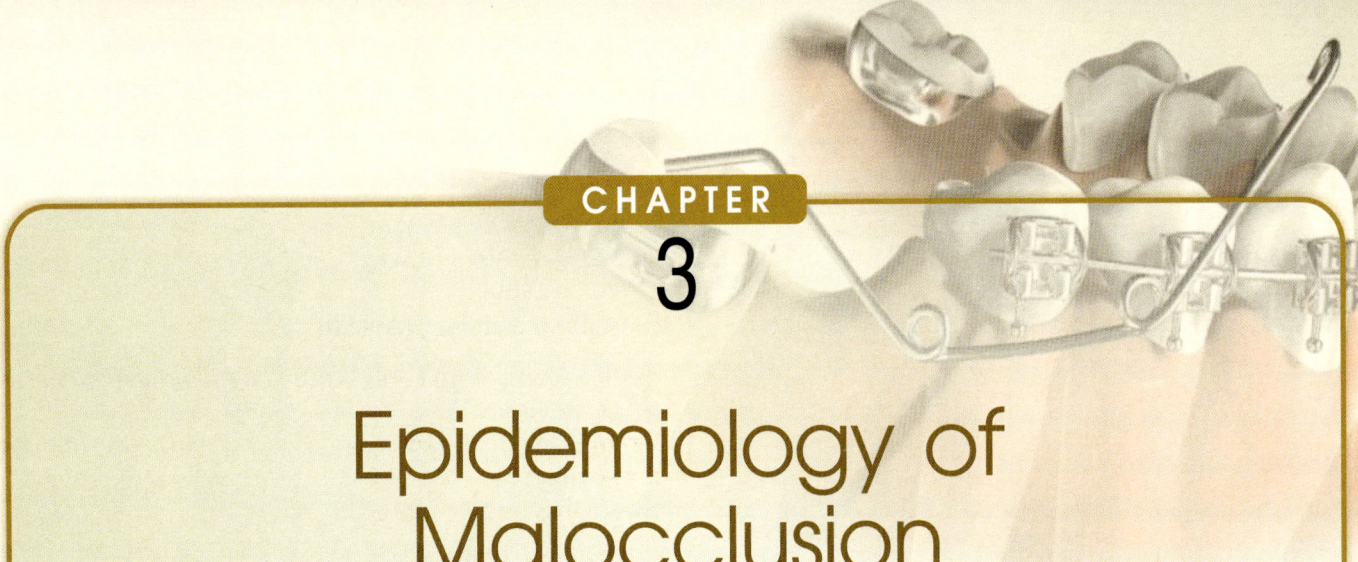

Epidemiology of Malocclusion

Chapter Outline

- Introduction
- Index of orthodontic treatment needs
- Peer assessment rating

- Index of complexity outcome and need (ICON)
- Handcapping labiolingual deviation index (HLD index)
- Dental aesthetic index (DAI)

INTRODUCTION

It is a branch of medical science that deals with the incidence, distribution and control of the disease in a population. It is derived from the Greek word, *Epi*—upon, *Demos*—people and *Logos*—study.

With the growing demand for orthodontic treatment, a variety of clinician-based indices have been developed to classify various types of malocclusion and determine their orthodontic treatment.

The most commonly employed malocclusion indices are the Dental Aesthetic Index (DAI), Index of Orthodontic Treatment Need (IOTN), Peer Assessment Rating (PAR) and Index of Complexity, Outcome and Need (ICON).

Generally, among the commonly used Indices, IOTN (AC, DHC), DAI and ICON are used to assess the orthodontic treatment needs while ICON and PAR are indices for the treatment outcome. In some ways, the indices of IOTN, DAI and ICON are similar. All include two components—morphological and esthetic. The difference is that for the IOTN, the esthetic component is separated from the dental health component. All the three indices measure similar traits, such as overjet, open bite, overbite, anteroposterior molar relationship and displacement. However, the weights of these traits are rated differently by each index. The five indices are described below.

Measurement of Malocclusion

- The measurement of malocclusion as a public health problem is difficult since most orthodontic treatment is undertaken for esthetic reasons.
- It is very difficult to estimate the extent to which malposed teeth or dentofacial anomalies constitute a psychological hazard by Russell.
- It is proved to be a difficult entity to define because individual perceptions of what constitute a malocclusion problem differ widely.
- Malocclusion indices have been used to categorize disorders for the purpose of epidemiology and research, in order to allocate patients into categories of treatment need and to compare the treatment success.

INDEX

A numerical value describing the relative states of a population on a graduated scale with a definite upper and lower limits which is designed to permit and facilitate comparison with other population classified by the same criteria and methods—by Russell AL.

Types of Index

1. Diagnostic index (Angle's classification).
2. Epidemiologic indices (Summer's Occlusal Index).

3. Treatment needs indices (Grainr's Treatment Priority Index—TPI).
4. Treatment outcome indices (Peer Assessment Rating Index—PAR).
5. The Index Orthodontic Treatment Need (IOTN).
6. Handicapping Labiolingual Deviation Index (HLD Index)

Requirements of Orthodontic Index

1. It should be simple, accurate, reliable and reproducible.
2. It should be objective and yield quantitative data which may be analyzed by current statistical methods.
3. It should differentiate between handicapping and non-handicapping malocclusions.
4. It should not be time consuming.
5. It should lend itself to modification for the collection of epidemiological data other than prevalence, incidence and severity.
6. Usable on both patients and study models.
7. It should measure the degree of handicap.

INDEX OF ORTHODONTIC TREATMENT NEEDS (IOTN)

Brook and Shaw in UK described in 1989. It determines the significance of various occlusal traits and perceived esthetic impairment. It has two components, namely:
1. Esthetic component
2. Dental health component

Esthetic Component

It consists of scale of 10 color photographs showing different levels of dental attractiveness which are also graded from score 1—the most esthetically pleasing and score 10—grades the least esthetically pleasing. The scores are categorized according to need for treatment as follows:

- Grades 1, 2, 3 and 4—no or slight treatment
- Grades 5, 6 and 7—moderate or borderline need for treatment.
- Grades 8, 9 and 10—need for orthodontic treatment.

Dental Health Component

It is a modification of treatment used by the Swedish Public Dental Health System and represents anatomical aspects of IOTN. Various occlusal traits:
1. Overjet
2. Reverse overjet
3. Overbite

4. Crossbite
5. Open bite
6. Displacement of tooth
7. Hypodontia
8. Defects of cleft lip and palate

Gradings

Grade-1: No treatment need. It shows extremely minor malocclusions including contact point displacements less than 1 mm.

Grade-2: Little need
2a. Increased overjet >3.5 mm but ≤6 mm with competent lips
2b. Reversed overjet >0 mm but ≤1 mm.
2c. Anterior or posterior crossbite with ≤1 mm discrepancy between retruded contact position and intercuspal position.
2d. Contact displacements >1 mm but ≤2 mm
2e. Anterior or posterior open bite >1 mm but ≤2 mm
2f. Increased overbite ≥3.5 mm without gingival contact
2g. Pre-normal or post-normal occlusions with no other anomalies

Grade-3: Borderline need
3a. Increased overjet >3.5 mm but ≤6 mm with incompetent lips. Reversed overjet
3b. Reversed overjet >1 mm but ≤3.5 mm
3c. Anterior or posterior crossbite with >1 mm but ≤2 mm discrepancy between retruded contact position and intercuspal position.
3d. Contact point displacements >2 mm but ≤4 mm
3e. Anterior open bite >2 mm but ≤4 mm.
3f. Deep overbite complete on gingival or palatal tissues but no trauma.

Grade 4: Need treatment
4a. Increased overjet >6 mm but ≤9 mm.
4b. Reversed overjet >3.5 mm with no masticatory or speech difficulties.
4c. Anterior or posterior crossbite with >2 mm discrepancy between retruded contact position and intercuspal position.
4d. Severe contact point displacement >4 mm
4e. Extreme lateral or anterior openbite >4 mm
4f. Increased and completed overbite with gingival or palatal trauma
4h. Less extensive hypodontia requiring pre-restorative orthodontic or orthodontic space closure to obviate the need for prosthesis
4i. Posterior lingual crossbite with no functional occlusal contact in one or both buccal segments

4m: Reversed overjet >1 mm, <3.5 mm with reported masticatory or speech difficulties

4t: Partially erupted, tipped and impacted against adjacent teeth

4x: Presence of supernumerary teeth

Grade 5: Need treatment

5a: Increased overjet >3.5 mm with reported masticatory or speech difficulties.

5h: Extensive hypodontia with restorative implication

5i: Impeded eruption of the teeth crowding, displacement, supernumerary teeth, retained deciduous teeth and pathological cause

5m: Reversed overjet >3.5 mm with reported masticatory or speech difficulties

5p: Defects of cleft lip and palate and other craniofacial anomalies

5s: Submerged deciduous teeth.

PEER ASSESSMENT RATING

It is referred to a quantitative occlusal index measuring how much a patient deviates from normal alignment and occlusion. It is designed to quantitate the outcome of the treatment by comparing the severity of occlusion on pretreatment and post-treatment casts. Unlike IOTN, the scores are cumulative. The features recorded are listed below, with the current weightings within parenthesis.

- Crowding—by contact point displacement (x1)
- Buccal segment replacement—in the anteroposterior, vertical and transverse planes (x1)
- Overjet (x6)
- Overbite (x2)
- Centerlines (x4)

The difference between pre- and post-treatment is calculated. The percentage change in score is determined to estimate the success of treatment. If the percentage is greater than 70%, it indicates a high standard of treatment. If a change of 30% or less, it indicates that no appreciable improvement has been achieved.

INDEX OF COMPLEXITY OUTCOME AND NEED (ICON)

The new index incorporates the features of both the Index of Orthodontic Treatment Need (IOTN) and the Peer Assessment Rating (PAR). The esthetic component of IOTN is included along with the scores for upper arch crowding/spacing, presence of crossbite; overbite/open bite and buccal segment relationship. As in the PAR < weightings are added to reflect current orthodontic opinion. The sum of the scores and their weightings gives a pre-treatment scores, which is said

to reflect the need for and likely complexity of the treatment required. Following treatment, the index is scored again to give an improvement grade (pre-treatment score − 4 × post-treatment score) and thus the outcome of treatment. This index is currently undergoing evaluation.

ICON Scoring Method

ICON score interpretation:

Need and acceptability	Threshold
Pretreatment need	>43
End treatment acceptability	<31 acceptable

Pretreatment complexity	Score value
Easy	<29
Mild	29–50
Moderate	51–63
Difficult	64–77
Very difficult	>77

Improvement grade	Score range
Pretreatment score − 4 × post-treatment score	
Greatly improved	>1
Substantially improved	−25 to 50
Moderately improved	−53 to −26
Minimally improved	−85 to −54
Not improved or worse	<−85

HANDICAPPING LABIOLINGUAL DEVIATION INDEX (HLD INDEX)

It was developed by Harry L. Draker in 1960. It is only applicable to the permanent dentition (the patient age should be at least 13 years). The main intention is to measure the presence or absence and the degree of handicapping malocclusion and dentofacial anomalies. It is commonly used index.

It measures the malocclusion in all three planes, namely vertical, sagittal and transverse planes. All measurements are made with a Boley gauge scaled in millimeters. Absence of any conditions must be recorded by entering −O. Any condition marked as −X without any further scoring indicates severe handicapping condition that is automatically considered to qualify for orthodontic services.

The modified component conditions of the HLD index can be entered as described below.

Category-1: *Cleft palate:* Mark X in the sheet and no further scoring as it is severe handicapping condition.

Category-2: *Craniofacial anomalies:* Indicate mark X in the sheet and should be supported with acceptable documentation by a craniofacial specialist.

Category-3: *Severe traumatic deviation:* Traumatic deviations are, for example, loss of a premaxilla segment by burns or by accident; the result of osteomyelitis or other gross pathology. Indicate an X on the score sheet and attach documentation and description of condition.

Category-4: *Deep impinging overbite:* Indicate X on the score sheet when lower incisors are destroying the soft tissue of the palate and tissue laceration and/or clinical attachment loss are present.

Category-5: *Crossbite of individual anterior teeth:* Indicate X on the score sheet when clinical attachment loss and recession of the gingival margin are present.

Category-6a: *Overjet >9 mm, mandibular protrusion (reverse overjet) >3.5 mm:* Overjet is recorded with the patient's teeth in centric occlusion. Indicate X and score no further (this condition is automatically considered to be a handicapping malocclusion without further scoring).

Category-6b: *Overjet ≤9 mm:* The measurement is rounded off to the nearest millimeter and centered on the score sheet.

Category-7: *Overbite in millimeters:* It is measured by rounding off to the nearest millimeter and entered on the score sheet. (Reverse overbite may exist in certain conditions and should be measured and recorded). The measurement is rounded off to the nearest millimeter and multiplied by 5 and recorded.

Category-9: *Open bite:* It is measured from incisal edge of a maxillary central incisor to incisal edge of a corresponding mandibular incisor, in millimeters. The measurement is entered on the score sheet and multiplied by four (4).

Category-10: *Ectopic eruption:* Count each tooth, excluding third molars. Each qualifying tooth must be more than 50% blocked out of the teeth. Enter the number of qualifying teeth on the score sheet and multiply by three (3).

Category-11: *Labiolingual spread:* A Boley gauge is used to determine the extent of deviation from a normal arch. The total distance between the most protruded and the most lingually displaced anterior is measured. In case of multiple anterior crowding, the most severe individual deviation should be entered on the score sheet.

Category-12: *Anterior crowding:* Only arch length insufficiency that is exceeding 3.5 mm should only be recorded. Enter five (5) points each separately for crowded maxillary arch and crowded mandibular arch. If ectopic eruption (condition category-10) exists in the anterior region of the same arch, count the condition that scores the most points. Do not count both conditions. However, posterior ectopic teeth can still be counted separately from anterior crowding when they occur in the same arch.

Category-13: *Posterior unilateral crossbite:* This condition involves two or more adjacent teeth, one of which must be a molar. The crossbite must be both palatal and buccal crossbites. The presence of posterior unilateral crossbite is indicated by a score of four (4) on the score sheet. No score for bilateral crossbite.

The following codes are used in the HLD index.
- O : Condition absent
- X : Condition present
- M : Mixed dentition (to be indicated, if present)
- A : Clinical approval
- D : Clinical disapproval

The categories or conditions: Category-1 to 6a which are marked as X automatically indicated handicapping condition. The remaining conditions should score at least 26 points to be qualified for orthodontic treatment. The HLD (Md) index is very similar to the original HLD index; however, the scoring cut off for constituting a handicap was raised from 13 to 15 points.

DENTAL AESTHETIC INDEX (DAI)

The Dental Aesthetic Index was developed by NC Cons, J Jenny and FJ Kohaut in 1986 to assess orthodontic treatment need. It is an orthodontic index, based on socially defined aesthetic norms.

It has been adopted by the World Health Organization as a cross-cultural index. It identifies deviant occlusal traits and mathematically derives a single score. Its structure consists of 10 occlusal features of malocclusion; overjet, underjet, missing teeth, diastema, anterior open bite, anterior crowding, anterior spacing, largest anterior irregularity (mandible and maxilla) and anteroposterior molar relationship. The 10 occlusal features are weighted on the basis of their relative importance according to a panel of lay judges. The codes and criteria are as follows:

- *Missing incisor, canine and premolar teeth:* The number of missing permanent incisor, canine and premolar teeth in the upper and lower arches should be counted and recorded.
- *Crowding in the incisal segments:* Both upper and lower incisal segments should be examined for crowding. Crowding in the incisal segments is recorded as following:

- 0—no crowding
- 1—one segment crowded
- 2—two segments crowded

- *Spacing in the incisal segments:* Both upper and lower incisal segments should be examined for spacing. Spacing in the incisal segments is recorded as following:
  - 0—no spacing
  - 1—one segment spaced
  - 2—two segments spaced
- *Diastema:* A midline diastema is defined as the space, in millimeters, between the two permanent maxillary incisors at the normal position of the contact points.
- *Largest anterior maxillary irregularity:* Irregularities may be either rotation out of or displacements from normal alignment. The four incisors in the maxillary arch should be examined to locate the greatest irregularity.
- *Largest anterior mandibular irregularity:* The measurement is the same as on the upper arch except that it is made on the mandibular arch.
- *Anterior maxillary overjet:* The largest maxillary overjet is recorded to the nearest whole millimeter.
- *Anterior mandibular overjet:* Mandibular overjet is recorded when any lower incisor is in crossbite.
- Vertical anterior open bite.
- Anteroposterior molar relation.

The right and left sides are assessed with the teeth in occlusion and only the largest deviation from the normal molar relation is recorded. The following codes are used:

- 0—normal
- 1—half cusp
- 2—full cusp

Calculation of DAI Scores

The regression equation used for calculating standard DAI scores is as follows:

Missing visible teeth × 6 + crowding + spacing + diastema × 3 + largest anterior maxillary irregularity + largest anterior mandibular irregularity + anterior maxillary overjet × 2 + anterior mandibular overjet × 4 + vertical anterior open bite × 4 + anteroposterior molar relation × 3 + 13. The severity of malocclusion is classified on the basis of the DAI scores as shown in Table 3.1.

Table 3.1: Severity of malocclusion and decision of treatment need

Severity of malocclusion	Treatment indication	DAI scores
No abnormality or minor malocclusion	No or slight need	<25
Definite malocclusion	Elective	26–30
Severe malocclusion	Highly desirable	31–35
Very severe or handicapping malocclusion	Mandatory	>36

BIBLIOGRAPHY

1. Brook PH, Shaw WC. The development of an index of orthodontic treatment priority. Eur J Orthod 1989; 11:309–20.
2. Daniels C, Richmond S. The development of the index of complexity, outcome and need (ICON). J Orthod 2000; 27:149–62.
3. Fox NA, Daniels C Gilgrass T. A comparison of the index of complexity outcome and need (ICON) with the peer assessment rating (Par) and the index of orthodontic treatment need (IOTN). Br Dent J 2002;193:225–30
4. Richmond S, Shaw WC, Roberts CT, et al. The PAR Index (Peer Assessment Rating): methods to determine outcome of orthodontic treatment in terms of improvement and standards. Eur J Orthod 1992; 14:180–7.

PREVIOUS YEAR'S UNIVERSITY QUESTIONS

Short Questions

- PAR index
- IOTN

MCQs

1. *HLD index stands for:*
   a. Handicapping labiolingual deviation index.
   b. Handy linguolabial deviation index.
   c. Hygiene labiolingual deviation index
   d. None of above   **(Ans: a)**

2. *HLD index was developed by:*
   a. Master and Frankel
   b. Vankirk and Pennel
   c. Poulton and Aaronson
   d. Harry L Draker   **(Ans: d)**

3. *HLD index is applicable to:*
   a. Only permanent dentition

b. Only deciduous dentition

c. Both permanent and deciduous dentition

d. None of the above   **(Ans: a)**

4. *Which index was the first index designed to meet the administrative needs of program planners?*

a. DAI

b. IOIN

c. HLD

d. TPI   **(Ans: c)**

5. *The HLD index is based on:*

a. 5 components

b. 7 components

c. 9 components

d. 6 components   **(Ans: b)**

6. *TPI stands for:*

a. Treatment priority index

b. Tendency priority index

c. Treatment prior index

d. Treatment priority improvement   **(Ans: a)**

7. *TPI was developed by:*

a. Grainger RM

b. Master and Frankel

c. Harry L Draker

d. Poulton and Aaronson   **(Ans: a)**

8. *Malalignment index was developed by:*

a. Master and Frankel

b. Vankirk and Pennel

c. Henry Draker

d. Poulton and Aaronson   **(Ans: b)**

9. *Occlusal index was developed by:*

a. Master and Frankel

b. Vankirk and Pennel

c. Poulton and Aaronson

d. Summers   **(Ans: d)**

General Principles of Growth and Development

Chapter Outline

- Definitions of growth and development
- Types of growth
- Factors affecting growth and maturation
- Methods of studying physical growth
- Modes of collection of growth data
- Basic tenets of growth: pattern, variability and timing

- Growth spurts
- Prenatal growth of craniofacial region
- Postnatal growth of craniofacial complex
- Postnatal growth of mandible
- Postnatal growth of nasomaxillary complex
- Clinical implications

DEFINITIONS OF GROWTH AND DEVELOPMENT

Growth

Todd: "Growth is an increase in size."
Krogman: "Increase in size, change in proportion and progressive complexity."
Huxley: "The self-multiplication of living substance."
Moss: "Change in any morphological parameter, which is measurable."
Moyers: "Qunatitative aspect of biologic development per unit of time."
Meridith: "Entire series of sequential anatomic and physiologic changes taking place from the beginning of prenatal life to senility."
Stewart (1982): "Developmental increase in mass".
Proffit (1986): "An increase in size or number".
Pinkham (1994): "Growth signifies an increase, expansion or extension of any given tissue".

Development

Todd: "Development is progress towards maturity."
Moyers: "All the naturally occurring unidirectional changes in the life of an individual from its existence as a single cell to its elaboration as a multinational unit terminating in death."

Prenatal growth: Prenatal growth is characterized by a rapid increase in cell numbers and fast growth rates.

Postnatal growth: It is characterized by declining growth rates and increasing maturation of tissues. It is the first 20 years of growth after birth.

The term growth and development are interrelated and some basic differences between the two can be appreciated. Growth is considered an anatomic phenomenon while development is a physiological and behavioral phenomenon. Growth is a change in size or quantity, i.e. growth is a measurable aspect of biologic life. Development on the other hand includes growth as well as differentiation.

The term "growth" simply means an increase in mass of life. However, the process of growth of cells and tissues is so complex that it is necessary to distinguish between different types of growth.

Generally, growth is irreversible. It is partially true as in the case of increase in the length of the body.

Growth may be reversible as seen in the case of increase in weight of the body.

Though growth is generally associated with an increase in size and unidirectional, yet some conditions involving regression are also considered to take place during growth, e.g. the atrophy of the thymus gland (Fig. 4.1).

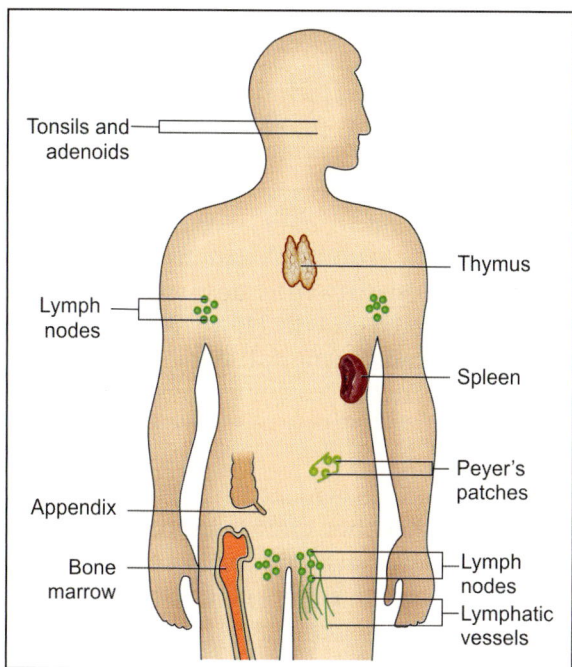

Fig. 4.1: Atrophy of thymus gland as regression during growth

Development is characterized by changes in complexity, a shift to fixation of function, and more independence, all of which is under genetic control, yet modified by the environment.

Development = Growth + differentiation + translocation

The changes associated with aging, i.e. degeneration and senility are considered by some as a part of maturation, while others consider it as part of development.

The stabilization of the adult stage brought about by the growth and development is called **maturation.**

Differentiation: Differentiation is the change from a generalized cell or tissue to one that is more specialized. Thus, differentiation is a change in quality or kind.

According to Todd, "growth and development relies on the other and under the influence of morphogenetic pattern; the threefold process works its miracles; self-multiplication, differentiation, organization—each according to its own kind! A fourth dimension is time".

Types of Growth

Growth at Cellular Level

Cellular hyperplasia: The phenomenon by which protein and DNA synthesis leads to an increase in cell number by mitotic division is known as cellular hyperplasia. For example, hyperplasia is seen during stages of embryogenesis, organogenesis, and growth in utero as well as in infancy and childhood.

Cellular hypertrophy: Here, synthesis of protein and cellular material without mitotic division leads to an increase in cell size. Thus, hypertrophic growth involves an increase in the size of the specific cells that characterize a tissue without their division. For example, it is usually seen in cells which can no longer divide like nerve cells and muscle fibers.

Growth at Tissue Level

- Accretionary growth
- Appositional growth
- Interstitial growth
- Meristematic growth
- Compensatory growth

Accretionary growth: In this type of growth, there is an increase in the amount of extracellular matrix between tissue cells rather an increase in cell number or cell size.

Appositional growth: It is the specific type of growth in which new generation of cells and extracellular matrix are added to the surface of the tissue by the repeated division of cells by a cambial layer that surrounds the tissue; e.g. periosteum and perichondrium.

Interstitial growth: Interstitial growth is seen where multiplication and sometimes accretionary growth continues throughout the thickness of a tissue mass which consequently grows as a whole and expands from within.

Meristematic growth: It describes growth from a tip that contains populations of dividing cells. As division occurs, the tip moves distally leaving behind populations of cells from its earlier divisions, e.g. growth seen in limb buds in which the progress zone first produces the cells of shoulder and then is moved distally to produce cell populations of the arm and so on.

Compensatory growth: A balance is maintained between losses through wear and tear the maintenance of functional tissue integrity. For example, the regeneration of liver gains its approximate original size after a major loss of its tissue.

Phases of Growth

Growth is continuous from conception to death, but it differs in rate and duration for various parts of body. Certain phases of growth can be identified as follows:

- *Prenatal growth:* It is characterized by a rapid rise in cell numbers and fast growth rates.

- *Postnatal growth:* It lasts for about the first 20 years of life and is characterized by declining growth rates and increasing the maturation of tissues.
- *Maturity:* It is a period of stability during which body achieves maximum function and growth processes are limited to the maintenance of an equilibrium state between cellular loss and gain.
- *Old age:* It is a period during which functional activity declines and growth processes slow down.

FACTORS AFFECTING GROWTH AND MATURATION

Growth during embryonic, fetal and postnatal periods is regulated by a variety of factors which are not completely understood. The following factors influence growth and maturation:

Genetic Factors

The genes have the basic control of growth including rate, timing and magnitude. However, the final outcome and growth depends on the interaction between the genetic potential and environmental factors.

Growth Hormones and Growth Factors

Probably all of the endocrine hormones have some influence on growth. In particular, postnatal growth is profoundly affected by the circulating concentration of growth hormone (somatotropin), growth hormone-releasing hormone and somatostatin. All tissues respond to growth hormone and produce a proportional body growth that slows after puberty when secretion of the hormone decreases. Lack of growth hormone causes dwarfism, whereas its continued secretion produces gigantism. Abnormal secretion of growth hormone after the epiphysis plates have fused, results in acromegaly.

Other growth factors affecting growth are:
- Insulin-like growth factor-I and II (IGF-I, IGF-II)
- Platelet-derived growth factor
- Epidermal growth factor
- Vascular endothelial growth factor (VEGF)
- Transforming growth factor B (TGF-B)

The hormones of thyroid gland, thyroxine and tri-iodothyronine, stimulate metabolism and are important in the growth of bones, teeth and brain. The changes seen at adolescence are caused by the secretion of androgens and gonadal hormones.

Nutrition

Poor nutrition at critical stages of life may permanently alter the normal development pattern of many organs and tissues. Proper nutrition is essential for normal postnatal growth. Apart from adequate supply of proteins, all diet should include vitamins, minerals, etc. Calcium, magnesium, phosphorus, manganese and fluorides are essential for proper bone and tooth growth. Vitamin A controls activities of both osteoclasts and osteoblasts, and its deficiency may be associated with defective bone growth. Vitamin C is necessary for proper bone and connective tissue growth. Malnutrition results in disordered growth. However, growth process accelerates when deficient nutrient is replaced during growth period, i.e. the "catching up" growth.

Secular Trends

There is considerable evidence that children today are growing faster than they grew in the past, for example, studies have shown that boys of 15 years of age are 5 inches taller than the same age group some decades earlier. Such secular trend may be due to decreased illness and improved health.

Illness

Prolonged and debilitating illness can have an adverse effect on growth. However, after the period of illness, "catch up" growth normally brings back to the predetermined growth curve.

Season and Circadian Rhythm

Growth in height is faster in spring than in autumn, while weight increase occurs faster in autumn than in spring. Growth also shows a circadian rhythm; growth in height and eruption of teeth appear to be greater at night than in daytime due to fluctuations in the hormone release.

Psychological Stress

Evidence shows that psychological stress can adversely affect growth by inhibiting hormone secretion.

METHODS OF STUDYING PHYSICAL GROWTH

The followings are the two major approaches of studying physical growth:
- Measurement approach
- Experimental approach.

Measurement Approach

This approach includes techniques that measure certain criteria on living animals/skeletal remains. These techniques are not invasive. Most growth studies on humans are conducted by measurement techniques. Various measurement techniques can be used on living individuals or the skeletal remains including:

- Craniometry
- Anthropometry
- Cephalometric radiography

Craniometry: It involves the measurement of human skulls of different age groups to appreciate the growth changes. Although it allows three-dimensional (3D) measurements, such studies can only be cross-sectional.

Anthropometry: It is a technique in which skeletal dimensions are measured on living individuals. Various standard landmarks established in the studies of dry skull are measured on living individuals by using soft tissue points overlying these bony landmarks. Although soft tissue thickness may vary, such techniques may be advantageous in that they allow longitudinal study of growth by repeated measurements of the same individual over a period of life.

Cephalometric radiography: This technique has contributed majorly in the study of growth and development before it became a routine practice to use the cephalogram for orthodontic diagnosis and planning. Standard cephalometric points are noted on serial radiographs of individuals and compared to analyze the growth changes occurring.

Experimental Approach

This approach includes techniques that may be manipulative and invasive in nature and thus may harm the animal. Such studies are carried out on experimental animals. Experimental methods of study growth include the following:
- Vital staining
- Radioisotopes
- Autoradiography
- Implant radiography

Vital Staining

Vital staining was introduced by John Hunter in the 18th century. Certain vital stains can be used to determine the sequence and amount of new bone formation as well as specific locations of bone growth by utilizing histologic sections. This method involves injecting the dyes that stain the mineralizing tissues. These stains get incorporated into the bones and teeth and thus allow the study of changes in bones and teeth. Experimental animals are then sacrificed and the mineralizing tissues are studied histologically.

By this method, detailed analysis of site, amount and rate of growth can be elicited. However, this does not allow longitudinal study. Repeated data of the same individual over time cannot be obtained. Examples of stains are *Alizarin S, Procion, Tetracycline, Trypan blue* and *Fluorochrome.*

Radioisotopes

Radioactive elements can be injected into tissues of experimental animals which get incorporated into the developing bone. Bone growth can be studied tracking the radioactivity emitted by those radioisotopes, e.g. *Calcium 45, Technetium 33.*

Autoradiography

It is a technique in which a film emulsion is placed over a thin section of tissue containing radioactive isotopes and then exposed in the dark by radiation. After the film is develoed, the location of the radiation that indicates where growth is occurring can be observed by looking at the tissue section through the film.

Implant Radiography (Fig. 4.2)

Metallic implants are used as radiographic markers in chemical and experimental work to study bone remodeling and displacement. The technique first introduced by Bjork (1955) involves the implantation of small pieces of inert alloys into the growing bone. These implanted alloys will act as radiographic reference points. By examining the position of these implants on serial radiographs taken at regular intervals, bone growth can be monitored.

Information, such as site of growth, amount of growth, rate of growth and direction of growth, can be elicited accurately using implant radiography. It allows longitudinal study of growth. However, this method allows only two-dimensional (2D) study of 3D growth process. Radiation hazard is another disadvantage of this method.

Sites of implantation
In mandible (Fig. 4.2c):
- Symphysis in the midline below roots (Fig. 4.2d).
- Right body of the mandible: One below first premolar and another below first molar
- Outer surface of the ramus on right side in level of occlusal plane.

In maxilla (Fig. 4.2a):
- Inferior to anterior nasal spine.
- Bilaterally in the zygomatic process.

In hard palate (Fig. 4.2b):
- Behind canines
- Front of first molar in the junction between alveolar process and palate.

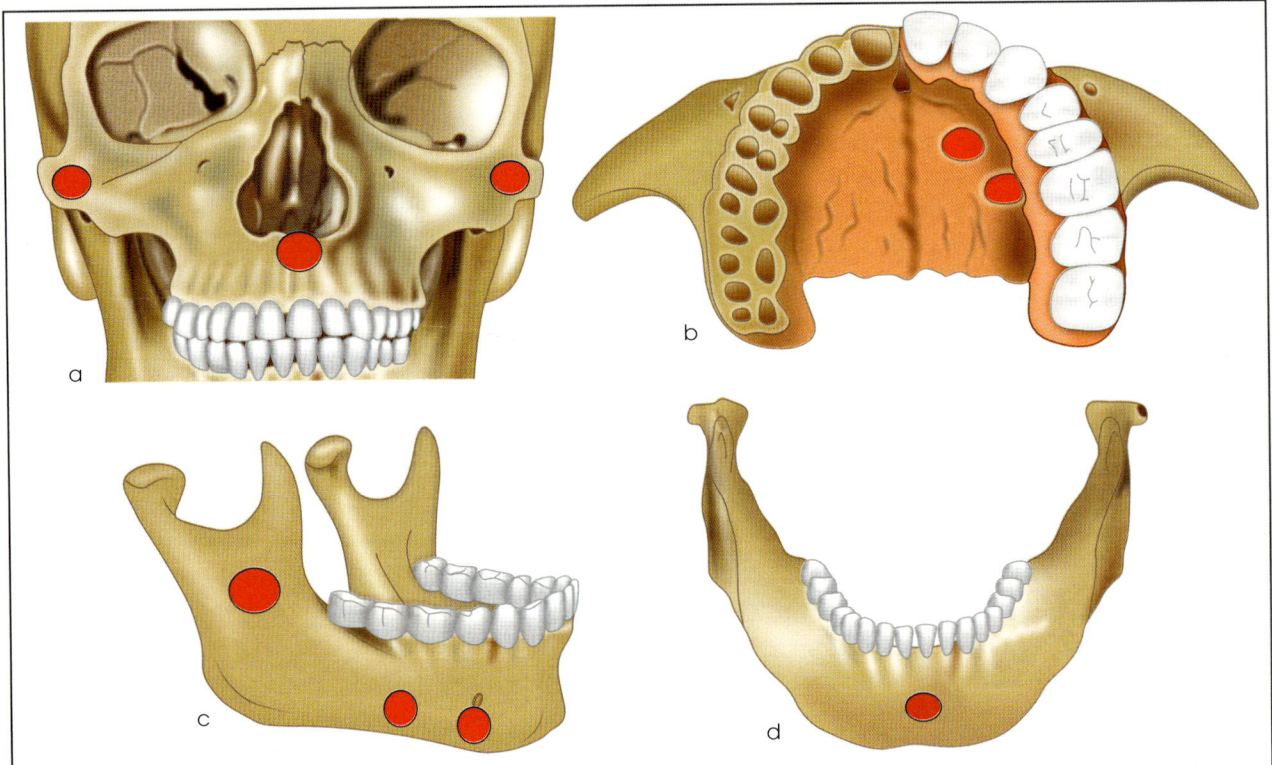

Fig. 4.2: Areas where implants are used: a. Maxilla; b. Hard palate; c. Mandible on right side; d. Midline of mandible (refer text)

Types of Growth Data

The following are the different types of growth data which can be used to study growth:

Opinion: It is a clever guess of an experienced person. It is not accurate and should be avoided.

Observations: These are useful in studying presence or absence of certain findings such as dental caries.

Ratings and rankings: They are used when it is difficult to quantify particular data. Rating uses a standard and conventionally accepted rate of classification while ranking involves arrangement of data in an orderly sequence based on the value.

Quantitative measurements: The data derived from accurate quantitative measurements are the most appropriate scientifically.

Measurements can be made in the following three ways:
1. Direct data is obtained from direct measurements on living individuals or skeletal remains using tapes and calipers.
2. Indirect data are the measurements obtained indirectly from images/reproduction of the individual, such as photographs, radiographs or dental casts.
3. Derived data are the measurements derived by comparison of two measurements, e.g. radiography and implant.

MODES OF COLLECTION OF GROWTH DATA

Growth studies are of three types:
1. Cross-sectional
2. Longitudinal
3. Mixed/semilongitudinal

Cross-sectional Studies

A large number of individuals of different age groups are examined at one occasion to develop information on growth attained at a particular age. In a short period of time, much information can be gathered about growth at many ages. The majority of information available about growth has been obtained using cross-sectional methods. It is less time consuming and a large sample size can be included in the study due to shorter span of time.

Although mean rate of growth for a population can be estimated, variability of growth in the subjects of the sample cannot be studied.

Longitudinal Studies

Longitudinal studies involve repeated examination and measurements of same subjects at regular intervals over a long period during active growth. As the same subjects are followed up over long periods, the velocity pattern of development of an individual can be studied.

Variability of individual growth can also be studied by this method.

Disadvantages include small sample size, difficulties in the maintenance of laboratory research, personal data storage over long periods and possible (sample decay) reduction in the sample size due to change of place and other reasons. Furthermore, inference of the study can only be obtained after analyzing the data at the end of the long study period.

Mixed/Semilongitudinal Studies

They are combinations of the cross-sectional and longitudinal types of studies to obtain the advantage of both methods of data collection.

Subjects at different age levels are seen longitudinally for shorter periods. For example, in a study of 6 years span, growth can be studied between birth and 6 years for 1 group, between 6 and 11 years for second group, between 10 and 16 years for the third group; and between 15 and 21 years in yet another age group. In this way, growth from birth to 21 years can be studied in only 6 years.

Interpretation of Growth Data

Growth data is presented in the form of graph to facilitate easy understanding of the findings. The rates of growth can be indicated by increments in body length or weight which when plotted form a growth curve. There are two basic curves of growth which are described below.

Distance curve/cumulative curve: It indicates the distance a child has traversed along the growth path. Data derived from the cross-sectional and longitudinal studies can be plotted as cumulative curve.

Velocity/incremental curve: It indicates the rate of growth of the child over a period of time. The velocity curve is drawn by plotting the increments in height or weight from one age to the next. For velocity curve, data is derived from longitudinal studies.

BASIC TENETS OF GROWTH: PATTERN, VARIABILITY AND TIMING

Concepts of Growth

Concept of Normality

- Normal refers to that which is usually expected, is ordinarily seen or is typical.
- The concept of normality must not be equated with that of the ideal. While ideal denotes the central tendency for the group.

- Normal refers to a range. Another aspect of craniofacial growth is that normality changes with age.

Variability

Rhythm of Growth

Hooton: Human growth is not a steady and uniform process wherein all parts die and body enlarge at the same rate and the increments of one year are equal to that of the proceeding or succeeding year.
- This growth rhythm is most clearly seen in stature or body height.
- The first "wave" of growth is seen in both sexes from birth to the fifth or sixth year

Pattern

Pattern of growth in human is allometric. There is a difference in the relative rates of growth between one part of the body and another. Different parts and organs of the body grow at different times and to different extents. This is termed as "differential growth."

Differential growth in humans is reflected in:
- Cephalocaudal gradient of growth
- Scammon's growth curve

Cephalocaudal Gradient of Growth

There are differences in the relative rates of growth between one part of the body and another. Overall proportions changes as one grows from fetal life to adulthood. There is an axis of increased growth extending from the head towards feet. The head is in advance of the trunk and the trunk in advance of the limbs regarding growth and maturity at all times. This axis of increased growth gradient extending from head towards the feet is called the cephalocaudal gradient of growth (Fig. 4.3).
- In fetal life, at around 2–3 months of intrauterine life, the head is nearly one-half of the total embryonic life. At this stage, limbs are rudimentary and trunk is underdeveloped.
- Subsequently, the head grows proportionally more slowly and limbs and trunk grow faster so that the proportion of entire body occupied by head is reduced to one quarter of the body length at birth.
- During childhood, this pattern of growth continues with lengthening of the torso and limbs. At adulthood, the head is reduced to one-eigth of the entire body length and lower limbs occupy one-half of the total length.

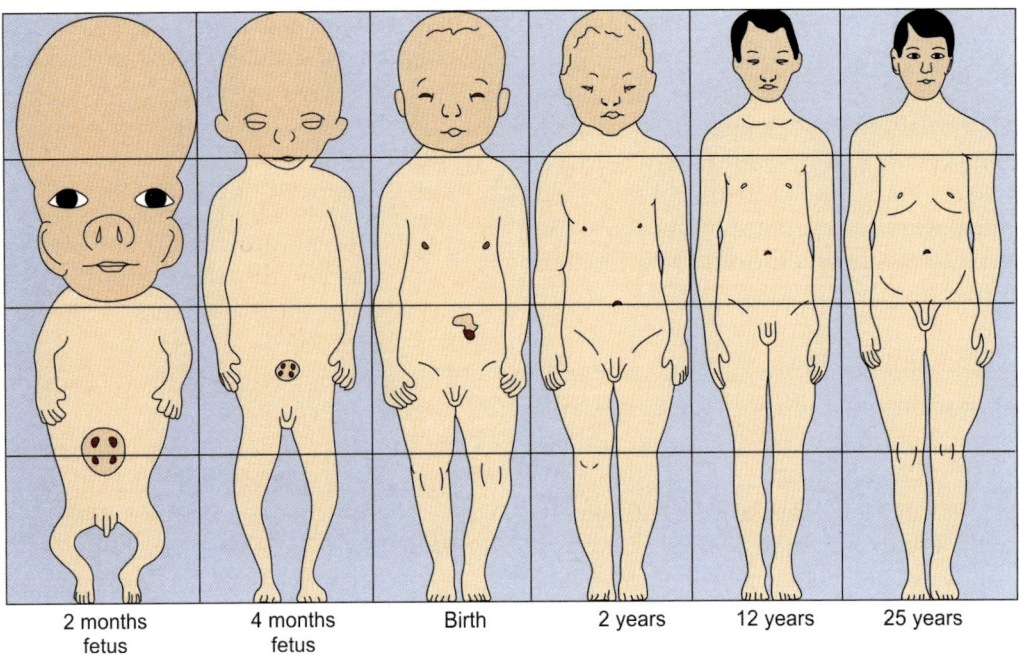

|2 months fetus|4 months fetus|Birth|2 years|12 years|25 years|

Fig. 4.3: Cephalocaudal gradient of growth

Cephalocaudal Growth in Face

- At birth, the face (nasomaxillary complex and mandible) is less developed with the cranium representing more than half of the total head.
- Maxilla being closer to the brain/head grows faster and its growth is completed before mandibular growth.
- Mandible being away from the brain completes its growth later than the maxilla.

Scammon's Growth Curve

Not all tissues of organs of the body grow at same time and to the same extent. Different body tissues show different growth rates. Richard scammon described four basic growth curves of the tissues of the body: Lymphoid, neural, general and genital. The curves span the entire postnatal period of 20 years. Normal adult size is regarded as 100% and starts from 0% at birth (Fig. 4.4).

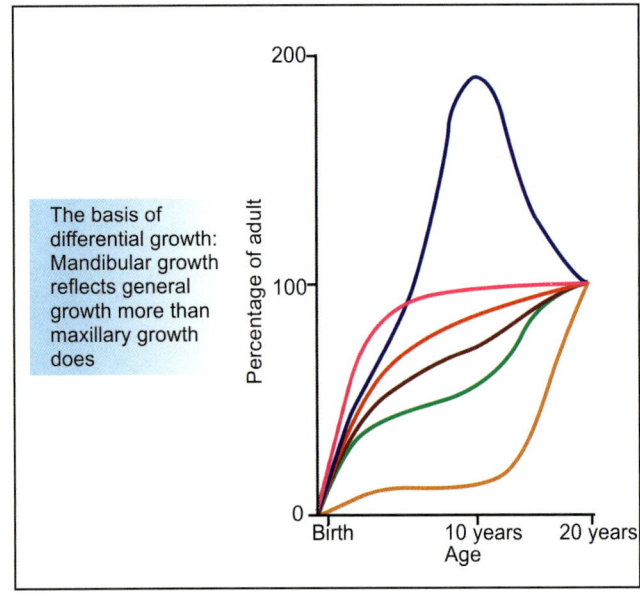

The basis of differential growth: Mandibular growth reflects general growth more than maxillary growth does

Fig. 4.4: Scammon's growth curve

Lymphoid Curve

- Lymphoid curve includes the thymus, pharyngeal and tonsillar adenoids, lymph nodes and intestinal lymphatic masses.
- Lymphoid tissues grow rapidly to reach 200% of adult size between 10 and 15 years of age. This is an adaptation to protect children from infections. Later their size is reduced from 200 to 100% at adult life.
- Reduction in the size is due to physiologic involution of the lymphoid tissues.

Neural Curve

- Neural curve includes brain, spinal cord, optic apparatus related bony parts of the skull, upper face and vertebral column.
- Neural curve rises strongly during childhood with the neural tissues growing very rapidly in early years of life.
- Brain is nearly 90% its adult size by 8 years of age. Growth in size is accompanied by growth in internal structure, enabling the 8-year-old child to function mentally at nearly the same level as an adult.

General Curve

- General curve/somatic tissues include musculature, bony skeleton, respiratory and digestive organs, kidneys, liver, and spleen and blood volume.
- The general tissues show an "S" shaped growth curve.
- The curve rises from birth to five years of age and then a plateau from 5 to 10 years followed by acceleration during puberty and then finally, it slows down in adulthood.

Genital Curve

- Genital curve includes the primary sex apparatus (ovary and testis) and all secondary sex characters/traits.
- Genital slow in the prepubertal period, but rapid at adolescence.

Effect of Scammon's Growth in Facial Region

- The maxilla follows neural growth pattern and its growth ceases earlier in life.
- Skeletal problems of the maxilla should be treated earlier than that of mandible. For example, growth modification procedures should be given earlier in life (6 years) to promote growth of maxilla.
- Mandibular growth follows general growth pattern. Its growth occurs until about 18–20 years in males. Growth modification treatment should be extended until cessation of mandibular growth so as to prevent relapse of Class III malocclusion due to continued growth of mandible.

Timing of Growth

A particular growth event may occur at different times in different individuals. Some children mature early. They are taller in childhood than average growers since they have matured faster than average, but they may not be particularly tall in adulthood. Late maturing children are shorter than average in childhood since they mature late.

One important factor in timing of growth is sex of the individual. Girls attain puberty earlier than boys. Timing of menarche (attainment of sexual maturity) in girls also shows a great variation. Some girls mature faster than others. Timing of growth modification procedures is considered in the treatment plan.

GROWTH SPURTS

There are periods of sudden accelerated growth. Such rapid increase in growth rate is termed as a "growth spurt". Three major growth spurts can be seen during postnatal development. The timing of growth spurts differ in boys and girls. Generally, girls precede boys in growth spurts by approximately two years.

- *Infantile/childhood growth spurt:* Up to 3 years in both sexes.
- *Mixed dentition/juvenile spurt:* 6–7 years in females; 7–9 years in males.
- *Adolescent growth spurt:* 10–12 years in females; 12–14 years in males.

Infantile growth spurt: Body length increases from a neonatal range of 48–53 cm to about 75 cm during first year after birth and increases by 12–13 cm in second year. Thereafter, 5–6 cm is added each year.

Childhood growth spurt: Growth rate at this period is less pronounced than the other two growth spurt.

Adolescent growth spurt: An increase in the velocity of growth occurs between 10 and 12 years in girls and 12 and 14 years in boys. This rapid increase in growth is termed as the "adolescent growth spurts". It occurs earlier in girls than in boys and it lasts for 2–2.5 years in both sexes. Rapid raise in growth during adolescence is most obvious in the increase in height, while weight gain is more variable.

Girls gain around 16 cm in height during the spurt with a peak velocity at 12 years of age. Growth rate reaches 10 cm increase in height per year. After peak height velocity (PHV) is attained, growth rate declines. The growth is stopped at 18 years in females and 20 years in males.

Clinical Significance of Growth Spurts

- Differences between the timing of growth spurt in males and females has to be kept in mind. More boys will have 2–3 peaks whereas girls show only two peaks. A few girls show mixed dentition period growth spurt, but all show pubertal growth spurt. Females mature earlier (2–3 years) than males, so early treatment is more critical in girls than in boys.
- During pubertal growth period, there is directional change from vertical to horizontal.
- Treatment of skeletal malocclusions by growth modification using orthopedic and functional appliances is best carried out during adolescent growth spurt.
- Rapid palatal expansion appliances respond well during adolescent growth spurt and the results are stable.
- Orthognathic surgery is best carried out after the cessation of active growth.

Growth Fields

The outside and inside surfaces of a bone are blanketed by a mosaic-like pattern of soft tissues, cartilage or osteogenic membrane called *growth fields*. When altered, it is capable of producing an alteration in the growth of the particular bone. About half of the periosteal surface of a whole bone has an arrangement of resorptive fields and the other half is covered by depository fields.

If a given periosteal area has a resorption type of field, the opposite inside (endosteal) surface of the same area has a depository field and vice versa. These combinations produce the drift of all parts of an entire bone.

All surfaces inside and outside of every bone are covered by an irregular pattern of growth fields comprised of various soft tissue, osteogenic membrane or cartilages. Hard bone tissue does not contain genetic program for growth rather the determinants of bone growth reside in the bone's investing soft tissue—muscle, mucosa, blood vessels and nerves. Varying activities and rates of growth of these fields are basis for different growth processes that produce bone of irregular shapes.

Growth Sites

Growth sites are growth fields that have a special significance in the growth of a particular bone, e.g. mandibular condyle and maxillary tuberosity. The growth sites may possess some intrinsic potential to growth (Table 4.1)

Mechanism of Bone Growth

The process of bone formation is called osteogenesis. It is of two types.
- Endochondral bone formation
- Intramembranous bone formation

Endochondral Bone Formation

The bone is not formed directly from the cartilage, it invades the cartilage and replaces it. The bone formation is preceded by the formation of a cartilaginous framework which provides support to the forming bone. This cartilage gets subsequently replaced by the bone. The cartilage grows both, interstitially by the cellular division of chondrocytes and appositionally, by the activity of chondrogenic membrane. As Moyers has explained, the endochondral bone formation is a form of morphogenetic adaptation which leads to continuous bone formation in the areas of high compression.

Following steps are followed during this process:
- Mesenchymal cells get condensed at the site of bone formation. It becomes the cartilage when some cells get differentiated into chondroblasts and lay down the hyaline cartilage framework.
- This cartilage is surrounded by a membrane called perichondrium which provides the osteogenic cells separated by intercellular substance.
- Cartilage cells secrete the matrix which gets calcified under the influence of enzyme alkaline phosphatase. It leads to the loss of nutritional supply to cartilage cells leading to their death. Thus, the empty spaces called primary areolae are formed. Further with advanced disintegration, it gets reduced to the bars and creation of larger empty spaces called secondary areolae.
- The blood vessels and osteogenic cells from perichondrium invade this disintegrating cartilaginous matrix. The osteogenic cells become osteoblasts and line these calcified bars. They start secreting the layers of unmineralized osteoid. With the growth of the osteoid, they start moving outward. This osteoid gets calcified to form a lamella. Then, another layer of osteoid is secreted to form new lamella. This process goes on.

In endochondral bone growth, the zone of reserved cartilage feeds new cells in the zone of cell division. Cells in this zone undergo rapid cell division and form the columns of chondrocytes. It leads to elongation of the bone. Further, these daughter cells undergo

Table 4.1: Differences between growth site and growth center	
Growth site	*Growth center*
• It is any location where growth takes place	• It is the site where genetically controlled growth occurs
• All growth sites are not the growth centers	• All growth centers are the growth sites also
• They do not control overall growth of bone	• They control overall bone growth
• They do not have independent growth potential	• They have independent growth potential
• When transplanted on other sites, they do not grow	• When transplanted, they can grow independently
• They are affected by external influences markedly	• They are mainly affected by functional needs
• They do not lead to growth of whole bone, but only some part of the bone	• They lead to growth of major parts of the bone

hypertrophy and calcification of the matrix occurs. It leads to cut-off of nutrition and disintegration of cells.

This calcified matrix gets partially resorbed by invading vascular channels which also carry osteoblast cells, which deposit the osteoids on the remnants of cartilage. With further growth, these osteoids get calcified and a new layer of osteoids is laid bone. In synchondrosis, the bone proliferates on both sides of the cartilaginous plate leading to lengthening of the cranial base bones.

Intramembranous Bone Formation

Here, the bone formation is not preceded by the formation of cartilaginous matrix. The bone is directly laid down in a fibrous membrane. The bone is formed as follows:

- Undifferentiated mesenchymal cells become condensed at the site of bone formation. Cells lay down the bundles of collagen fibers leading to formation of a membrane.
- Some cells change in osteoblasts which secrete osteoid around the collagen fibers. This osteoid gets calcified to form lamella. The original blood vessels remain near the forming trabeculae.
- The osteoblasts move away from this lamella and lay another layer of osteoid which gets calcified to form new lamella. In this process, some cells get entrapped between two lamellae and become osteocytes. Blood vessels also become enclosed in fine cancellous spaces which also have osteoblast, fibers and connective tissue cells.
- Bone tissue is laid down by periosteum, endosteum, PD membrane, sutures are all intramembranous type of bone formation. This is a more rapid type of bone formation.

Primary and Secondary Cartilages

Primary cartilage: It is derived from the primordial cartilage. It has an intrinsic growth potential and can grow independently, if transplanted to other sites. Primary cartilage is the tissue which has the capacity to grow from within (interstitial growth) and hence the growth is 3D. It is identical to the growth-plate cartilage of long bones. It has genetic predisposition for growth and acts as an autonomous tissue for growth. Here, the chondroblasts divide and synthesize intercellular matrix, the chondroblasts are surrounded by cartilaginous matrix.

In primary cartilages, the cartilaginous matrix isolates the dividing chondroblasts from local factors which are able to restrain or stimulate the cartilage growth rate, so the growth of primary cartilages is not affected by the external influences. These cells are arranged in a columnar fashion. They are not influenced by local factors, e.g. environment, etc. They act as the genetic pacemakers of growth. Examples of primary cartilages are spheno-occipital and other synchondrosis, nasal septal cartilage and epiphyseal cartilages of long bones.

Secondary cartilage: It does not have an intrinsic growth potential and its growth is influenced by external influences, local and environmental factors. There is no intercellular matrix and the prechondroblasts are not surrounded by cartilaginous matrix. The cells arranged in haphazard manner. They show peripheral growth only and help in regional adaptive growth only.

In secondary cartilages, the dividing cells are not surrounded by the cartilaginous matrix and thus not isolated from the influence of local factors. Secondary cartilages are coronoid, condylar, angular and those in some craniofacial sutures.

Growth Rotation

Growth of jaws is not uniform but some directional movements occur within and on the surface of the jaws due to bone remodeling which change the orientation of bone. These changes are termed as rotations. Pattern of growth rotation depends on the growth pattern of face and it affects the facial heights, profile, anchorage requirements, and treatment planning and extraction decisions.

Forward Rotation

It is seen in horizontal growth patterns. The posterior growth is greater than anterior growth. The increase in posterior facial height is more than anterior facial height and it leads to an anticlockwise rotation of mandible in an upward and forward direction. It thrusts the mandible in the upper arch and leads to development of deep bite (both skeletal and dental nature). Other features are prominent chin, short face height, pursing of lips, and straight profile. The masticatory muscles in such cases are stronger. Such cases should be treated by non-extraction method as far as possible, since space closure and anchorage loss is difficult. Extreme forward rotation leads to short face syndrome.

Backward Rotation

It occurs in vertical growth patterns. Here, the posterior growth is less than the anterior growth leading a clockwise rotation of mandible in a downward and backward direction. It rotates the mandible away from the upper arch leading to development of open bite which includes skeletal and dental open bite. Other features are deficient chin, increased face height, long face, incompetent lips, convex profile, etc.

The masticatory muscles in such cases are weaker. Such cases generally need extraction of teeth for treatment. The anchorage requirements are more in these cases, since there are more chances of anchorage loss. Extreme backward rotation leads to long face syndrome.

If increase in anterior and posterior heights of mandible is proportionate, there is no abnormal rotation. Normally, the growth of posterior facial height keeps pace with the growth of anterior facial height. Growth of alveolar processes and eruption of teeth adapt to the growth in intermaxillary space so that normal growth takes place.

PRENATAL GROWTH OF CRANIOFACIAL REGION

Prenatal period is a dynamic phase of development which starts with fertilization of ovum which gets implanted in the uterine wall. Face and neck development of the embryo refers to the development of the structures from 3rd to 8th week that give rise to the future head and neck. They consist of three layers—the ectoderm, mesoderm and endoderm which form the mesenchyme (derived from the lateral plate and paraxial mesoderm), neural crest and neural placodes (from the ectoderm).

- The paraxial mesoderm forms structures named somites and somitomeres that contribute to the development of the floor of the brain and voluntary muscles of the craniofacial region.
- The lateral plate mesoderm consists of the laryngeal cartilages.

The three tissue layers give rise to the pharyngeal apparatus formed by 6 pairs of pharyngeal arches, a set of pharyngeal pouches and pharyngeal grooves which are the most typical feature in development of the head and neck.

The formation of each region of the face and neck is due to the migration of the neural crest cells which come from the ectoderm. These cells determine the future structure to develop in each pharyngeal arch. Eventually, they also form the neuroectoderm which forms the forebrain, midbrain and hindbrain, cartilage, bone, dentin, tendon, dermis, pia mater and arachnoid mater, sensory neurons and glandular stroma.

The prenatal life is broadly classified into the following three phases (Flowchart 4.1).

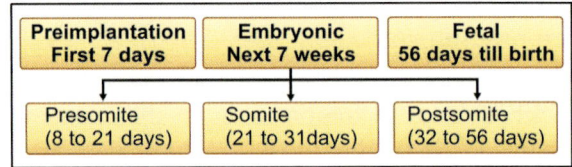

Flowchart 4.1: Prenatal growth phases

Period of ovum: This period extends to approximately 2 weeks from the time of fertilization. During this period, from the single cell stage of fertilized ovum to the cleavage of ovum and then implantation of the fertilized ovum to intrauterine wall occurs. After approximately 3 days of fertilization, the cells of the embryo divide to form a 16-cell morula (Figs 4.5–4.7).

Note: The morula transforms into a blastocyst containing a cavity called blastocele.

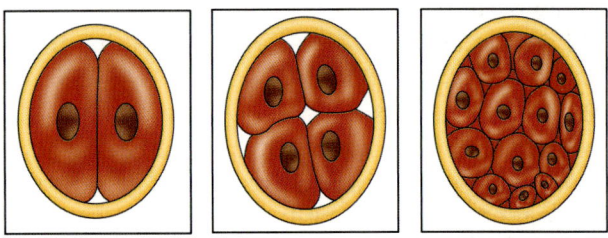

Fig. 4.5: Preimplantation period—cleavage

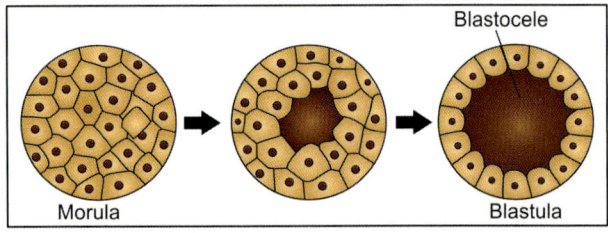

Fig. 4.6: Preimplantation period

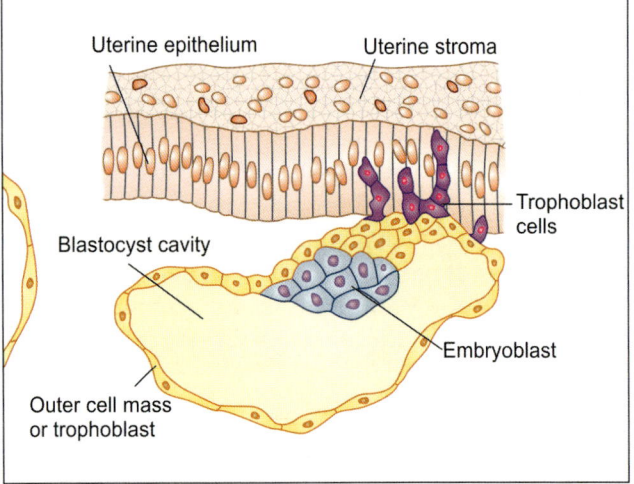

Fig. 4.7: Preimplantation period—chorionic connection (7 days)

Period of embryo: It extends from 14th to 56th day. This is the period of most rapid growth and cellular differentiation, and their allocation of the function occurs. It is one of the most crucial periods of development. During this period, major parts of craniofacial region develop. Any disturbance during this period may lead to development of craniofacial defects.

Period of fetus: It extends from 56 days till birth.

Pharyngeal Arches (Fig. 4.8)

Pharyngeal arches are formed during the 4th week. Each arch consists of a mesenchymal tissue covered on the outside by ectoderm and on the inside by epithelium of endodermal origin. In human embryology, there are six arches which are separated by pharyngeal grooves externally and pharyngeal pouches internally. These arches contribute to the physical appearance of the embryo because they are the main components that build the face and the neck. In addition, the muscular components of each arch have their own cranial nerve and wherever the muscle cells migrate, they carry their nerve component with them and each arch has its own arterial component. When the neural cells migrate to the arches and surround them, they begin to increase in size. The six pharyngeal arches give rise to much of the skeletal and muscle tissue in the head and neck region. When the embryo is 42 weeks old, the mesenchmal arches can be recognized with its corresponding cranial nerve (Table 4.2).

- *First pharyngeal arch:* It forms maxillary and mandibular processes. It is innervated by the trigeminal nerve and molds muscles related to mastication such as temporal, masseter, medial, lateral, pterygoid bones, tensor palatini and tensor tympani. This arch originates maxillary and mandibular prominences, part of the temporal bone and Meckel's cartilage (malleus and incus).
- *Second pharyngeal arch:* It is innervated by the facial cranial nerve. Muscles that arise from the arch are those involved with facial expression and the posterior diagastric muscles. Skeletal structures that originate here are the cervical sinus, Reichart cartilage (stape), the styloid process of the temporal bone, the lesser cornu and the thyroid bone.
- *Third pharyngeal arch:* It is innervated by glosso-pharyngeal nerve. It molds the stylopharyngeous muscle and forms the skeletal structures of the greater horn and lower portion of body hyoid bone.
- *Fourth and sixth arches:* They are innervated by the vagus cranial nerve. Both arches will fuse to form the laryngeal cartilages.
- *Fifth cartilage:* It does not appear to have any contribution to adult anatomy and disappears.

Pharyngeal Pouches

The pouches penetrate the surrounding mesenchyme but do not establish communication with the pharyngeal grooves. They appear simultaneously with the development of the arches.

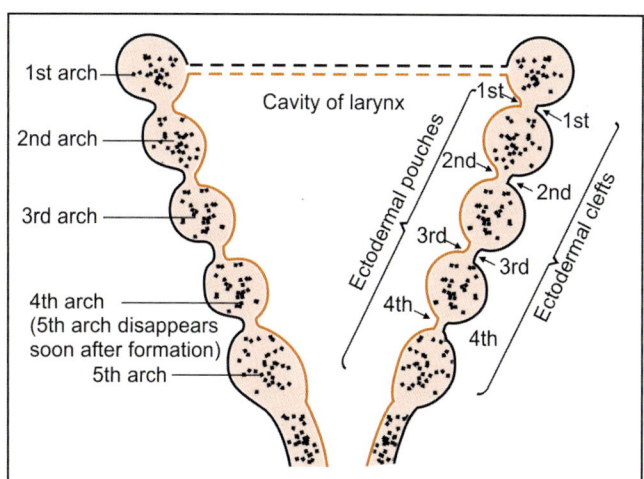

Fig. 4.8: Formation of pharyngeal arches

Table 4.2: Derivatives of pharyngeal arches				
Arches	Nerves	Muscles	Skeletal	Artery
I—Maxillary arch	Trigeminal	MOM	Mandible, maxilla, incus, malleus	Maxillary
II—Hyoid	Facial	Muscles of facial expression	Stapes, styloid process, lesser cornu and upper part of body of hyoid	Stapedial (embryonic) Corticotypanic (adult)
III—Greater corn and lower part of hyoid	Glossopharyngeal	Stylopharyngeus	Gr. corn and lower part of body of hyoid	Common carotid
IV—Thyroid cartilage and VI	Sublaryngeal and recurrent laryngeal	Intrinsic muscles of larynx, pharynx, levator palatini	Thyroid, cricoid, arytenoid, corniculate, cuneiform	IV—Rt subclavian VI—pulmonary

- *First pharyngeal pouch:* However, it does not disappear and eventually forms the Eustachian tube.
- *Second pharyngeal pouch:* It develops differently from the first onenmainly because most of it disappears leaving the tonsillar fossa.
- *Third pharyngeal pouch:* It gives rise to the inferior parathyroid gland and thymus.
- *Fourth and fifth pharyngeal pouch:* It develops as a unique structure in that molds the superior parathyroid and parafolicular cells of thyroid gland.

Pharyngeal grooves: Initially, pharyngeal grooves consist of four bars of mesenchymal tissue that separate pharyngeal nerves. Most of these structures obliterate. Its only remain left is the external auditory meatus.

Development of Tongue

In the fourth week of pregnancy, the structures develop from the first pharyngeal arch are two lingual lateral prominences and one in the middle which does not develop and disappears.

- A second prominence, the hypobrachial eminence comes from the second, third and fourth pharyngeal arches.
- A third prominence that comes from the fourth arch develops the epiglottis. The laryngeal orifice is behind the third prominence which is surrounded by the arytenoid prominences.
- Later, the lateral and middle prominences join forming the first of the three parts of the tongue. The sulcus terminalis linguae is a V-shaped line that separates the body of the tongue from the posterior part. The corresponding nerve for the three prominences of the anterior tongue is the trigeminal nerve. The posterior tongue is innervated by the glossopharyngeal nerve. The muscles of the tongue are innervated by the hypoglossal nerve.

Development of Thyroid

The thyroid appears as an epithelial proliferation in the pharynx floor between the copula linguae and the tuberculum impar. This point later will be the foramen cecum. Later, the thyroid descends in front of the pharyngeal gut when it already has a bilobed diverticulum shape. The thyroglossal duct keeps the thyroid until it disappears. The thyroid keeps descend in front of the hyoid bone until finally it affixes to the front of the trachea in the seventh week. The thyroid starts working in the third month when the first follicles are visible and start producing colloid. The parafollicular cells come from the ultimobranchial body and produce calcitonin.

Cranium: Development of the Skull

At the beginning of the 3rd month, the head constitutes half of overall length. At the beginning of 5th month, head is one-third of the total length and at birth, it is one-fourth of the total length (Fig. 4.9).

Approximately, 110 ossification centers appear in the embryonic human skull. Many of these centers fuse to produce 45 separate bones in the neonatal skull. In the young adult, 32 separate skull bones are recognized. Centers of ossification within the basal plate, commencing with the basioccipital in the 10th week IU lay the basis for the endochondral bone portions of the occipital, sphenoid and temporal bones and for the wholly endochondral ethmoid and inferior nasal concha bones.

The bones of skull can be divided into viscerocranium which supports the nasal passages, oral cavity, the pharynx and forms the face and the neurocranium which surrounds the brain. The neurocranium can be subdivided into the cranial base/chondrocranium and calvaria (cranial vault/desmocranium). Cranial base is chondrocranium (cartilages), cranial vault is desmocranium (flat bone) and cranium is neurocranium (having neural tissues, neurocranial capsule). The bones of the skull base are formed mainly by endochondral ossification and the cartilaginous joints between the bones are called synchondroses. The bones of the cranial vault and face are primarily formed by intra-membranous ossification. The skull is formed from the mesenchymal connective tissue around the developing brain.

Cranial Vault

The sites of intramembranous ossification that appear in the mesenchyme covering the brain are termed as

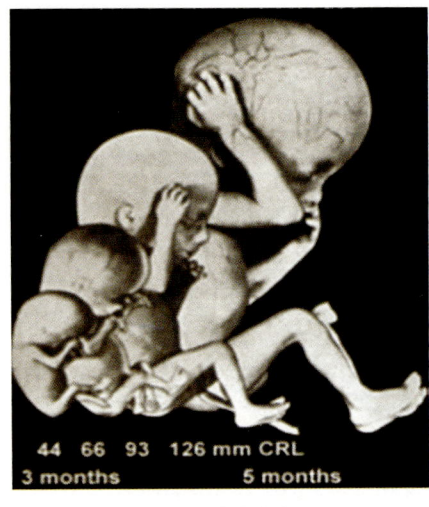

Fig. 4.9: Fetal size

membranous neurocranium or desmocranium. The cranial vault is formed by intramembranous bone formation without any cartilage precursor.

- These cites first appear at 8th week of IUL, the beginning of fetal period, as ossification centers. The membranous neurocranium gives rise to the flat bones of the calvaria including the superior portion of the frontal, parietal and occipital bones.
- The calvarial bones are separated by dense connective tissue sutures and six large fibrous areas called fontanelles; these fontanelles enable the skull to undergo shaping during birth which is called molding.

Cranial Base

The cartilaginous neurocranium, i.e. cranial base, is also called chondrocranium. It consists of several cartilages which fuse and undergo endochondral ossification to give rise to the cranial base. The junctions between two bones are called synchondroses as they contain intervening cartilage. The occipital bone is formed first, followed by the body of sphenoid bone and then the ethmoid bone. Chondrocranium also forms the vomer bone of nasal septum and petrous and mastoid parts of the temporal bone.

During fourth week IU, mesenchyme condenses between the developing brain and the foregut to form the ectomeningeal capsule around the cranial base. Its base gives rise to future cranial base. It is the earliest evidence of skull formation. Ectomeningeal mesenchyme starts changing into cartilage at around 40th day in different areas which later on fuse together to form a single cranial base which is the beginning of chondrocranium. These chondrification centers appear in four regions which are:

- Parachordal chondrification
- Hypophyseal cartilages
- Nasal cartilage
- Otic cartilages

Parachordal Chondrification

The centers forming around the cranial end of notochord are called parachordal cartilages.

Hypophyseal Cartilages

At the level of oropharyngeal membrane, the hypophyseal pouch gives rise to anterior lobe of pituitary gland. On either side, the post-sphenoid cartilages appear which fuse together and form posterior body of sphenoid bone. Cranial to pituitary gland, two cartilages develop and fuse to form anterior part of sphenoid bone.

Presphenoid cartilage gives rise to a vertical plate called mesethmoid cartilage which forms the perpendicular plate of ethmoid bone and crista galli. Mesethmoid cartilage is very important for the growth of the middle third of face. On the lateral side of pituitary gland, the chondrification centers appear which form the greater and lesser wings of sphenoid bone. So, sphenoid bone, ethmoid bone and crista galli are endochondral bones.

Nasal Cartilage

A nasal capsule develops around nasal sense organs which chondrifies and gets fused to cartilages of cranial base.

Otic Cartilages

A capsule forms around the vestibule cochlear sense organs. It chondrifies and ossifies to form mastoid and petrous parts of temporal bone. It also fuses with cranial base. These separate areas of chondrification in cranial base.

Origin of Mandible

The mandible has its origin in the mandibular processes of the first branchial arches around the 40th day of intrauterine life. It begins to form lateral to Meckel's cartilage and develops inward medial to the dental and incisal nerves. With these, centers of ossification are formed the angle, coronoid process, inner alveolar wall and alveolar borders.

By the 42nd day, the ramus and alveolar process may be distinguished. At 55 days, the beginning of the coronoid process and condyles is seen. By the middle of the 3rd month, the mandible reaches its characteristic shape.

Ossification of the Mandible

Centers of ossification can be seen in the mandible on the 39th day. During the 6th week of intrauterine life, a center of ossification appears at the angle. Bone formation spreads rapidly beginning with the 7th week and continues forward towards the midline and backwards. Meckel's cartilage supports the mandibular processes prior to ossification and union of the two sides of the mandibular bone. Ossification stops at this point which will later become the mandibular lingual and the remaining part of the Meckel's cartilage continues on its own to form the sphenomandibular ligament and spinous process of the sphenoids.

Secondary accessory cartilages appear between the 10th and 14th weeks IU to form the head of the condyle,

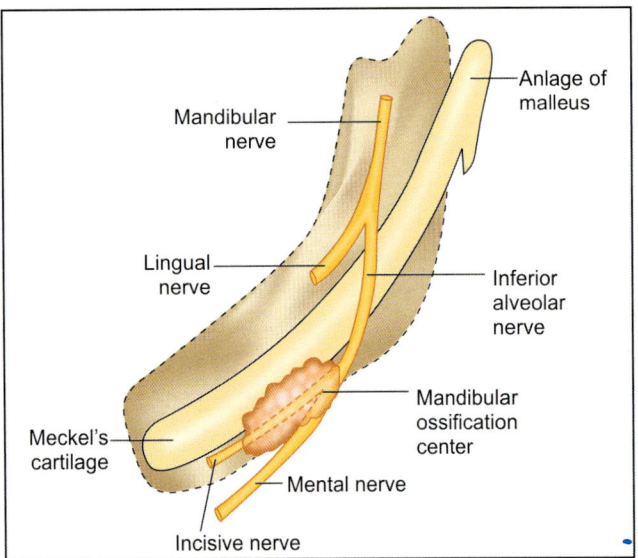

Fig. 4.10: Center of ossification of mandible lateral to Meckel's cartilage at the bifurcation of the inferior alveolar nerve

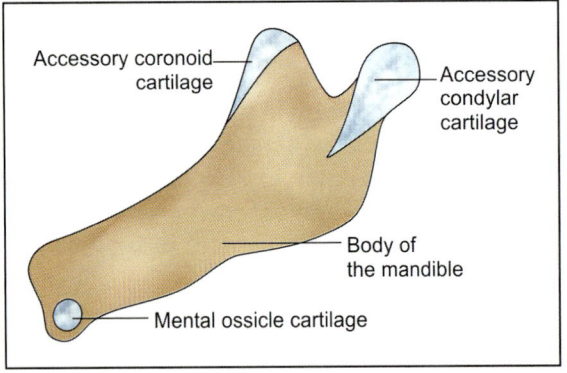

Fig. 4.11: Accessory cartilages of the fetal mandible

part of the coronoid process and the mental protuberance (Figs 4.10 and 4.11).

Maxilla

A primary intramembranous ossification center appears for each maxilla in the 8th week IU at the termination of the infraorbital nerve just above the canine tooth dental lamina. Secondary cartilages appear at the end of the 8th week IU in the regions of the zygomatic and alveolar processes that rapidly ossify and fuse with the primary intramembranous center. Two further intramembranous premaxillary centers appear anteriorly on each side in the 8th week IU and rapidly fuse with the primary maxillary center.

Single ossification centers appear for each of the zygomatic bones and the squamous portions of the temporal bones in the 8th week IU.

Palate

Development of Palate (Figs 4.12 and 4.13)

There are two parts of two different embryonic origins:
1. *Primary palate:* The triangular part of hard palate anterior to incisor foramen which originates from the premaxilla (frontonasal prominences). It develops between 4th and 8th week of gestation.
2. *Secondary palate:* Remaining part of the hard palate and all soft palate posterior to incisor foramen which comes from palatine shelves of the maxillary prominences. It develops between 8th and 12th week of gestation.

The three elements responsible to make up the secondary definite palate are:
- Lateral maxillary processes (left and right side).
- Primary palate of the frontonasal process.

These are initially widely separated due to the vertical orientation of the lateral shelves on either side of the tongue. Later in the 7th week IU (between 47th and 54th day), a remarkable transformation in position of the lateral shelves takes place, when they alter from vertical to horizontal, as a prelude to their fusion and partitioning the oronasal chamber.

Ossification of the palate proceeds during the 8th week IU from the spread of the bone into the mesenchyme of the fused lateral palatal shelves and from trabeculae appearing in the primary palate as premaxillary centers, all derived from the single primary ossification centers of the maxillae.

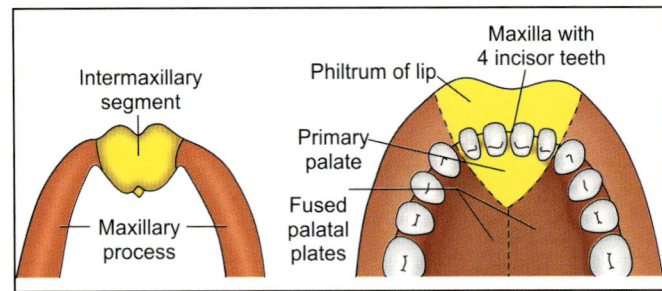

Fig. 4.12: Development of palate

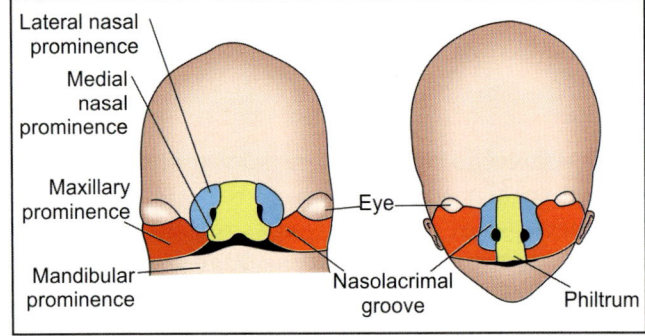

Fig. 4.13: Development of palate

Posteriorly, hard palate is ossified from the trabeculae spreading from the single primary ossification centers of each of the palatine bones. Mid-palatal sutural structure is first evident at around 10th week IU when an upper layer of fiber bundles develops across the midline. In most posterior part of the palate, ossification does not occur giving rise to the region of soft palate.

A cleft of the palate occurs, if the palatal shelves fail to fuse together as may happen, if the tongue fails to descent due to underdevelopment of the mandible. Incomplete penetration of the mesoderm into the palatal shelves can give rise to a submucous cleft palate. Thus, the formation of a cleft of palate and alveolus (primary palate) occurs between 4th and 8th week after conception and clefts of the hard and soft palate (secondary palate) occur between 8th and 12th week. A complete cleft of the lip, alveolus and palate would, therefore, suggest a continuation of the effects of the etiological factors over all these weeks while clefts of the primary or secondary palate alone would imply its restriction to the appropriate weeks.

The reasons for cleft palate are:
- Defective growth of the palatine shelves
- Failure of elevation of the shelves
- Failure of fusion of the shelves
- Postfusion rupture of the shelves
- Micrognathia as in Robin complex

POSTNATAL GROWTH OF CRANIOFACIAL COMPLEX

The whole craniofacial complex skull is divided into the neurocranium and viscerocranium. The growth of craniofacial complex can be studied by noting the changes occurring in the following areas:
- Neurocranium
  - The cranial vault
  - The cranial base
- Viscerocranium (face)
  - The nasomaxillary complex
  - The mandible

The cranial vault and face are formed by intramembranous ossification where bone is directly formed from undifferentiated mesenchymal tissue with no cartilaginous precursor.

On the other hand, the cranial base undergoes endochondral ossification where a precursor/primary cartilage is converted into bone. The membranous bones may develop secondary cartilages to provide rapid growth.

Cranium and facial skeleton grow at different rates. Growth of cranium being intimately associated with growth of the brain follows the neural growth curve where most of the growth occurs in first few years of life. Growth of facial skeleton follows the general growth curve. Remodeling and growth occurs primarily at periosteum-lined contact areas between adjacent skull bones, called the skeletal sutures at birth, the flat bones of the skull are rather widely separated by relatively loose connective tissues. These open spaces, the fontanelles, allow considerable amount of deformation of skull at birth—a fact which is important in allowing the relatively large head to pass through the birth canal.

After birth, apposition of bone along the edges of the fontanelles eliminates these open spaces fairly quickly, but the bones remain separated by a thin periosteum-lined suture for many years, eventually fusing in adult life.

The newborn not only has his frontal bone separated by the soon to close metopic suture, but also has no frontal sinuses. Both the inner and outer surfaces are quite parallel and quite close to each other. With the general growth and thickening of the cranial vault, there is an increase in the distance between the internal and external plates in the supraorbital region. This may be seen on the external surface as a ridge. The spongy bone between the external plates is gradually replaced by the developing frontal sinus (Fig. 4.14).

Postnatal Growth of the Cranial Vault

Cranial vault covers the upper and outer surfaces of the brain. It consists of a number of flat bones which are formed from intramembranous ossification.

Adaptive growth occurs at the coronal, sagittal, parietal, temporal and occipital sutures to accommodate the rapidly expanding brain. As the brain expands, the separate bones of the cranial vault are displaced the outward direction. This intramembranous sutural growth replaces the fontanelles that are present at birth.

Apart from growth at sutures, growth also occurs by periosteal and endosteal remodeling. Resorption at the endosteal lining and apposition at the periosteum leads to an increase in the overall thickness of the medullary space between the inner and the outer tables.

Cranial vault following the neural growth curve achieves most of its growth during first few years of life with over 90% of growth by 5 years and 98% by 15 years of age.

Postnatal Cranial Base

Contrary to the cranial vault, the bones of the cranial base are formed by ethmoid, sphenoid and occipital

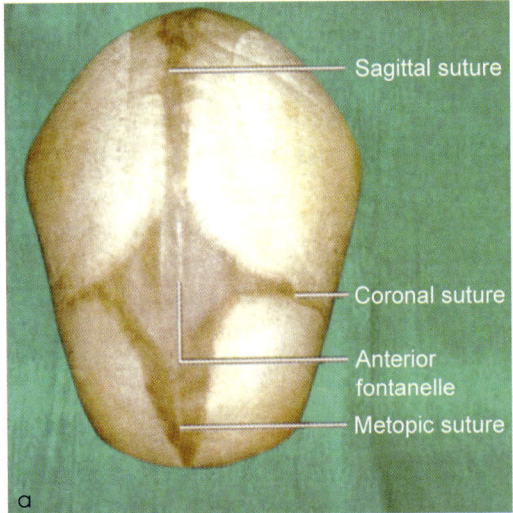

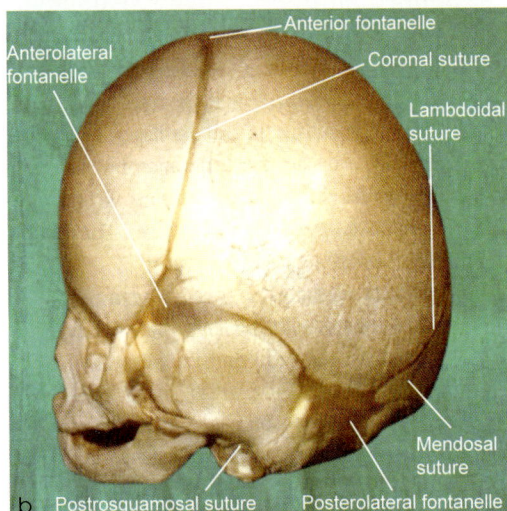

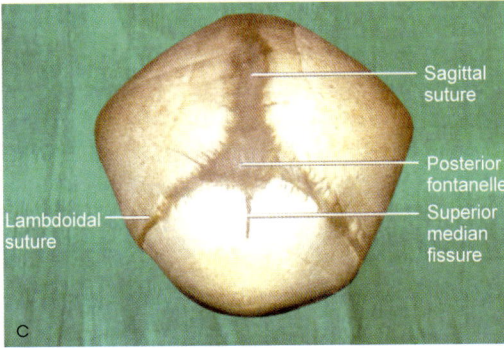

Fig. 4.14: Location of various fontanelles: (a) Superior view; (b) Lateral view; (c) Posterior view

Elongation at Synchondroses

It is a major contributor in the postnatal growth. It fuses at 12–13 years in girls and 14–15 years in boys and ossifies at 20 years of age. Most of the bones of the cranial base are formed by a cartilaginous process. Later, the cartilage is replaced by bone. Certain bands of cartilage remain at the junctions of various bones. These areas are called synchondroses. They are important growth sites of the cranial base.

The cranial base grows by cartilage growth in the sphenoethmoidal, intersphenoethmoidal, sheno-occipital and intraoccipital synchondroses. It follows a neural growth curve, but partially the general growth curve.

- Activity at intersphenoidal synchondroses disappears at birth.
- Interoccipital synchondrosis closes in third to fifth years of life.
- Spheno-occipital synchondrosis does not ossify until 13–15 years of age and close at 20 years (Fig. 4.15).
- Endochondral ossification does not stop here until 20th year of life.

Growth Theories

Genetic Theory (Brodie)

It is controlled by genetic influence and is preplaned. Genes are a basic participant in the operation of any given cells organelles leading to the expression of that cell's particular function. The DNA content of all cells in the body is identical.

It is the RNA which determines the cell's intracellular and extracellular proteins and ultimately the functions of that cell. The role of genetic tissues in growth is controlled by epigenetic influences from other tissue groups and their functional, structural and developmental input signals. However, this theory is referred to as the sutural dominance theory with proliferation of connective tissue and its replacement by bone in the sutures being a primary consideration.

bones. The changes in the cranial base occur primarily as a result of endochondral growth through a system of synchondroses. A synchondrosis is a cartilaginous joint where the hyaline cartilage divides and subsequently is converted into bone. A series of synchondroses occurs within and between the three bones of cranial base and cartilage growth at these synchondroses leads to the growth of cranial base.

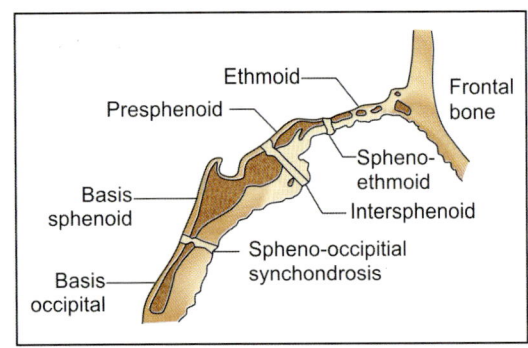

Fig. 4.15: Spheno-occipital synchondrosis

Sutural Theory (Weinmann and Sicher)

Sicher believed that craniofacial growth occurs at the sutures. According to him, the facial areas are attached to the skull and the cranial base region by paired parallel sutures. These sutures push the nasomaxillary complex forwards to pace its growth with that of the mandible. This theory is also based on genetic control of growth.

Cartilagious Theory (Scott)

The Irish anatomist James H Scott proposed the nasal septal theory. He viewed the cartilaginous sites throughout the skull as primary centers of growth. According to this theory, sutures play little or no direct role in the growth of the craniofacial skeleton, but cartilage and periosteum play primary role in the craniofacial growth.

Scott concludes that various craniofacial regions are dependent primarily on the cartilage and secondarily on the sutures.

Example:
- The condylar cartilages are growth centers for the growth of the mandible as they push the mandible downward and forward.
- Synchondroses in the cranial base are the primary cartilages for the calvaria growth and sutures of cranial vault are secondary.
- Nasal septal cartilage is responsible for midface growth in the prenatal and postnatal periods up to 4 years of age in humans. The nasal septal cartilage situated against the cranial base drives the midface downward and forward.

Functional Matrix Concept (Melvin Moss)

He introduced the theory in 1962. It was developed based on the original concept of functional cranial component by Van der Klaauw (1952). This is widely accepted growth theory. He stressed the dominance of non-osseous structures of the craniofacial complex over the skeletal components.

Skeletal unit: The totality of all the soft tissues, organs and functioning spaces associated with a single function is taken as a whole, comprising the functional matrix. The corresponding skeletal tissues which support and protect this related specific functional matrix comprise the skeletal unit.

According to the functional matrix hypothesis, the origin, form, position, growth and maintenance of all skeletal tissues and organs are always secondary, compensatory and mechanically. In this view, the soft tissues grow and both bone and cartilage react and are grown in response to the growth of soft tissue.

All the skeletal tissues associated with a single function is called the skeletal unit. The skeletal unit may be comprised of bone, suture, cartilage, synchondroses and tendinous tissue. The skeletal unit is made up of several small contiguous skeletal units (microskeletal unit). When adjoining portions of a number of microskeletal units work in tandem to carry out a single cranial component, it is termed as a macroskeletal unit. Thus, macroskeleton is composed of small microskeletal units. The different microskeletal units may form anatomically different macroskeleton.

Functional component: Head is a composite structure; number of relatively independent functions is operating in the craniofacial region. These include respiration, olfaction, vision, hearing, balance, chewing, digestion, swallowing, speech and neural integration. Each of these functions is accomplished by certain tissues and spaces in the head. All tissues, organs, spaces and skeletal parts necessary to carry out a given single function have been termed as "functional cranial component".

The functional cranial component is divided into functional matrix, and skeletal unit.

There are two types of functional matrices:
- Periosteal matrix
- Capsular matrix

Periosteal matrix: These matrices act directly and actively on adjacent skeletal units. With the direct action, the skeletal tissue undergoes transformatory changes by deposition and resorption process. Ultimately, the periosteal matrix is to alter the form of that particular skeletal unit. The periosteal matrices include the muscles, blood vessels, nerves and glands.

Capsular matrix: It is defined as the organs and spaces that occupy a broader anatomical complex. The capsular matrix unlike periosteal matrix acts indirectly and passively on their related skeletal units producing a secondary translation in space. These alterations in spatial position of skeletal units are brought about by the expansion of the orofacial capsule within which the facial bones arise, grow and are maintained. No deposition and resorption occurs.

Examples:
- Neurocranial capsule
- Orocranial capsule

Each of these capsules is an envelop which contains a series of functional cranial components which as a whole are sandwiched in between two covering layers.

Neurocranial capsule: It comprises brain and covering layers, aponeurosis, dura mater, and skin. This cover consists of the skin and the dura mater.

Orocranial capsule: It comprises spaces, like oropharynx, and nasopharynx which arise within the facial bones are maintained. In the orofacial capsule, the skin and mucosa form the covering. These two capsular units expand, allowing the skeletal units to move and translate. These capsular units do not cause deposition or resorption like periosteal unit as mentioned above.

Van Limborgh's Theory

A multifactorial theory which has given a new view to the morphogenesis of skull was put forward by Van Limborgh in 1970. This synthesis is essential from the three basic theories of craniofacial growth namely Scott's, Sicher's and Moss's functional matrix theories. The drawbacks of the above theories were left unanswered to a large extent. He suggested following the essentials of the entire three hypotheses. He lists the essentials of the entire three hypotheses.

Servosystem Theory

A new concept in understanding the process of controlling postnatal craniofacial growth is the servosystem theory by Petrovic and Stutzman in 1980.

It is based on "Cybernetic concept". Cybernetic concept states that everything affects everything and living organisms never operate in open loop mechanism. In an open loop mechanism, the input/ stimulus leads to a response and there is no feedback or regulation.

Closed loop mechanism can be of two types:
- Regulator system in which the main input is constant.
- Servosystem/follow-up system in which the main input varies rather than being constant.

Components of servosystem
- *Command:* It is a signal established independently of the feedback system under scrutiny. It affects by the consequences of this behavior, e.g. somatotropic hormone, growth hormone, testosterone and estrogen.
- *Reference input elements:* Establish the relationship between the command and reference input. It includes septal cartilage, septopremaxillary ligament.
- *Reference input:* It is the signal established as a standard of comparison sagittal position of maxilla.
- *Comparator:* The configuration between the position of the upper and lower dental arch is the comparator of the servosystem.

- *Actuating signal:* Activity of the retrodiscal pad and lateral pterygoid constitutes the actuating signal. The elastic meniscotemporal and mensicomandibular frenums of the condylar disc from the retrodiscal pad.
- *Controlled system:* It is between the articulator and controlled variable, e.g. growth of condylar cartilage through the retrodiscal pad stimulation.
- *Controlled variable:* It is the output signal of the servo system. Best example is sagittal position of mandible.

How the servosystem theory explains the growth of jaws?
According to the servosystem theory, the influence of somatotropic hormone on growth of primary cartilages, i.e. nasal septum, sphenooccipital synchondrosis, and other synchondroses, has a cybernetic form of a "command". Growth-related hormones have a direct influence on the growth of primary cartilages. On the other hand, these hormones have both direct and indirect effects on the growth of secondary cartilages, e.g. condylar, coronoid cartilages of mandible, suture and some craniofacial sutures. The growth of secondary cartilages corresponds to local epigenetic and environmental factors.

In the development of jaws and face, the upper arch acts as a constantly changing reference input and the lower arch is the controlled variable. Any disturbance or confrontation between the respective positions of the upper and lower arch acts as the peripheral comparator and sends activating signals through the stimulation of retrodiscal pad and lateral pterygoid muscles.

This affects the output signal, i.e. the final sagittal position of the mandible. The inference is that, the final sagittal position of the mandible depends on the modifications of condylar growth by the activity of retrodiscal pad and lateral pterygoid muscle stimulation.

Other Theories Related to Craniofacial Growth

Expanding "V" Principle by Enlow

The concept of expanding "V" principle was put forward by Enlow. The "V" principle is an important facial skeletal growth mechanism since many facial and cranial bones have a "V" configuration or "V" shaped regions.

Expanding "V" principle: In "V" shaped bones/areas, bone resorption occurs on the outer surface of the "V", and deposition on the inner surface. As the remodeling continues, the "V" moves away from its tip and enlarges simultaneously giving rise to simultaneous growth as well as movement of the bone.

In this way, growth as well as movement of the bone occurs simultaneous movement of the bone in the shape of "V" is called the expanding "V" principle.

Such a growth process results in:
- Enlargement in overall size of the "V" shaped area.
- Movement of the entire "V" structure towards its own wider end.
- Continuous relocation.

Most of the craniofacial bones including mandible, maxilla and palate grow on an expanding "V" growth of the palate is one of the best examples of expanding "V" principle. Deposition occurs on the palatal periosteal surface and resorption occurs on the side of nasal floor. In this way, palate expands on lateral direction and also moves downwards.

It is easier to visualize mandible as a "V" shaped bone than maxilla because of its horseshoe shape. Ramus of the mandible grows on an expanding "V" and internal width of the mandible also increases by expanding "V" principle. The condyle remodels according to the expanding "V" principle and the neck of the condyle gets lengthened.

Enlow expanding principle: Many facial bones or parts of bone have a 'V' shaped pattern of growth. Bone deposition occurs on the inner side of the wide end of the 'V' and bone resorption on the outer surface (Fig. 4.16).

Enlow's counter-principle
a. Amount of growth between the counterparts
b. Direction of growth between the counterparts
c. Time of growth between the counterparts

Mutual counterparts—maxillary and manibular arch, bone and corpus of mandible.

Nasomaxillary complex relates to anterior cranial fossa, middle cranial fossa, maxillary tuberosity and lingual tuberosity.

POSTNATAL GROWTH OF MANDIBLE

Intramembranous ossification:
- Whole body of mandible except the anterior part
- Ramus of mandible as far as mandibular foramen

Endochondral ossification:
- Anterior portion of the mandible (symphysis)
- Part of ramus above the mandibular foramen
- Coronoid process
- Condylar process

Of all the facial bones, the mandible undergoes the most growth postnatally and evidences the greatest variation in morphology.

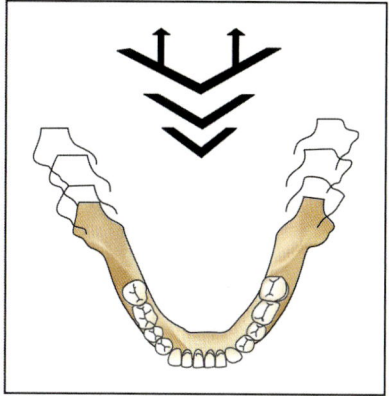

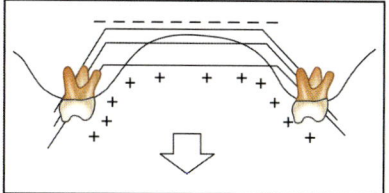

Fig. 4.16: Enlow's expanding principles

Of the facial bones, mandible exhibits greatest amount of postnatal growth. Mandible grows in a downward and forward direction and the growth rate follows the general growth curve with significant growth spurts during puberty.

Growth of mandible largely occurs due to intramembranous ossification. However, a few secondary cartilages, especially the condylar cartilage, accelerate its growth postnatally.

Although a single bone, the mandible, can be divided into functionally and developmentally into several subunits. Postnatal development can be better understood by studying the growth of these units, which include body of mandible, alveolar process that is attached to the body, condyles, rami and lingual tuberosity with chin and angular and coronoid processes (Fig. 4.17).

Mandible at Birth

At birth, the mandible is made of two halves, as it is not united at the midline. By the end of first year, the two halves get united to form a single mandibular bone. The rami are short and condylar development is minimal at birth (Figs 4.17 and 4.18).

Mandibular growth from infancy to adolescence is seen in Fig. 4.19.
- *6 months–4 years* symmetric broadening posteriorly, downward and forward.
- *Till 4 years of age,* there is rapid growth in all three dimensions. After 4 years, transverse growth occurs only in the posterior segment and it slows by 8 years.

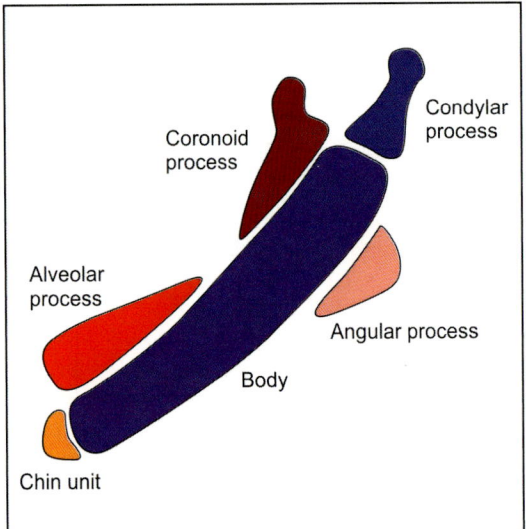

Fig. 4.17: Skeletal units

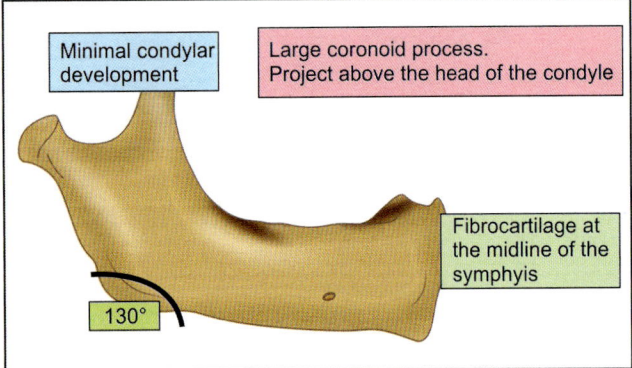

Minimal condylar development

Large coronoid process. Project above the head of the condyle

Fibrocartilage at the midline of the symphyis

130°

Fig. 4.18: Mandible at birth

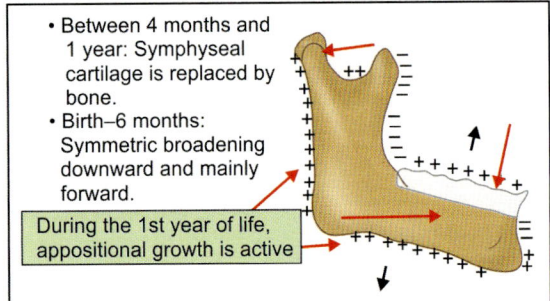

- Between 4 months and 1 year: Symphyseal cartilage is replaced by bone.
- Birth–6 months: Symmetric broadening downward and mainly forward.

During the 1st year of life, appositional growth is active

Fig. 4.19: Mandibular growth from infancy to adolescence

- *4–8 years* broadening at condyles, downward and forward.
- *8 years* onwards downward and forward.
- Vertical and posteroanterior growth continues till 20 years of age.
- On average:
  - Ramus height increases 1–2 mm/yr, and
  - Body length increases 2–3 mm/yr.

Ramus

Bone resorption at the anterior border and deposition at posterior border of the ramus accounts for the anteroposterior growth of the ramus and the body of the mandible. Such remodeling converts former ramal bone into the posterior part of the body and thereby increasing the length of mandibular arch to accommodate the erupting permanent molars. Drift of the ramus in a posterior direction also provides area for insertion of the increasing mass of masticatory muscles (Figs 4.20 and 4.21).

The most important structural part as:

- It positions the dental arch and corpus in occlusion with the upper arch.
- It is continuously adaptive to the multitude of changing craniofacial proportions.
- Remodels in the posterosuperior manner. As it is relocated in a posterior direction—posterior lengthening of the corpus and dental arch occurs.

Ramus Uprighting

During development, ramus becomes more vertically aligned (Fig. 4.22).

It occurs by posterior direction of growth and relocation. It results in remodeling rotation of the ramus.

Vertical lengthening continues even after horizontal ramus growth ceases. This is to match the continued vertical growth of the midface.

In order to achieve this, condylar growth become vertically directed and reverse remodeling patterns of ramus occur (Fig. 4.23).

- Results in:
  - More upright alignment, and
  - A longer vertical dimension without increase in breadth.
- *It is referred to as:* Developmental 'compensation' at work—to retain constant positional relationships

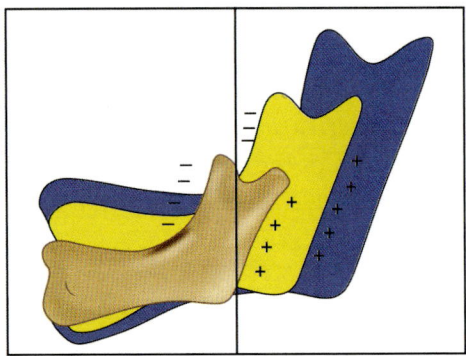

Fig. 4.20: Drift of ramus in posterior direction

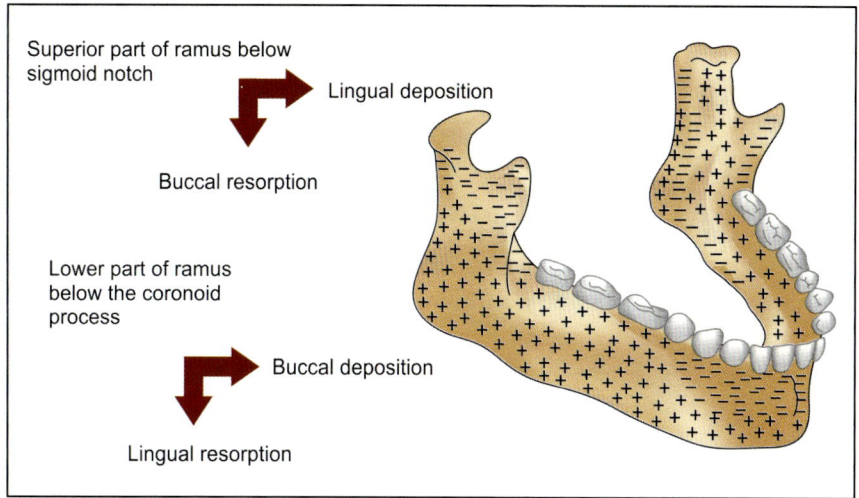

Fig. 4.21: Increase in the length of mandibular arch to accommodate permanent molars

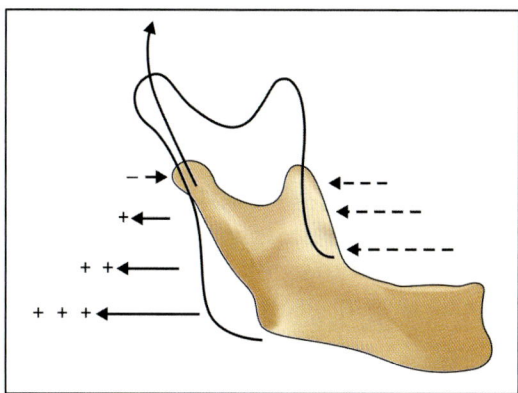

Fig. 4.22: Ramus uprighting

between the upper and lower arches without increase in the breadth of the ramus.

Body of Mandible

The body of the mandible maintains a relatively constant angular relationship to the ramus throughout life. As the ramus drifts in a posterior direction, the length of the body of mandible increases at its posterior aspect. This increase in the length of mandible provides room for erupting permanent molars (Fig. 4.24).

Angle of Mandible

Selective bone remodeling at the angle of mandible causes flaring of the angle as age advances. On the lingual side of angle of mandible, resorption occurs on the posteroinferior aspect while deposition occurs on the anterosuperior aspect. On the buccal aspect, resorption occurs on the anteroposterior aspect while deposition takes place on the posterosuperior aspect causing flaring of the angle of mandible.

- The gonial angle closes with growth in order to prevent change in the occlusal relationship between the upper and lower arches. Thus, the gonial angle, which is obtuse (140° or more) in infants, changes to about 110° in adults (Fig. 4.25).
- The gonial region is anatomically variable in the pattern of growth.

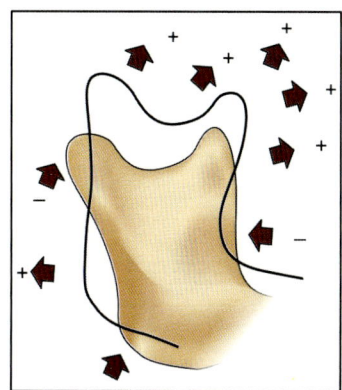

Fig. 4.23: Vertical direction of condylar growth

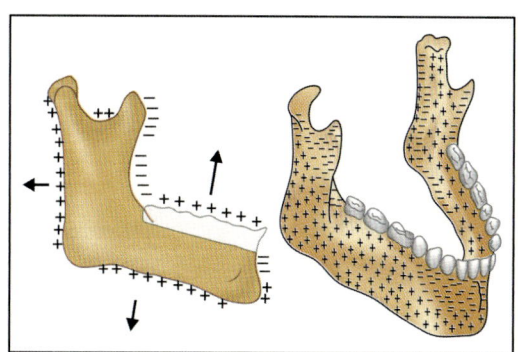

Fig. 4.24: Increase in the length of mandible

- Depending on the presence of inwardly or outwardly directed gonial flares, the buccal side can be either depository or resorptive, with the lingual side having the converse type of growth.

Antegonial Notch (Fig. 4.26)

A single field of resorption is present on the inferior edge of the mandible at the ramus–corpus junction.

This forms the antegonial notch by remodeling from the ramus behind it as the ramus relocates posteriorly.

- The size of the antegonial notch is determined by:
  - The ramus–corpus angle (gonial angle), and
  - By the extent of bone deposition on the inferior margin of the corpus just posterior or anterior to the notch.
- Antegonial notch is less prominent when gonial angle becomes closed and more prominent when gonial angle becomes opened.
- When the growth of the mandibular condyle fails to contribute to the lowering of the mandible, the masseter and medial pterygoid, by their continued

growth, cause the bone in the region of the angle to grow downward, producing antegonial notching.

- There is pronounced apposition beneath the angle with excessive resorption under the symphysis. The resultant upward curving of the inferior border of the mandible anterior to the angular process is known as antegonial notch.

Mandibular Foramen

The mandibular foramen maintains its relative position by "drifting" in a posterior and upward direction through resorption in the post-lingular fossa and periosteal addition on the lingula (Fig. 4.27).

Mandibular Condyle (Fig. 4.28)

The condyle shows minimum growth at birth. It is an anatomic part of special interest because it is a major site of growth of mandible having considerable clinical significance. Growth of the condylar cartilage would increase the length and height of the mandible.

There are two major schools of thought about the role of condyle:

1. The condyle is considered as the major growth center of mandible with an intrinsic genetic potential. Others thought that the condylar cartilage was analogous to an epiphyseal cartilage. As the condyle pushes against the cranial base, the entire mandible gets displaced in a forward and downward direction.

2. Secondly, the growth of soft tissues, including muscles and connective tissues (functional matrix), carries the mandible forward and downward with growth expansion of the soft tissue matrix associated with it. The condylar remodeling is not a driving force of growth, but it is rather an adaptive change

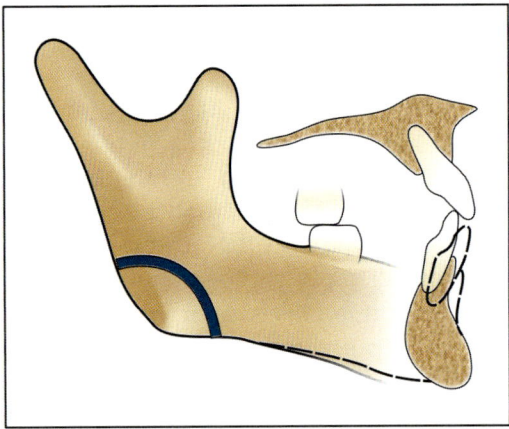

Fig. 4.25: Gonial angle change

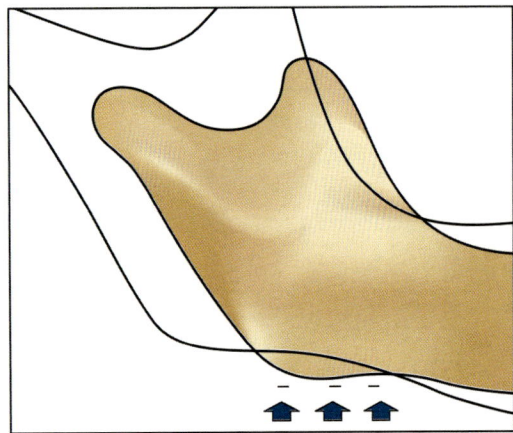

Fig. 4.26: Antegonial notch development

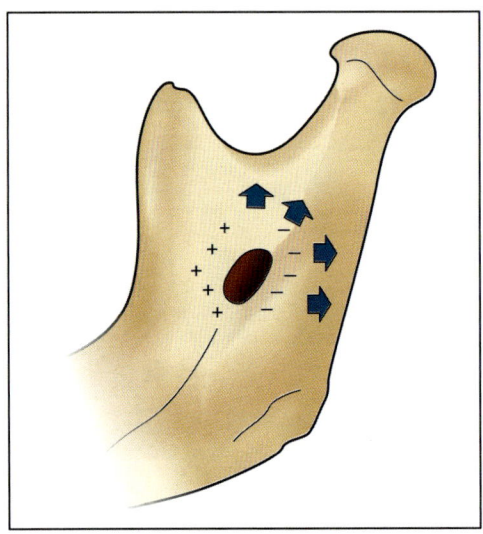

Fig. 4.27: Growth around mandibular foramen

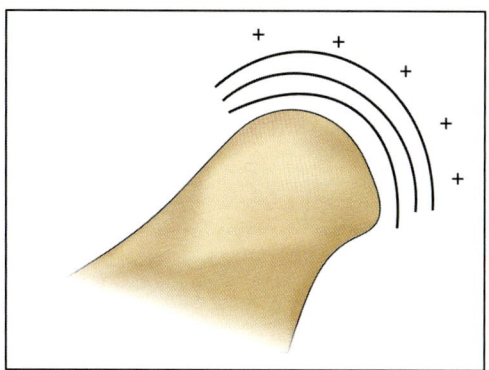

Fig. 4.28: Mandibular condyle development

secondary to the displacement of mandible by the functional matrix. Thus, as the mandible is displaced away from its basocranial articular contact, the condyle, and whole ramus secondarily remodels towards the cranial base, thereby closing any potential space without an actual gap being created.

It contributes to the overall size of the mandible through a process of endochondral replacement of proliferating condylar cartilage by bone tissue. As the mandible grows in a generally posterior direction, the condyle grows in a posterior direction.

Coronoid Process (Fig. 4.29)

Growth of the coronoid process follows the expanding "V" principle. A vertical section through the ramus, coronoid process shows a characteristic growth pattern involving periosteal deposition on the lingual surface of coronoid processes together with resorption from buccal surface. Basal part of ramus shows deposition on the buccal side with contralateral resorption from

the lingual surface. This remodeling causes an increase in height of coronoid process with their apices growing further apart.

The lingual surface of the coronoid process faces three general directions: Cephalic, posterior and medial.

This arrangement produces three corresponding results as the mandible grows in overall size.

Lingual Tuberosity (Fig. 4.30)

- It directs anatomic eqivalent of maxillary tuberosity
- Major growth and remodeling site
- It is an effective boundary between ramus and corpus.

Alveolar Process

Alveolar growth occurs around the tooth buds. As the teeth develop and begin to erupt, the alveolar process increases in size and height. This continued growth of alveolar bone with developing dentition increases the height of the mandibular body. The alveolar process grows upward and outward on an expanding arch. This permits the dental arch to accommodate the larger permanent teeth.

- Formation of the alveolar process is controlled by dental eruption and it resorbs when teeth are exfoliated or extracted.
- It serves as a "buffer zone" and helps to maintain occlusal relationships during differential mandibular and midface growth.
- Vertical alveolar growth persists even after corpus growth is over, to compensate for the occlusal wear of teeth. This helps to maintain the occlusal height in adulthood.
- Adaptive remodeling of the alveolar process makes orthodontic tooth movements possible.

The Chin (Fig. 4.31)

The chin is not well developed at birth. Significant growth of the chin occurs at puberty as age advances and is influenced by sexual and genetic factors. Chin becomes prominent at puberty especially in male by selective bone remodeling. Bone resorption occurs in

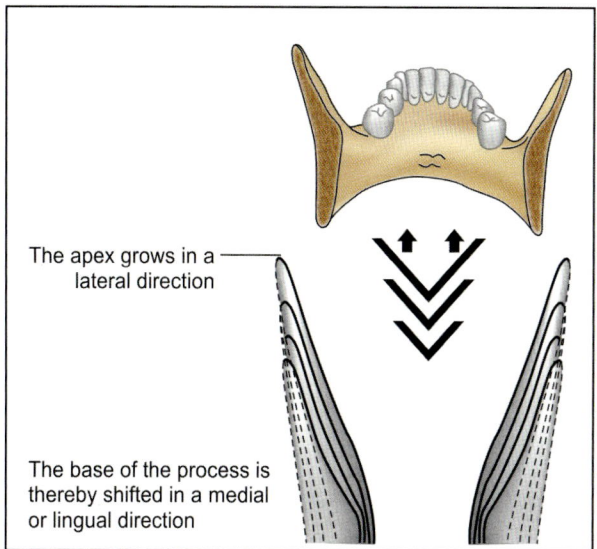

The apex grows in a lateral direction

The base of the process is thereby shifted in a medial or lingual direction

Fig. 4.29: Coronoid process development

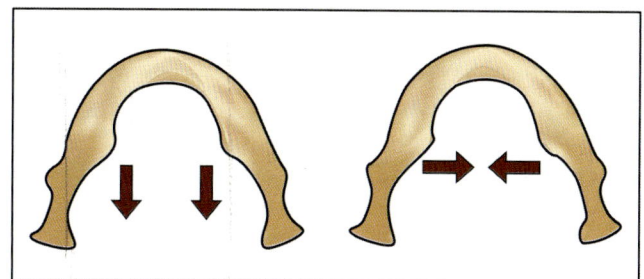

Fig. 4.30: Lingual tuberosity direction

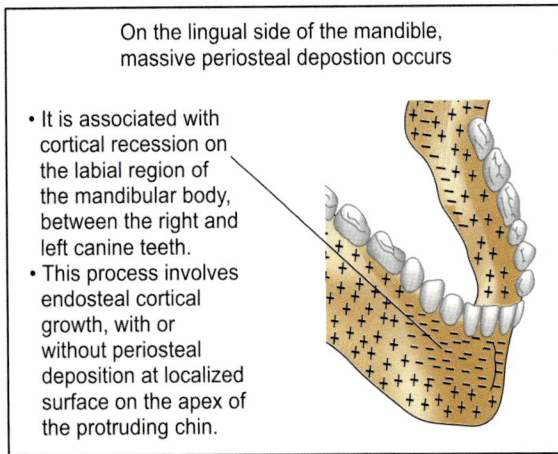

On the lingual side of the mandible, massive periosteal depostion occurs

• It is associated with cortical recession on the labial region of the mandibular body, between the right and left canine teeth.
• This process involves endosteal cortical growth, with or without periosteal deposition at localized surface on the apex of the protruding chin.

Fig. 4.31: The chin

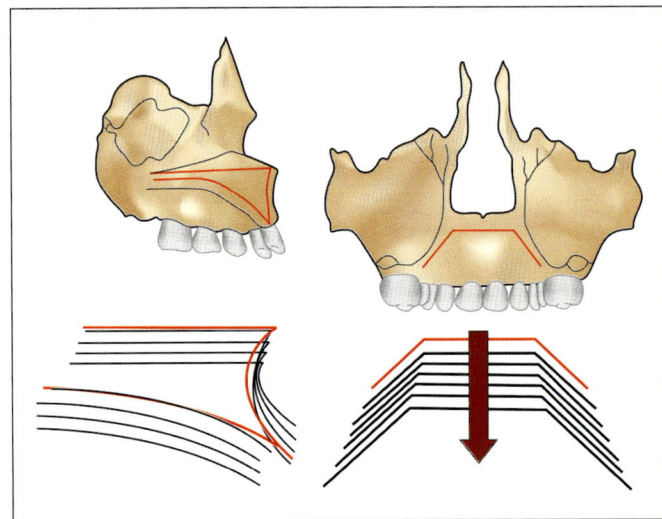

Fig. 4.32: Expanding 'V' principle in nasomaxillary complex

the alveolar region above the prominence creating a concavity. Apposition occurs at the inferior aspect.

POSTNATAL GROWTH OF NASOMAXILLARY COMPLEX

The cranium and the facial skeleton grow at different rates. By this differential growth, the face appears to literally emerge from beneath the cranium. The upper face under the influence of cranial base inclination, moves upward and forward while the lower face moves downward and forward on the expanding "V" (Fig. 4.32).

As maxilla is joined to the cranial base, its growth is strongly influenced by the changes occurring at the cranial base. Thus, the position of the maxilla is dependent on the growth of the cartilaginous nasal septum, which carries the nasomaxillary complex downward and forward.

Growth of nasomaxillary complex can be attributed to the following mechanisms:
• Translation/displacement
  – Primary
  – Secondary
• Growth at sutures
• Surface remodeling

Primary Translation/Displacement

Primary translation occurs where actual enlargement of the bone will change its position in space. In other words, primary displacement of the bone is brought about by its own enlargement.

Primary displacement of maxilla in a forward direction occurs due to the growth of maxillary tuberosity in a posterior direction. The amount of anterior displacement is equal to the amount of posterior lengthening. Periosteal surface of the

tuberosity receives continuous deposits of new bone and the results in horizontal lengthening of the maxillary arch.

Secondary Translation

It occurs when the growth of one bone results in a change in the spatial position of an adjacent bone. Nasomaxillary complex grows by secondary translation during primary dentition period.

As the maxilla is attached to the cranial base, the growth occurring at cranial base produces a passive/secondary displacement of the nasomaxillary complex in a downward and forward direction (Fig. 4.33).

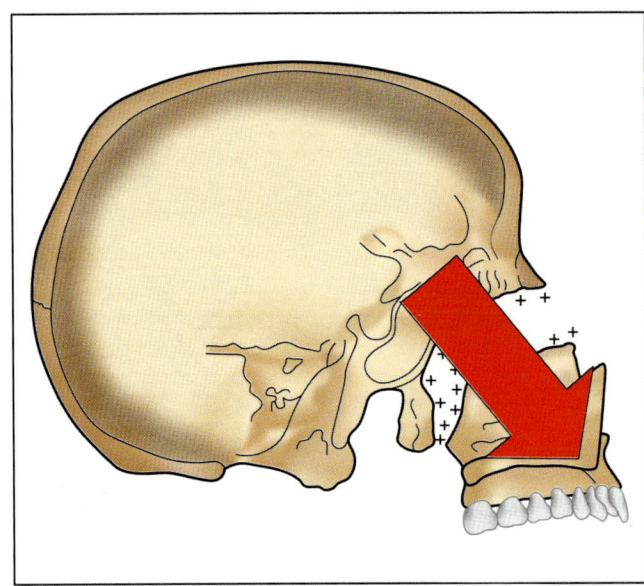

Fig. 4.33: Secondary displacement of the nasomaxillary complex

Growth at Sutures

The nasomaxillary complex is surrounded by a system of sutures that allows for the growth of various bones both anteroposteriorly and laterally. These sutures include:

- Frontomaxillary sutures
- Zygomaticotemporal suture
- Zygomaticomaxillary suture
- Pterygopalatine suture

These sutures are oblique and more or less parallel with each other. Tension produced by the downward and forward displacement of the maxillary bone stimulates the sutural bone growth at these sutures. New bone is formed on either side of the suture as a response to the tendency to displacement. Thus, the entire maxilla is carried forward and downward by displacement, the osteogenic sutural membranes form new bone tissues that enlarges the overall size of the maxilla, while constantly maintaining the bone to bone sutural contact (Fig. 4.34).

Surface Bone Remodeling

In addition to the specific sites of bone formation, all bony surfaces undergo selective bone remodeling through deposition and resorption along with endosteal and periosteal surfaces of bone. Along with an increase in size, bone remodeling brings about changes in shape and functional relationship of the bone (Fig. 4.35).

Maxillary Sinus

It is rudimentary at birth. Its postnatal increase in size contributes significantly to the development of nasomaxillary complex. The cortical surface of maxillary sinus is all resorptive except the medial nasal wall which is depository, because it remodels laterally to accommodate nasal expansion.

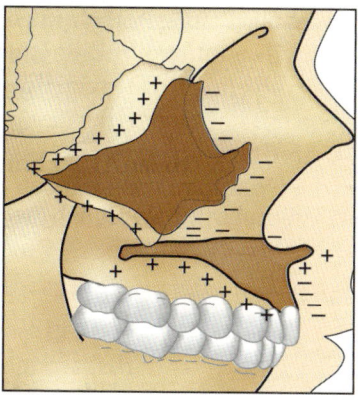

Fig. 4.35: Surface bone remodeling in maxilla

Nasal Cavity

The resorption occurs on its lateral walls of nasal cavity. The nasal wall is lowered by resorption of floor of nasal cavity. This is accompanied by bone deposition on the oral side of palatal vault.

Orbit

Widening of orbit occurs by resorption of inner surface of the lateral rim. Compensatory deposition occurs on the outer surface of the lateral rim and on the medial wall of the orbit.

Maxillary Tuberosity

Deposition of periosteal bone on the posterior surface of the tuberosity increases the length of maxillary arches and provides room for erupting molars. The endosteal surface is resorptive and this contributes to maxillary sinus enlarging (Fig. 4.36).

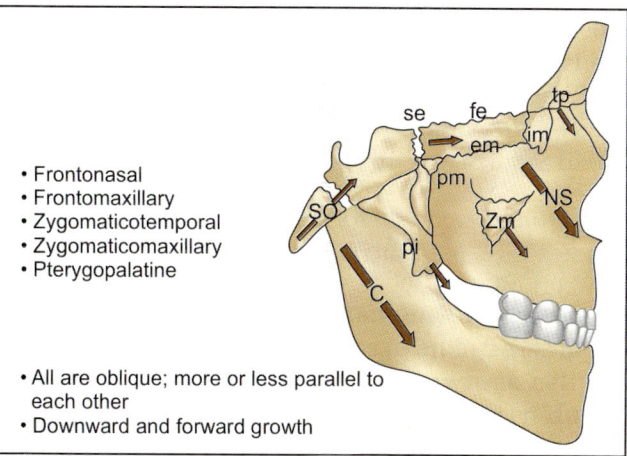

- Frontonasal
- Frontomaxillary
- Zygomaticotemporal
- Zygomaticomaxillary
- Pterygopalatine

- All are oblique; more or less parallel to each other
- Downward and forward growth

Fig. 4.34: Growth at sutures

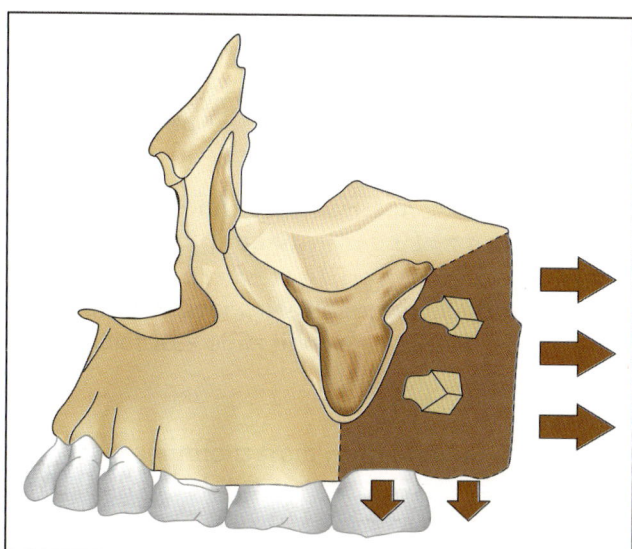

Fig. 4.36: Increase the length of maxillary arch

Zygoma

The zygomatic arch moves laterally and posteriorly by deposition of bone on lateral and posterior surfaces. Compensatory resorption occurs on medial and anterior surfaces.

Palatal Remodeling and Increase in Maxillary Height

The palatal growth follows the principle of the expanding "V". Resorption occurs on the floor of the nasal cavity and deposition on the oral side of the palatal vault. This moves the palate in a downward direction. However, depth of palatal vault continues to increase with age expanding in a "V" shape. This is a result of growth of alveolar process that accompanies the eruption of primary and permanent teeth.

Increase in Maxillary Height

Increase in the height of maxillary complex is mainly due to continued apposition of alveolar bone on the free borders of the alveolar process as the teeth erupt.

Increase in Maxillary Width

Growth in width occurs during the first 5 years of life, mostly at intermaxillary and midpalatal sutures. Later, any additional increase in the width of the maxilla occurs as a result of bone deposition on the outer surface of maxilla and by the buccal eruption of permanent teeth.

Neurotropic Process in Orofacial Growth

It is a non-impulse transmitting neural function that involves axoplasmic transport and provides for long-term interaction between neurons. Different types of neurotrophic mechanisms are:

1. *Neuroepithlial trophism:* Epithelial mitosis and synthesis are eutrophically controlled; the normal epithelial growth is controlled by release of neurotropic substance.
2. *Neurovisceral trophism:* Embryonic myogenesis is independent of neural innervation and trophic control.
3. *Neuromuscular trophism:* Salivary glands, fat tissue and other organs are trophically regulated.

To conclude, the different mechanisms of bone growth are as follows:

- Bone deposition and resorption—known as bone remodeling.
- Cortical drift—combination of bone deposition and resorption resulting in a growth movement toward the depository surface.
- Displacement—is the movement of whole bone as a unit. It is due to pull or push of different soft and bone tissues as they all continue to enlarge.
- Primary or active displacement—i.e. if the bone gets displaced due to its own growth. For example, growth at maxillary tuberosity pushes maxilla anteriorly.
- Secondary or passive displacement—i.e. if the bone gets displaced due to growth and enlargement of an adjacent bone.
- Sutural growth
- Enlow's expanding-V-princilple—many bones/parts of the bone have V-shape pattern of the growth, which occurs toward wider ends of the v due to selective apposition and resorption.
- Enlow's counterpart principle—states that the growth of any given facial or cranial part relates specifically to other structural and geometric counterparts in face and cranium.
- Neurotrophism—is a nonimpulse transmitting neural function which involves axoplasmic transport and provides for long-term interaction between neurons and innervated tissues, which homeostatically regulates the morphological, compositional and functional integrity of these tissues.

CLINICAL IMPLICATIONS

Growth of the craniofacial complex is a dynamic phenomenon. It is not uniform throughout life and occurs in phases known as growth spurts and differential growth. There are phases of rapid growth and slow growth. Any intervention done during the period of active growth helps in redirection of the growth to achieve a state of balance.

- *Timing of growth:* Most important growth spurts occur during preadolescent and during adolescent years of age. These are the periods when maximum advantage of natural growth can be obtained through well-timed treatment procedures to stimulate or to redirect growth.
- The growth of parts of face which are near to cranium gets completed first. So, it is sure that the growth of maxilla will get completed before mandible. So any treatment modality for growth redirection of maxilla has to be used at an early age as compared to mandible.

Also, the sequence of timing of growth completion is different in different planes of space. The growth in transverse dimension is first to be completed and then in sagittal and lastly in the vertical plane. Hence, the transverse growth of maxilla gets completed first. In addition to that, during preadolescent, growth spurt is observed at around 8 years of age. It is the right time to achieve a skeletal expansion of maxilla. The mid-palatal suture can also be easily activated and opened with normal physiological expansion forces. With age, the suture gets more interdigitated and becomes difficult to open with normal forces. The skeletal effects diminish with age and dental effects start coming more.

Treatment of sagittal dimension of maxilla also needs an early intervention. A maxillary deficiency needs protraction therapy which is best done during the early age of 8–9 years, to obtain maximum advantage of ensuing active maxillary growth.

If maxilla is protrusive, it has to be restricted with the help of headgear forces to prevent its further growth in sagittal direction during early or mild mixed dentition period.

Excessive vertical growth of the maxilla leading to gummy smile and bite problems (deep bite if anterior region grows more, open bite if posterior region grow more), should also be addressed in early mixed dentition period to control the active maxillary growth. It can be done with the help of high-pull headgears.

Role of Growth Pattern on Treatment Decisions

Growth patterns have been divided into horizontal, average and vertical types. They influence the extraction decisions and anchorage planning. Horizontal growth pattern leads to development of skeletal deep bite, increased mandibular and ramal lengths, flat basal plane angle, short and strong masticatory musculature. These factors provide a strong anchorage and thus loss of anchorage in such cases is extremely difficult. During anchorage loss, the molar has to walk along a straight path, under strong muscles, which is very difficult. Thus, such cases should be treated on non-extraction basis.

In vertical growth pattern, there is skeletal open bite, decreased mandibular and ramal lengths, steep basal plane angle, long face and weaker masticatory musculature. These factors provide a weak anchorage and thus loss of anchorage in such cases is very fast. During anchorage loss, the molar has to walk along a slope/inclined path and muscular forces are weak, which do not prevent any movement of molar, thus leading to an easy mesial movement of molars. Thus, such cases generally are treated on extraction basis depending on space requirements and they need anchorage reinforcement by various methods.

Myofunctional Treatment

Since mandible follows cephalocaudal gradient of growth, it is the bone of face which grows till a later age. It follows a growth spurt in adolescent period of growth. If proper functional appliance is placed, it can lead to enhanced growth of mandible.

BIBLIOGRAPHY

1. Enlow DH, Harris DB. A study of postnatal growth of human mandible. Am J Orthod 1964; 50:25–50.
2. Graber TM. Orthodontics: Principles and Practice, 3rd Ed. WB Sounders. 1988.
3. Proffit WR. Concepts of growth and development. In: Contemporary Orthodontics, 2nd edition. StLouis: Mosby Yearbook, 1999;24–62.
4. Enlow DH, Marks Hans. Handbook of facial growth. 2nd Ed, 2008. WB Saunders Company.
5. Melvin L Moss. The unitary logarithmic curve descriptive of human mandibular growth. Acta A."lat 1971;78:532–542.
6. Ricketts RM. Principle of apical growth of the mandible. Angle Orthod 1972;42:368–386.
7. Moss ML. Neurotrophic regulation of craniofacial growth. J Dent Res l 971;50:192.
8. Moss ML, Letty Moss-Salentijin, Ostreicher HP. The logarithmic properties of active and passive mandibular growth. Am J Orthod 1974; 66 (6):645–664.
9. Moyers RE. Handbook of Orthodontics. 4th Ed., 1988, Year Book Medical Publishers.

PREVIOUS YEAR'S UNIVERSITY QUESTIONS
Essay

1. Clinical implications of growth and development.
2. Enumerate different growth theories. Explain functional matrix theory in detail.
3. Define growth and development. Explain postnatal growth of maxilla.
4. Enumerate various methods of studying growth. Explain growth spurts.

Short Notes

1. Sphenooccipital synchondrosis
2. Fontanelle
3. Rotation of jaw bases
4. Nasal septal cartilage
5. Cephalocaudal growth gradient
6. Expanding V principle
7. Endochondral bone formation
8. Growth charts
9. Meckel's cartilage factors affecting growth
10. Drift vs displacement

MCQs

1. *The daughter cells formed from cleavage of the zygote are known as:*
   a. Gastrula
   b. Morula
   c. Blastula
   d. Blastomeres   **(Ans: d)**

2. *Sixteen cell stage is called:*
   a. Zygote
   b. Morula
   c. Blastula
   d. Gastrula **(Ans: b)**

3. *What are three successive prenatal phases in human development?*
   a. Period ovum, embryo, morula
   b. Period of embryo, ovum, fetus
   c. Period of ovum, embryo, fetus
   d. Fetus, embryo, ovum **(Ans: c)**

4. *Period of ovum in prenatal development of human spans from:*
   a. Ovulations to 14th day
   b. Fertilization to 3 weeks
   c. Fertilization to 14 weeks
   d. Implantation to 2 weeks **(Ans: c)**

5. *Period of embryo in prenatal development of human spans from:*
   a. 4 to 8 weeks
   b. 5 to 9 weeks
   c. 6 to 10 weeks
   d. 3 to 8 weeks **(Ans: d)**

6. *Period of fetus in prenatal development of human spans from:*
   a. 80 days to birth
   b. 56 days to birth
   c. 50 days to birth
   d. 55 days to birth **(Ans: b)**

7. *Notochord develops from:*
   a. Primitive yolk sac
   b. Trophoblast
   c. Amniotic cavity
   d. Anterior extremity of primitive streak **(Ans: d)**

8. *The primordial of the craniofacial complex develops from:*
   a. Hensen's node
   b. Notochordal process
   c. Cloacal membrane
   d. Blastopore **(Ans: b)**

9. *During which period of human prenatal development does the congenital defects occur?*
   a. Period of ovum
   b. Period of embryo
   c. Period of morula
   d. Period of fetus **(Ans: b)**

10. *What are the causes for congenital defects during the period of embryo?*
    a. Virus infection
    b. Bacterial
    c. Drugs
    d. Both A and C **(Ans: d)**

11. *Most of the mesenchymal structures of the face are formed from:*
    a. Ectoderm
    b. Endoderm
    c. Neural crest cells
    d. Mesoderm **(Ans: c)**

12. *Which of the following cells are responsible for embryo proper?*
    a. Inner cell mass/embryoblast
    b. Myeloblast
    c. Trophoblast
    d. Blastocyte **(Ans: a)**

13. *How many pharyngeal arches are seen during embryonic development of humans?*
    a. 12
    b. 6
    c. 8
    d. 5 **(Ans: b)**

14. *Which of the pharyngeal arch completely regresses without contribution to development of any structures during development in humans?*
    a. IV
    b. V
    c. VI
    d. III **(Ans: b)**

15. *First arch is also called:*
    a. Hyoid arch
    b. Mandibular arch
    c. Maxillary arch
    d. Pharyngeal arch **(Ans: b)**

16. *Second arch is also called:*
    a. Hyoid arch
    b. Mandibular arch
    c. Maxillary arch
    d. Pharyngeal arch **(Ans: a)**

17. *Which specific nerve passes through the first arch or mandibular arch?*
    a. Vagus nerve
    b. Glossopharyngeal
    c. Trigeminal nerve
    d. Facial nerve **(Ans: c)**

18. *Which specific nerve passes through the second arch or hyoid arch?*
    a. Vagus nerve
    b. Glossopharyngeal
    c. Trigeminal nerve
    d. Facial nerve **(Ans: d)**

19. *Gastrulation refers to the following:*
    a. Trilaminar embryo is converted into bilaminar embryo
    b. Bilaminar embryo is converted into trilaminar embryo
    c. Myeloblast embryo is converted into bilaminar embryo
    d. Embryoblast embryo is converted into trilaminar embryo **(Ans: b)**

Development of Dentition and Occlusion

Chapter Outline

- Introduction
- The Deciduous dentition stage
- The Mixed dentition period
- Dimensional changes in the dental arches
- Occlusion

INTRODUCTION

Dental occlusion undergoes significant changes from birth until adulthood and beyond. This continuation of changes in the dental relationship during various stages of the dentition can be divided into four stages:
- *Gum pads stage:* 0–6 months
- *Deciduous dentition:* 6 months–6 years
- *Mixed dentition:* 6–12 years
- *Permanent dentition:* 12 years and beyond.

There are different phases of teeth development:
- *Pre-eruptive phase:* From the initiation of tooth development to completion of the crown.
- *Pre-functional phase:* It begins once roots begin to form
- *Functional phase:* After teeth have emerged, it is concerned with development and maintenance with occlusion.

The stages of occlusal development are classified as follows:
- 1st stage—3 years: Primary dentition
- 2nd stage—6 years: Eruption of first permanent molars
- 3rd stage—6–9 years: Exchange of the incisors
- 4th stage—9–12 years: Eruption of the cuspids and bicuspids
- 5th stage—12 years: Eruption of the second molar

Periods of Growth and Dental Development (Hellman)

Stage I: It is the period of early infancy before the completion of the deciduous dentition.

Stage II: It is the period of late infancy at the completion of the deciduous dentition.

Stage III: Childhood when the first permanent molars are erupting or have taken their positions.

Stage IV: It is the period of pubescence when the second molars are erupting or have taken their positions.

Stage V: It is the period of adulthood when the third molars are erupting or have taken their place.

Stage VI: It is the period of old age when the occlusal surfaces of molars are worn off the extent of obliterating the pattern of the grooves.

Stage VII: It designates the period of senility.

Natal and Neonatal Teeth

Occasionally, a child is born with teeth usually lower incisors called natal teeth. The teeth that erupts within first 30 days after birth are called neonatal teeth. This causes difficulty in feeding. This may cause ulcers on the breast of the feeding mother.

Riga-Fede disease: Early eruption of teeth (natal or neonatal) causes ulceration on the ventral surface of the tongue by the sharp edges of the tooth.

Gum Pad Stage

The basic form of gum pads is determined by 4th month of IUL. The upper gum pad is horseshoe shaped and the lower is "U" shaped. They are horseshoe shaped and develop in two parts. First the gum pads differentiate into a labial-buccal portion and later lingual portion.

The labial-buccal portion is divided into 10 transverse grooves, each corresponding to one developing deciduous tooth sac. The gingival groove separates the gum pad from palate and floor of the mouth in the corresponding upper and lower jaws.

The transverse groove between canine and deciduous molar is referred to as lateral sulcus. The lateral sulci are useful in judging the interarch relationship at a very early stage. The lateral sulcus of the mandibular arch is normally most distal to that of the maxillary arch.

The lingual portion is separated from labial-buccal portion by dental groove which is the site of origin of dental lamina. It starts from incisive papilla running backward to merge with gingival groove in the canine region and extends laterally up to molar region.

Relationship of Gum Pads

Infantile open bite: The upper and lower gum pads are identical to each other. The upper gum pad is both wider as well as longer than the mandibular gum pad. Thus, when the upper and lower gum pads are approximated, there is a complete overjet all around. When gum pads are in contact, they occlude only in the posterior region. Thus, anterior open bite exists; the tongue protrudes anteriorly through this space. This infantile open bite is considered normal and it helps in suckling. This is a self-correcting anomaly which closes by eruption of primary teeth (Fig. 5.1).

Growth of Gum Pads

At birth, gum pads are long enough only to accommodate all primary teeth, if they were to erupt at the same time. However, the width of the gum is just adequate to accommodate the incisors. In the first few months after birth, the growth of gum pads is rapid. Transverse dimensions of the gum pads increase with the growth of the jaws. With the development of the deciduous tooth, the segments of each gum pad become prominent. The eruption of deciduous teeth commences at six months of age.

Gum Pad Classification (1932)

Type 1: Anterior margin of the mandibular 1st molar segment lies slightly anterior to the anterior margin of the maxillary 1st molar segment.

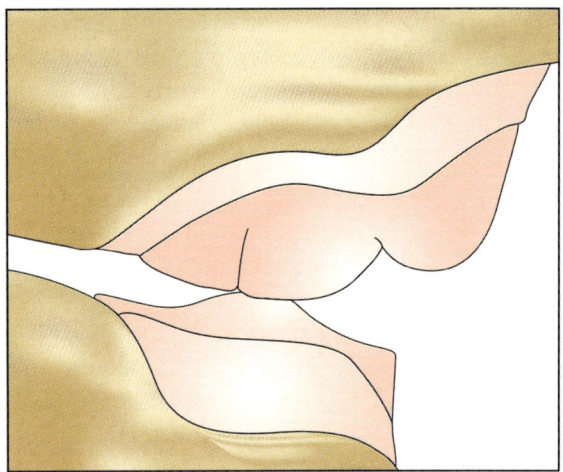

Fig. 5.1: Relationship of gum pad

Type 2: The relationship is slightly distal.

Type 3: The relationship is markedly distal.

THE DECIDUOUS DENTITION STAGE

This stage starts from eruption of first deciduous mandibular central incisors (around 4–6 months) and ends with the eruption of first permanent molar. The deciduous dentition is initiated during the first six weeks of intrauterine life. The primary teeth begin to erupt at the age of about 6 months. By 12 to 18 months, the first molars erupt resulting in a vertically supported occlusal contact between the two arches. The eruption of all primary teeth is completed by 2½–3½ years of age when the second deciduous molars reach into occlusion. The deciduous mandibular central incisors are the first teeth to erupt into the oral cavity. The mandibular eruption precedes maxillary dentition. Deciduous dentition completes by three years with root formation and attains function fully (Fig. 5.2).

Developmental Spacing (Table 5.1)

Physiologic spacing: Spaces present between deciduous teeth are often referred to as physiologic spacing. Sufficient interdental space is needed for the permanent teeth to erupt into an uncrowded condition and for the establishment of their proper alignment. If there is no space in the deciduous dentition, it will lead to crowding in the permanent dentition (Fig. 5.3).

Primate spaces: It is otherwise called anthropoid spaces or Simian spaces. It is presented mesial to the upper canine and distal to the lower canine. Such spaces, originally described by Lewis and Lehman (1929), are a normal feature of the permanent dentition in the higher apes (primates) and are present in the human

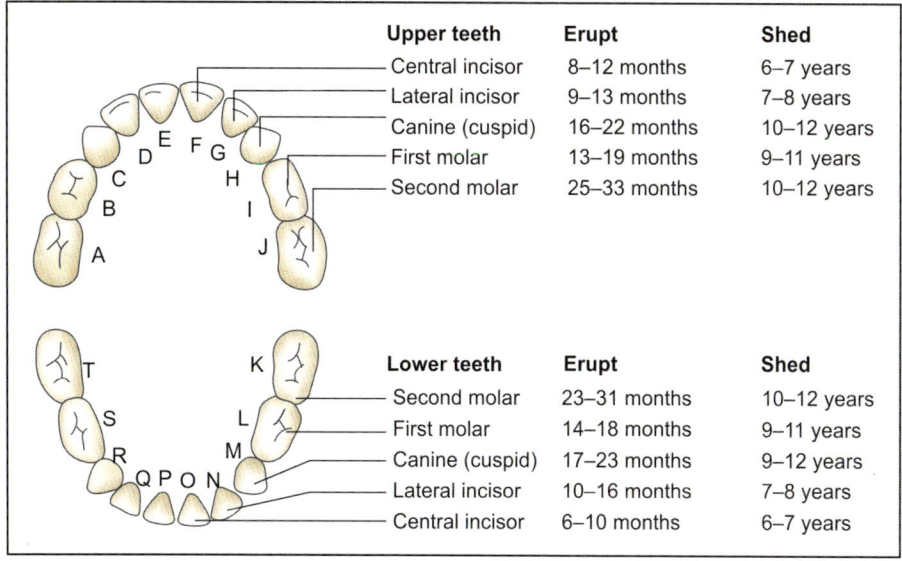

Upper teeth	Erupt	Shed
Central incisor	8–12 months	6–7 years
Lateral incisor	9–13 months	7–8 years
Canine (cuspid)	16–22 months	10–12 years
First molar	13–19 months	9–11 years
Second molar	25–33 months	10–12 years

Lower teeth	Erupt	Shed
Second molar	23–31 months	10–12 years
First molar	14–18 months	9–11 years
Canine (cuspid)	17–23 months	9–12 years
Lateral incisor	10–16 months	7–8 years
Central incisor	6–10 months	6–7 years

Fig. 5.2: Sequence of eruption of deciduous teeth

Table 5.1: Self-correcting anomalies during development of occlusion

1. Pre-dental period

Anomalies

- Retrognathic mandibular gum pad
- Anterior open bite
- Infantile swallow

Time of self-correction, factors involved

- Corrected with forward growth of the mandible
- Eruption of deciduous anterior teeth
- When children are fed with solid food at the end of first year

2. Primary dentition

- Anterior deep bite
- Flush terminal plane

- Spacing

- Eruption of primary molar and attrition of anterior teeth.
- Shift early and establish Class I molar relation utilizing generalized spaces; late shift establish utilizing leeway space to establish Class I molar relation
- Eruption of permanent teeth

3. Mixed dentition

- Ugly duckling stage
- End-on molar
- Anterior deep bite

- With eruption of maxillary permanent canine
- Tongue pressure and spaced primary dentition
- With late shift utilizing leeway space—Class I molar relation established

4. Early permanent dentition

- Increased overjet and overbite

- Decreases with eruption of all posterior teeth and downward, forward growth of the mandible

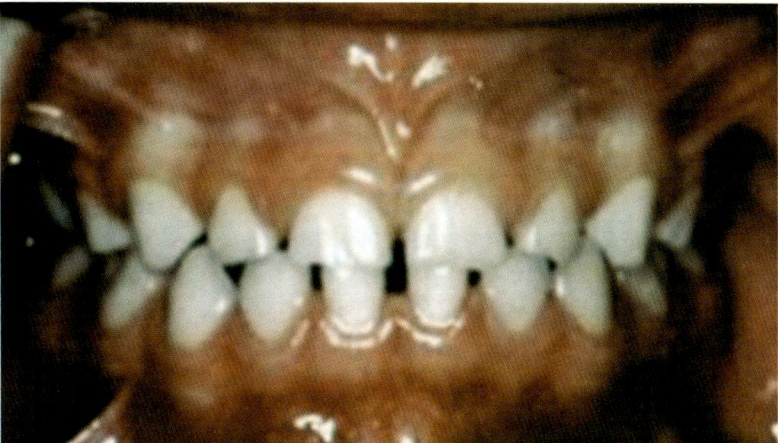
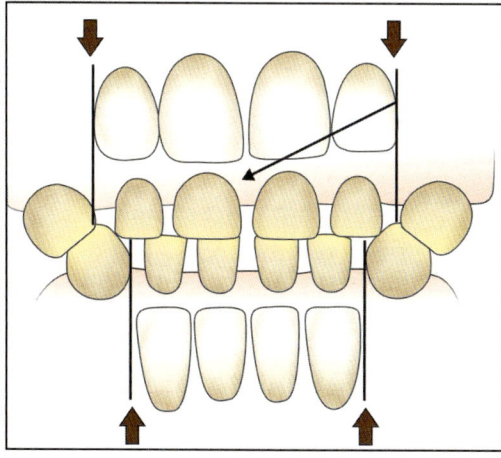

Fig. 5.3: Spacing in the deciduous dentiton

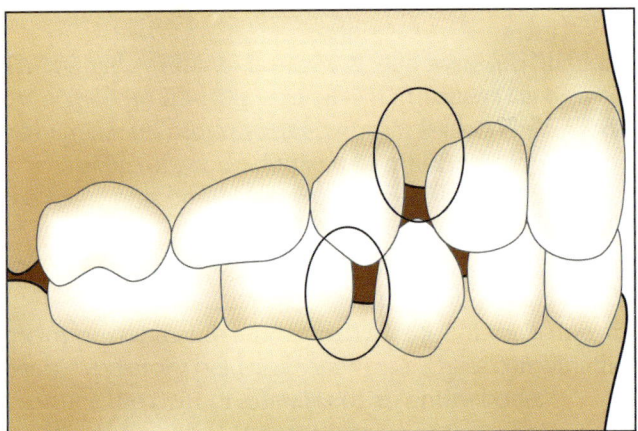

Fig. 5.4: Primate space

primary dentition. Thus it is referred to as the anthropoid spaces (Fig. 5.4).

Significance of Anthropoid Spaces

Following eruption of primary first molars, when canine teeth erupt and reach occlusion, the primate spaces facilitate proper interdigitation of the opposing canines into Class I canine relationship.

Incisor Relationship

Incisor relationship in deciduous dentition normally show:
- Increased deep bite
- Increased overjet

Deep Bite

An increased overbite is usually seen in the initial stages of development with the deciduous mandibular incisors contacting the cingulum area of the deciduous maxillary incisors in centric occlusion. Deep bite may be due to the fact that the primary incisors are more vertically placed than the permanent incisors.

The ideal position of the deciduous incisors has been described as being more vertical than the permanent incisors, with a deeper incisal overbite. This deep bite later gets self-corrected by:
- Attrition of incisors
- Eruption of deciduous molars. It is also called natural bite opener. Natural bite opening occurs at 6, 12, 18 years of age with eruption of permanent molars. There are 3 periods of natural bite opening according to Schwarz.
  – At 6 years, when first molar erupts
  – At 12 years when 2nd molar erupts
  – At 18 years when 3rd molar erupts.
- Differential growth of the alveolar processes of the jaws.

Increased Overjet

Excessive incisal overjet is often observed in deciduous dentition. Excessive overjet usually gets corrected later by forward growth of the mandible.

THE MIXED DENTITION PERIOD

This is the period where both deciduous and permanent teeth are present in the oral cavity. This is also the most important period of development of normal dentition and occlusion. During the mixed dentition period, various malocclusions are encountered. It is an ideal time for functional appliances (Fig. 5.5).

It is divided into two periods:
- Early mixed dentition—6–9 years
- Late mixed dentition—9–12 years

It is further subdivided into following stages:
- First transitional period (6–9 years)
- Intertransitional period
- Second transitional period

First transition period:
- Emergence of first permanent molar
- Incisors transition
- Establishment of occlusion

Intertransition period:
- Both sets of teeth present
- 4 permanent incisors and 1st permanent molars present
- Deciduous canine, 1st and 2nd molars

Second transition period:
- Emergence of bicuspids, cuspids and second permanent molar
- Establishment of occlusion

First Transition Period

The location and relationship of 1st permanent molar which is the first permanent tooth to erupt depends much upon the distal surface relationship between upper and lower second deciduous molars. The mesiodistal relationship of the distal surface of upper and lower second deciduous molars can be of three types. It has been mentitioned in the next page as straight, mesial/distal step.

Second Transitional Period

It starts after the emergence of the first premolars or lower canine in girls and upper first premolar in boys at the age of 9.5 years.

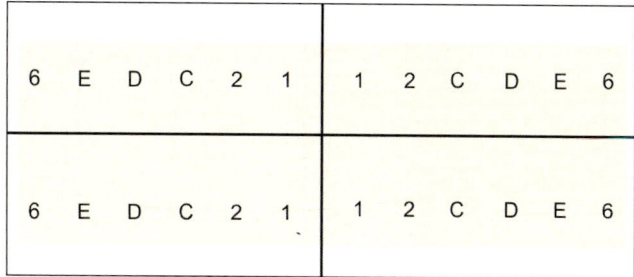

6	E	D	C	2	1	1	2	C	D	E	6
6	E	D	C	2	1	1	2	C	D	E	6

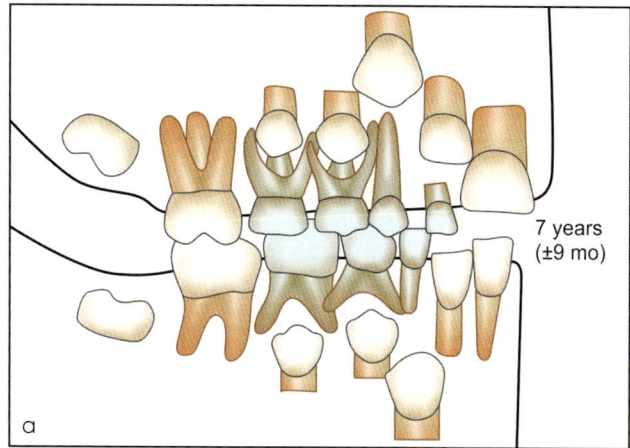

7 years
(±9 mo)

a

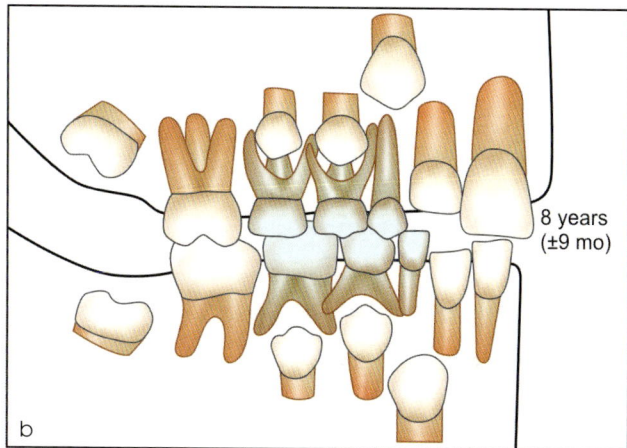

8 years
(±9 mo)

b

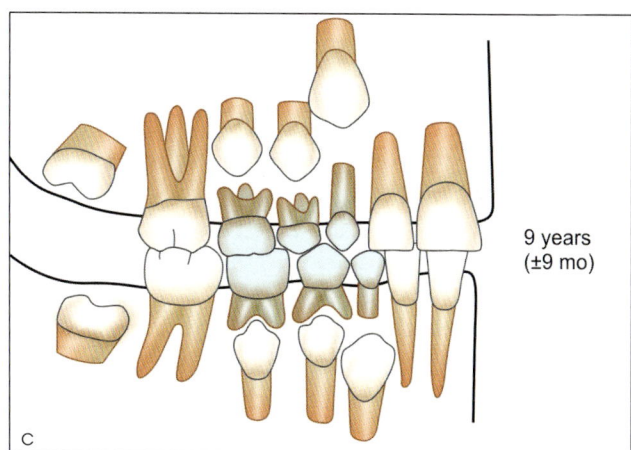

9 years
(±9 mo)

c

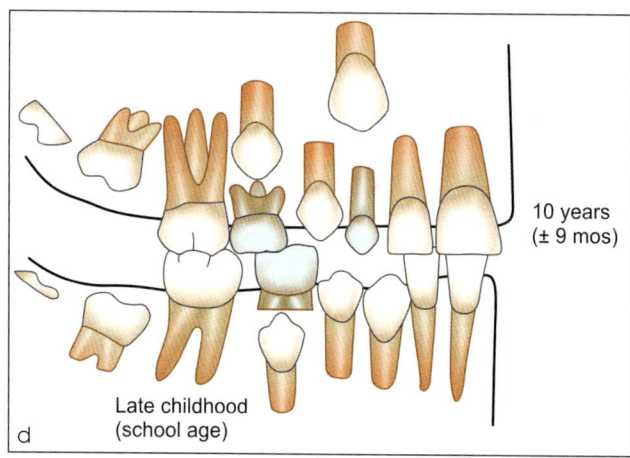

10 years
(± 9 mos)

Late childhood
(school age)

d

Fig. 5.5: Teeth present during mixed dentition

Flush Terminal Plane

The mandibular second primary molar has a greater mesiodistal diameter than the maxillary second primary molar. This difference in the dimensions makes the distal surfaces of both maxillary and mandibular deciduous second molars to fall in same vertical plane in centric occlusion. Such an arrangement is called flush terminal plane (Fig. 5.6).

Moyers described 3 types of primary molar relationship:
- Straight
- Mesial step
- Distal step

Straight flush terminal plane: The distal surfaces of the maxillary and molars are in the vertical plane.

Mesial step: The distal surface of the mandibular deciduous second molar is more mesial to the distal surface of the maxillary deciduous second molar.

Distal step: The distal surface of the mandibular deciduous second molar is more distal to the distal surface of the maxillary deciduous second molar.

Significance of flush terminal plane: It is of great importance because the erupting first permanent molars are guided by the distal surfaces of the second primary molars as they erupt into occlusion. Thus, the

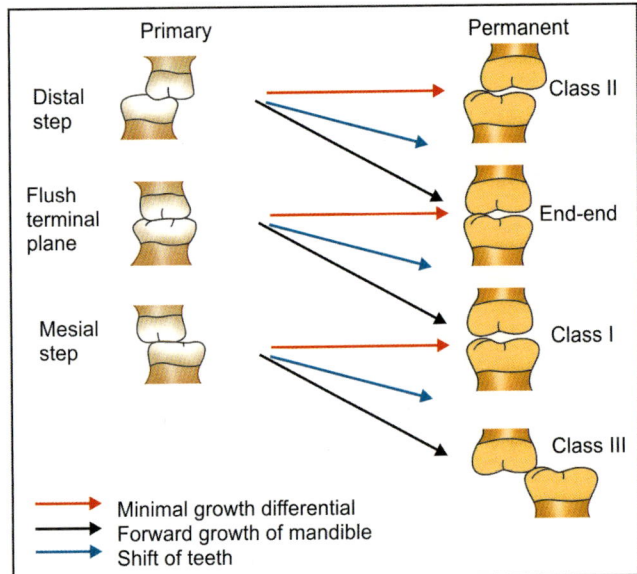

Fig. 5.6: Flush terminal plane

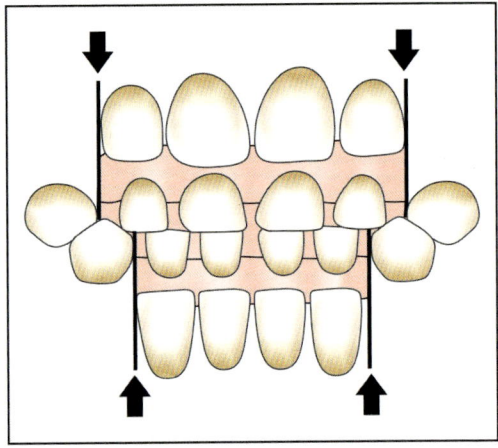

Fig. 5.7: Incisor liability

terminal plane relationship of primary dentition largely determines the type of molar relationship in the permanent dentition to be achieved later.

Incisor Liability by Warren Mayne

Normally, in the anterior segment, the incisor liability plays an active role whereas in the posteriors, the leeway space of Nance helps in the resolution of any crowding.

Incisor liability in the anterior occurs due to the greater mesiodistal dimensions required by the permanent incisors as compared to their deciduous predecessors. Due to the same, the crowding may further accentuate especially in a non-spaced dentition and where primate spaces are absent. In such clinical conditions, the mandibular lateral incisors may erupt more palatally or labially. The deciduous permanent tooth size differential averages 6–7 mm. Mayne in 1965 listed the mechanisms by which incisor liability is resolved by the growth and development of occlusion.

According to black

- Incisor liability in the maxillary arch is about 7.6 mm—i.e. the maxillary permanent incisors are larger than their predecessors by 7.6 mm.
- Incisor liability in mandibular arch is about 6 mm—i.e. mandibular permanent incisors are 6 mm larger than their predecessors.

The mesiodistal crown dimensions of permanent incisors are considerably greater than that of the primary incisors. This difference in the mesiodistal crown dimension between the primary and permanent incisors is termed as incisor liability by Warren Mayne (Fig. 5.7).

The following factors govern the incisor liability:

- **Utilization of physiological spacing** in the primary dentition by 2–3 mm. Incisor liability is partly compensated by the developmental spaces that exist in the primary dentition. Anterior crowding of permanent dentition may develop in the absence of interdental spacing.
- **Increase in the intercanine arch width about 3–4 mm.** Continuing growth of the jaws often results in an increase in the intercanine arch width during the mixed dentition period. This may significantly contribute to accommodate bigger permanent incisors in the arches.
- **Change in the incisor inclination:** Permanent incisors are labially placed which tend to increase dental arch perimeter. It gives 2–3 mm.

Intertransitional Period

This is the most stable period of mixed dentition. This stage is marked by the presence of both the permanent and primary dentition in both arches. The deciduous canines and molars are present in between the newly erupted permanent incisors and first molars. It persists for an average of 1.5–2 years. Any asymmetry in emergence and corresponding differences in the height levels or crown length between the right and left side teeth are made up. Root formation of the emerged incisors, canines and molar continues, along with the concomitant increase in alveolar process height. Resorption of the roots of deciduous molars is noticed. This phase prepares for the second transitional phase (Fig. 5.8).

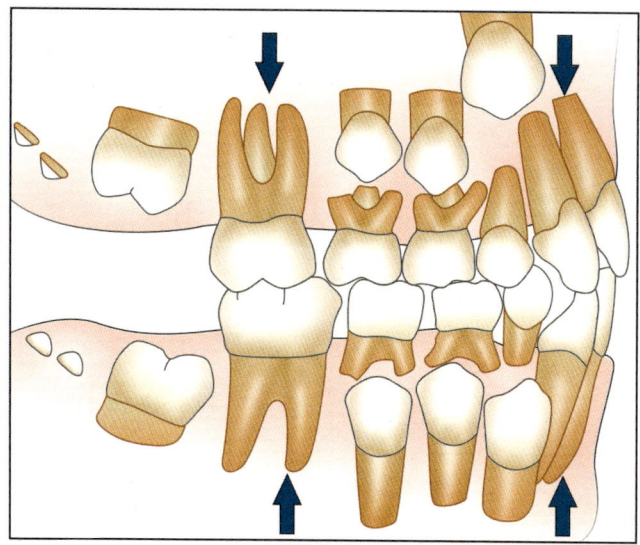

Fig. 5.8: Intertransitional period

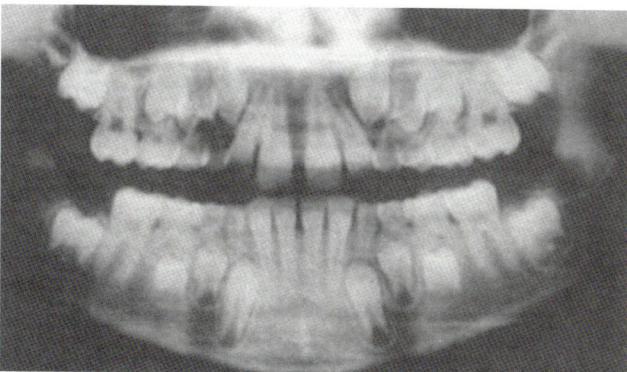

Fig. 5.9a: A ugly duckling stage

Ugly Duckling Stage (Table 5.1)

A transient malocclusion with appearance of midline diastema and flaring of upper incisors is often observed to develop in the maxillary anterior region during 8 to 12 years of age. As the upper canine slide over the distal slope of upper lateral incisor and erupts into occlusion, the ugly duckling stage disappears. The erupting canine pushes the lateral incisors toward midline. Thus flaring of upper incisors is corrected and spacings get closed. It is described by Broadbent and hence it is also known as Broadbent phenomenon. It is a self-correcting anomaly and it does not require any treatment (Fig. 5.9a and b).

E-space: It is the space provided by the primary mandibular second molar when the second premolar erupts after its shedding. It is approximately 3 mm.

Leeway Space

The combined mesiodistal crown dimension of the primary canine and primary first and second molars is greater than the combined mesiodistal crown dimension of their successors namely permanent canine, first and second premolars. The amount of space gained by this difference in the posterior segments is termed as the Leeway space of Nance and present in both arches (Fig. 5.10).

In maxilla
- Leeway space in maxilla in each quadrant is about 0.9 mm.
- The total leeway space in maxlla is 1.8 mm.

In mandible
- Leeway space in each quadrant of the mandible is about 1.7 mm
- The total leeway space in the mandible is 3.4 mm.

Significance of leeway space of Nance:
- It allows mesial movement of the permanent molars.
- It is more in the lower arch because of the primary mandibular molars are wider than primary maxillary molars allowing mandibular molars to move mesially than maxillary permanent molar. Such arrangement changes the end on molar relationship in the early mixed dentition to Class I relation at the late mixed dentition period (late mesial shift).

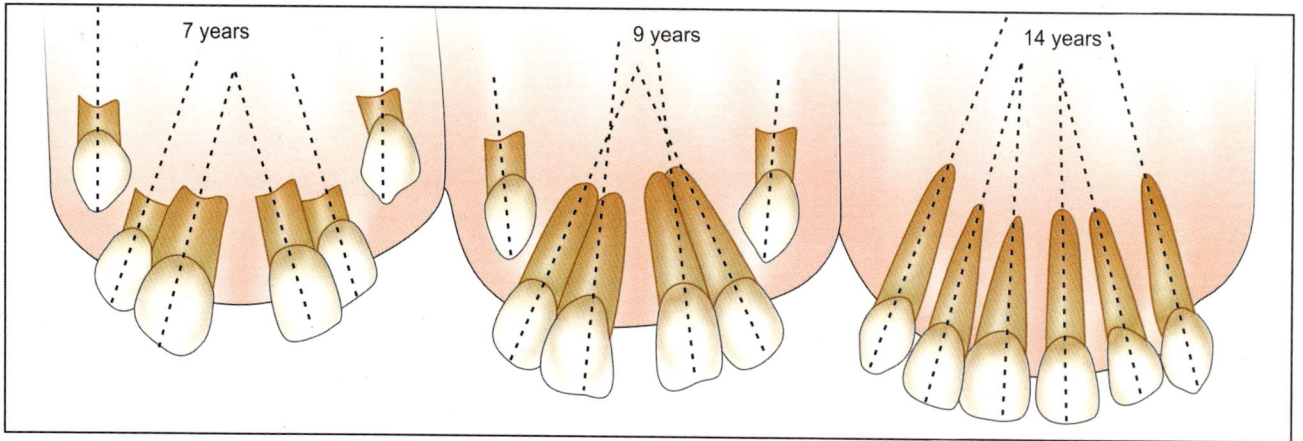

Fig. 5.9b: Ugly duckling stage (schematic)

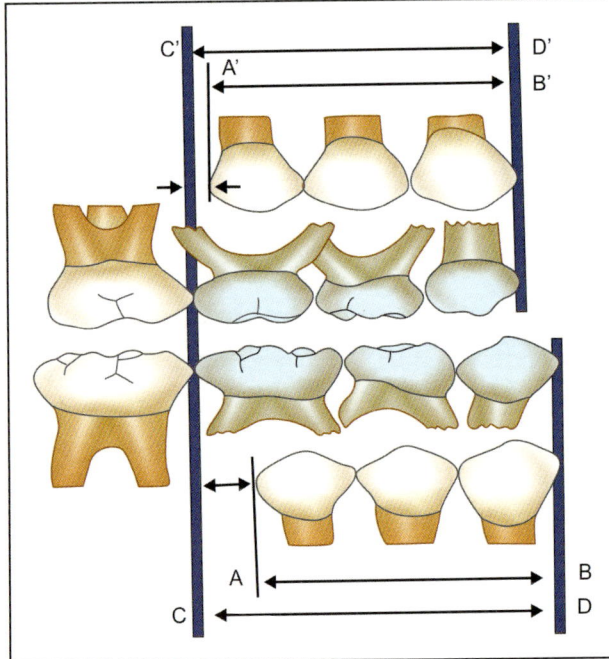

Fig. 5.10: Leeway space

This is described in two ways.

- *Early mesial shift:* Early mesial shift of lower permanent first molar occurs by utilization of the physiologic spaces present between primary incisors and the primate spaces. The eruptive force of permanent molars push the deciduous molars forward into the spaces, there by establishing Class I mixed dentition, the shift is called "early mesial shift" (Fig. 5.11).
- *Late mesial shift:* In the absence of sufficient developmental spaces in primary dentition, the erupting permanent first molars may not be able to establish Class I relationship in early mixed dentition period. In such cases, Class I molar relationship can

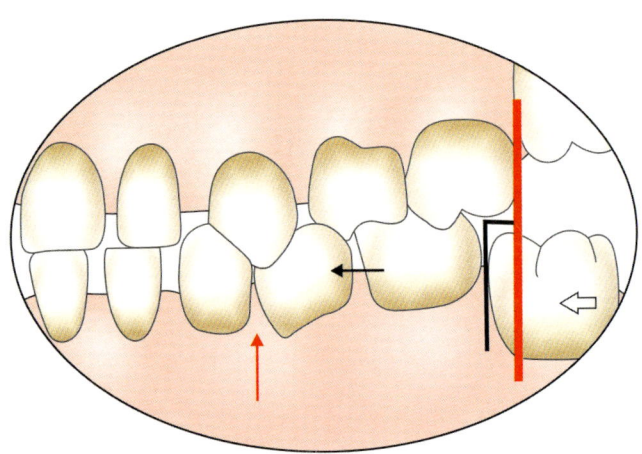

Fig. 5.11: Early mesial shift

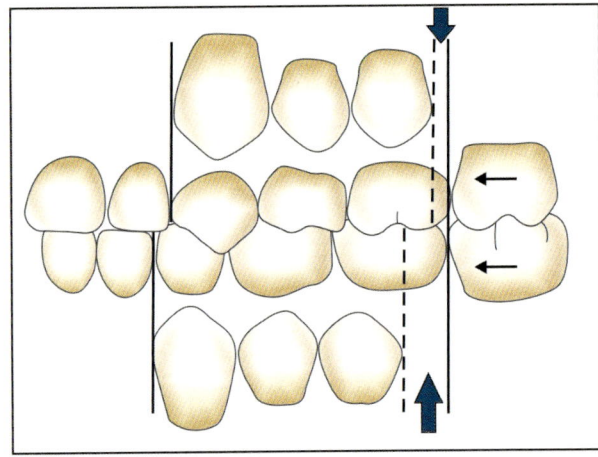

Fig. 5.12: Late mesial shift

be established following the exfoliation of primary second molars; by utilizing leeway space. As this occurs in late mixed dentition, it is called the "late mesial shift" (Fig. 5.12).

DIMENSIONAL CHANGES IN THE DENTAL ARCHES

The transition from the primary dentition stage to the permanent dentition has an impact on dental arch length, circumference and intermolar and intercanine widths.

Changes in the Maxillary Arch

The intercanine width increases by an average of 6 mm in a child between 3 and 13 years of age. It continues to increase between 13 and 45 years of age by approximately 1.7 mm. In the primary dentition stage there is an increase of intermolar width of 2 mm between 3 and 5 years of age. The first permanent intermolar width increases by 2.2 mm between 8 and 13 years of age and decreases by 1 mm by 45 years of age. There is a slight decrease in arch length with age because of the uprighting of the incisors.

Changes in the Mandibular Arch

Between 3 and 13 years of age, the intercanine width increases by an average of 3.7 mm.

Then, between 13 and 45 years of age, the intercanine width decreases by 1.2 mm. It should be noted that after the eruption of the mandibular incisors, there is little change to be expected in the intercanine width.

In the primary dentition stage, there is an increase of intermolar width of 1.5 mm between 3 and 5 years of age. The first permanent intermolar width increases by 1mm between 8 and 13 years of age and then decreases by 1 mm by age 45.

The arch length decreases in the mixed and permanent dentition stages as a result of the uprighting of the incisors and the loss of the leeway space by the mesial movement of the first permanent molars.

Safety Valve Mechanism

The intercanine width of maxilla acts as "safety valve". Postnatally, the mandible grows comparatively more than maxilla. However, inter-canine width of mandible is completed earlier to that of maxilla which may extend up to 12–16 years. This may check any abnormal horizontal growth of mandible that occurs up to 18 years of age.

OCCLUSION

An understanding of the principles and the relationship to oral health and disease is of paramount importance. There is a balance of forces of tongue, lips and cheeks at rest creating a neutral zone. This allows for the proper alignment of the teeth, development of dental arches and normal facial development.

Angle defined occlusion as normal relation of the occlusal inclined planes of the teeth when jaws are closed. But, occlusion is a complex phenomenon involving the teeth periodontal ligament, the jaws, the TMJ, muscles and the nervous system.

Definitions

Occlusion (Oc—up, clusion—closing) can be defined as the relationship of the maxillary and mandibular teeth, as they are brought into functional contact (Fig. 5.13).

The static relationship between the incisal or masticating surfaces of the maxillary or mandibular teeth or tooth analogues.

It may be defined also as the contact at an occlusal interface, but also to all those factors concerned with the development and stability of the masticatory system and with the use of the teeth in the oral motor behavior (Wheelers).

Ideal Occlusion

The important aspect of ideal occlusion now includes functional harmony, health and stability of stomatognathic system. Houston et al (1920) suggested the following concepts of ideal occlusion in permanent dentition.

a. Each arch is regular; the teeth have ideal mesiodistal and buccolingual inclination; and correct approximal relationship with each other.

b. The arch relationships are such that each lower tooth (except the central incisor) contacts the corresponding upper tooth and the tooth anterior to it. The upper arch overlaps the lower arch anteriorly and laterally.

c. In maximum intercuspation of teeth when the mandible is in centric relation, i.e. both mandibular condyles are symmetrical retruded unstrained positions in the glenoid fossae.

d. During mandibular movements, the functional relationships are correct. In particular, during lateral excursions, there should be either group function or a canine protected/rise on the working side with no occlusal contact on the non-working side; while in protrusion, the occlusion should be on incisor teeth while buccal segment should disocclude.

Physiologic occlusion: This refers to an occlusion that deviates in one or more ways from ideal yet it is well adapted to that particular environment, is esthetic and shows no pathologic manifestation or dysfunction.

Balanced occlusion: An occlusion in which balanced and equal contacts are maintained throughout the entire arch during all excursions of the mandible.

Functional occlusion: It is defined as arrangement of teeth which will provide the highest efficiency during all the excursive movements of the mandible which are necessary during function.

Therapeutic occlusion: Traumatic occlusion that has been modified by appropriate therapeutic modalities in order to change a non-physiologic occlusion to one that is at least physiologic, if not ideal.

Traumatic occlusion: Traumatic occlusion is an abnormal occlusal stress which is capable of producing or has produced an injury to the periodontium.

Trauma from occlusion: It is defined as periodontal tissue injury caused by occlusal forces through abnormal occlusal contacts.

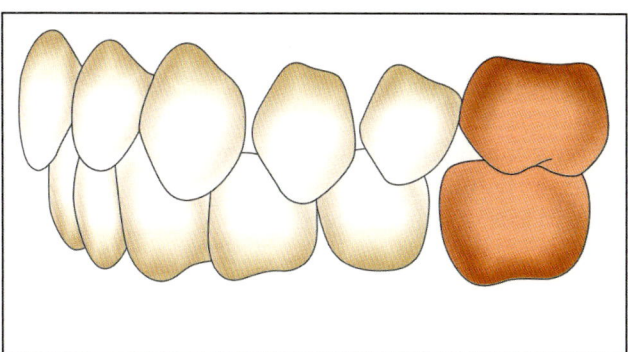

Fig. 5.13: Normal occlusion

Classifications of Occlusion

The important classifications are:
1. Based on the mandibular position
2. Based on relationship of first permanent molar
3. Based on organization of occlusion
4. Based on pattern of occlusion

Based on the Mandibular Position

Centric occlusion: It is the occlusion of the teeth when the mandible is in centric relation.
1. *Lateral occlusion:* It is defined as the contact between opposing teeth when the mandible is moved either right or left of the midsagittal plane.
2. *Protruded occlusion:* It is defined as the occlusion of the teeth when the mandible is protruded, i.e. the position of mandible is anterior to centric relation.
3. *Retrusive occlusion:* It is the occlusion of the teeth when the mandible is retruded, i.e. position of mandible is posterior to centric relation.

Based on Relationship of First permanent Molar

Refer to Angle's classification

Based on the Organization of Occlusion

1. *Canine guided or protected occlusion:* During lateral movements, only working side canine comes into contact with the other. This results in distocclusion of all posterior teeth, i.e. on both working and balancing side. This is because the mandible moves away from the centric occlusion. Here the tip or the buccal incline of the lower canine is seen to slide along with palatal surface of the upper canine.
2. *Mutually protected occlusion:* Occlusal scheme in which the posterior teeth prevent excessive contact of the anterior teeth in maximum intercuspation. Also, the anterior teeth disengage the posterior teeth in all mandibular excursive movements.
3. *Group function occlusion:* It is defined as the multiple contact relationship between the maxillary and mandibular teeth, in lateral movements of the working side; whereby simultaneous contacts of several teeth is achieved and they act as a group to distribute occlusal forces.

Based on Pattern of Occlusion

There are two types:
a. *Supporting cusps:* They fit in central fossae and marginal ridges of opposing teeth. They are also called centric holding cusps or stamp cusps, e.g. lower buccal and upper palatal cusps. They help in maintaining the vertical dimension of occlusion and should not be reduced during occlusal equilibration.

b. *Non-supporting cusps or shearing cusps:* They are also called guiding cusps. They contact and guide mandible during lateral movements and help in shearing food, e.g. lower lingual and upper buccal cusps.

Occlusal Interdigitation

It is of two types:
a. Cusp-to-fossa relation
b. Cusp-to-embrasure relation

Cusp-to-Fossa Relation

The cusps of opposing teeth occludes in fossae of opposing teeth. This is a one tooth to one tooth relation. Advantages of cusp-fossa arrangement over cusp embrasure arrangement are that the occlusal forces are directed towards the long axis of teeth in a better way. It leads to greater stability of the arch and the chance of food impacting in the embrasures is less.

Cusp-to-Embrasure Relation

Here, one stamp cusp occludes in the fossa of opposing tooth, and another cusp of the same tooth occludes into the embrasure area of two opposing teeth. This is a one tooth to two teeth relation occlusion.

BIBLIOGRAPHY

1. Bishara SE Hoppens BJ, Jakobsen JR Kohout FJ. Changes in molar relationships between the deciduous and permanent dentitions: a longitudinal study. Am J Orthod Dentofac Orthoped 1988; 93:19.
2. Inuzuka K. Changes in molar relationships between the deciduous and permanent dentitions: a longitudinal study. Am J Orthod 1990; 93:18.
3. Moorrees C. The dentition of the growing child: a longitudinal study of dental development between 3 and 18 years of age, Cambridge, Mass, 1959, Harvard University presses.
4. Sillman JH. Dimensional changes of dental arches: longitudinal studies from birth to 25 years. Am J Orthod 1964; 50:824–42.

PREVIOUS YEAR'S UNIVERSITY QUESTIONS
Short Questions

1. Ugly duckling stage
2. Gum pads
3. Transient malocclusion
4. Incisor liability
5. Early loss of primary teeth

MCQs

1. *Calcification of first permanent molar begin*
   a. Before birth
   b. At birth

c. 1 year after birth
d. 2 years after birth   **(Ans: a)**

2. *First tooth to erupt in primary dentition is*
   a. First premolars
   b. Mandibular central incisors
   c. 1 year after birth
   d. 2 years after birth   **(Ans: b)**

3. *Ugly duckling stage was termed by*
   a. Broadbent
   b. Nance
   c. Lawrence F Andrews
   d. Calvin Case   **(Ans: a)**

4. *Leeway space was determined by*
   a. Nance
   b. Angle
   c. Calvin Case
   d. Martin Dewey   **(Ans: a)**

5. *Ugly duckling stage*
   a. Needs fixed appliance at a later stage
   b. Self correcting
   c. Transient
   d. Both B and C   **(Ans: d)**

6. *Incisor liability is corrected by*
   a. Utilization of interdental spaces
   b. Increase in intercanine width
   c. Change in incisor inclination
   d. All of the above   **(Ans: d)**

7. *Early mesial shift utilizes*
   a. Primary space
   b. Leeway space
   c. Both a and b
   d. None of the above   **(Ans: a)**

8. *Eruption sequence of deciduous dentition is*
   a. A-B-C-D-E
   b. D-A-B-C-E
   c. E-A-B-D-C
   d. A-B-D-C-E   **(Ans: d)**

9. *Alveolar processes at the time of birth is known as*
   a. Gingival pads
   b. Gum pads
   c. Oral cavity
   d. Gums   **(Ans: b)**

10. *Teeth which erupt during first month of age are*
    a. Prenatal teeth
    b. Neonatal teeth
    c. Natal teeth
    d. All of the above   **(Ans: b)**

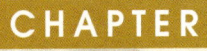

Functions of Stomatognathic System

Chapter Outline

- Definition and Introduction
- Trajectories of the mandible
- Buccinator mechanism
- Functional development

DEFINITION AND INTRODUCTION

Salzmann's Definition

Stomatognathics is the approach to the practice of orthodontics which takes into consideration, the interdependence of form and function of the teeth, jaw relationship, temporomandibular articulation, craniofacial conformation and dental occlusion.

Introduction

Stomatognathics deals with the functional anatomy. Stability of the orthodontically moved teeth depends on the integration of the stomatognathic components.

The dentist and orthodontist should have sound-knowledge and understand the importance of the stomatognathic system. Until we know what is normal, we will not be able to recognize aberrancy.

The SS is a functional unit characterized by several structures: Skeletal components (maxilla and mandible), dental arches, soft tissues (salivary glands, nervous and vascular supplies), and the temporo-mandibular joint and masticatory muscles (MM). These structures act in harmony to perform different functional tasks (to speak, to break food down into small pieces, and to swallow). In particular, the temporomandibular joint makes muscular and ligamentary connections to the cervical region, forming a functional complex called the "cranio-cervico-mandibular system.

The development of the greatest amount of patient's stomatognathic system occurs during the first 14 to 18 years of life and its development occurs in the transverse, vertical and sagittal dimensions.

The different functions of stomatognathic system are:

- Mastication
- Deglutition
- Speech
- Respiration

Benninghoff (1925) did extensive studies on dried craniofacial bones. He found that the architecture of the cranial and facial skeleton is built in such a way so as to resist the functional stresses. These functional stress-bearing areas of the bone are known as Benninghoff's lines or trajectories of bone. The maximum pressure and tension are dissipated through these pathways of trajectories. These trajectories are seen in both spongy and compact bone.

Wolff's Law of Transformation of Bone

In 1870, Julius Wolff, the German physiologist, stated that external morphology and internal architecture of bone are directly proportional to the functional forces acting upon it. According to Wolff, the trabecular pattern of a bone is related to stress trajectories and this can be correlated with its function in a mathematical way. This is called *law of orthogonality*. In the early 1900s, Wolff demonstrated that bone trabeculae were arranged in response to the stress lines on the bone (the internal architecture of the head of the femur is the classic example, and condylar process of the mandible also follows the Wolff's law of bone).

Koch described the concept of the laws of bone architecture. Laws of force described by him are as follows:

a. Inner structure and external form of human bones are closely adapted to mechanical conditions which exist at every point in the bone.

b. Inner architecture is determined by the definite and exact requirements of the mathematical and mechanical laws to produce maximum strength with minimal of material.

c. There is a close relationship between form and function of the bone. Any continued deviation from the normal function must be followed by a continuous structural adaptaion to the altered functions.

The masticatory forces are dissipated through the trajectories by three components.

• *Anterior component:* It is dissipated through the contact point and when it comes to the midline, it gets nullified.

• *Horizontal component:* It is dissipated through the cusp and plane.

• *Vertical component:* It is dissipiated through the periodontal ligament and from the apex, it goes to the trajectories and gets dissipiated at the lower border of mandible which is thick in nature

The accessory trajectories include the symphysis, gonial angle, vertical pillar from coronoid process into the ramus and the body of the mandible.

In the maxilla: There are two types of trajectories in the maxilla (Fig. 6.1)

1. Vertical trajectories
   i. Frontonasal buttress

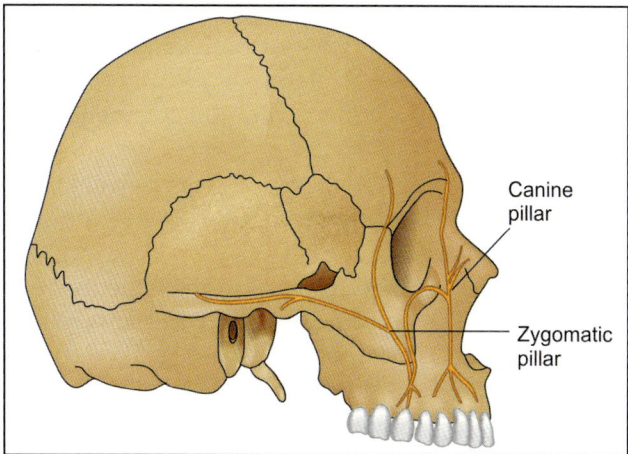

Fig. 6.1: Trajectories in the maxilla

Canine pillar

Zygomatic pillar

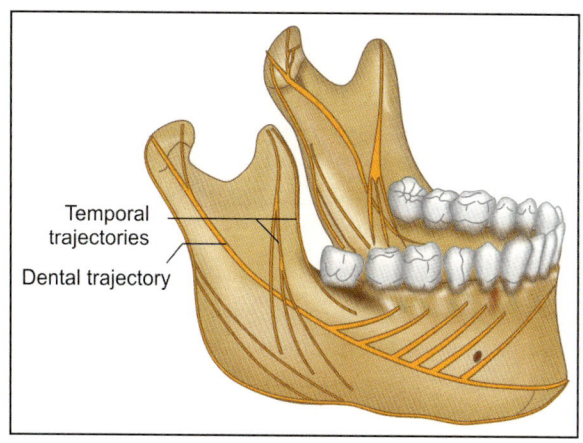

Fig. 6.2: Trajectories in the mandible

Temporal trajectories

Dental trajectory

ii. Zygomatic buttress
iii. Pterygoid buttress

2. Horizontal buttress

Vertical trajectories: All three above said trajectories arise from alveolar process and end in the base of the skull. These trajectories curve around the sinuses, nasal and orbital cavities.

i. *Frontonasal buttress:* It projects from the incisors, canines and first upper premolar and spreads cranially along the sides of piriform aperture, the crest of the nasal bone and terminates in the frontal bone.

ii. *Zygomatic buttress:* Zygomatic buttress transmits stress from the posterior teeth in three pathways which are as follows:

• It arises from the second premolars and partly molars and eminates in the cranium and this trajectory transmits the stress pathways from the buccal group of teeth:
  – Through the zygomatic arch to the base of the skull.
  – Upward to the frontal bone through the lateral walls of the orbit.

• It runs cranially and mesially, along the lower orbital margin to join the upper part of the frontonasal buttress and terminates in the frontal bone

• Along the lower orbital margin to join the upper part of the frontonasal buttress.

iii. *Pterygoid buttress:* This trajectory transmits the stress from the nasal bone, 2nd and 3rd molars. It ends in the middle portion of the base of the skull.

TRAJECTORIES OF THE MANDIBLE (Fig. 6.2)

Mandible has major and minor trajectories to withstand the occlusal stresses.

Major trajectories: Trabecular lines originate from beneth the teeth in the alveolar process and join together into a common stress pillar or trajectory system. Mandibular canal and nerve are protected by this concentration of trabeculae. The thick cortical layer of trabeculae along the lower border of the mandible offers high resistance to bending forces.

Minor trajectories: These accessory trajectories are produced due to the effect of muscle attachment. They are seen at symphysis and gonial angle. One trabecular line is also seen running downwards from the coronoid process into the ramus and body of the mandible.

BUCCINATOR MECHANISM

It is a continuous band of muscles that encircles the dentition and is firmly anchored at the pharyngeal tubercle of the occipital bone.

Buccinator mechanism starts with the decussating fibers of the orbicularis oris joining the right and left fibers of the lip which constitute the anterior component of the buccinator mechanism.

It then runs laterally and posteriorly around the corner of the mouth, joining other fibers of the buccinator muscle which get inserted into the pterygomandibular raphe.

Here it mingles with the fibers of superior constrictor muscle and runs posteriorly and medially to get fixed to the pharyngeal tubercle (Fig. 6.3).

Equilibrium Theory

The teeth are well aligned and well balanced at the summit of the alveolar bone between the tongue inside and the buccinators mechanism outside. This is called the equilibrium theory.

- If the musculature of tongue is predominating, the buccal teeth move laterally causing the buccal crossbite.
- If the musculature of buccinators is predominating than the tongue, the teeth move towards the tongue causing the constriction of the arch as in Class II division 1 malocclusion.
- The teeth will move towards least resistance the arch as in Class II division 1 malocclusion.

FUNCTIONAL DEVELOPMENT

Orofacial region is associated with a variety of functions such as mastication, deglutition, respiration (ventilation) and speech. Since the functions are interrelated, normal development of orofacial region depends on normal functions.

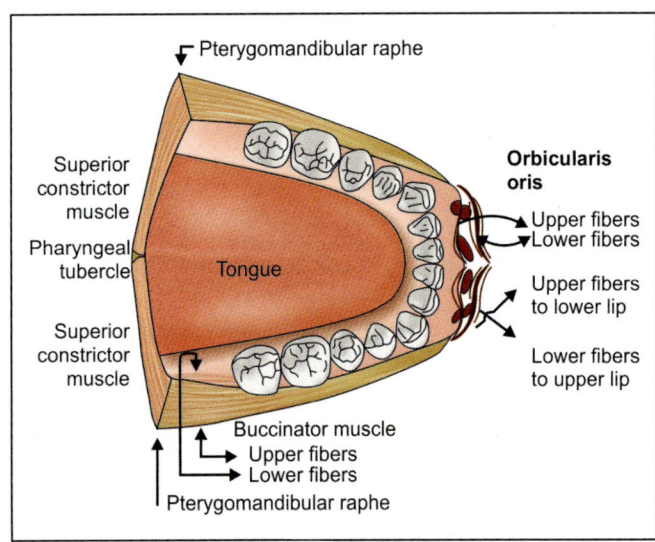

Fig. 6.3: Buccinator mechanism

Mastication

Mastication is the process whereby ingested food is cut or crushed into small pieces, mixed with saliva and formed into a bolus in preparation for swallowing. Mammals are heterodonts, i.e. possess teeth of different forms adapted to the communition of food. Thus the process of mastication is a characteristic feature of mammals. In non-mammalians, teeth are mainly used for withholding their prey before swallowing as a whole.

In humans, the process of mastication is associated with various functions, such as:

- It enables the food bolus to be easily swallowed.
- It decreases the size of food particles so that the surface area is increased for enzyme activity.
- It stimulates secretion of saliva and gastric juices by reflex action.
- It mixes food with saliva, thus initiates digestion by the activity of salivary amylase.
- It prevents irritation of gastrointestinal system by large food masses.
- It ensures healthy growth and development of the oral tissues.

Mastication occurs by the convergent movements of maxillary and mandibular teeth. During chewing cycle, two processes occur:

1. Food is first crushed by vertical movements of the mandible. The initial crushing of food does not require full occlusion of teeth.
2. After the food is softened well by initial crushing, maxillary and mandibular teeth meet in full occlusion. The food is then sheared by lateral to medial movement of the mandible to make a bolus.

Once the cusps interdigitate the ridges on the slopes of the cusps shear the food as the mandibular teeth move across the maxillary teeth. Food is ground in the manner of mortar and pestle when the cusps move across the fossae of the opposing teeth.

Control of Mastication

Mastication is dependent upon a chain of events to produce rhythmic opening and closing movements of the jaws and correlated tongue movements. Several theories are proposed to explain the origin and control of the rhythmic activity of the jaws during mastication.

1. *Cerebral hemisphere theory:* This theory proposed that mastication was a conscious act, a patterned set of instructions originating in the higher center of the CNS (motor cortex) and descending directly to trigeminal, facial and hypoglossal motor nerves.

2. *Reflex chain theory:* It is held that mastication involved a series of interacting chains of reflexes. It is negated because mastication involved prolonged bursts of muscle activity and not the brief and abrupt behavior usually associated with reflex action of muscle.

3. *Rhythm (pattern) generation theory:* This theory is now generally accepted. It advocates that there are central pattern generators (CPGs) within the brainstem which on being stimulated from either higher centers (motox cortex) or sensory inputs in the mouth (teeth, periodontal ligament), are driven into rhythmic activity.

Deglutition (Swallowing)

Deglutition involves an ordered sequence of events that carry food or saliva from the mouth into the stomach. Humans swallow approximately 600 times in a day; about 150 times for swallowing foods or drinks and the rest of the times for clearing saliva from the mouth.

The swallowing pattern in infants is different from that of adults. Persistence of infantile swallow in children is a common cause of tongue thrusting habit which may lead to malocclusion. Humans show two types of swallow pattern:

- Infantile and neonates swallow
- Mature/adult swallow

Infantile Swallow

It is characterized by:
- Active contraction of the lip muscles.
- Tongue placed between the gum pads and tongue tip is brought forward by pharyngeal muscle activity.

- Little posterior tongue activity/pharyngeal muscle activity.
- Tongue to lower lip posture adopted by infants at rest.
- Contraction of lips and facial muscles helps to stabilize the mandible.
- Vigorous mandibular thrust

Physiologic transition of swallow begins during the first year of life and continues for several years. Infantile swallow is mainly carried out by the facial nerve.

Mature Swallow

It is seen usually by 4–5 years. Maturation of swallow pattern occurs with the addition of semisolid and solid foods to the diet. Increasing activation of the elevator muscles of mandible is seen. When sucking activity stops, a continued transition of swallow leads to acquisition of adult pattern of swallow. This swallow is characterized by:

- Cessation of lip activity, i.e. lips relaxed.
- Placement of tongue tip against the palate and behind upper incisors.
- Posterior teeth into occlusion during swallow.
- Downward and forward mandibular growth increases intraoral volume and vertical growth of the alveolar process changes tongue posture.
- Mandible stabilized by contraction of muscles of mastication. Thus mature swallow is controlled through the trigemminal nerve activity.

The process of swallowing is classically divided into the following three stages for descriptive convenience:

1. *Oral stage:* Food bolus enters pharynx from mouth.
2. *Pharyngenal stage:* Bolus enters esophagus from pharynx.
3. *Esophageal stage:* Bolus enters stomach from esophagus.

Stage 1: Oral stage
- It is voluntary stage.
- Anterior oral seal is established by elevation of the mandible by masseter and temporalis muscles and approximation of lips by circumoral muscles.
- A longitudinal furrow is formed in the posterior dorsum of the tongue and bolus is positioned in this furrow, it is called the "preparatory position".
- The tongue is then elevated against the palate by the action of mylohyoid muscles and groove in the tongue is progressively emptied from before backwards, moving the bolus towards the pharynx.
- Airway remains open at this stage.

Stage 2: Pharyngeal stage
- It is involuntary.
- In this stage, the bolus is pushed from oropharynx into the esophagus
- As the bolus reaches pharynx, a wave of contraction within the pharyngeal constrictor muscle arises and moves the bolus into the esophagus.
- Food entering back into the nasopharynx is prevented by elevation of the soft palate.
- Movement of bolus into larynx is prevented by approximation of vocal cords, elevation of larynx and backward movement of epiglottis to seal the laryngeal opening.
- The airway is thus closed and there is temporary arrest of breathing at this stage.

Stage 3: Esophageal stage
- It is also involuntary.
- When bolus reaches the esophagus, peristaltic waves are initiated which propels the bolus into the stomach.
- The passage of bolus into the stomach requires relaxation of the lower esophageal sphincter.
- Soft palate, epiglottis and tongue return to their normal positions and the airway is re-established.

Respiration

Respiration is an inherent reflex process that begins at birth. Breathing is evoked spontaneously at birth and is facilitated by posture of the mandible and hyoid bone. Establishment of normal nasal respiration is important for normal development of orofacial structures.

Partial or total nasal obstruction may lead to mouth breathing habit in some children. Such an alteration in breathing pattern disturbs the orofacial muscular balance because of lowered mandibular and tongue position. This may adversely affect the development of dental arches. Narrowed maxillary arch and posterior open bite are commonly observed in mouth breathers.

Speech

Coordinated activity of respiration, laryngeal behavior and oral structures are essential to produce effective speech.

Sounds are produced initially in the larynx by the coordinated movements of normal, thoracic and laryngeal muscles. This is called "phonation". The laryngeal note has a thin and reedy quality. This basic laryngeal sound is then modified within the resonating chambers of pharyngeal, oral and nasal cavities by the action of lips, tongue and soft palate to produce meaningful speech. This is called "articulation".

Muscles Involved in Speech

Although all oral structures are important, tongue has a significant role in speech. The highly complex nature of speech process is indicated by the number of muscles and nerves involved and the large areas of cerebral hemispheres of brain involved with speech. The muscles involved in speech include:
- Muscles of chest that control breathing.
- The intrinsic muscles of the larynx that are concerned with phonation.
- Muscles in the pharynx and soft palate that help in resonance.
- Muscles of the tongue, palate, jaws and facial musculature that produce meaningful speech.

Although altered speech may not cause malocclusion, certain malocclusions and skeletal abnormalities (e.g. open bite, increased overjet, reverse overbite, cleft palate, etc.) may cause altered phonation of consonants and can adversely affect speech.

BIBLIOGRAPHY

1. Graber Tm Orthodontics: Principles and Practice, 3rd Ed. WB Sounders. 1988.
2. Proffit WR. Concepts of growth and development. In: Contemporary Orthodontics, 2nd edition. St Louis: Mosby Yearbook, 1999;24–62.

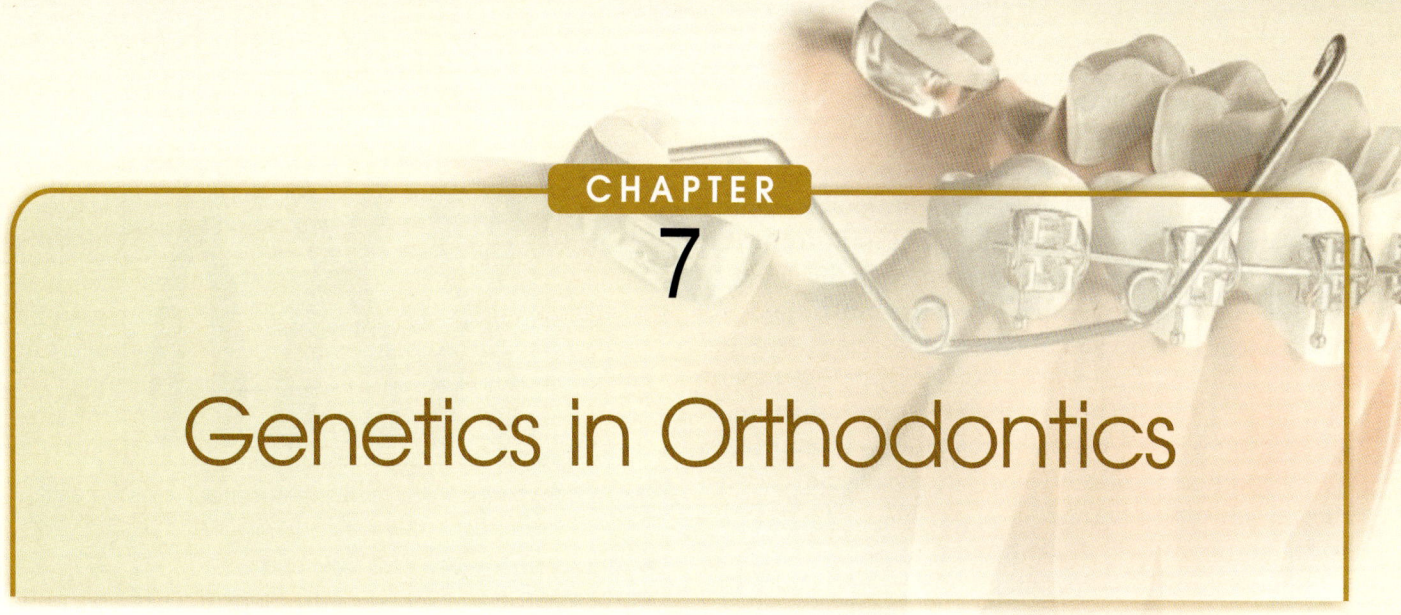

CHAPTER

7

Genetics in Orthodontics

Chapter Outline

- History/Introduction
- Clinical Implications of genetics in orthodontics
- Genetic disorders

- Methods of studying role of genes
- Genetics and malocclusion

HISTORY/INTRODUCTION

It was **Regnier de Graaf** who was the first to put forth the idea both the male and the female parents transmit genetic characteristics to the off spring. In the early 1700s, **Pierre Louis Moreau de Maupertuis** was the first to propose that there were certain hereditary particles. Two such particles—one from each parent. One particle might dominate the other recessive. But in the chapter, the genetics is explained with the work of **Gregor Mendel**. Gregor Mendel worked on various varieties of garden peas (*Pisum sativum*).

Depending on the findings, Mendel proposed three laws:

Mendel's 1st law—the law of segregation: There are two factors which determine a specific character:

- The parent transmits only one of the pair to the offspring.
- It is only a matter of chance as to which of the transmitted pairs unites.

Before Mendel's time, it was believed that the characteristics of parents blended into the offspring.

Mendel's 2nd law—the law of unit inheritance:

- Mendel clearly stated that blending did not occur.
- The characteristics of one parent may not appear in one generation but may reappear in the next generation.

Mendel's 3rd law—law of independent assortment:

- Members of different gene pairs assort to the gametes (sex cells) independently of one another.

- There is a random recombination of paternal and maternal chromosomes in the gametes.

Mendel's contribution went unnoticed for a long time. In the year 1900, three independent workers—Vriesin Holland, Correns in Germany and Tschermak von Seysenegg in Austria rediscovered Mendel's laws and that heralded the beginning of genetics as a science. In 1903, Sutton and Boveri, independently proposed that it was the interaction between these chromosomes that lead to the phenomenon of inheritance called "The Chromosome Theory of Inheritance".

Human Chromosomes

There are 46 chromosomes in the normal human—23 pairs.

22 pairs are alike in males and females which is known as autosomes and 1 pair differs which is called the sex chromosomes.

When prepared for analysis, the chromosomes appear under the microscope as **achromosome spread**. The chromosomes are then cut out from a photomicrograph and arranged in pairs in a standard classification. This process is called karyotyping. The complete picture is called the **karyotype**.

In 1960, at a conference in **Denver,** a classification system was devised to distinguish 7 chromosome groups (A through G) based on length and entromere position (Figs 7.1a and b).

73

The members of each pair match with respect to the genetic information they carry. One chromosome of the pairs inherited from the father, and one from the mother, and further, one is transmitted to the child.

The members of a pair of chromosomes are microscopically indistinguishable and this is true for the all chromosomes except male sex chromosomes. In the male, there is one X chromosome and one Y chromosome which is smaller than the X chromosome.

The location of the centromere can be used to classify the chromosomes Fig. 7.2.

- Metacentric—central centromere
- Submetacentric—off-center

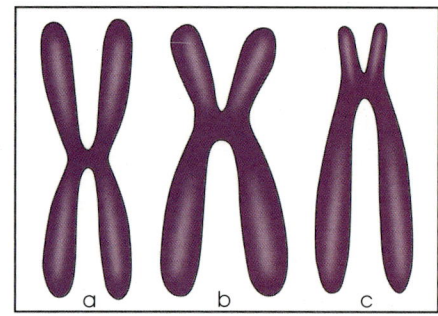

Fig. 7.2: (a) Metacentric; (b) Submetacentric; (c) Acrocentric

- Acrocentric—towards one end
- Telocentric—terminal centromere (does not occur in man)

Structure of Nucleic Acid

Nucleic acid was first isolated as early as 1869 by a Swiss doctor named **Meicher**, from pus-soaked bandages of wounded solders. He found a compound which was very rich in phosphorus and it was quite unique. Initially, he named it nuclein. He had even postulated in 1892 that this might be the actual hereditary factor. Nucleic acid is composed of long chains of molecules called **nucleotides**.

Each nucleotide is composed of:
- A sugar molecule
- A nitrogenous base
- A phosphate molecule

Sugar molecule: It is of two types:
- Ribose sugar
- Deoxyribose sugar

The nitrogenous bases: They are of two types:
- Purines
- Pyrimidines.

The purines include:
- Adenine
- Guanine

The pyrimidines include:
- Cytosine
- Thymine and
- Uracil.

The first stage in the formation of nucleotide or nucleic acid is the combination of
- One molecule of phosphoric acid,
- One molecule of deoxyribose, and
- One of the four nitrogen bases

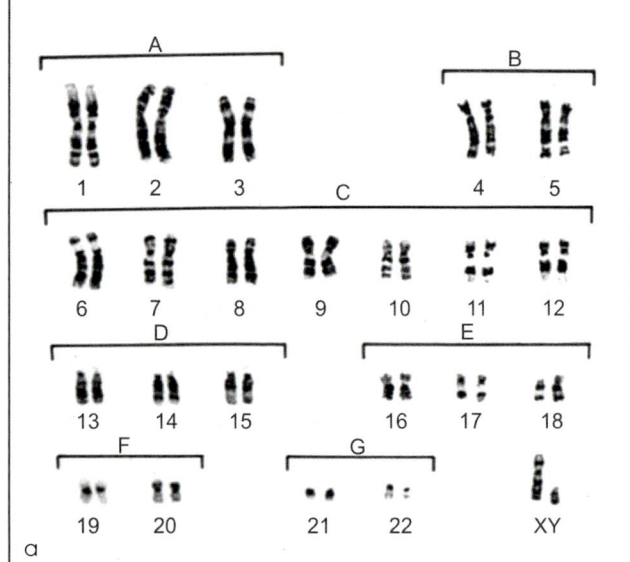

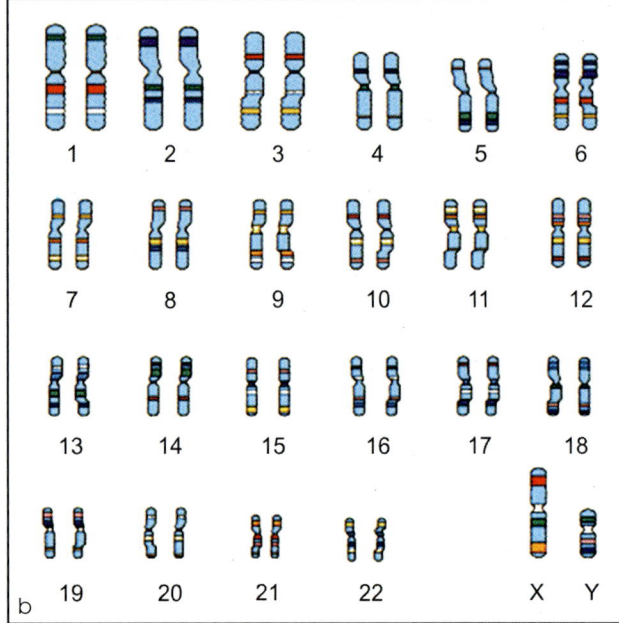

Figs 7.1a and b: Chromosome groups

Four separate nucleotides are thus formed, one for each of the four bases:

- Deoxyadenylic
- Deoxythymidylic
- Deoxyguanylic
- Deoxycytidylic

The nucleic acids can further be of 2 types depending on the sugar molecule:

- Sugar-ribose → Ribonucleic acid (RNA)
- Sugar-deoxyribose → Deoxyribonucleic acid (DNA)
- RNA is found in the nucleolus and in the cytoplasm.
- DNA is found mainly in the chromosomes.

Structure of DNA: The structure of DNA was suggested by Wilkins, Watson and Crick (Fig. 7.3).

Requirements of DNA

1. Structure should be sufficiently versatile to account for the great variety of different genes.
2. Should be able to reproduce itself in such a manner that an identical replica is formed at each cell division.

The DNA molecule is composed of two chains of nucleotides arranged in a double helix. The backbone of each chain is formed by the sugar-phosphate molecules.

The two chains are held together by hydrogen bonds between the nitrogenous bases which point in towards the centre of the helix (Fig. 7.4).

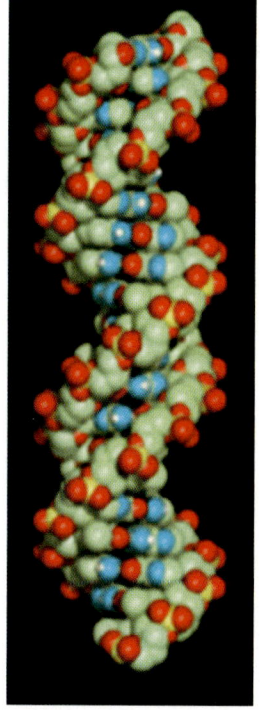

Fig. 7.3: Structure of DNA

Two chains have opposite orientation, and are said to be in an **antiparallel orientation**.

Pairing of the nitrogenous bases always occurs as:

- Purine with pyrimidine.
- Guanine with cytosine
- Adenine with thymine

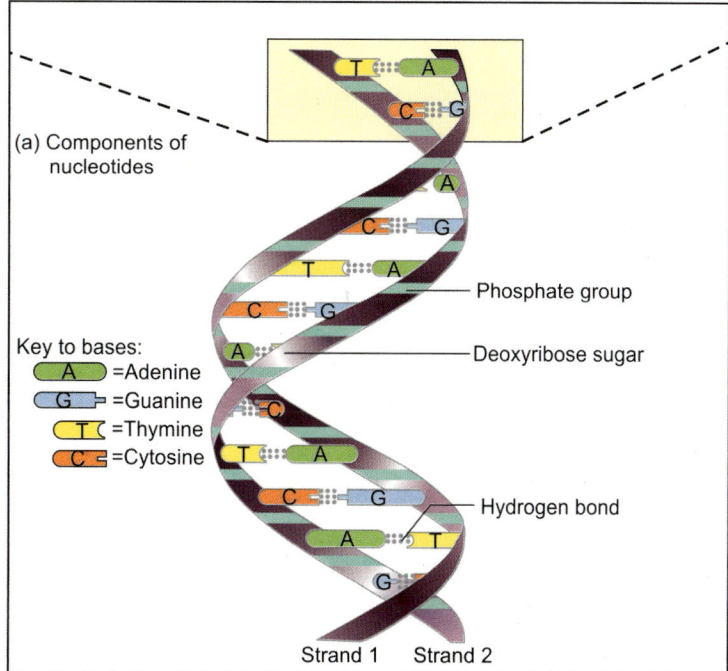

Fig. 7.4: Portion of DNA molecule

The bases are bound together by very loose hydrogen bonds between A and T two bonds and between G and C three bonds are formed.

Because of the looseness of these bonds, the two strands can pull apart with ease, and they do so many times during the course of their function in the cell.

There are three types of RNA:

1. *Messenger RNA:* Which carries the genetic code to the cytoplasm.
2. *Transfer RNA:* Which transports activated amino acids to the ribosomes.
3. *Ribosomal RNA:* Which, along with about 75 different proteins, forms the ribosomes, the physical and chemical structures on which protein molecules are actually assembled.

Replication of Nucleic Acid

Replication of the DNA molecule occurs in what is termed as the semi-conservative method. The individual chains divide at multiple sites, and on account of the specific base pairing, the complementary chain is formed. So the daughter cell has one parent strand and one new strand.

Genetic Code within the DNA Molecule

The Watson and Crick model of the DNA molecule also helps to explain the genetic code. The ability of DNA to control the formation of other substances in the cell lies in its ability to generate what is called genetic code. Function of genes is to synthesize proteins. Genes actually code the sequence of the amino acids needed to produce each protein.

There are 20 different amino acids. The arrangement of the nitrogenous bases is what gives the code for the amino acids. Since there are 4 bases and 20 amino acids, it can be calculated that groups of 3 bases are essential for coding the amino acids. The triplet code for one amino acid is called a codon (triplet codon) (Table 7.1).

When the two strands of a DNA molecule are split apart, this exposes the purine and pyrimidine bases projecting to the side of each strand. It is these projecting bases that form the code. The genetic code consists of successive "triplets" of bases that is each group of three successive bases is a code word. The successive triplet will eventually control the sequence of amino acids in a protein molecule synthesized in the cell.

Protein Synthesis

DNA is located in the nucleus of the cell. But most of the functions of the cell are carried out in the cytoplasm which is in turn controlled by DNA. The control is

Table 7.1: Amino acids	
Essential	*Non-essential*
• Arginine	• Glycine
• Histidine	• Proline
• Threonine	• Alanine
• Methionine	• Serine
• Valine	• Cysteine
• Phenylalanine	• Aspartic acid
• Leucine	• Asparagine
• Isoleucine	• Glutamic acid
• Tryptophan	• Glutamine
• Lysine	• Tyrosine

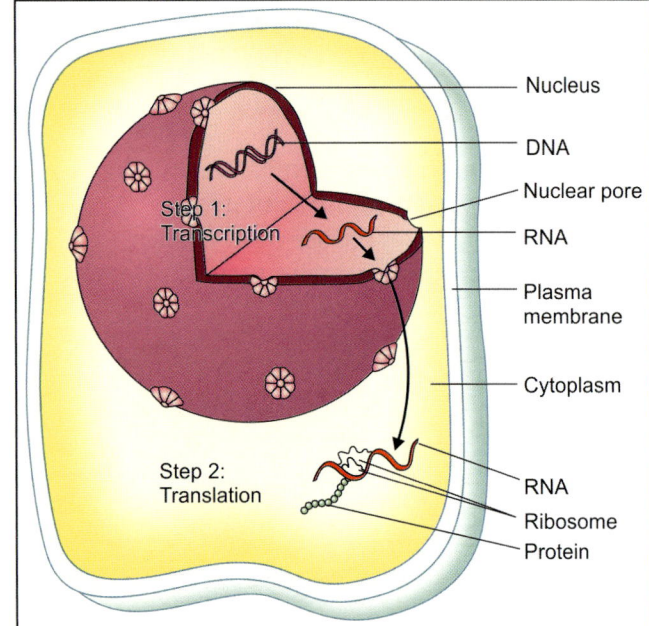

Fig. 7.5: Steps of protein synthesis

achieved by the formation of another type of nucleic acid called RNA, the formation of which is controlled by the DNA of the nucleus.

Steps involved in protein synthesis are (Fig. 7.5):
1. Transcription
2. Translation
   – Initiation
   – Elongation
   – Termination

Transcription

Formation of the RNA molecule from activated nucleotides using the DNA strand as a template is called "transcription". Initiation takes place under the influence of the enzyme RNA polymerase (Fig. 7.6).

When the RNA polymerase reaches the end of the DNA gene, it encounters a new sequence of DNA

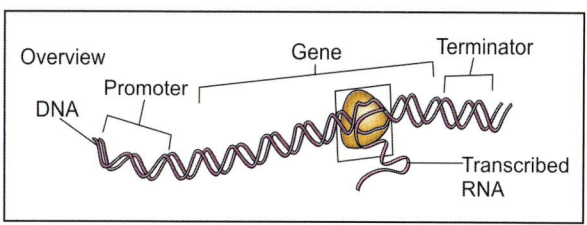

Fig. 7.6: Transcription

nucleotides called the chain-terminating sequence. This causes the polymerase to break away from the DNA strand and at the same time the RNA strand which is formed released into the nucleoplasm.

Translation

The process of formation of proteins in the ribosome are given in Figs 7.7a to f and 7.8.

CELL DIVISION

There are two types of cell division:

1. **Mitosis** (somatic cells): Normal cell division, by virtue of which the body grows. It results in two daughter cells, identical to the parent cell in genetic makeup, and number of chromosomes.
2. **Meiosis** (germ cells): This results in the production of reproductive cells (gametes). Each of which have only 23 chromosomes.

Mitosis

The cytoplasm of the cell apparently simply cleaves into two approximately equal halves. The nuclear division is more complicated. Four stages are:

1. Prophase
2. Metaphase
3. Anaphase
4. Telophase

Interphase (Fig. 7.9)

This is the resting stage when the cell is not dividing and the chromosomes are difficult to visualize. It is divided into three phases:

G1 (Gap 1): Stage just after previous mitosis. After mitosis, the cell enters a post-mitotic period during which there is no DNA synthesis.

S-phase: In this phase, replication of all DNA in the chromosomes occurs. The DNA begins to be duplicated some 5 to 10 hours before mitosis, and this is completed in 4 to 8 hours. DNA is replicated in much the same way that RNA is transcribed by DNA except for a few important differences.

Prophase

The chromosomes can be seen and easily discerned. The two chromatids can be seen. The centriole, which is an organelle outside the nucleus, duplicates itself and each one migrates to the opposite pole of the cell. The nuclear membrane disappears and the nucleus begins to loose its identity.

Metaphase

During this phase, the chromosomes are maximally contracted, and hence most deeply staining. They move to the centre of the cell, or the "equatorial plane". The chromosomes are now arranged in an almost two-dimensional metaphase plate and most easily studied and also the spindle is now formed. This is formed by microtubules of protein (spindle fibers) which extend from the centrioles at either pole of the cell up to the equatorial plane up to the kinetochores (sites of attachment at the centromere) (Fig. 7.10).

Anaphase

The centromeres divide, and the paired chromatids separate becoming daughter chromosomes. The spindles contract and draw the chromosomes, centromere to the respective poles of the cell. The mechanism is not fully understood, but it is probably due to actin–myosin interactions (Fig. 7.11).

Telophase

The daughter chromosomes arrive at the poles of the cell. Cytokinesis (division of the cytoplasm) occurs at this stage. The chromosomes unwind and stain less deeply. They get enclosed in a nuclear membrane, and the cell division is complete (Fig. 7.12).

Meiosis

This takes place when the gametes are formed. The number of the chromosomes is halved, each gamete receiving only a haploid set of chromosomes. It takes place in two phases:

- Meiosis I: The reduction division
- Meiosis II: An ordinary mitosis, without DNA replication.

Meiosis I

Prophase I: The prophase is very long and divided into several stages in meiosis.

Leptotene: Chromosomes begin to condense. Unlike the chromosomes in mitosis, they are not smooth in outline, but consist of alternating thick and thin regions. Thick

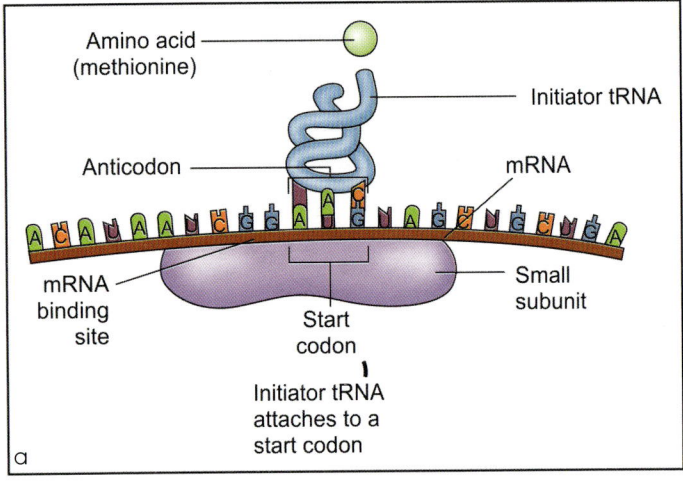

a

Initiator tRNA attaches to a start codon

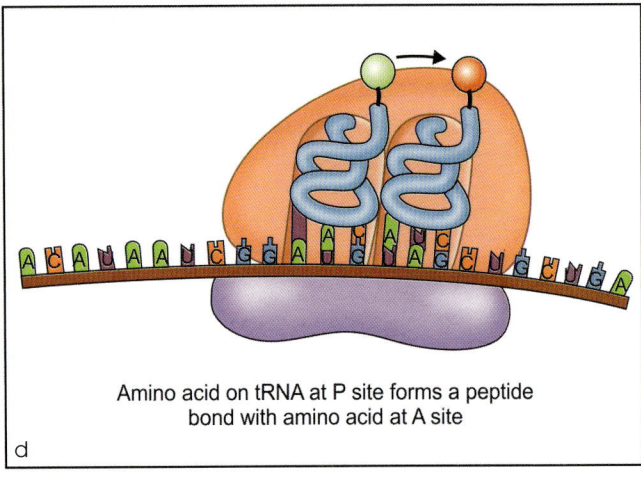

d

Amino acid on tRNA at P site forms a peptide bond with amino acid at A site

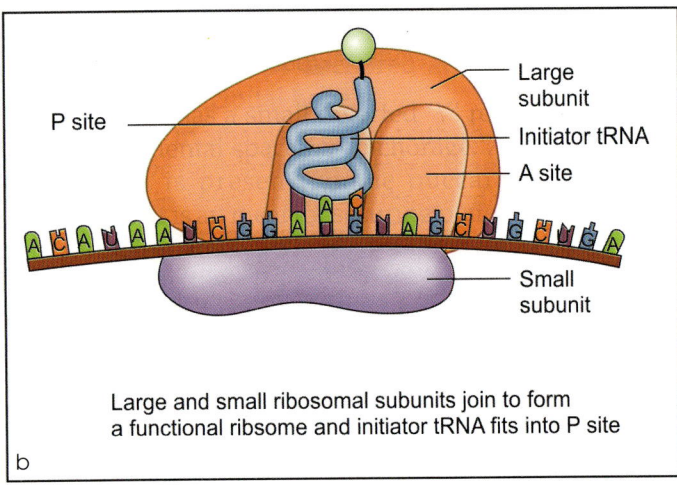

b

Large and small ribosomal subunits join to form a functional ribsome and initiator tRNA fits into P site

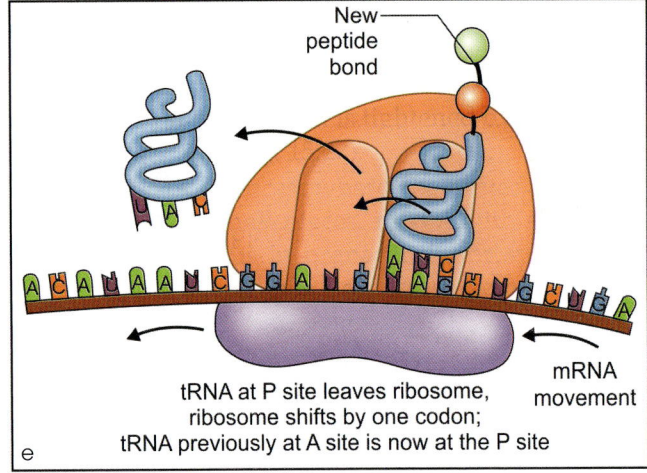

e

tRNA at P site leaves ribosome, ribosome shifts by one codon; tRNA previously at A site is now at the P site

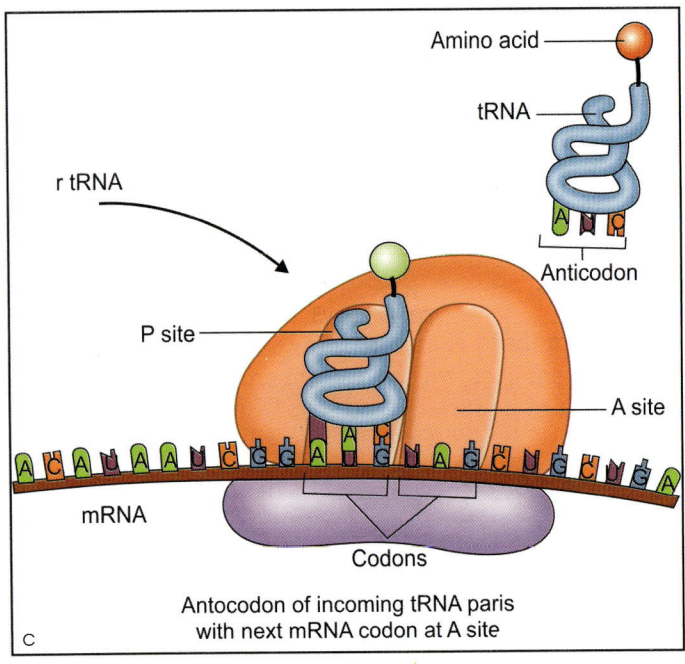

c

Antocodon of incoming tRNA paris with next mRNA codon at A site

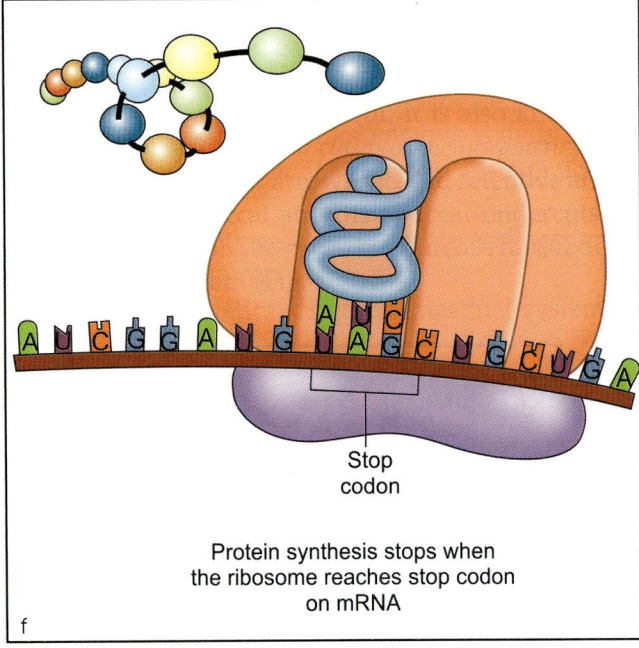

f

Protein synthesis stops when the ribosome reaches stop codon on mRNA

Fig. 7.7: Process of formation of protein

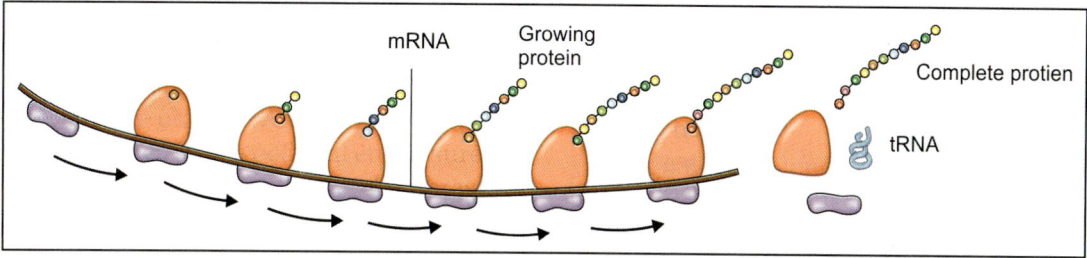

Fig. 7.8: Summary of movement of ribosome along mRNA

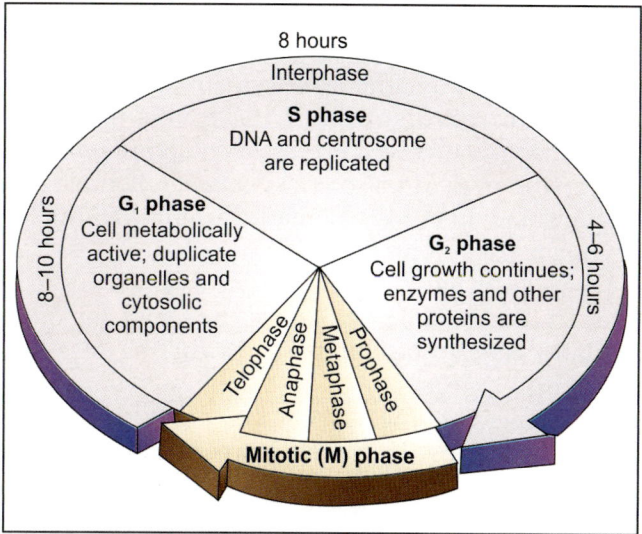

Fig. 7.9: Interphase

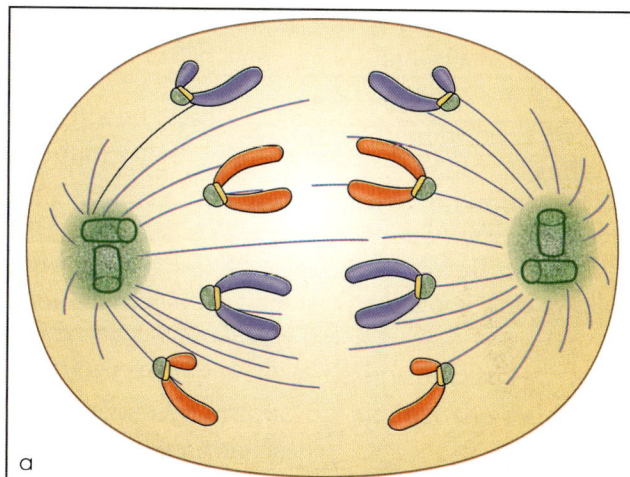

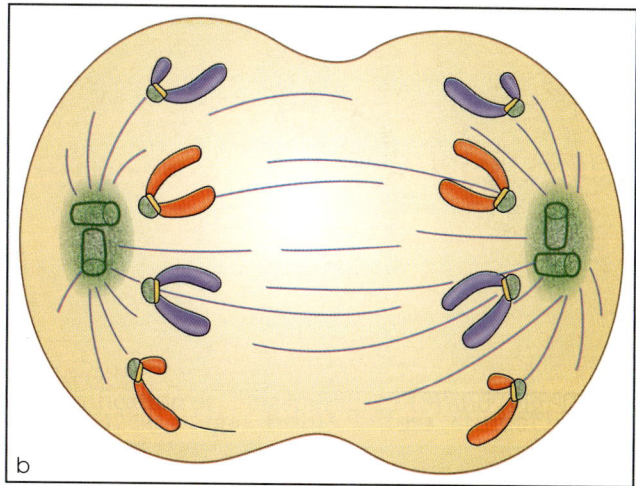

Fig. 7.11: Anaphase

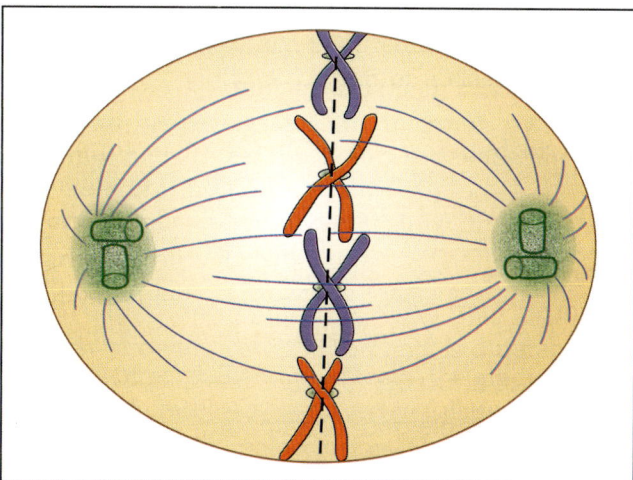

Fig. 7.10: Metaphase

regions are known as chromomeres, and are characteristic for each chromosome.

Zygotene: The pairing (synapsis) of homologous chromosomes takes place. The chromosome pairs lie parallel to each other in point for point association to form bivalents. This does not occur in mitosis (Fig. 7.13).

Pachytene: The chromosomes coil more tightly, and stain more deeply, and the chromomeres become more prominent. The bivalent is in close association, and is actually a tetrad—2 chromosomes of 2 chromatids each. This is the stage at which crossing over occurs.

Diplotene: During this phase, the two components of the bivalent begin to separate. The centromere of each chromosome remains intact, so the 2 chromatids are together. During the separation, the chromatids seem to be contact at several places, called chiasmata. These are sites of crossovers.

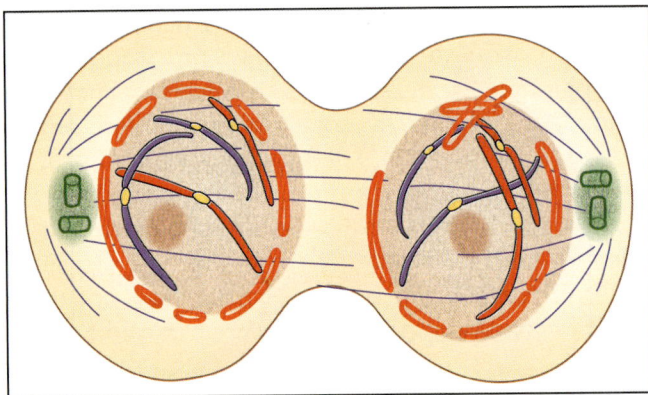

Fig. 7.12: Telophase

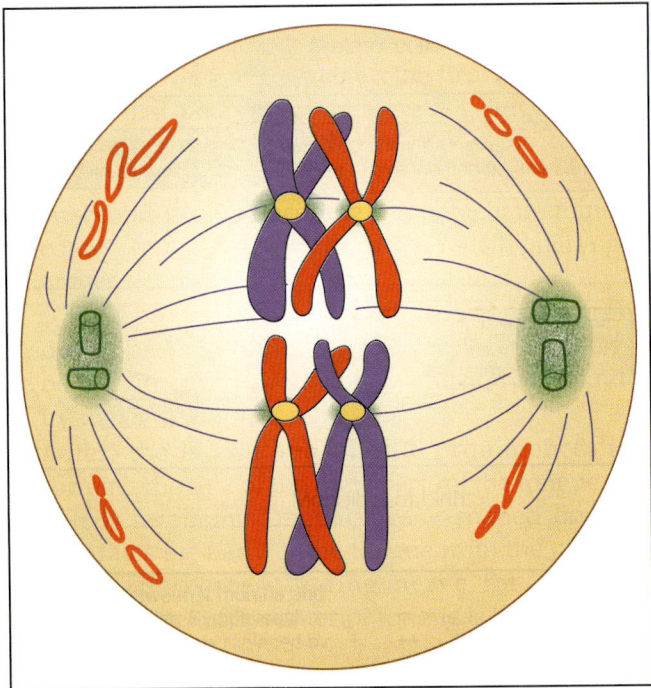

Fig. 7.13: Crossing over

Diakinesis: This is the final stage of the prophase, the chromosomes condense even more and become even deeper staining.

Metaphase I: The nuclear membrane disappears, and the chromosomes move to the equatorial plane.

Anaphase I: The two members of the bivalent disjoin, and one member goes to each pole. The bivalents get randomly assorted, so that each pole receives a random arrangement of paternal and maternal chromosomes. The first meiotic division provides the physical basis for Mendelian inheritance. At the end of meiosis I, each product has a haploid number of chromosomes.

Meiosis II

This follows meiosis I immediately, without DNA replication, and without an interphase. The centromeres divide, and the sister chromatids disjoin, passing to opposite poles and produce two daughter cells.

Crossing over: The crossing over, in effect, causes a reorganization of genes among the chromosomes, and hence increases genetic variability. The chiasmata of the chromosome mark the sites where the chromosomes have exchanged segments by breakage and recombination.

Only two chromatids take part in any crossover. But all four chromatids of the bivalent may be simultaneously involved in crossovers at different sites.

Crossing over can also occur between homologous chromosomes in mitosis **(somatic recombination)**. But it is much less common than in meiosis.

This could have an important effect in case of heterozygous cells. The crossover can cause one of the resultant cells to be homozygous for the recessive character.

Sometimes crossing over can also occur between the sister chromatids. It is seen increasingly in **Bloom syndrome**—where there is **growth retardation**—prenatally and postnatally, and a butterfly rash is seen on the face (Fig. 7.14).

Inheritance

- Chromosomes exist in pairs so our cells contain two copies of each gene, although they may be alike or may differ in their substructure.
- The two genes at the locus or position on the chromosome are called **alleles**. If both genes are identical, the individual is described as **homozygous** for that trait, while if they differ, it is **heterozygous**.
- The exception to this rule that all cells contain pairs of chromosomes are gametes i.e. sperm and ovum which are haploid in number i.e. contain only one set of chromosome.

Genetic Disorders and Inheritance

Genetic disorders can be of three main types:
- *Single gene disorders:* These occur due to mutations of single genes. They show typical pedigree patterns and are rare—1 in 2000 or less.
- *Chromosome disorders:* The disorder occurs due to an excess or deficiency of whole chromosomes or chromosome segments. More common than single gene disorders—7 in 1000 births.
- *Multifactorial inheritance:* These are caused due to a combination of genetic and environmental factors.

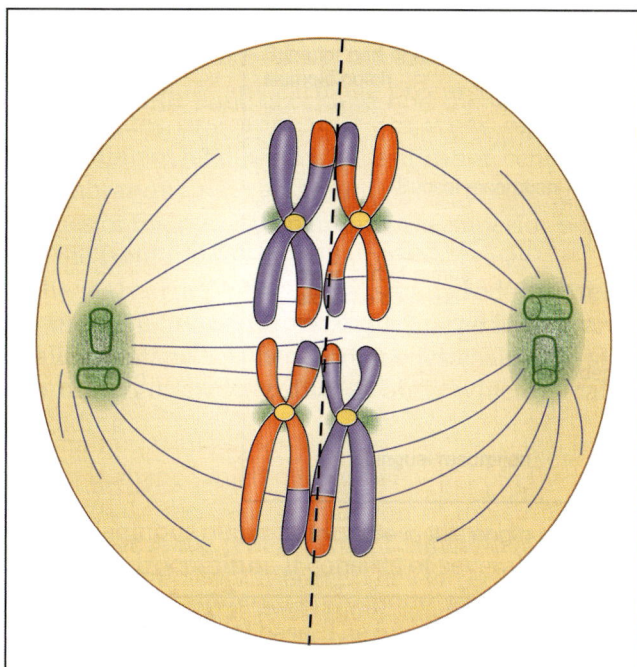

Fig. 7.14: Zygotene

They are the most common of the genetic disorders and do not show the typical pedigree patterns on single gene disorders.

Single Gene Disorders

These can be:
- Autosomal dominant
- Autosomal recessive
- Sex-linked (gonosomal) dominant
- Sex-linked (gonosomal) recessive

The science of genetics is concerned with the inheritance of traits, whether normal or abnormal and with the interaction of genes and the environment. The orthodontists are interested in genetics to understand why a patient has a particular occlusion.

CLINICAL IMPLICATIONS OF GENETICS IN ORTHODONTICS

Importance of Genetics

Genes

- Control heredity from parents to children.
- Control the reproduction.
- Control the day by day function of all cells.
- Control growth and development.
- Helps in early diagnosis and treatment of diseases.

How will genetics help us?

- The popular thinking since dentoalveolar structures adapt very readily to environmental factors, so local malocclusions are primarily acquired and are not related to heredity.
- But the similarity of sibling pair in tooth malpositions and malocclusions shows the presence of genetic component.
- It is also important to remember that soft tissue morphology and behavior have a genetic component and so siblings are likely to respond to environmental factors in similar fashion and so may have similar dentoalveolar morphology.
- In clinical orthodontics, each malocclusion occupies its own distinctive slot in the genetic/environmental spectrum, and therefore, the diagnostic goal is to determine the relative contribution of genetics and the environment.
- The greater the genetic component, the worse the prognosis for successful outcome by means of orthodontic intervention.
- Whatever it is for all practical purpose, the bottom line is that it is seldom possible to determine the precise contribution of heredity and environmental factors in a particular case.
- It is possible to influence the dentoalveolar regions of the jaws within certain parameters using environmental factors, but what evidence is available from human studies to date tends to support the genetic determination of craniofacial form with a lack of evidence to show any significant long-term influence on mandibular or maxillary skeletal bases using orthopedic appliances.
- The malocclusions of genetic origin (skeletal discrepancies), when detected in growing period, are being successfully treated using orthopedic and functional appliances.
- Examination of parents and older siblings can give information regarding the treatment need for a child and treatment can be begun at an early age.
- They affect growth, development and function of orofacial structures.
- Helps to diagnose, treat or to probably prevent malocclusion from occurring in the next generation

GENETIC DISORDERS

- Numerical disorders
- Structural disorders

Numerical Disorders

There is a change in the number of chromosomes within the cell, e.g.
- Polyploidy
- Monosomy

- Trisomy
- Turner's syndrome
- Klinefelter's syndrome

Trisomy

An autosomal disorder: Person has 3 homologous chromosomes instead of 2 homologous chromosomes. It often dies between conception (when sperm meets egg) and 1-year-old (Fig. 7.15).

Structural Disorders

There is change in basic composition and structure of chromosomes, e.g.

- Translocation
- Deletions
- Ring chromosomes

Patterns of Genetic Transmission

- Repetitive traits
- Discontinuous traits
- Variable traits

Repetitive traits: Recurrence of single dentofacial deviation within the immediate family and in the progenitors is seen generation after generation

Discontinous traits: Tendency of a malocclusal trait to reappear in the family background over several generations is seen in family but not in all generations

Variable traits: Occurrence of different but related type of malocclusion is seen within several generation of same family. Traits are seen with variable expression, e.g. missing teeth, commonly seen feature in some families, but the same teeth may not be missing in different generations or within the same generation

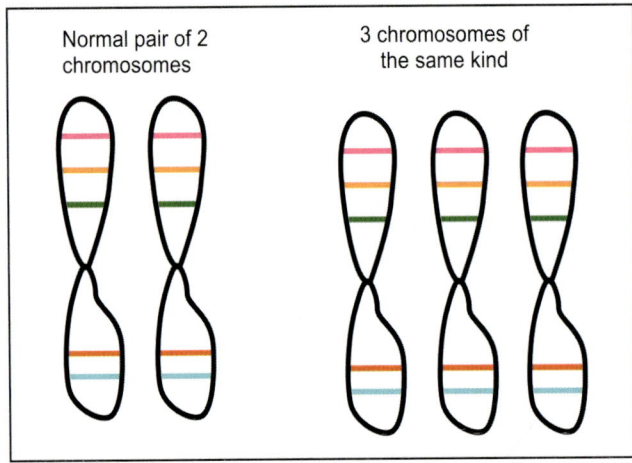

Normal pair of 2 chromosomes

3 chromosomes of the same kind

Fig. 7.15: Trisomy

Methods of Studying Role of Genes

- Twin studies
- Tracing the gene in family pedigree studies
- Inbreeding

Twin Studies

Twin studies are done by analyzing monozygotic and dizygotic twins in a specific manner.

They help us to study the expression of the genetic factor and at the same time the environmental influences on this genetic expression. Human twins are of two types:

- Monozygotic twins
- Dizygotic twins

Monozygotic twins: Two individuals developed from single fertilized ovum, which divides into two at an early stage of development. They have a genetic make-up identical to each other.

Dizygotic twins: Two individuals developed from two separate ova, ovulated and fertilized by two different sperms.

Not genetically identical as they develop from two different embryos.

Tracing the Gene in Family Pedigree Studies

- Autosomal dominant inheritance
- Autosomal recessive inheritance
- Sex-linked recessive inheritance
- Sex-linked dominant inheritance
- Polygenic disorder and multifactorial inheritance

Autosomal Dominant Inheritance (Flowchart 7.1)

It arises due to defect in at least one gene out of a pair of genes. Distinguishning features are:

- In this the mutant gene manifests itself in the homozygote or in heterozygote.
- These disorders are quite rare
- Usually the person is heterozygous and one of the parents is affected.
- Disease usually appears in each generation.
- Delayed age of onset
- Vertically transmitted
- Mostly involve structural proteins.
- Male and female siblings are equally affected.
- It is inherited as a simple Mendelian dominant factor.
- Autosomal dominant characteristics can also occur as new mutations
- Capability of transmission is the same in both the affected parents

- Each child of an affected parent is at 50% risk of inheriting the abnormal gene.
- Autosomal dominant disorders variable in clinical manifestation, e.g. polydactyl
- Sometimes the gene may not express itself at all in one generation, which is known as non penetrance.
- Some autosomal genes are expressed more frequently in one sex than another. This is called sex influence, e.g. gout and baldness in males.
- In absence of male-to-male transmission, an autosomal dominant trait cannot be distinguished from an X-linked dominant inheritance.
- In absence of male-to-male transmission, an autosomal dominant trait cannot be distinguished from an X-linked dominant inheritance.

Autosomal Recessive Inheritance (Flowchart 7.2)

- Trait appear in every generation
- An affected child must have at least one affected parent.
- About one-half of the offspring of an affected person are affected.
- Both male and female are affected.
- Autosomal recessive inheritance.
- Abnormal recessive genes are affected through heterozygote.
- The trait visible only in siblings but not in their parents and relatives.
- Parents of an affected person may be blood relatives.
- About one-fourth of children are affected.
- Recurrence risk—25%.
- Equal male female predilection.

Sex-linked Recessive Inheritance

- Mostly X-linked
- Male predilection
- Heterozygous females are carriers expected to produce normal and affected sons in ratio of 1:1
- Affected male parent cannot transmit the trait directly to his sons, i.e. trait will skip a generation

Sex-linked Dominant Inheritance

- Affected male parent transmits the trait to his daughter but not to son.
- When affected females are homozygous they transmit the trait to all children irrespective of their sex.
- When affected females are heterozygous only 50% of children of both sexes have a chance of being affected.

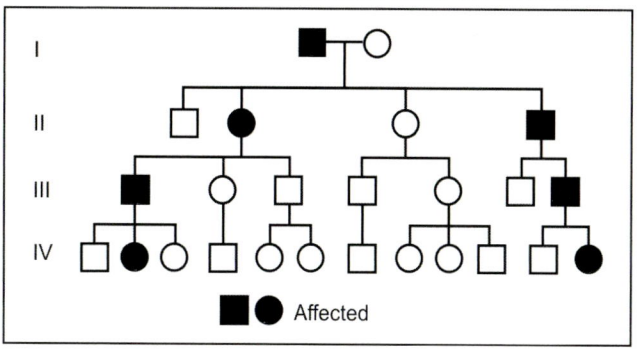

Flowchart 7.1: Pattern of autosomal dominant inheritance

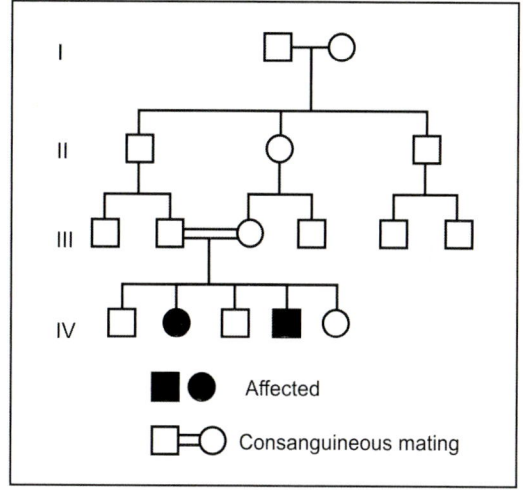

Flowchart 7.2: Pattern of autosomal recessive inheritance

Polygenic Disorder and Multifactorial Inheritance

Cumulative effects of all polygene or local or general environmental factor.

For example:
- Cleft lip and cleft palate
- Inbreeding and consanguineous marriages
- Inbreeding—mating between close relatives
- Genetic consequence of inbreeding
- Increase in proportion of homozygote thus recessive genes are more easily expressed
- Unmasking of a hidden recessive genes
- Occurrence of malocclusion and cleft lip and cleft palate is more in offspring of inbreeding marriages
- Dental and skeletal characteristics inherited
- Developmental hereditary characteristics are influenced by local and general environmental factors and their penetrance and expressivity can be greatly modify by these influence
- Occlusal variations are polygenic, i.e. control by many genes and various environmental factors
- Extreme deviation are due to chromosomal or single gene effect

Genetics and Malocclusions

- Down's syndrome
- Cleft lip and palate
- Bimaxillary protrusion
- Bimaxillary atresia
- Retarded eruption of teeth
- Hypodontia, anodontia, oligodontia
- Abnormal overjet and overbite
- Open bite
- High-arched palate
- Abnormal number and arrangement of teeth
- Micrognathia
- Macrognathia
- Gardners syndrome
- Marfan's syndrome
- Cherubism
- Cleidocranial dysplasia
- Mandibulofacial dysplasia
- Osteogenesis imperfect

GENETIC INFLUENCES ON TOOTH SIZE, NUMBER, MORPHOLOGY

Position and Eruption

Tooth Size

Twin studies have shown that tooth crown dimensions are strongly determined by heredity. Butler's field theory, explained later in this chapter. As dietary habits in humans adapt from a hunter/gatherer to a defined food culture, evolutionary selection pressures are tending to reduce tooth volume, which is manifested in third molar, second premolar and lateral incisor "fields". Hypodontia of the above mentioned teeth shows a familial tendency and fits polygenic models of inheritance.

Tooth Number

The supernumerary teeth, most frequently seen on premaxillary region, also appear to be genetically determined. Mesiodens are most commonly present in parents and siblings of the patients who exhibit them. Hereditary nature of hypodontia is revealed in familial and twin studies. Maxillary lateral incisor, most common tooth to be congenitally missing next to third molars, often exhibits familial occurrence.

Abnormal Tooth Shape

Abnormalities in lateral incisor region varies from peg-shaped to microdontia, missing teeth, all of which have familial trends, female preponderance and association with other dental anomalies (missing teeth, ectopic canines, transposition), suggesting a polygenic etiology. Carabelli trait also appers to be strongly influenced by genes.

Ectopic Maxillary Canine

Various studies have indicated a genetic tendency for ectopic maxillary canine. Pecketal (1991) concluded that palatally ectopic canines have an inherited trait, being one of the anomalies in a complex and genetically related dental disturbances, often occurring in combination with missing teeth, microdontia, supernumerary teeth and other ectopically positioned teeth. In addition, tooth transposition most commonly affects maxillary canine/first premolar class position and shows a familial occurrence.

Submerged primary molars: Primary molars, especially in mandibular arch, are the commonly submerged teeth.

HEREDITABILITY AND FUNCTIONAL COMPONENT OF OCCLUSION

Balance between external and internal functional matrices is important for the establishment of normal occlusion. During diagnostic process, it is also important to consider the possible role of functional components of occlusion.

Soft tissue morphology and behavior have a genetic component and they have a significant influence on the dentoalveolar morphology, e.g. in Class II division 1, a short upper lip and low lip level with flaccid lip tone will favor proclination of upper incisors. The external matrix (lip morphology and behavior, cheeks) is thought to be strongly genetically determined, while internal matrix (tongue posture and behavior) can be influenced by both genetic and environmental factors.

Butler's Field Theory

According to this theory, mammalian dentition can be divided into several developmental fields. The developmental fields include molar/premolar field, the canine field and the incisor field. Within each developmental field, there is a key tooth, which is more stable developmentally and on either side of this key tooth, the remaining teeth within the field become progressively less stable.

Example-1: Within Molar/Premolar Field

Within molar/premolar field, according to Butler's field theory, maximum variability will be seen for the third molars. Third molars are the most common teeth to be congenitally absent and to be impacted.

Variability of third molars includes:

- *Variable in size:* Third molars can be small appearing as microdonts. They can have small roots and small cusps.
- *Variable in form:*
  1. They may have well-formed cusps or several small tubercles.
  2. Some maxillary third molars may not resemble any of the teeth and appear like abnormalities.
  3. The roots can be very short, long often fused, may be separate and sometimes an extra root can be seen.

Second molar can also show variation, such as microdontic tooth. When premolars are congenitally absent, the second premolars are more commonly affected than the first premolars.

Example-2: Within Incisor Field

Within incisor field, according to Butler's theory, the maximum variability will be seen for the lateral incisor. Variability of lateral incisor includes:

a. Peg-shaped lateral incisor
b. Congenitally missing laterals

Example-3: Within the Canine Field

Canines especially in maxillary arch can be impacted or ectopically erupted.

BIBLIOGRAPHY

1. Horowitz SL, Osborne RH, Degeorge FV. A Cephalometric Study of Craniofacial Variation in Adult Twins. Angle Orthod 1960; 30:1–5
2. King L, Harris EF, Tolley EA. Heritability of skeletal-dental relationships. Am J Orthod 1993; 121–31.
3. Litton Sf, Ackerman LV, Isaacson RJ, et al. A genetic study of Class III malocclusion. Am J Orthod 1970; 58:556–77.

PREVIOUS YEAR'S UNIVERSITY QUESTIONS

Short Questions

1. Butler's field theory
2. Genetic disorders
3. Twin study
4. Mendalian disorders
5. Pedigree studies

MCQs

1. *Who is called founder of human genetics?*
   a. Adam Joseph
   b. Gregor Mendel
   c. Charles Darwin
   d. Pythagoras   **(Ans: a)**

2. *Who is called father of modern genetics?*
   a. Adam Joseph
   b. Gregor Mendel
   c. Charles Darwin
   d. Pythagoras   **(Ans: b)**

3. *Gregor Mandel was a*
   a. Scientist
   b. Scholar
   c. Monk
   d. Dentist   **(Ans: c)**

4. *Who proposed the structure of DNA molecule?*
   a. Watson and Crick
   b. Finch and Klung
   c. Sulton and Boveri
   d. Adam Joseph   **(Ans: a)**

5. *Number of chrosomes present in every cell of an organism:*
   a. Constant
   b. Changes from one species to another
   c. Both A and B
   d. None of theabove   **(Ans: c)**

6. *Hapsburg jaw refers to:*
   a. Class I malocclusion
   b. Class III malocclusion with prognathic mandible
   c. Class II malocclusion
   d. Both b and c   **(Ans: b)**

7. *According to Butter's field theory, the stable key tooth in molariform field is:*
   a. 1st premolar
   b. 1st molar
   c. 3rd molar
   d. 2nd molar   **(Ans: b)**

8. *Which of the below is numerical disorder of chromosome?*
   a. Klinefelters syndrome
   b. Turner's syndrome
   c. Trisomy and monosomy
   d. All of the above   **(Ans: d)**

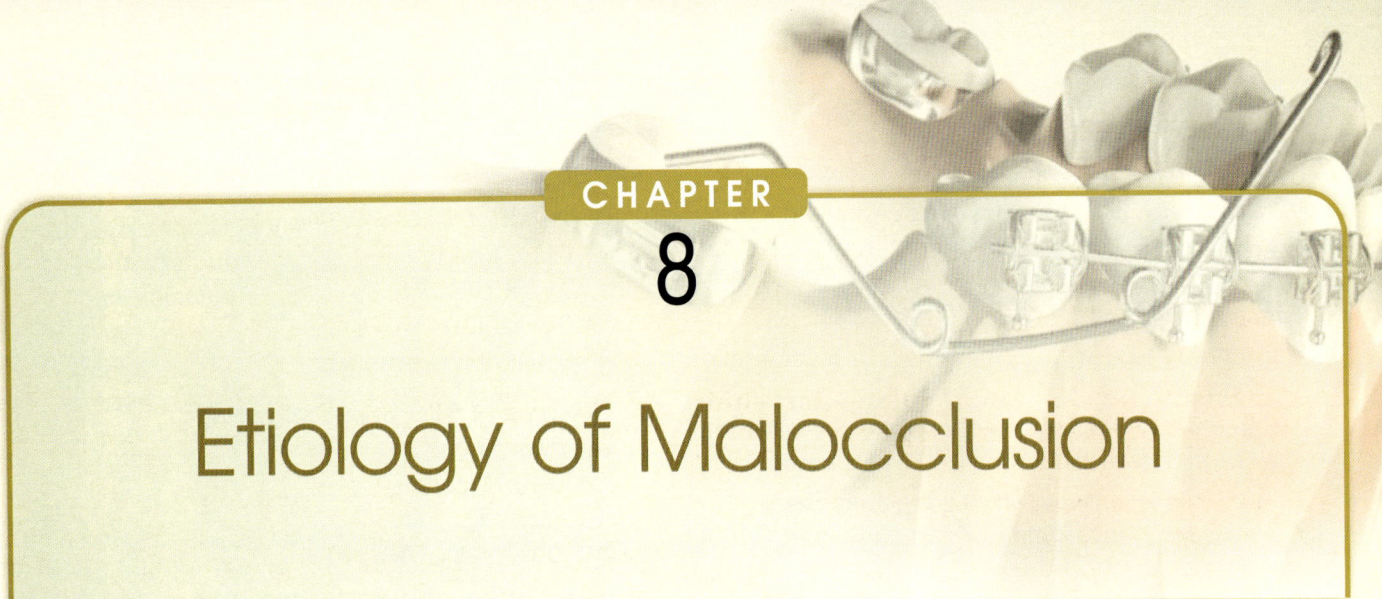

Etiology of Malocclusion

Chapter Outline

- Introduction
- Classifications

- General factors
- Local factors

INTRODUCTION

Several methods have been used to categorize the etiologic factors of malocclusion. One classification refers to *inherited and congenital* as one group and another group as *acquired*.

Inherited and congenital group lists such factors as characteristic inherited from parents, problems of tooth number and size, congenital deformities, conditions affecting mother during pregnancy and fetal environment.

Acquired factors include premature loss and prolonged retention of deciduous teeth, habits abnormal function, diet, trauma, metabolic and endocrine disturbances.

Another approach is indirect or predisposing causes and direct or determining causes.

Indirect: It would be heredity, congenital defects, prenatal abnormalities, acute or chronic infectious and deficiency diseases, metabolic disturbances, endocrine imbalance and unknown causes.

McCoy lists the following as *direct* causes: The missing teeth, supernumerary teeth, transposed teeth, malformed teeth, abnormal labial frenum, intrauterine pressure, sleeping habits, posture, abnormal muscular habits, malfunctioning muscles, premature shedding of deciduous teeth, prolonged retention of deciduous teeth, premature loss of deciduous teeth, loss of permanent teeth and improper dental restorations.

Moyers lists seven causes and clinical entities:

1. Heredity
   a. Neuromuscular system
   b. Bone
   c. Teeth
   d. Soft parts
2. Developmental defects of unknown origin
3. Trauma
   a. Prenatal trauma and birth injuries
   b. Postnatal trauma
4. Physical agents
   a. Prenatal
   b. Postnatal
5. All abnormal pressure habits
6. Disease
   a. Systemic disease
   b. Endocrine disorders
   c. Local disease
7. Malnutrition

CLASSIFICATIONS

Salzman's Classification

A modification of Salzman's representation of the etiologic factors in malocclusion embodies prenatal and postnatal factors. It shows well the genetic, differentiate and congenital factors that make up the prenatal elements of causation which can influence any one or all of the postnatal developmental, functional and environmental.

Graber's Classification

General Factor

- Heredity (inherited pattern)
- Congenital defects (cleft palate, torticollis, cleidocranial dysostosis, cerebral palsy, syphilis, etc.)
- Environment
- Prenatal (trauma, maternal diet, maternal metabolism, German measles, etc.)
- Postnatal (birth injury, cerebral palsy, TMJ injury).
- Predisposing metabolic climate and disease:
  a. Endocrine imbalance.
  b. Metabolic disturbance.
  c. Infectious diseases (poliomyelitis).
- Dietary problems (nutritional deficiency).
- Abnormal pressure habits and functional aberrations).
- Abnormal sucking (forward mandibular posture, non-physiologic nursing, excessive buccal pressures, etc.).
- Thumb and finger sucking.
- Tongue thrust and tongue sucking.
- Lip and nail biting.
- Abnormal swallowing habits.
- Speech defects.
- Respiratory abnormalities (mouth breathing).
- Tonsils and adenoids (compensatory tongue position).
- Psychogenetic and bruxism.

Local Factors

- *Anomalies of number:*
  1. Supernumerary tooth
  2. Missing tooth (congenital absence or loss due to accidents, caries, etc.)
- Anomalies of tooth size
- Anomalies of tooth shape
- Abnormal labial frenum and mucosal barriers.
- Premature loss
- Prolonged retention of tooth
- Delayed eruption of permanent teeth.
- Abnormal eruptive path.
- Ankylosis.
- Dental caries
- Improper dental restoration.

Although there are drawbacks to this approach, it is easiest one to use. It works well if at all times the reader remains aware of the interdependence of general and local factors. But, there are a few local factors that are not modified by one or more general influences. These correlations will be pointed out in the discussion of specific causes of malocclusion.

GENERAL FACTORS

The offspring inherits a few attributes from his/her parents. These factors or these attributes may be modified by prenatal and postnatal environment, by physical entities, by pressures, abnormal habits, nutritional disturbances, cerebral palsy, torticollis, cleidocranial dysostosis, congenital syphilis produce demonstrable abnormalities that require dental guidance.

Environment

Uterine posture and fibroids of mother cause marked cranial or facial asymmetries that are apparent at birth, but disappear after first year of life. Thus the deformity is temporary. Even in cases of so-called micromandible or Pierre Robin syndrome and Treacher-Collins syndrome, there are tremendous increments of adjective growth that are largely eliminate the original malformation.

Amniotic Lesion

- **Maternal diet and metabolism.** It appears to be unlikely causes of developmental deformity.
- Since fetus is well cushioned by the amniotic fluid, minor injury to the mother is unlikely to affect the child.
- German measles as well as medications taken during pregnancy cause gross congenital deformities including malocclusion.

Postnatal Influences

Birth injury: It is certainly possible to injure the infant at birth with a high forceps delivery.

Disabling accidents
- It produces undue pressures on the developing dentition.
- Falls that produces condylar fractures causing facial asymmetries.
- Extensive scar tissue from burns may also produce malocclusion.

Predisposing Metabolic Climate and Disease

- Exanthematous fevers are known to upset the developmental timetable and often they leave their permanent marks on the surface of the teeth.

- Acute fibril diseases may temporarily slow down the pace of growth and development.
- Endocrinologic diseases may be potent makers of malocclusion.
- Diseases with a paralytic effect such as poliomyelitis are capable of producing bizarre malocclusions.
- Diseases with muscle malfunction such as muscular dystrophy and cerebral palsy have characteristic deforming effects on the dental arch.
- Hypothyroidism produce abnormal resorption patterns, delayed eruption patterns and gingival disturbances, retained deciduous teeth and individualized malposed teeth.

Dietary Problems (Nutritional Deficiency)

Disturbances such as rickets, scurvy and beriberi can produce severe malocclusions upsetting the dental developmental time tables. The resultant premature loss, prolonged retention, poor tissue health and abnormal eruptive paths cause malocclusion.

Abnormal Pressure Habits

A wide variety of oral habits in infants and young children have been the center of much controversy for many years. Orthodontists, parents, pediatricians, psychologist, speech pathologist and pedodontists have discussed and argued the significance of these habits each from the view point of their own expertise and responsibility.

While orthodontist, pedodontist and speech pathologist are more interested in oral structural changes resulting from prolonged habit patterns, Pediatricians, psychologist place more importance on the deeper seated behavioral problems of the child, of which oral habit may be only a symptom.

Most oral habits exert abnormal forces on the teeth and perioral structures, thus it adversely affect the optimum growth and development of the dentoalveolar structures. The facial bones are not densely calcified in early childhood, so the abnormal pressures from oral habits can create abnormal developmental forces, which result in malocclusion.

Damaging oral habits that may interfere with growth and development and it should be treated early. Otherwise the problems become progressively worse and more difficult to manage. Further, these habits may be initiated to complicate the deformity and add to the difficulty of treatment.

Trident of Habit Factors

- Duration
- Frequency
- Intensity

The severity of malocclusion due to finger and thumb sucking habit depends on trident factor as mentioned above.

LOCAL FACTORS

Anomalies in Tooth Number

If the number of teeth presents increases or size of teeth is abnormally large, it can cause crowding or hamper the eruption of succedaneous teeth in their ideal positions. Similarly, if the number of teeth present is less than normal then gaps will be seen in the dental arch. It can be of two types:

- Increased number of teeth or supernumerary teeth
- Less number of teeth or missing teeth.

Supernumerary Teeth

Supernumerary teeth are defined as teeth in excess of the normal series. Males are twice as commonly affected than females with the following reported prevalence. Paul of Aegina was the first to mention supernumerary (Figs 8.1 and 8.2):

- 0.3–0.8% in the primary dentition
- 0.1–3.8% in the permanent dentition

Supernumerary teeth occur 10 times more frequently in the maxilla than in the mandible, with the premaxilla being most commonly affected followed by the mandibular premolar region.

Etiology: Both genetic and environmental factors are probably involved in the development of supernumerary teeth. Developmentally, these teeth are thought to form due to hyperactivity of the dental lamina.

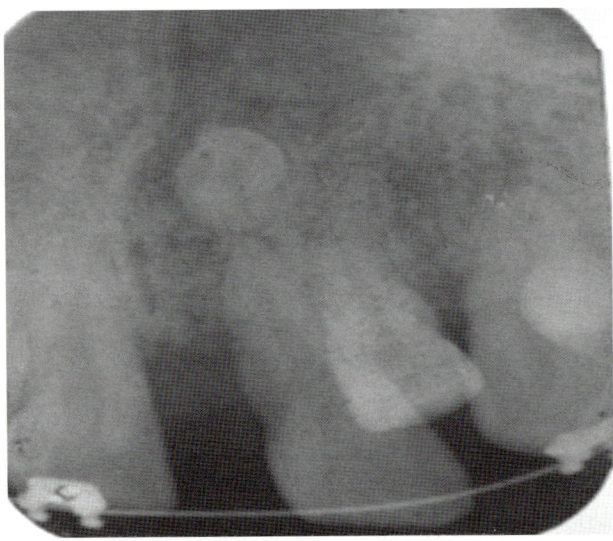

Fig. 8.1: Supernumerary tooth

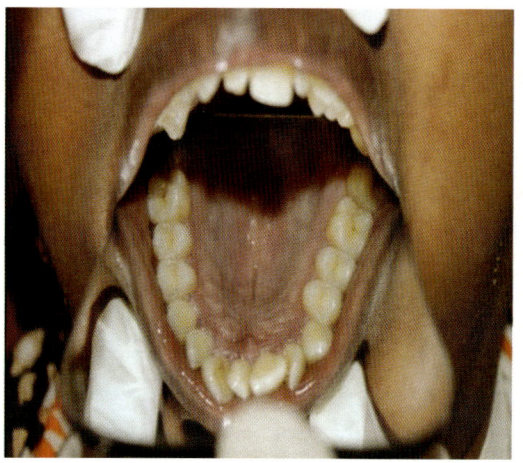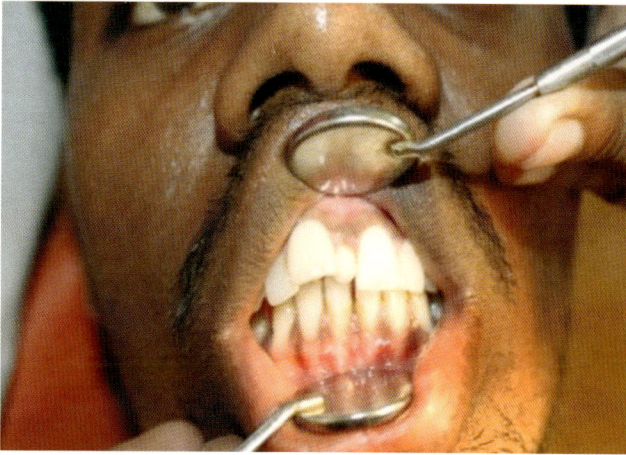

Fig. 8.2: Supernumerary teeth seen clinically

Classification (Flowchart 8.1 and Table 8.1): Super-numerary teeth can be classified into four groups based on their morphology

- Conical
- Tuberculate
- Supplemental
- Odontomes

Clinical features: Supernumerary teeth may remain unnoticed or present as incidental radiographic findings. Sometimes a complication due to their presence may be a presenting feature.

Complications include:
- *Failure of eruption:* Any tooth can be affected where a supernumerary tooth lies in the path of eruption. This is the most common cause of failure of eruption of maxillary central incisors.
- *Formation of midline diastema:* A mesiodens may prevent approximation of the central incisor roots with resultant diastema formation.
- *Crowding:* Erupted supernumerary teeth may take up arch space and evidence suggests that there is a generalized increase in tooth size in patients with supernumerary teeth.

Flowchart 8.1: Classification of supernumerary

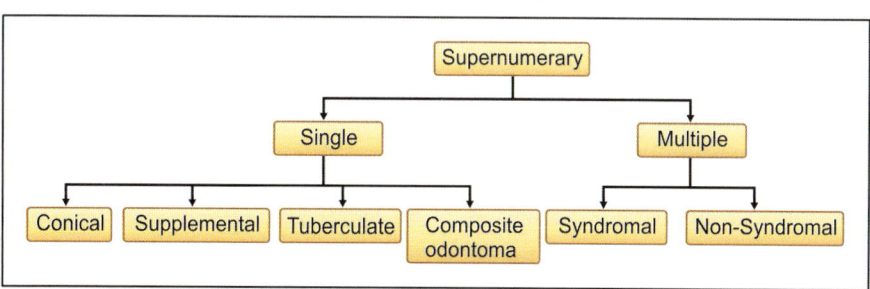

Table 8.1: A comparison of the different types of supernumerary teeth

	Conical	Tuberculate	Supplemental	Odontomes
Occurrence	75%	12%	7%	6%
Shape	• Conical shape called mesiodens • Complete roots	Barrel-shaped, consists of multiple tubercles	Resemble normal teeth	Irregular mass or denticles
Site	• Anterior maxilla • Usually solitary • Usually paired	• Anterior maxilla	• Commonly the upper lateral incisors • Lower premolars	• Anterior maxilla • Posterior mandible
Features	• Commonly unerupted • May be inverted or may erupt	Impede incisor eruption	May erupt	• Remain unerupted • Can impede eruption

- Displacement or rotation of adjacent teeth
- Root resorption of neighboring teeth.
- Cystic change within the follicle of the supernumerary tooth and/or migration into adjacent structures.
- *Prevention of tooth movement:* The presence of a supernumerary tooth may prevent orthodontic movement of adjacent teeth, be a rare cause of incomplete space closure or damage the roots of colliding teeth.

A number of conditions may be associated with the presence of supernumerary teeth:
- Cleft palate and cleft lip
- Cleidocranial dysplasia
- Gardner's syndrome

Missing Teeth

Anodontia is a genetic or congenital absence of one or several temporary of permanent teeth. The upper lateral incisors are among the teeth that are most often congenitally missing. Several environmental factors like virus infections, toxins and radio or chemotherapy may cause missing of permanent teeth. However, most of the cases are caused by genetic factors.

Besides an unfavorable appearance, patients with missing teeth may suffer from malocclusion, periodontal damage, insufficient alveolar bone growth, reduced chewing ability, inarticulate pronunciation. Treatment might be usually multidisciplinary.

Anomalies of Tooth Shape

Tooth fusion is defined as union between two or more separate developing teeth. The union may be between enamel or enamel and dentin. The terms such as synodontia, connate teeth, joined teeth or double formations are often used to describe fused teeth. Fusion most commonly occurs in the anterior region of primary dentition. It may be seen in unilateral or bilateral region. Usually fusion occurs between two normal teeth and sometimes it is seen between normal tooth and supernumerary tooth.

Fusion can be classified as complete and incomplete type based upon the stage of tooth development. Complete fusion takes place, if the contact occurs before the calcification stage, whereas incomplete fusion takes place at the root level after the formation of crown. The prevalence of fusion in the primary, permanent and supernumerary teeth is 0.5%, 0.1% and 9.1%, respectively.

This developmental anomaly may cause clinical problems including esthetic impairment, pain, caries and tooth crowding. Treatment of fused teeth usually requires multidisciplinary approaches.

Anomalies of tooth shape include true fusion, germination, concrescence, talon cusp and dens in dente. Dilaceration is also an anomaly of the tooth shape in which there is a sharp bend or curve in the root or crown. It generally does not affect orthodontic treatment planning but may complicate the extraction of the affected tooth. In congenital syphilis, Mulberry molars/Moon's molar is noticed which causes irregular occlusal surface of molars that prevents intercuspation of posteriors.

Treatment

Three ways of treating incomplete fusion are as follows:
- Crown width of the fused teeth reduced by selective grinding
- Surgical sectioning followed by restoration of teeth structures to normal size
- Separation and extraction of the anomalous tooth with orthodontic closing of the space and reshaping of the teeth (Fig. 8.3).

Anomalies of Tooth Size

It may occur in two forms: Macrodontia (Fig. 8.4) and microdontia (Fig. 8.5).

The most commonly seen form of localized microdontia involves the maxillary lateral incisors. The tooth is called peg-shaped lateral and the mesial and distal sides converge incisally. The root may be shorter and a more cylindrical than normally seen.

Premature Loss of Deciduous Teeth

Deciduous teeth may be lost prematurely due to dental caries, and trauma. Premature loss of deciduous teeth before their permanent successors cause delaying, preventing and deviating the path of eruption of the succeeding permanent tooth (Figs 8.6 and 8.7).

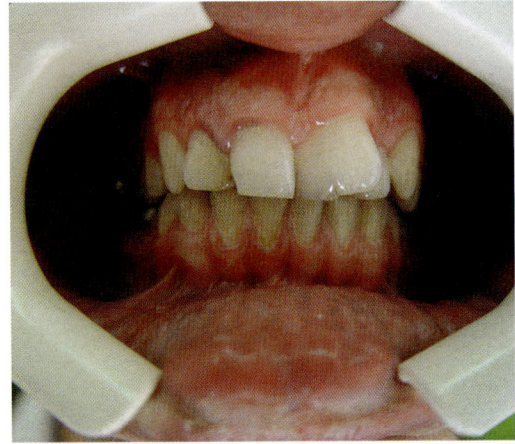

Fig. 8.3: Change in the shape of tooth

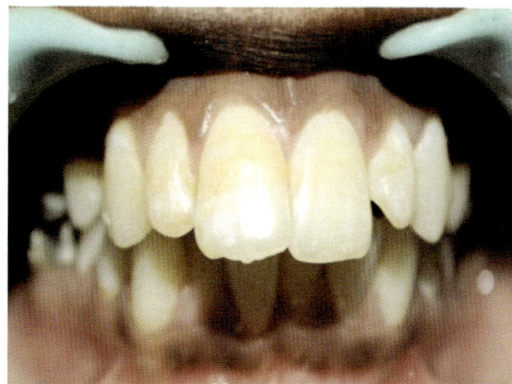

Fig. 8.4: Macrodontia

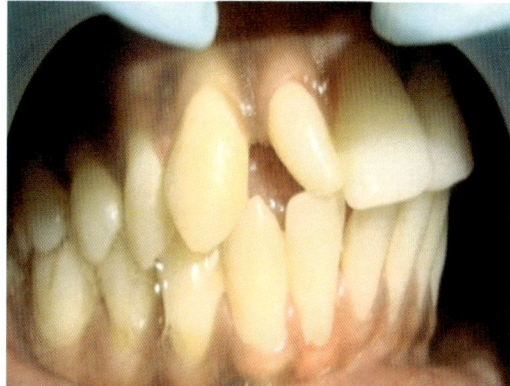

Fig. 8.5a: Ped-shaped lateral—microdontia

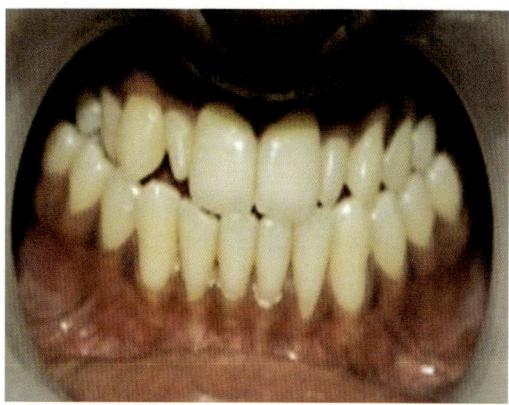

Fig. 8.5b: Bilateral peg-shaped lateral with posterior crossbite

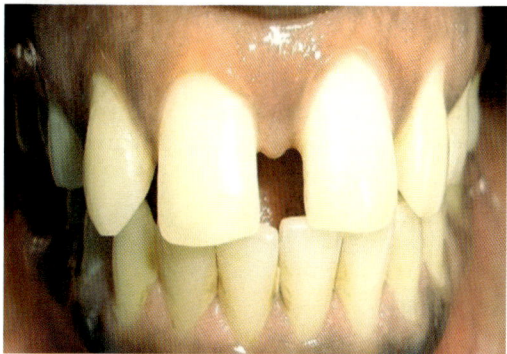

Fig. 8.6a: Congenital missing laterals high

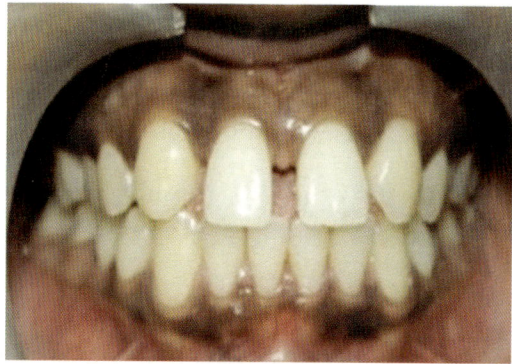

Fig. 8.6b: Congenital missing laterals with frenal attachment

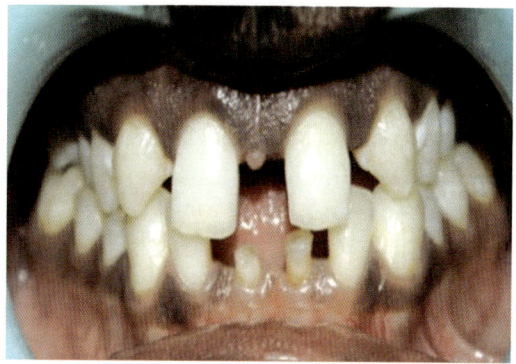

Fig. 8.7: Bilateral congenital missing of laterals with retained deciduous lower teeth

Prolonged Retention of Deciduous (Fig. 8.8)

There are number of causes for prolonged retention of deciduous teeth as listed below:

- Absence of underlying permanent tooth.
- Nonvital deciduous tooth, which fails to resorb
- Ankylosed deciduous tooth that does not resorb
- Endocrinal disturbances, for example hypothyroidism

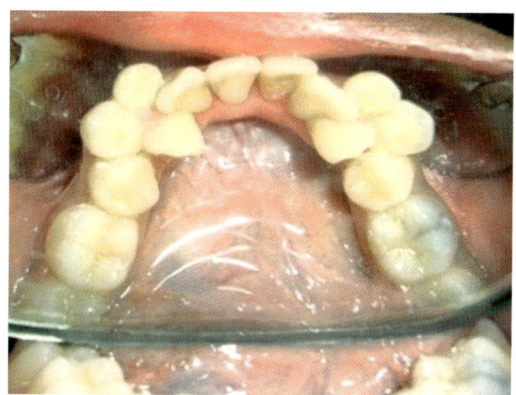

Fig. 8.8: Multiple retained deciduous teeth

Delayed Eruption of Permanent Teeth

Some of the common causes of delayed eruption of permanent teeth are listed below:
- Mesiodens can delay eruption of maxillary central incisors
- Retained deciduous root fragments in the jaw may delay or displace the erupting successor tooth.
- Presence of thick mucosal barrier overlying the erupting permanent teeth.
- Premature loss of deciduous tooth can delay eruption of its successor due to formation of bony barrier
- Ankylosed deciduous tooth that does not resorb can delay eruption of its successor.
- Endocrinal disturbances like hypothyroidism.

Abnormal Eruptive Path

Some of the factors causing delayed eruption of permanent teeth may also deviate their path of eruption.
- Trauma to the tooth during development.
- Presence of supernumerary tooth.
- Prolonged retention of deciduous teeth.
- Retained deciduous root fragments.
- Deficiency of arch length and excess of tooth material.

Maxillary canine often shows an abnormal eruptive pathway possibly due to following factors:
- It has to travel a long distance from its developmental position near the floor of the orbit to its final position in the oral cavity.
- The sequence of its eruption is after the eruption of one or both of the maxillary premolars
- After premature loss of primary canines, the premolars may migrate mesially depriving the canine of its erupting space.

Abnormal eruptive path of one or more teeth can cause:
- Crowding in the arch
- Crossbite when more anterior erupt palatally.

Ankylosis

The tooth is said to be ankylosed when a part or whole of its root surface is directly used to the bone without intervening periodontal ligament. The term submerged teeth often refers to the ankylosed deciduous teeth. Deciduous second molars are most commonly affected.

Ankylosed deciduous teeth prevent their natural exfoliation and replacement by their successional permanent teeth. Once the adjacent permanent teeth erupt to their normal level, the ankylosed tooth appears to be submerged below the level of occlusion. This occlusion is created due to:
- Continued growth of alveolar process in relation to adjacent permanent teeth.

- Smaller crown height of deciduous tooth when compared to that of adjacent permanent teeth.

The antagonistic tooth may supraerupt leading to malocclusion.

Dental Caries

Dental caries is one of the most common local causes of malocclusions. Proximal caries cause the following effects:
- Proximal caries can cause drifting of adjacent teeth into space created with resultant loss of arch length.
- Premature loss of affected tooth leads to abnormal inclination of adjacent teeth.
- Over eruption of opposing tooth.

Improper Restoration

Improper restoration of proximal contours may result in an increased arch length and occlusal irregularities.

Overcontoured proximal restorations lead to increase arch length and elongation of restored tooth or adjacent teeth.

Abnormal Labial Frenum

At birth, the labial frenum is attached to the alveolar ridge, with fibers running into the lingual interdental papilla. As the teeth erupt and as alveolar bone is deposited, the frenum attachment migrates superiorly with respect to the alveolar ridge. In some cases, fibers may persist below the maxillary central incisors and in the "V" shaped intermaxillary suture.

Abnormal labial frenum attachment can be diagnosed clinically by blanch test. When upper lip is pulled forward and upward, a blanching of the tissue just lingual to the maxillary central incisors in the region of incisive papilla is observed.

Radiologically, a notch-like radiolucency is seen interdentally between two maxillary centrals near the alveolar crest (Fig. 8.9). Presence of an abnormal labial frenum attachment prevents the approximation of two central incisors leading to spacing between these two teeth called midline diastema (Fig. 8.10).

Dilaceration

Dilacerated tooth often fails to erupt to proper level and can thus interfere with norml occlusion. They may also complicate extraction of teeth and may interfere with tooth movement and alignment (Fig. 8.11).

Dens Evaginatus

A developmental condition appears clinically as an accessory cusp or a globule of enamel on the occlusal

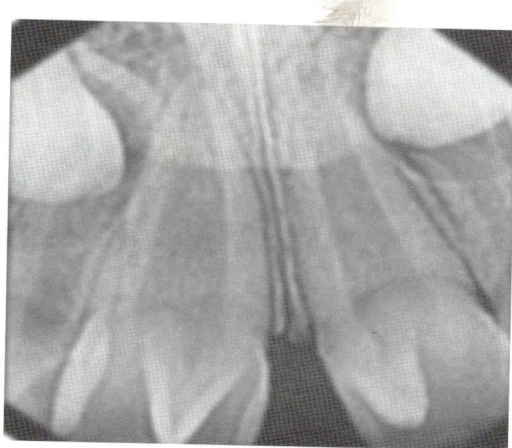

Fig. 8.9: Notch seen

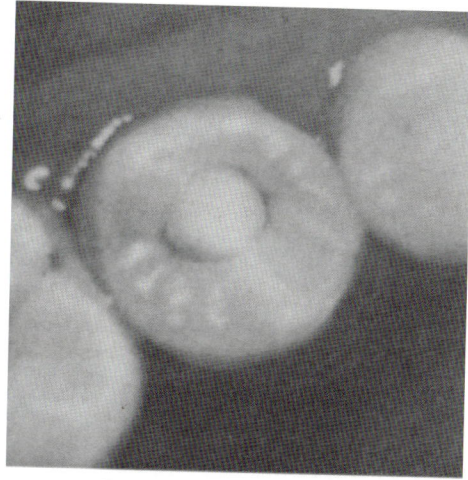

Fig. 8.12: Dens evaginatus

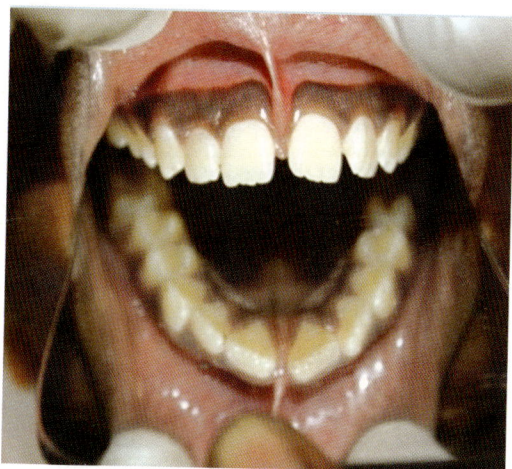

Fig. 8.10: High frenal attachment

surface between the buccal and lingual cusps mainly of premolars. It may result in incomplete eruption, displacement of teeth and may interfere with normal occlusion (Fig. 8.12).

BIBLIOGRAPHY

1. Graber TM. Orthodontic: Principles and Practice. WB Saunders, 1998.
2. Moyers RE. Handbook of orthodontics, 3rd edn. Year book, Chicago; 1973.
3. Tomita NE, Bijella VT, Franco LJ. The relationship between oral habits and malocclusion in preschool children. Rev Saude Publica 2000;34:299–303
4. Khinda V, Grewal N. Relationship of tongue thrust swallowing andanterior open bite with articulation disorders. J Ind Soc of Pedo Prev Dent 1999; 17:33–39.
5. Michael Speidel, Robert J Isaacson, Frank W Worms. Tongue thrust therapy and anterior dental open bite: A review of new facial growth data. Am J Orthod, 1972;62:287–295.
6. M Bhargava, D Chaudhary and S Aggarwal, "Fusion presenting as germination: a rare case report", Journal of Oral and Maxillofacial Pathology, vol. 3, pp. 211–214, 2012.

PREVIOUS YEAR'S UNIVERSITY QUESTIONS

Essay

1. Classify the etiology of malocclusion. Write in detail about the environmental factors causing malocclusion.
2. Write in detail about the general factors.

Short Questions

1. Prenatal cause of malocclusion
2. Supernumerary tooth
3. Delayed eruption
4. Abnormal shape of tooth
5. Congenitally missing tooth

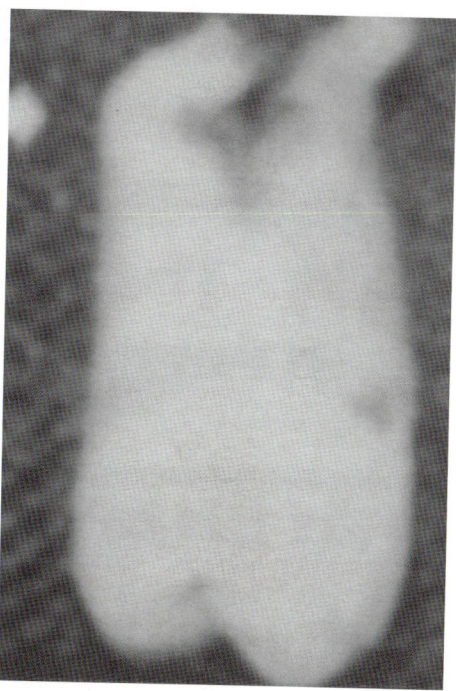

Fig. 8.11: Dilacerated tooth

MCQs

1. *Which is the most common type of supernumerary teeth seen?*
   a. Paramolar
   b. Mesiodens
   c. Both a and b
   d. None of the above   **(Ans: b)**

2. *Most common site of supernumerary teeth is:*
   a. In the midline between two maxillary central incisors
   b. In the midline between two mandibular central incisors
   c. In the midline between two deciduous maxillary central incisors
   d. In the midline between two deciduous mandibular central incisors   **(Ans: a)**

3. *Extra tooth adjacent to molar is called:*
   a. Paramolar
   b. Distomolar
   c. Combination of a and b
   d. None of the above   **(Ans: a)**

4. *Occurrence of congenitally missing teeth may be:*
   a. Single or multiple
   b. Unilateral or bilateral
   c. In maxilla or mandible
   d. All of the above   **(Ans: d)**

5. *True fusion can cause:*
   a. Spacing
   b. Complicate its movement by orthodontic means
   c. Both a and b
   d. None of the above   **(Ans: c)**

6. *Peg-shaped lateral incisor can be:*
   a. Associated with congenital syphilis
   b. Can cause spacing in the arch
   c. Commonly associated with maxillary lateral incisor
   d. All of the above   **(Ans: d)**

7. *Dilacerated tooth:*
   a. Is an anomaly of the tooth
   b. Is a sharp bend or curve in the root of crown
   c. Can complicate the orthodontic treatment
   d. All of the above   **(Ans: d)**

8. *Prenatal trauma:*
   a. Is often associated with hypoplasia of the mandible
   b. Associated with facial asymmetries
   c. Both a and b
   d. None of the above   **(Ans: c)**

Diagnosis and Diagnostic Aids

9.1 CASE HISTORY AND CLINICAL EXAMINATION

Chapter Outline

- Introduction
- Definition
- Essential diagnostic aids
- Supplemental diagnostic aids

- Case history
- Clinical examination
- Functional analysis

INTRODUCTION

Diagnosis in orthodontics requires the collection of an adequate database of information about the patient and the formulations of a problem list from the database. Diagnosis is a Greek word; *Dia*—Apart and *gnosis*—to come to know.

The task of treatment planning is to synthesize the possible solutions to these specific problems into a specific treatment strategy. The process of orthodontic diagnosis and treatment planning is called the problem-oriented approach. In this approach, diagnosis and treatment planning are carried out in a series of logical steps.

DEFINITION

Graber and Rakosi defined orthodontic diagnosis as "The recognition and systemic designation of anomalies, the practical synthesis of the findings, permitting therapy to be planned and indication to be determined".

For orthodontic purposes, the database may be collected from major sources.

- Patient questioning

- Clinical examination of the patient
- Evaluation of diagnostic records including dental casts, radiographs and photographs.
- Since all possible diagnostic records will not be observed.

ESSENTIAL DIAGNOSTIC AIDS

Essential diagnostic aids are considered essential for the diagnosis of an orthodontic case. These include the following:

- Case history
- Clinical examination
- Study models
- Certain radiographs:
    - Periapical radiographs
    - Lateral radiographs
    - Orthopantomograms
    - Bitewing radiographs
- Facial photographs

These diagnostic aids are simple and easy to obtain, except for OPG and lateral cephalograms where a specialized radiographic set up might be required.

SUPPLEMENTAL DIAGNOSTIC AIDS

These diagnostic aids may be required only in certain cases and may require specialized equipment which might not be available in every dental clinic. It includes:

- Specialized radiographs like occlusal views of maxilla and mandible:
  - Selected lateral jaw views
  - Lateral cephalogram
- Electromyographic examination of muscle activity
- Hand-wrist radiographs
- Cone beam computed tomography (CBCT)
- Computed axial tomography (CT scan)
- Magnetic resonance imaging (MRI)
- Endocrine tests and other blood tests
- Estimation of the basal metabolic rate
- Occlusograms

CASE HISTORY

A complete case history includes all the relevant information derived from the patient and the parents and is an essential prerequisite for planning and executing any orthodontic treatment. The case history must include the following data.

Name

- Knowing the patient's name is the important step towards understanding patient's concern and treatment needs.
- It gives a good rapport by calling the patient by his/her name but also imparts confidence in the patient's mind about the clinician.

Age

The patient's chronological age should be recorded for diagnosis, treatment planning as well as the outcome of planned treatment.

Chronologic and dental age is synchronous in the normal patient. A child is labeled as an early or late developer, if there is a difference of ±2 years from the average value. If the chronologic age of the patient is younger than the dental age, one can rely on increased growth to a greater degree than when dental age is retarded in relation to the chronologic age.

Dental age can be determined by two different methods;

1. Stage of eruption.
2. Stage of tooth mineralization on radiograph. This is dealt in development of dentition chapter.

For age determination, one does not rely on the last stage tooth formation but on the entire process of dental mineralization. This renders the estimation of age more accurate.

Sex

The patient's sex should be recorded in the case history. Sex is important in planning treatment as the timing of growth events such as growth spurts is different in males and females. Girls mature earlier than boys. The growth spurts, eruption of teeth and onset of puberty are different in males and females.

Address and Occupation

These are important for communication assessing the socioeconomic status as well as for record purpose. This also helps in future correspondence, if any long-term and short-term study and research purpose.

Chief Complaint

The patient's chief complaint should be recorded in his/her own words. This helps the clinician in identifying the priorities and expectations of the patient.

Family History

Skeletal Class II and Class III malocclusions, generalized congenital conditions such as cleft lip and palate, have genetic predisposition. Thus, it is mandatory to record all the details of malocclusion existing in other members of the family for 3 successive generations

Medical History

A thorough medical history should be taken. Conditions which might affect orthodontic treatment include the following:

1. Rheumatic fever
2. Epilepsy
3. Juvenile diabetics
4. Hemophilia
5. Handicapped children

The orthodontic treatment should be delayed or removable orthodontic appliance should be recommended instead of fixed appliance.

Dental History

The patient's past dental history should include the details of any previous appliance therapy, relapsed occurred, discontinuation of previous orthodontic therapy, etc.

Prenatal History

- The condition of the mother during pregnancy must be recorded. Infections like German measles and

intake of certain drugs like thalidomide may cause congenital deformities in child.
- Type of delivery must also be noted as injury to TMJ by way of forceps delivery may affect mandibular growth of patients leading ankylosis.

Postnatal History

Type, duration of feeding, milestones of normal development and presence of any habits such as thumb sucking, tongue thrusting and lip biting must be recorded.

CLINICAL EXAMINATION

General Examination

It includes general appraisal of the patient which begins as soon as the patient enters the clinic.

Height and weight: Recording of the weight and height aids in assessing the physical growth and maturation of the patient.

Gait: Any abnormality in gait is recorded.

Posture: Abnormal posture of patient may be accentuating the existing malocclusion.

Extraoral Examination

Physique

The physique of an individual may fall into one of three categories in either of the classifications given below.

According to general classification:
- Athletic—average physique with normal sized dental arches.
- Plethoric—short physique with broad dental arches
- Esthetic—thin physique with narrow dental arches

According to Sheldon:
- Mesomorphic—average physique
- Endomorphic—short and obese physique
- Ectomorphic—tall and thin physique

Cephalic and Facial Examination

The shape of head and facial form may give an idea about the dentoalveolar archform of an individual. Martin and Saller in 1957 formulated cephalic and facial indices to evaluate shape of the head and the facial form, respectively.

Shape of Head (Cephalic Index)

$$\text{Cephalic index} = \frac{\text{Maximum skull width}}{\text{Maximum skull length}}$$

Depending on the cephalic index value, the shape of the head may fall into three categories:
- Mesocephalic—normal or average sized head
- Brachycephalic—short and broad
- Dolichocephalic—long and narrow

Facial Form

Facial index value = Morphologic facial height (distance between nasion and gnathion)/bizygomatic width (distance between the zygomatic points).

Depending on facial index values obtained, facial form of an individual may be categorized into one of the following types:
- Mesoprosopic—average facial form
- Euryprosopic—short and broad facial form
- Leptoprosopic—long and narrow facial form

Assessment of Facial Asymmetry

Gross asymmetry of the face may occur in the following conditions:
- Hemifacial hypertrophy
- Hemifacial atrophy
- First arch syndrome
- Congenital defects such as cleft lip and palate
- Unilateral condylar hyperplasia
- Unilateral ankylosis
- Facial palsy

The symmetry of the face can be assessed by drawing an imaginary line connecting from trachion, glabella, the tip of the nose and the chin as reference line. There are three parameters with which the asymmetry can be assessed.
- *Intercanthus line:* The intercanthus lines of right and left eyes coincide with alar of the nose.
- *Interpupillary lines:* They join with commissure of the oral cavity
- Interzygomatic distances

The distance between the midline of the face and intercanthus and interpupillary lines of both right and left side of the face should be equal. The distance is reduced in affected sides.

Facial Profile

The profile is examined from the side by making the patient view at a distant object, with FH plane parallel to the floor. Clinically, the profile can be obtained by joining two reference lines:
- Line joining forehead and soft tissue point A
- Line joining point and soft tissue pogonion: Three types of profiles are seen (Fig. 9.1):
  - *Straight/orthognathic profile:* The two lines form an almost straight line.

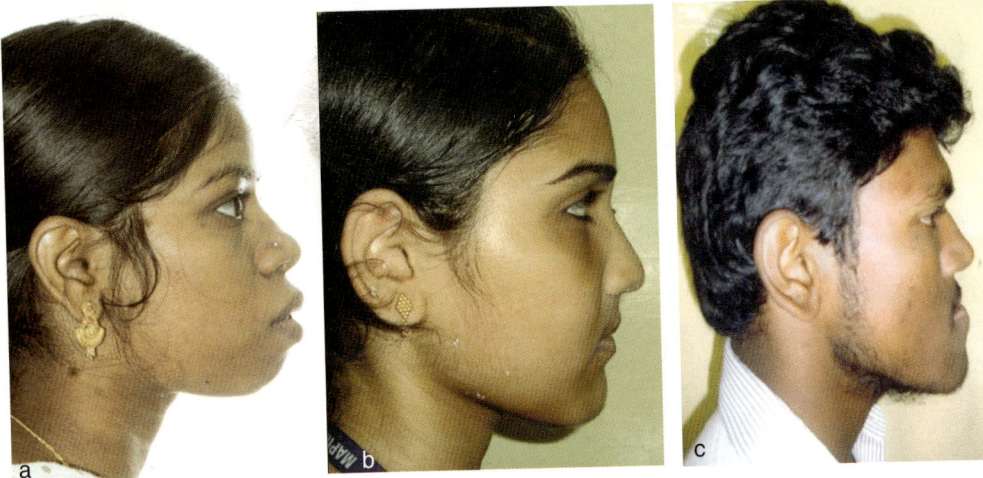

Fig. 9.1: (a) Convex profile; (b) Straight profile; (c) Concave profile

– *Convex profile:* The two lines form an acute angle with concavity facing the tissues. This type of profile is seen in Class II division 1 patients due to either a protruded maxilla or a retruded mandible.

– *Concave profile:* The two lines form an obtuse angle with the convexity facing the tissues. This type of profile is seen in class III patients due to either a protruded mandible or a retruded maxilla.

Facial Divergence

It is defined as an anterior or posterior inclination of the lower face or chin point relation to the forehead. The facial divergence can be evaluated clinically or on photographs. The divergence was described by Milo Hellmano.

Method

A line is drawn from the forehead to the chin to determine whether the face is:

- *Straight or orthognathic:* The line between the forehead and chin is straight or perpendicular to the floor.
- *Anterior divergent:* A line drawn between the forehead and the chin is inclined anteriorly towards the chin.
- *Posterior divergent:* A line drawn between the forehead and chin slants posteriorly towards the chin.

An imaginary line is drawn vertically downwards tangent to the forehead preferably through nasion.

- If the chin is ahead of this line, it is called anterior divergent.
- If the chin is far behind this line, it is called posterior divergent.
- If the chin is in line +2 mm with this line, it is called orthognathic.

Assessment of Anteroposterior Jaw Relationship

Two-Finger Method by Mill

This can be assessed by placing the index finger at point A (deepest point in curvature of upper lip) of maxilla and middle finger at point B (deepest point in curvature of lower lip) of the mandible (Fig. 9.2).

Inference

- If the index finger is 2 to 3 mm ahead of mandibular skeletal base, it indicates Class II skeletal base pattern.
- If the middle finger is ahead of the index finger, it indicates Class III skeletal base pattern.

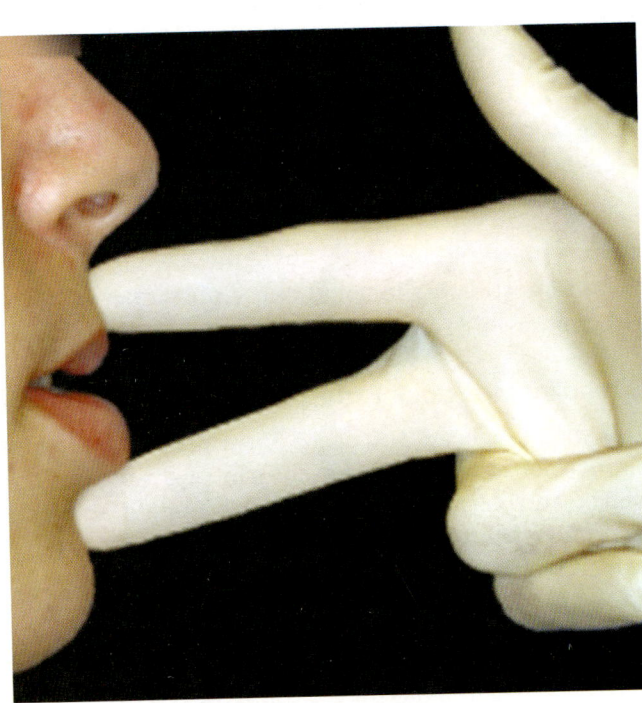

Fig. 9.2: Two-finger method

Assessment of Vertical Skeletal Relationship

- This can be done by assessing either of the relationship between upper facial height (UFH) and lower facial height (LFH).
- Upper facial height (UFH) is the distance between the glabella and subnasale.
- Lower facial height (LFH) is the distance between subnasale to the gonion.

In normal vertical relationship, the ratio of LFH: UFH is 55:45. In other words, LFH is almost equal to the upper facial height.

Reduced lower facial height is associated with deep bite while the increased lower facial height is seen in anterior open bite.

Clinical Frankfort Mandibular Plane Angle (FMA)

The vertical skeletal relationship can also be assessed by studying the angle FMA. It is an angle formed between the mandibular plane and the Frankfort horizontal plane. The normal range of this angle is measured cephalometrically ranging from 17° to 32° with an average of 25°.

This angle can be assessed clinically also.

- In normal growth pattern, two planes meet beyond the occipital region indicating horizontal growth pattern.
- In high angle, the two planes meet anterior to the occipital region indicating vertical grower.

The examination of profile divergence, vertical facial proportions, lip posture, incisor protrusion and clinical FMA constitute the facial profile analysis. It is also called "Poor man's cephalometric analysis".

Evaluation of Facial Proportions

The face can be divided into one-third by using 4 horizontal planes passing at the level of hairline, the supraorbital ridge, the base of the nose and inferior border of chin. A well-proportioned face has all the three vertical thirds in equal proportion.

For a face to be harmonious, the height of the forehead (distance from hairline to glabella), the height of mid-third (glabella to subnasale) and lower third (subnasale to mental) should be proportionate and equal (Fig. 9.3).

Forehead

The profile is influenced by the shape of the forehead and the nose which determines the esthetic prognosis of the orthodontic case.

In the frontal view, the forehead is considered in its relationship to the bizygomatic width to describe it as narrow or wide. The lateral forehead contour can be flat, protruding or oblique. In case with a steep forehead, the dental bases are more prognathic than in cases with a flat forehead.

Nose

The size, shape and position of the nose determine the esthetic appearance of the face. Besides the contour of the bridge and the tip of the nose, size and the shape and width of the nostrils as well as the position of the nasal septum should be assessed. These findings can indicate impairment of nasal breathing. If the nasal profile is not improved by orthodontic procedures, the rhinoplasty may be necessary.

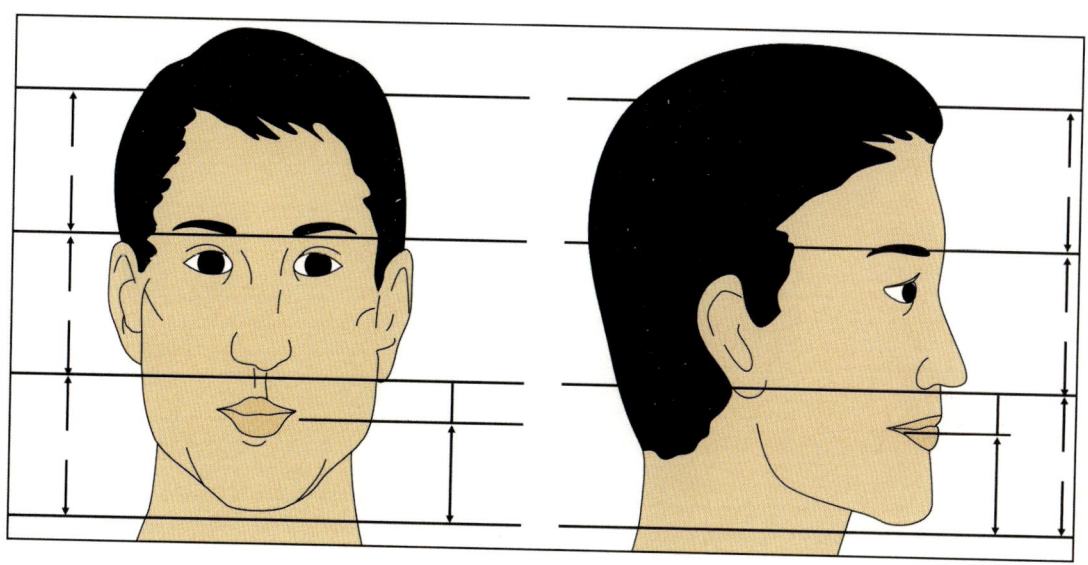

Fig. 9.3: Vertical facial proportion

Size of nose: The vertical nasal length measures one-third of total face height (distance from hairline to gnathion).

Nostrils: The width of the nostrils (ala base) is approximately 70% of the length of nose (distance from nasion to tip of nose).

Nasolabial angle: It is the angle formed at tangent to the base of the nose and a tangent to upper lip (Fig. 9.4).
- Normal angulation is 110°.
- Increased NLA shows the retrusive position of upper lip to nose. There is retroclination of upper incisors (Fig. 9.5).
- Decreased NLA with proclination of upper incisors (Fig. 9.5).

Lips

The configuration of the lips can be assessed by the following criteria: Lip length, width and curvature.

Length of upper lip: In balanced situation, the length of the upper lip measures one-third, the lower lip and the chin two-thirds of lower face height. In addition, the length of the upper lip should be assessed in relation to the position of upper incisal edges.

Lip protrusion: It is influenced by the thickness of the soft tissues, the tone of the orbicularis oris muscle, the position of the anterior and the configuration of underlying bony structures.

Lip step according to Korkhaus (Fig. 9.6)
- Protrusion of lower lip in relation to upper lip indicative of Class III malocclusion.
- Normal lip profile—upper lip protrudes slightly in relation to lower lip.

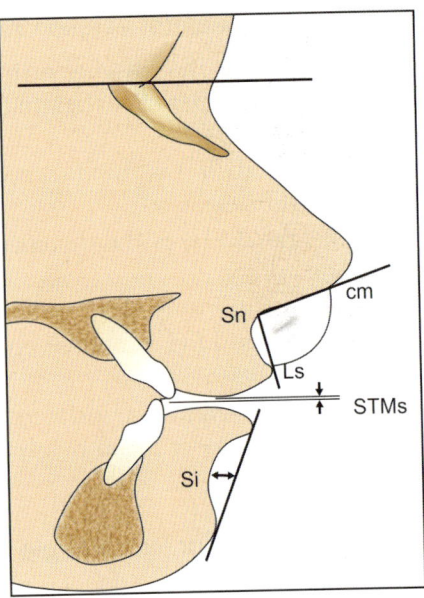

Fig. 9.4: Nasolabial angle

- Marked retrusion of the lower lip indicative of Class II malocclusion.

Lip seal

Anterior seal: The approximation of upper and lower lips when all the muscles of mastication are in relaxed condition and the teeth are in centric occlusion. This is called competency of the lips.

Middle oral seal: This seal is formed between the dorsum of the tongue and the vault of the palate.

Posterior oral seal: It is formed between soft palate and the root of the tongue.

If the anterior lip seal is broken, then it is called incompetency of the lips. In case of incompetent lips, the interlabial distance exceeds 4 mm at rest.

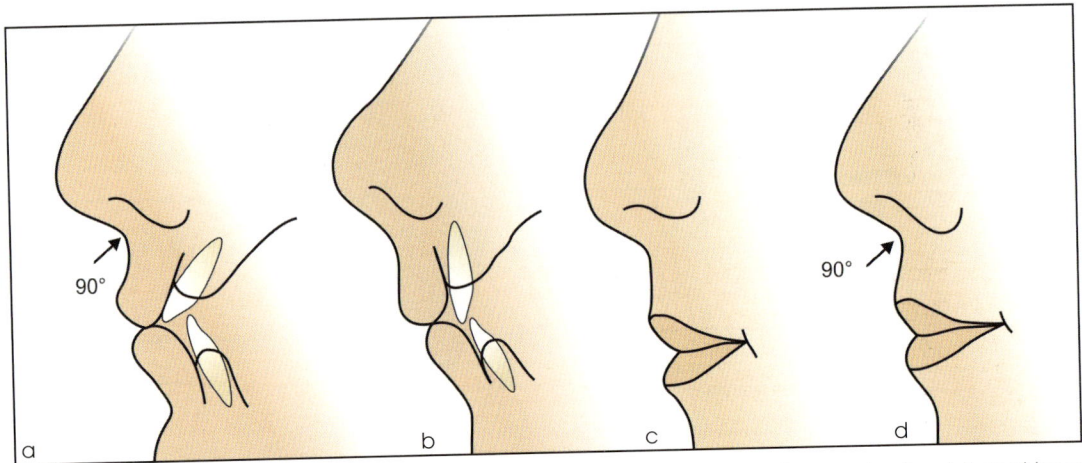

Fig. 9.5: (a) When the teeth are proclined, nasolabial angle is 90° or less; (b) When the teeth are retroclined, it must be more than 90°; (c) When the columella is prominent and the ala is high, it must be more than 90°; (d) When the columella is prominent and the ala is at the same level, it must be 90°

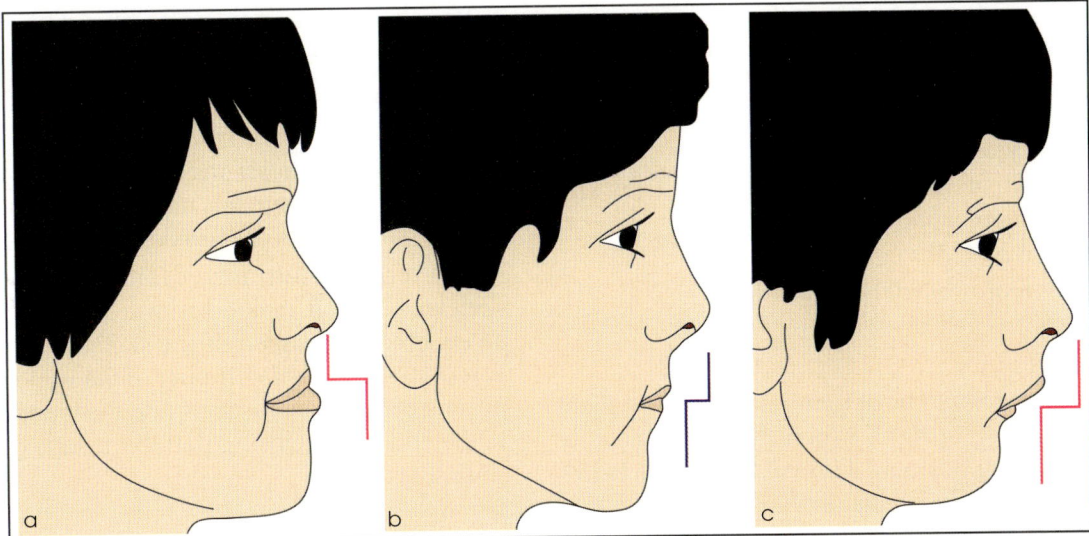

Fig. 9.6: (a) Positive lip step; (b) Slightly negative lip step (normal cases); (c) Marked negative lip step

Incompetent lips are morphologically short lips which do not form a lip seal in relaxed state. Lip seal is achieved only by active contraction of orbicularis oris and circumoral muscles in cases of short upper lip.

The lips are normally developed but the patient is unable to approximate the lips at rest due to upper incisors proclination.

Lip trap: In severe Class II division 1 cases, the lower lip tugs behind the upper incisors and prevents proper lip seal.

Based on the lip seal, the lips are classified into:
- Competent (Fig. 9.7)
- Incompetent (Fig. 9.7)
- Potentially incompetent

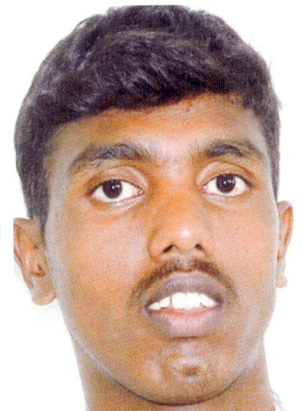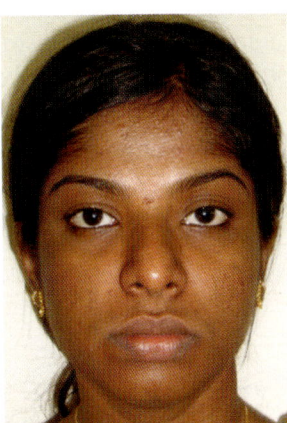

Fig. 9.7: (a) Incompetent lips; (b) Competent lips

Powell's Aesthetic Triangle

This triangle analyzes in a simple way: Forehead, nose, lips, chin and neck using interrelated angles.

Nasal Evaluation

Different methods of evaluation are:
- Baum's method
- Goode's method
- Simon's method
- Changes in nose projection may be assessed on the basis of Powell's triangle. It is always appropriate to cross-check them by means of methods that evaluate the nose length: Base ratio (Baum's and Goode's methods) and nose projection and the upper lip length (Simon's method).

Baum's method: A vertical line is drawn from nasion to subnasale and horizontal line is drawn perpendicular to the vertical line and goes through the tip of the nose. The ratio between both lines 2:1.

Goode's method: The vertical line is drawn from the point where the nasion crosses the alar canal. The dorsum is measured from nasion to tip. The ratio between ala–tip and nasion–tip is 0.55 to 0.60.

Simon's method: It establishes a 1:1 ratio the nose between the length of the upper lip and the base of the nose. The upper lip is measured from subnasale to the mucocutaneous edge of the upper lip (upper vermillion), while the base of the nose is measured from subnasale to the tip of the nose. However, this method has one limitation as the different lip lengths prevent any adjustments of nose projection.

FUNCTIONAL ANALYSIS

Functional analysis constitutes a considerable part of the clinical examination. It is not only significant for the etiologic evaluation of the malocclusion but also for determining the type of orthodontic treatment indicated.

The three most important aspects of orthodontic functional analysis are:
- Examination of the postural rest position and maximum intercuspation.
- Examination of TMJ
- Examination of orofacial dysfunctions

Rest Position

The rest position should be determined with the patient relaxed and sitting upright. When the mandible is in the postural resting position, it is usually 2–3 mm below and behind the centric occlusion.

The space between the teeth, when the mandible is at rest, is referred to as the freeway space or inter-occlusal clearance. Several methods can be used to determine the rest position during clinical examination:
- Phonetic method
- Command method
- Non-command method
- Combined method

Phonetic method: The patient is told to pronounce certain consonants or words repetitively (M or Mississippi). The mandible returns to the postural resting position 1–2 seconds after the exercise.

Command method: The patient is commanded to perform selected functions (e.g. swallowing) after which the mandible spontaneously returns to the rest position.

Non-command method: The patient is distracted (the clinician talks to the patient) so as not to perceive which type of examination is being carried out. While being distracted, the patient relaxes, causing the musculature to relax as well and the mandible reverts to the postural rest position.

Combined methods: These methods of determining the rest position are the most suitable for functional analysis in children. The patient is first observed during swallowing and speaking. The patient is then distracted, similarly to when using the non-command method.

Class III Malocclusion

The functional relationships of Class III cases determine the orthodontic treatment possibilities and the prognosis of the malocclusions. The closing path of the mandible from the rest position can be divided into three types.

- Rotational movement without sliding action
- Rotational movement with anterior sliding action.
- Rotational movement with posterior sliding action

With this functional analysis, the true forced bite with its favorable prognosis and the pseudo forced bite with its unfavorable prognosis must be differentiated as far as cepholometric is concerned.

The term pseudo forced bite includes those true skeletal Class III malocclusions due to partial dento-alveolar compensation of the skeletal dysplasia in the anterior region (labial tipping of the upper and lingual tipping of the lower incisors) and the mandible occludes at the end of the closing path by means of an anterior sliding action.

Evaluation of the Relationship between Rest Position and Habitual Occlusion in the Vertical Plane

This analysis is of particular importance to cases with a deep overbite. This is divided into two types:
1. *True deep overbite:* The true deep overbite with a large freeway space is caused by infraocclusion of the molars. The prognosis for successful therapy with functional methods is favorable. As the interocclusal clearance is large, sufficient freeway space will remain after extrusion of the molars.
2. *Pseudo deep overbite:* It has a small freeway space. The molars have erupted fully. The deep overbite is caused by overeruption of the incisors. The prognosis for elevating the bite using functional appliances is unfavorable. If the freeway space is small, extrusion of the molars adversely affects the rest position and may create TMJ problems or cause a relapse of the deep overbite.

Evaluation of the Relationship between Rest Position and Habitual Occlusion in the Transverse Plane

The position of the mandible is observed while the jaw is moved from the postural rest to habitual occlusion. This analysis is particularly relevant for the differential diagnosis of cases with unilateral crossbite. Depending on the functional analysis, two types of skeletal mandibular deviation can be differentiated:
1. *Laterognathy:* The center of the mandible is not aligned with the facial midline in rest and in occlusion. This dysplasia constitutes anatomical asymmetry. A lateral crossbite with laterognathy is termed true crossbite. The prognosis is unfavorable.
2. *Laterocclusion:* The skeletal midline shift of the mandible can be observed only in occlusal position; in postural rest, both midlines are well aligned. The deviation is due to tooth guidance.

Methods of Tongue Examination

Various methods can be used to examine tongue dysfunctions. The different types of clinical examination are:

- Electronic recordings
- Electromyographic examination
- Roentgenocephalometric analysis
- Cineradiographic
- Palatographic
- Neurophysiologic examination

The position and size of the tongue in relation to the available space can be assessed using roentgenographic cephalometrics. However, in most cases, registering the position of the tongue is more important than determining its size.

Mouth Breathing

The mode of respiration is examined to establish whether the nasal breathing is impeded or not. Chronically disturbed nasal respiration represents a dysfunction of the orofacial musculature. It can restrict development of the dentition and hinders the orthodontic treatment. The following are the clinical findings:

- High palate
- Narrowness of the arch
- Crossbite
- Poor oral hygiene
- Hyperplasia of the gingiva
- Adenoid facies

Tongue Posture in Oronasal Respiration

- *Type-1:* The tongue is flat and its tip is behind the lower incisors. This type is often encountered in conjunction with an anterior crossbite.
- *Type-2:* The tongue is flat and retracted. This type of abnormal tongue posture is common in cases with oral respiration and distocclusion.

Various clinical methods of examination in oronasal obstruction are:

- Mirror test
- Cotton pledge test
- Observation of nostrils

Differential diagnosis: It must be used to determine whether the problems in nasal respiration are due to an obstruction of the upper nasal passages or to habitual oral respiration. In the first case, an operation by an ENT specialist is indicated, i.e. in the case of allergic rhinopathy, medication should be applied. Otherwise, pre-orthodontic therapy should be carried out to treat the restricted nasal breathing. This may include breathing exercises or incorporation of a perforated oral screen.

The Smile

During clinical examination, it is important to differentiate between the two primary smile types—the social smile and the enjoyment smile.

The smile is a voluntary smile developed by the patient in posing for photographs or social settings. The enjoyment smile is an involuntary smile and represents the emotion (e.g. laughing).

In assessing smile dynamics, the social smile in most cases represents a repeatable smile. It is important that the maturation of the social smile occurs at different ages; therefore, the social smile in preadolescent patients may not be consistent over time. The range of variation in lip–teeth–gingiva relationships during the social and enjoyment smiles should be assessed in the clinical examination.

Smile Style

Three styles of the dynamic social smile are:

- The commissure smile
- The canine smile
- The complex smile

In the commissure smile, the corners of the mouth turn upward, followed by elevation of the upper lip due to the pull of the zygomaticus major muscles.

In the canine smile, the upper lip is elevated uniformly without the corners of the mouth turning upward.

In the complex smile, the upper lip moves superiorly as in the canine smile but the lower lip also moves inferiorly in similar fashion.

Vertical Smile Traits

The gingival margins of the maxillary anterior teeth should be coincident with the upper lip in the social smile. However, this is a function of the age of the patient, because children often show more teeth at rest and more gingival display on smile than do adults. These are the following dentofacial traits.

- *Philtrum height:* The philtrum height is measured in millimeters from the base of the nose at the midline to the most inferior portion of the upper lip on the vermilion. The linear measurement of this trait is not as important as its relationship to maxillary incisor display and the height of the commissures of the mouth. In the adolescent, it is common to find the philtrum height less than the commissure height.

- *Commissure height:* The commissure height is measured vertically from a line constructed at the alar base of the nose to a parallel line passing through the commissures.
- *Interlabial gap:* The interlabial gap is the distance in millimeters between the upper and lower lips at rest or during smile.
- *Amount of incisor shown at rest:* The amount of maxillary incisor shown at rest is an age-dependent dentofacial trait. One of the characteristics of aging is diminished maxillary incisor shown at rest and during smile.
- *Amount of incisor display on smile:* When smiling, patients will either show their entire maxillary incisors or part of those incisors. Measurement of part of incisor diplay, when combined with the crown height measured next, aids the orthodontist's decision as to how much vertical tooth movement is required to attain the appropriate tooth display for the patient.
- *Crown height:* The vertical height of the maxillary central incisors in the adult is measured in millimeters and is normally between 9 and 12 mm, with an average of 10.6 mm in males and 9.6 mm in females. The patient's age is a factor in measuring crown height because of the apical migration of the gingival tissues seen in adolescence.
- *Gingival display:* A mildly gummy smile is often judged more pleasing than a smile with insufficient tooth display. The following are possible etiologies contributing to excessive gingival display during smile:
  1. Vertical maxillary excess
  2. Short philtrum
  3. Excessive upper lip animation
  4. Short clinical crown height
- *Smile arc:* The smile arc is defined as the relationship of the curvature of the incisal edges of the maxillary teeth to the curvature of the lower lip in the social smile. The constant smile arc exhibits the maxillary incisal edge curvature parallel to the curvature of lower lip on smile. A flat or reverse smile arc is characterized by the maxillary incisal curvature being flatter or concave relative to the curvature of the lower lip on smile.

Transverse Smile Traits

Three interrelated factors affecting the appearance of transverse smile traits are arch form, buccal corridor and the transverse cant of maxillary occlusal plane.

Arch form: In patients in whom the arch forms are narrow or collapsed, the smile may appear narrow and present inadequate tooth display transversely. Orthodontic expansion and widening of a collapsed arch form can dramatically improve facial appearance and smile by increasing tooth mass projected laterally in the buccal corridors. Although a transverse increase in the dental arch may fill the buccal corridors, two undesirable side effects may result.

First, full obliteration of the buccal corridor will create a denture-like smile.

Second, when the anterior sweep of the maxillary arch is broadened, the smile arc is often flattened.

Anteroposterior Smile Traits

In clinical examination, it is important to visualize the maxilla relative to the lower lip. The maxilla may be canted anteroposteriorly in a number of orientations. Deviations in maxillary orientation include a downward cant of the posterior maxilla, upward cant of the anterior maxilla or variations of both.

The anteroposterior dental traits that affect the smile are overjet and incisor angulation.

OTHER DIAGNOSTIC AIDS

- Lip prints and skeletal malocclusion
- Dermatoglyphics and skeletal malocclusion

Lip Print and Skeletal Malocclusion

In orthodontics, apart from essential diagnostic aids, there are so many soft tissue analyses in which lips are major part of concern. Recently, the lip prints can be used as evidence in personal identification and criminal investigation in forensic dentistry. The relationship between the skeletal malocclusions and lip prints has been an area of vast research in contemporary orthodontics.

Lip prints are normal lines and fissures in the form of wrinkles and grooves present in the zone of transition of human lip between inner labial mucosa and outer skin. The study of lip prints is referred to as cheiloscopy.

Lip prints are unique to an individual just like the fingerprints and shows strong heredity pattern.

There are different methods of recording lip prints like lipstick-paper-cardboard method, photography, lipstick-paper method, lipstick cellophane method or using dental impression materials to make three-dimensional casts of the lips. The most commonly used lipstick-cellophane technique (Fig. 9.8).

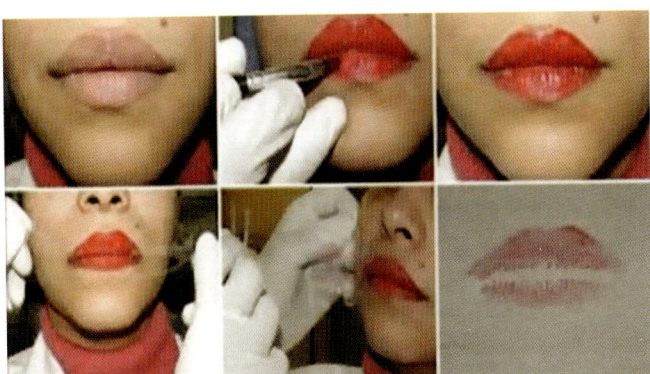

Fig. 9.8: Lipstick-cellophane tape technique

Classification of Lip Print Patterns as Proposed by Tsuchihashi (Fig. 9.9)

Type-I: Clear cut vertical grooves that run across the entire lips.

Type-I': Straight grooves that disappear half way into lip instead of covering the entire breadth of the lip or partial length groove of type I.

Type II: Branched grooves (Branching Y shaped pattern)

Type III: Intersected grooves (criss-cross pattern, transverse grooves)

Type IV: Reticular grooves

Type V: Undetermined (grooves do not fall into any of the type I–IV and cannot be differentiated morphologically).

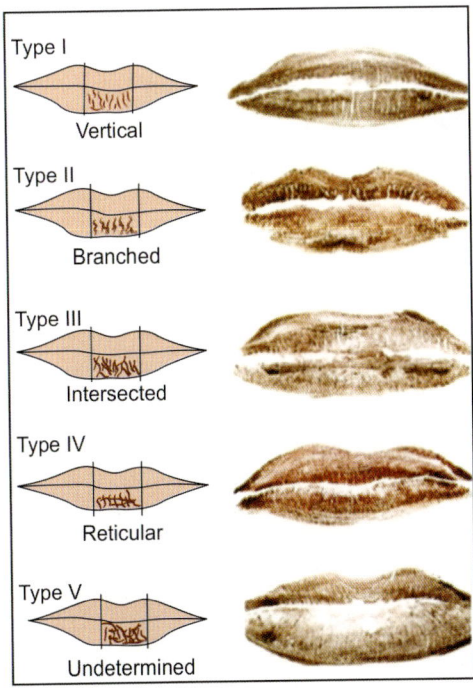

Fig. 9.9: Lip print pattern

For classification, the middle part of the lower lip (10 mm wide) is taken as study area. The lip print pattern is determined by counting highest number of lines in this area.

Research reveals that a significant correlation is found between vertical lip pattern and skeletal Class III malocclusion. If lip print records are available, then dental profiling could be done by skeletal malocclusion only and help in determining possible identity of the victim (Fig. 9.10).

Dermatoglyphics and Skeletal Malocclusion

Dermatoglyphics is derived from the Greek word '*Derma*' meaning skin and '*Glyphic*' meaning carvings.

Embryogenesis

The development of dermatoglyphic patterns begins with the appearance of fetal pads in the 6th week of gestation and ends with the appearance of finished patterns on the surface of the skin in the 24th week of gestation. From this stage onwards, they are unaffected by the environment, and this explains their unique role as an ideal marker for individual identification and the study of populations, as well as detection of defects due to intrauterine irregularities in the early weeks of pregnancy.

Significance of left and right hands: The left hand is the one we are born with, and right is what we have made of it. The future is shown in the right, the past in the left. The left hand is controlled by the right brain (pattern recognition, relationship understanding) reflects the inner person, the natural self, the anima and the lateral thinking. It could be even considered to be a part of person spiritual and personal development. It is the "yin" of personality (feminine and receptive).

The right hand is controlled by the left brain (logic, reason, and language), reflects the outer person, objective self, influence of social environment, education and experience. It represents linear thinking. It also corresponds to the "yang" aspect of personality (masculine and outgoing).

Advantages of Dermatoglyphics

The major advantages of the dermatoglyphics are:
1. The epidermal ridge of the palms fingers are fully developed at birth and thereafter remain unchanged for life.
2. Scanning of recording of their permanent impressions (i.e. prints) can be accomplished rapidly, inexpensively and without causing any trauma to the patient. The scanning and recording is better in children as they are fine in them.

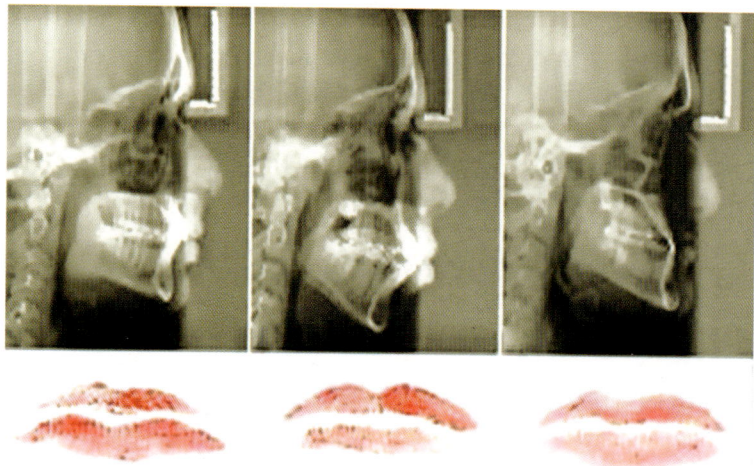

Fig. 9.10: Lip prints of subjects having different skeletal malocclusion. **Note:** Intersected (transverse) lip pattern in skeletal Class I, branched lip pattern in skeletal Class II and Vertical lip pattern in skeletal Class III malocclusion

Anatomy of the fingerprints: A fingerprint is an individual characteristic, and has yet been found to possess identical ridge characteristics. It is raised ridges of skin on the hairless surfaces of hands and feet (dermal ridges). Also found on palms and soles of the feet.

Fingerprints are a reproduction of friction skin ridges found on the palms of the fingers and thumbs. It is designed for firmer grasp and resistance to slippage. It is the shape and form of skin ridges seen as black times of an inked fingerprint.

Dermatoglyphic Patterns

Dermatoglyphic patterns are studied by rolling complete palm and fingerprints of both hands on a smooth white paper by ink and roller method as suggested by Cummins and Midlo. The palm and fingerprints of the individuals are studied under the following headings:

1. Type of pattern on the fingers of both right and left hands (Fig. 9.11)
2. Total finger ridge count (TFRC)
3. A-t-d angle of each hand (Fig. 9.12)
4. T-a-b angle of each hand
5. A-b ridge count of each hand
6. Presence or absence of patterns in hypothenar area, thenar or first interdigital area and i2, i3 and i4 interdigital areas.

When compared with normal occlusion, Class I and Class II malocclusions are associated with an increased frequency of whorls at the expense of ulnar loops and Class II division 1 malocclusions are associated with an increased frequency of ulnar loops at expense of whorls. Both Class I and Class II division 1 malocclusions are associated with an increased frequency of radial loops and arches. While the arches decrease in Class III

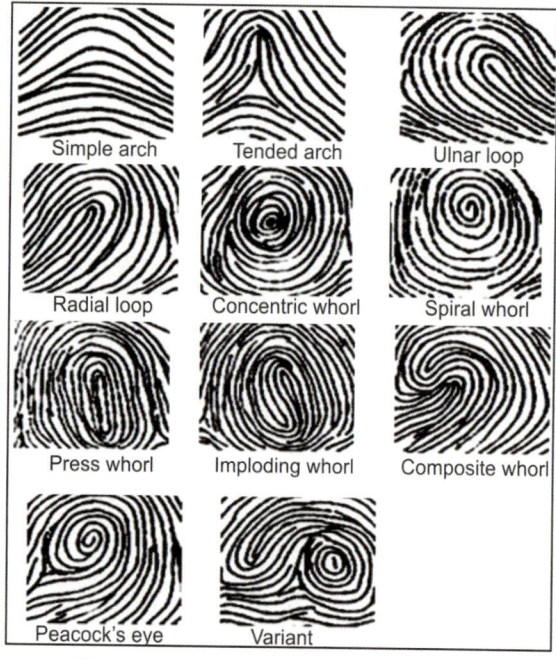

Fig. 9.11: Different types of finger pattern

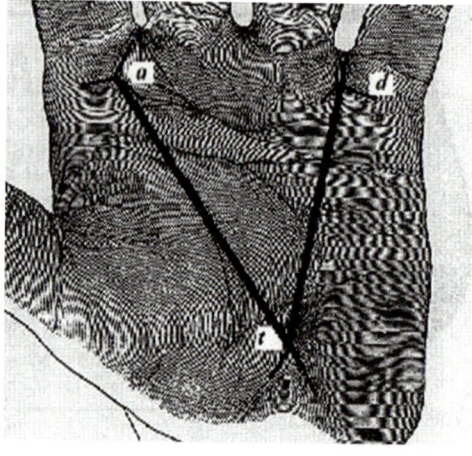

Fig. 9.12: A-t-d angle

malocclusions, the radial loops remain the same (Fig. 9.11).

There is an increased frequency of patterns in the hypothenar area in all the malocclusion groups as compared to normal occlusion.

BIBLIOGRAPHY

1. Graber TM. Diagnosis and panoramic radiography. Am J Orthod 1967;53:799–821.
2. Graber TM. Orthodontics: Principles and Practice, 3rd edition, WB Saunders; 1988.
3. Moorees CFA, Gron Am. Principles of orthodontic diagnosis. Angle Orthod. 1966;36:258–62.
4. Moyers RE. Handbook of orthodontics, 3rd edn. Year book, Chicago; 1973.

PREVIOUS YEAR'S UNIVERSITY QUESTIONS

Essay

1. Mention about the essential diagnostic aids and write about the role of orthodontic study models to aid in treatment planning.
2. Classify and enumerate the various diagnostic aids in orthodontics. Explain in detail about Carey's analysis.

Short Questions

1. Cephalic index.
2. Poor man's cephalometry
3. Assessment of facial asymmetry
4. Facial divergence
5. Assessment of skeletal pattern
6. Evaluation of facial proportions
7. Nasolabial angle
8. Functional analysis
9. Mouth breaking

MCQs

1. *According to general classification, aesthetic physique refers to:*
   a. Tall and thin physique
   b. Average physique
   c. Short and obese physique
   d. None of the above   **(Ans: a)**

2. *The term plethoric physique refers to:*
   a. Average physique
   b. Tall and thin
   c. Short and obese physique
   d. None of the above   **(Ans: c)**

3. *The term athletic physique refers to:*
   a. Average physique
   b. Tall and thin
   c. Short and obese physique
   d. None of the above   **(Ans: a)**

4. *Who classified the general body built?*
   a. Sheldon
   b. Saller
   c. Martin
   d. None of the above   **(Ans: a)**

5. *Facial divergences refer to:*
   a. Anterior or posterior inclination of the lower face relative to the forehead.
   b. Anterior inclination of the lower face relative to the forehead.
   c. Posterior inclination of the lower face relative to the forehead.
   d. All of the above   **(Ans: d)**

6. *Normal nasolabial angle is:*
   a. 110°
   b. 90–110°
   c. 112°
   d. 113°   **(Ans: b)**

7. *Increased nasolabial angle is seen in:*
   a. Patients with retrognathic maxilla or retroclined maxillary anteriors
   b. Patients with prognathic maxilla
   c. Combination of a and b
   d. None of all   **(Ans: a)**

8. *Decreased nasolabial is seen in:*
   a. Patients with retrognathic maxilla or retroclined maxillary anterior
   b. Patients with prognathic maxilla
   c. Combination of a and b
   d. None of all   **(Ans: b)**

9.2 CEPHALOMETRIC ANALYSIS

Chapter Outline

- Introduction
- Uses and limitations of cephalometry
- Tracing technique
- Cephalometric landmarks and planes
- Steiner's analysis

- Tweed's analysis
- Wits appraisal
- Down's analysis
- Bjork-Jarabak analysis
- Superimposition

INTRODUCTION

Cephalometric is the backbone of orthodontic diagnosis and treatment planning. The term cephalometric is used to describe the analysis and measurements made on the cephalometric radiographs.

DEFINITION

"Cephalometric analysis includes measurements, description and appraisal of the morphological configuration and growth changes in skull by ascertaining the lines, angles and planes between anthropometric landmarks established by physical anthropologists and points selected by orthodontists".

Cephalogram

A cephalogram is a two-dimensional projection of the skull. Types include frontal, lateral and oblique cephalograms.

Cephalostat

It is an instrument for holding the patients head and the X-ray film in a desired relation to each other and to the central ray of the X-ray machine. Cephalostat consists of two ear rods. The functions of ear rods are to prevent the movement of the head in the horizontal plane. The distance between the X-ray source and the mid-sagittal plane of the patient in cephalometric radiograph should be 5 feet (Fig. 9.13).

HISTORY

The beginning of modern cephalometric might be attributed to Van Loon of Holland. He was first to introduce cephalometric to orthodontics when he applied anthropometric procedures in analyzing the facial growth.

In 1931 Broadbent of USA and Hofrath of Germany developed a device or head holder called cephalostat, to standardize cephalometric technique.

USES AND LIMITATIONS OF CEPHALOMETRY

Uses of Cephalometry

- Study of craniofacial growth (comparing to the same individual)
- Diagnosis (comparing to standards)
- Planning orthodontic treatment
- Evaluation of treated cases
- Monitor the changes occurring due to growth
- Cephalometric superimposition
- Research activities

Limitations of Cephalometry

- Radiation hazards
- Image enlargement and distortion
- Equipment limitations
- Patient's education is tough

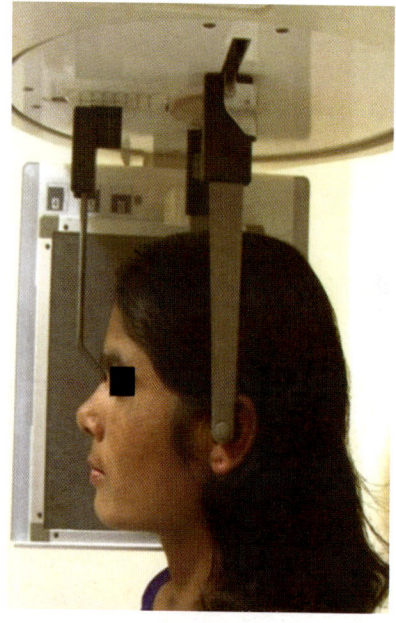

Fig. 9.13: Cephalostat

- It is only two-dimensional data registration of three-dimensional structures
- Technique sensitivity
- Time
- Growth prediction errors

Tracing Supplies and Equipment

- Lateral cephlogram usual dimensions are 8 × 10 inches.
- Acetate matte tracing paper 0.003 inch.
- A sharp 3H pencil or a very fine felt-tipped pen.
- Masking tape
- Protractor and tooth symbol tracing template
- Dental cast
- View box

TRACING TECHNIQUE

Masking tape is used to attach the cephalometric X-ray to the acetate tracing paper sheet. Tracing is done on the frosted surface of the acetate tracing sheet.

It is done by marking the hard tissue and soft tissue points needed for analysis.

Soft tissue profile is traced; sella turcica going forward to plenum sphenoidal along the floor of anterior cranial fossa of the shadows of the greater wing of sphenoid bone are traced.

The anterior part frontal and nasal bones are traced following by the outline of maxilla from ANS to floor of nasal cavity.

The distance between the X-ray source and patient is fixed as 5 feet.

CEPHALOMETRIC LANDMARKS AND PLANES

Cephalometric Landmarks (Fig. 9.14)

Nasion (N): The most anterior point on the frontonasal suture in the mid-sagittal plane.

Sella (Se): Sella is the midpoint of pituitary fossa (sella turcia).

Anterior nasal spine (ANS): The anterior tip of the sharp bony process of the maxilla at the lower margin of the anterior nasal opening.

Posterior nasal spine (PNS): The intersection of a continuation of the anterior wall of the ptrygopalatine fossa and floor of the nose marks the dorsal surface of the maxilla at the level of the nasal floor.

Gonion (Go): A point on the curvature of the angle of the mandible located by bisecting the angle formed by lines tangent to the posterior ramus and inferior border of the mandible.

Gnathion (Gn): A point located by taking the midpoint between the pogonion and menton points on the bony chin.

Menton (Me): The lowest point on the symphyseal shadow of the mandible seen on the lateral cephalogram.

Orbitale (Or): The lowest point on the inferior bony orbit.

Pogonion (Pog): The most anterior point on the chin.

Point A (subspinale): The most posterior midline point in the concavity between the anterior nasal spine and the prosthion.

Point B (supramentale): The most posterior midline point in the concavity of the mandible between the most superior point on the alveolar bone overlying the incisors.

Pterygomaxillary (Ptm): The contour of the pterygo-maxillary fissure formed by the retromolar tuberosity of the maxilla and posteriorly by anterior curve of Spee of the pterygoid process of the sphenoid bone.

Planes and Lines

- Sella-nasion (S-N)—a line connecting S to Na
- Frankfort horizontal (FH)—a line connecting Po to Or
- Mandibular plane (MP)—a line connecting Go to Me
- Y-axis (Y)—a line connecting Se to Pg
- Upper anterior facial height (UAFH)—a line connecting Na to ANS
- Lower anterior facial height (LAFH)—a line connecting ANS to Me
- Nasion-A point (Na-A)—a line connecting Na to A
- Nasion-B point (Na-B)—a line connecting Na to B
- Upper incisor (UI)—a line connecting the incisal edge and the root apex of the most prominent maxillary incisor
- Lower incisor (LI)—a line connecting the incisal edge and the root apex of the most prominent lower incisor

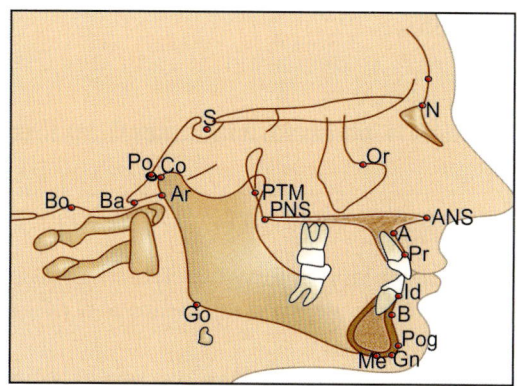

Fig. 9.14: Cephalometric landmarks

STEINER'S ANALYSIS

It is introduced by Cecil C. Steiner in 1953. He proposed a "three-way analysis" including:

- Skeletal
- Dental
- Soft tissue

The reference plane in Steiner's analysis is sella-nasion plane (Fig. 9.15).

Following are the parameters of skeletal analysis:

- SNA angle
- SNB angle
- ANB angle
- Mandibular plane angle
- Occlusal plane angle

SNA angle is formed by SN horizontal plane and NA vertical plane. The SNA angle is noted to determine whether the maxilla is positioned anteriorly or posteriorly to the cranial base (Fig. 9.16)

- Normal value—80°
- SNA >82°—relative forward positioning of the maxilla.
- SNA >82°—relative backward positioning of the maxilla (Fig. 9.17)

SNB Angle

Point B is regarded as the anterior limit of the mandible apical base. It determines whether the mandible is located anterior or posterior to the cranial base (Fig. 9.18). SNB angle is formed by the intersection of SN and NB plane

Mean SNB: 80°

- >80°—indicates prognathic mandible.
- <80°—indicates retrognathic mandible.

ANB Angle (Fig. 9.19)

ANB angle is defined as the mutual relationship in sagittal plane of the maxillary and mandibular bases.

- Normal value is 2°.
- If ANB angle is decreased, it indicates Class III skeletal tendency.
- If ANB angle is increased, it indicates Class II skeletal tendency.

Mandibular Plane

The mandibular plane is drawn between gonion (Go) and gnathion (Gn). It gives an indication of growth pattern of an individual.

Steiner chose the **GoGn line** for representing the mandibular plane because it more nearly represents the

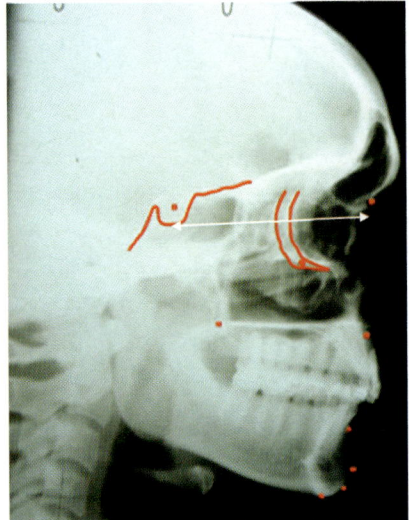

Fig. 9.15: Sella-nasion line

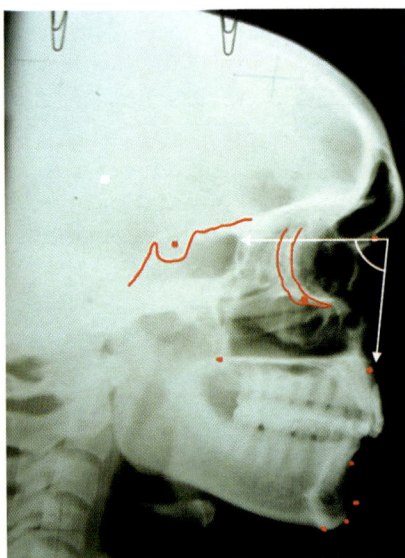

Fig. 9.16: Skeletal SNA angle

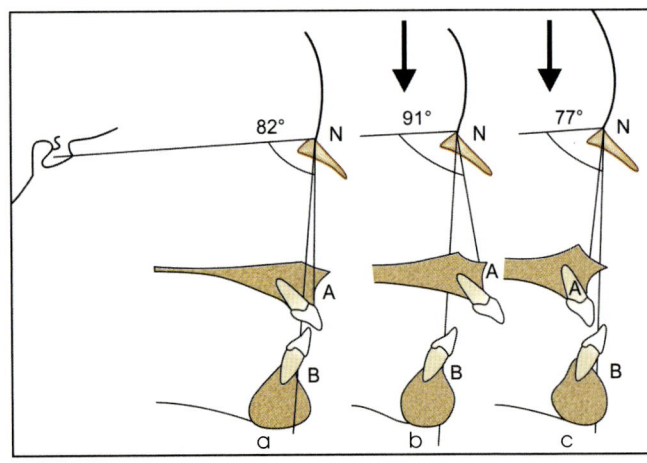

Fig. 9.17: (a) Normal SNA; (b) 91° SNA angle suggestive of protrusive maxilla; (c) 77° SNA angle suggestive of recessive maxilla

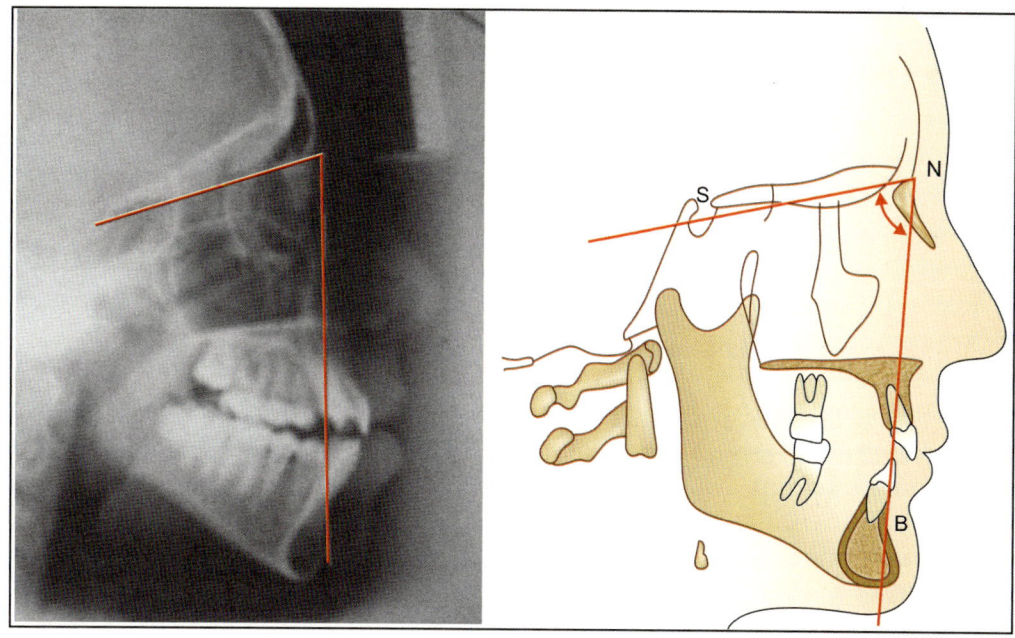

Fig. 9.18: SNB angle

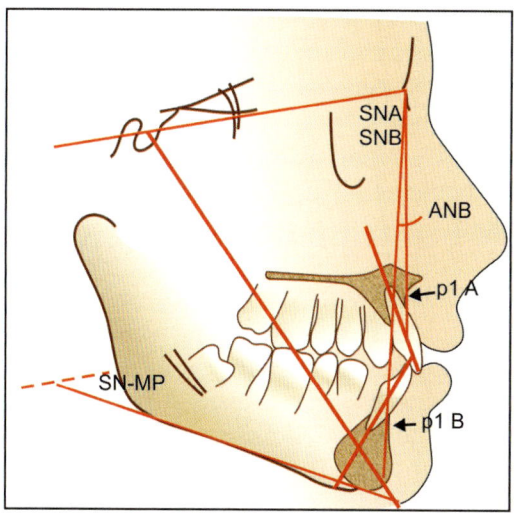

Fig. 9.19: ANB angle

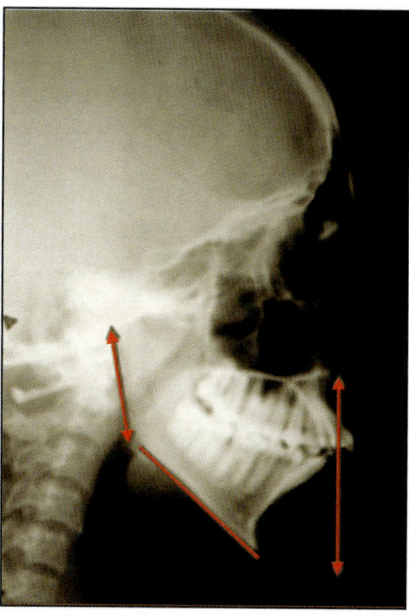

Fig. 9.20: Cephalometric finding showing small size of ramus of mandible

mass of the body of the mandible, rather than its lower border (which is curved) (Fig. 9.19)

- Normal value is 32°.
- If it is increased, it indicates vertical growth pattern.
- If it is decreased, it is suggestive of horizontal growth pattern.

Cephalometric findings indicating Class II due to mandibular deficiency: Downward and backward rotation of mandible caused by small size of ramus and body of mandible (Fig. 9.20).

- Decreased posterior facial height.
- Steep mandibular plane angle.
- Increased ANB angle
- Increased angle of convexity.

Occlusal Plane Angle

Occlusal plane angle indicates the relation of the occlusal plane to the cranium and face. It is the angle formed between SN plane and the occlusal plane.

Occlusal plane: It represents a line passing through the overlapping cusps of first premolars and first molars.

- *Normal value—14°*
- *Increased occlusal plane angle:* Indicates vertical growth pattern.
- *Decreased occlusal plane angle:* Indicates horizontal growth pattern.

Dental Analysis

Maxillary incisor position: The parameters used in dental analysis are:

- Upper incisor to NA angle
- Upper incisor to NA linear
- Lower incisor to NB angle
- Lower incisor to NB linear
- Interincisal angle

The upper incisor to NA angle is formed by the long axis of upper central incisors and the line joining nasion to Point A.

The upper incisor to NA linear is a measurement between the labial surface of upper central incisors and the line joining nasion to point A. It helps in determining the upper incisor position.

Linear measurement: Mean: 4 mm

Angular measurement: Mean: 22° (Fig. 9.21)

- If the upper incisor to NA angle is increased, it indicates as proclined upper incisors.
- If the upper incisor to NA angle is decreased, it indicates as retroclined upper incisors.

Mandibular incisor position: The lower incisor to NB angle is formed between the NB plane and the long axis of lower incisors.

- If the lower incisor to NB plane angle is increased, it indicates the proclination of lower incisors.
- If the lower incisor to NB plane angle is decreased, it indicates the retroclination of lower incisors.

  Mean LI-NB (degrees)—25°

  Mean LI-NB (linear)—4 mm (Fig. 9.22)

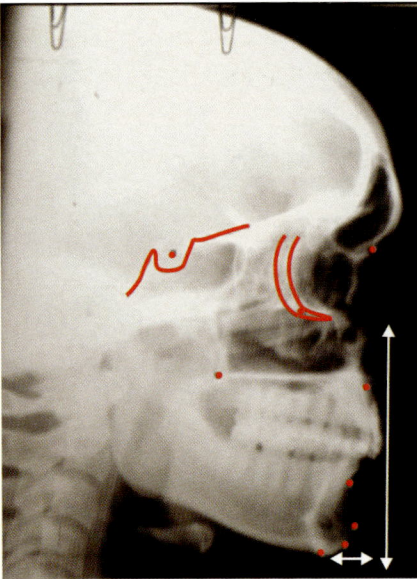

Fig. 9.22: NB (linear)

Interincisal Angle (Fig. 9.23)

This relates the relative position of the upper incisor to that of the lower incisor. Mean UI-LI—130°

UI-LI <130°—denotes upper and/or lower incisors require uprighting.

UI-LI >130°—denotes upper and/or lower incisors require advancing anteriorly or correcting of the axial inclinations.

Soft Tissue Analysis

The soft tissue analysis is a graphic record of the visual observations made in the clinical examination of the patient. It includes an appraisal of the adaptation of soft tissue to the bony profile with consideration to the size, shape and posture of the lips on the lateral cephalogram. The thickness of the soft tissue over the symphysis mentalis and the nasal structure as it relates to the lower face is also analyzed.

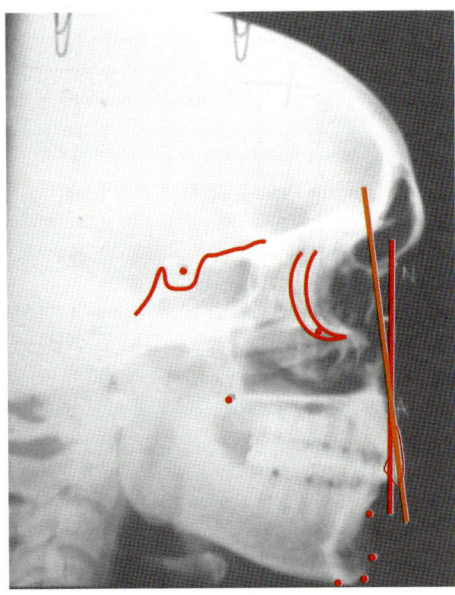

Fig. 9.21: UI-NB angle

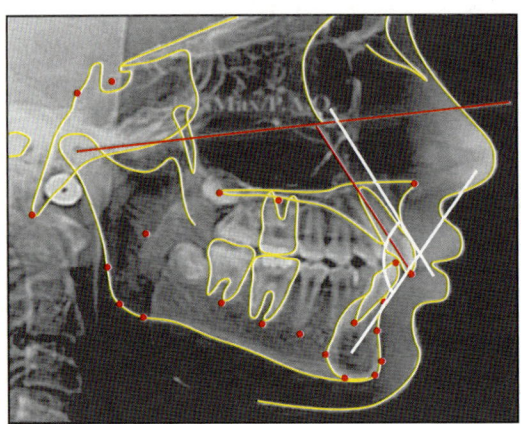

Fig. 9.23: Interincisal angle

Reference line of Steiner's analysis is the line joining from center point of the "S" shaped curve between the tip of nose and subnasale to the lower point (soft tissue pogonion) (Fig. 9.24).

Interpretation of soft tissue analysis: This line is the **S-line**.

- If the lips located beyond this line, it tends to be protrusive.
- If the lips are positioned behind this line, the patient's profile is interpreted as 'concave'.

Cephalometric Findings of Bimaxillary Protrusion

- Decreased interincisal angle
- Increased incisor mandibular plane angle
- Increased SNA and SNB angle

Cephalometric Findings of Class III Malocclusion

1. *Dentoalveolar class III*
   a. No apparent sagittal skeletal discrepancy (normal ANB angle)
   b. Tipping of incisors: Upper—lingual; lower—labial.
2. *Skeletal class III*
   a. Negative to 0 ANB angle
   b. Increased mandibular length and more obtuse gonial angle
   c. Tipping of incisors: Upper—labial; lower—lingual
3. *Pseudo class III*
   a. Cephalometric values intermediate to Class I and III

Different vertical facial patterns are noticed in skeletal Class III malocclusion as shown in Fig. 9.25.

TWEED'S ANALYSIS

He placed esthetics first in his list of treatment objectives and to achieve this he resorted to extraction of teeth.

He stated "My conviction are the acceptance of 25° for Frankfort-horizontal plane angle, 87° for incisor mandibular plane angle and 69° for Frankfort mandibular incisor angle. It will result in more ideally proportioned facial esthetics and give more stable results." Tweeds diagnostic facial

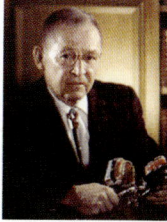
Charles H Tweed

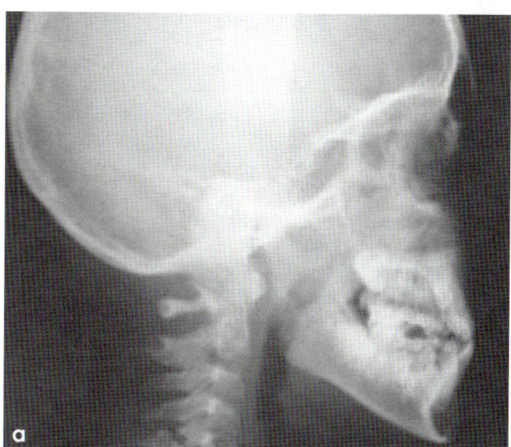
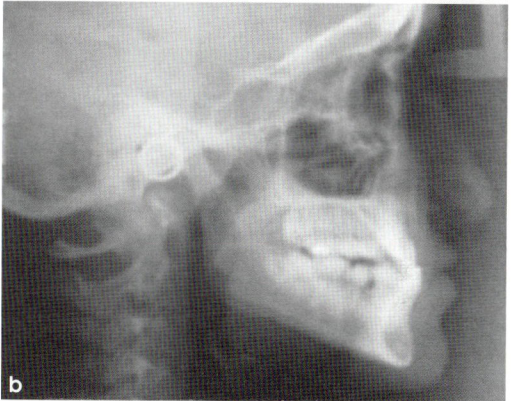
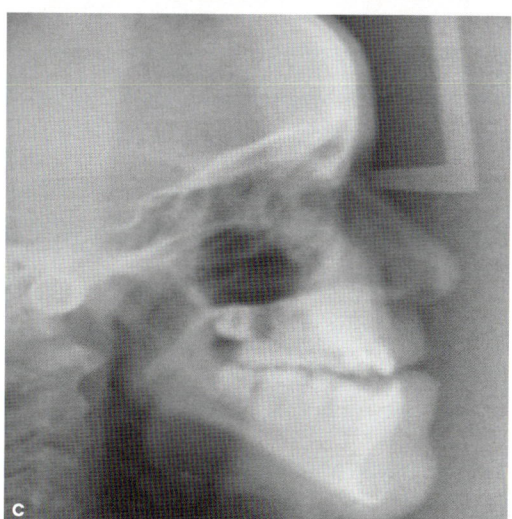

Fig. 9.25: Different vertical facial patterns: (a) Mesofacial; (b) Brachyfacial; (c) Dolichofacial

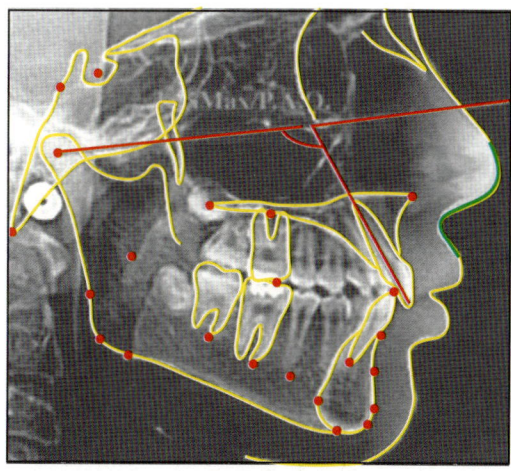

Fig. 9.24: Steiner's soft tissue analysis

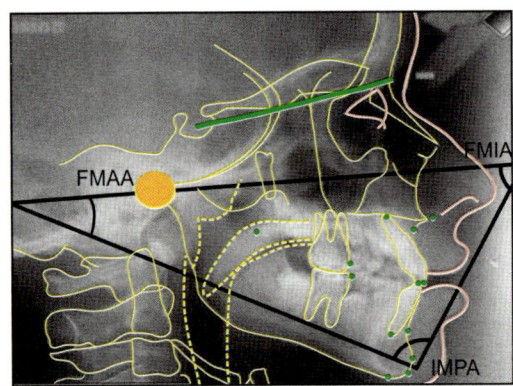

Fig. 9.26: Tweed's diagnostic tringle

triangle is not a complete analysis in itself. It provides information about the skeletal pattern for diagnosis and treatment planning.

This analysis, popularly known as "Tweed's Diagnostic Triangle", consists of three planes forming the three sides of a triangle and the three angles of the triangle make up a sum of 180° (Fig. 9.26).

The three planes are:
- The Frankfort horizontal plane
- A line passing through the long axis of the lower incisor crown
- The mandibular plane

FMA: The angle between the mandibular plane and the Frankfort horizontal.

FMIA: The angle between the long axis of the incisor and the Frankfort plane.

IMPA: The angle between the long axis of the lower incisor and the mandibular plane.

Objectives of This Analysis

- To determine the position of the lower incisor should occupy at the end of the treatment. Predetermination of this relationship provides useful treatment planning information especially in extraction cases.
- A prognosis on the treatment result, based on the configuration of the triangle
- Frankfort mandibular plane angle (FMPA): Normal value—16–35°
- Incisor mandibular plane angle (IMPA)—85–95°
- Frankfort mandibular incisor plane angle (FMIA)—60–75°
  - Decreased IMPA—indicates lower incisor retroclination.
  - Increased IMPA—indicates lower incisor proclination.
  - Decreased FMIA—indicates lower incisor proclination.
  - Increased FMIA—indicates lower incisor retroclination.
  - Decreased FMIA—indicates lower incisor proclination.
  - Increased FMIA—Indicates lower incisor retroclination.

The basis is the FMA angle and the following can be derived from the change in its value as:
- If FMA 16 to 28°:
  - Prognosis is good at 16°.
  - IMPA should be 90 + 5 = 95 at 22°
  - IMPA should be 90 at 28°
  - IMPA should be 90 – 5 = 85°.

Approximately 60% malocclusions have FMA between 16° and 28°.
- If FMA from 28 to 35°:
  - IMPA should be 90–5 = 85°. Extractions necessary in majority of cases at 35°
  - IMPA should be 80 to 85°
- If FMA is above 35 degree: Prognosis is bad. Extractions frequently complicate problems. Tweed stressed the importance of FMIA angle, recommending that it be maintained at 65 to 70°.

Tweed's Growth Trends

- Two cephalograms are taken at a gap of 12–18 months.
- They are then superimposed on S-N keeping S as the reference point.
- Three types of growth are seen.
- Tweed classified it into:
  - Type A: Subdivision
  - Type B
  - Type C

Type A

- Middle and lower third grew forward and downward in unison.
- The ANB value remains constant.
- If the ANB value does not exceed 4.5° and case is having a molar relation of Class I, then is type A.
- If molar relation is of Class II and ANB is more than 4.5°, then is called as Type A subdivision.
- 25% of patients are in this category.

Type B

- There is a change in ANB reading in pre- and post-radiographs.
- The growth trend is in downward and forward direction with middle face growing more rapidly than the lower face.

- In cases of ANB of less than 4°, the prognosis is fair while in cases with an increased ANB of 7° or beyond, the prognosis is poor.
- 15% patients belong to this category.

Type C

- In case the lower face is growing downward and forward more rapidly than the middle face.
- The ANB decreases.
- The mandibular incisors usually get tipped lingually and get crowded or the max incisors get tipped labially.
- 60% patients belong to this category.

WITS APPRAISAL

Wits (abbreviation for university of Witwatersrand, Johannesburg, South Africa). Jacobson described Wits appraisal (Fig. 9.27).

According to Jacobson, It is not an analysis per se; rather it is intended as a diagnostic aid whereby the severity or degree of A-P disharmony can be measured. It is measured of extent to which jaws are related to each other A-P, independent of relationship to cranial landmarks.

More recently it has been claimed that the ANB angle is affected by several environmental factors and thus a diagnosis based on this angle may give false results.

The following factors have been reported to affect the ANB angle:
- The patient's age: The ANB angle has a definite tendency to decrease with increasing age.
- The change of the spatial position of the nasion either in the vertical or anteroposterior direction or both.
- The upward or downward rotation of the SN line.
- The upward or downward rotation of the jaws.
- The change in the angle between the SN and the occlusal plane.
- The degree of facial prognathism.
- Effect of short and long cranial bases on ANB angle (Figs 9.28 and 9.29)

Measurement and Interpretation

- Occlusal plane is drawn through the region of overlapping cusps of premolars and molars.
- Perpendiculars are drawn on occlusal plane from points A and B. Contact points labelled as AO and BO.
- If the point is located behind the point AO, it denotes skeletal class II jaw dysplasia
- If the point is ahead than the point AO, it denotes skeletal class III jaw dysplasia

DOWN'S ANALYSIS

It is one of the most frequently used analyses in orthodontics. It consists of the following five parameters:
- Facial angle
- Angle of convexity

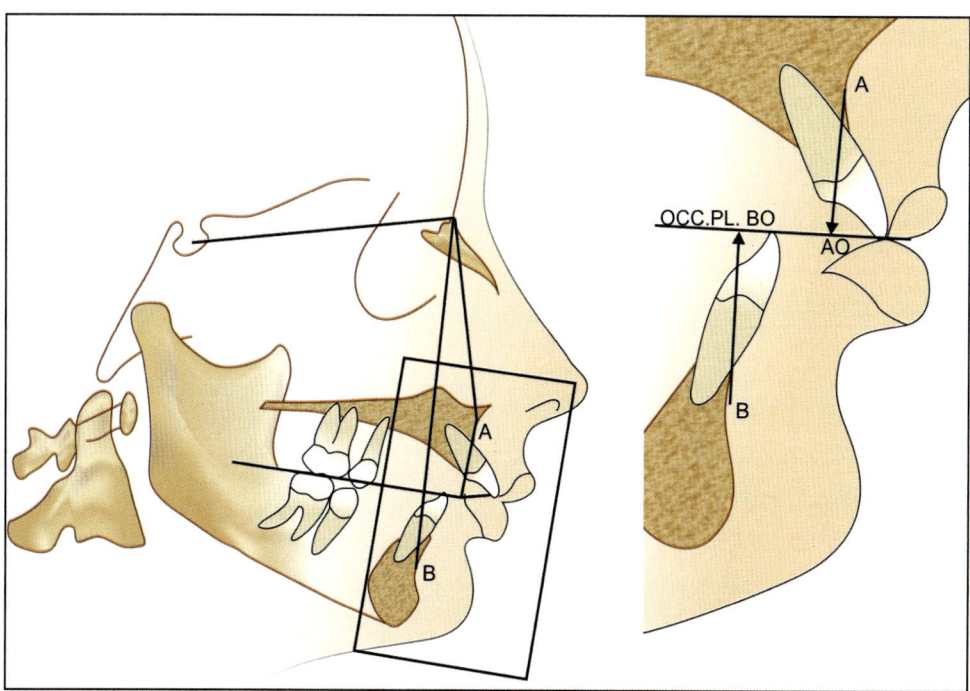

Fig. 9.27: Wit's appraisal

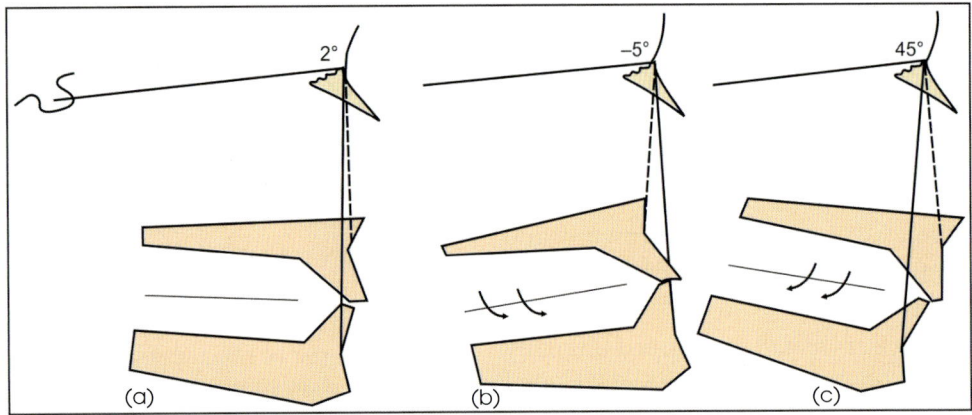

Fig. 9.28: Effect of angulation of jaws, occlusal plane on ANB angle: (a) Normal relationship; (b) Effect of counterclockwise rotation of face; (c) Effect of clockwise rotation of face

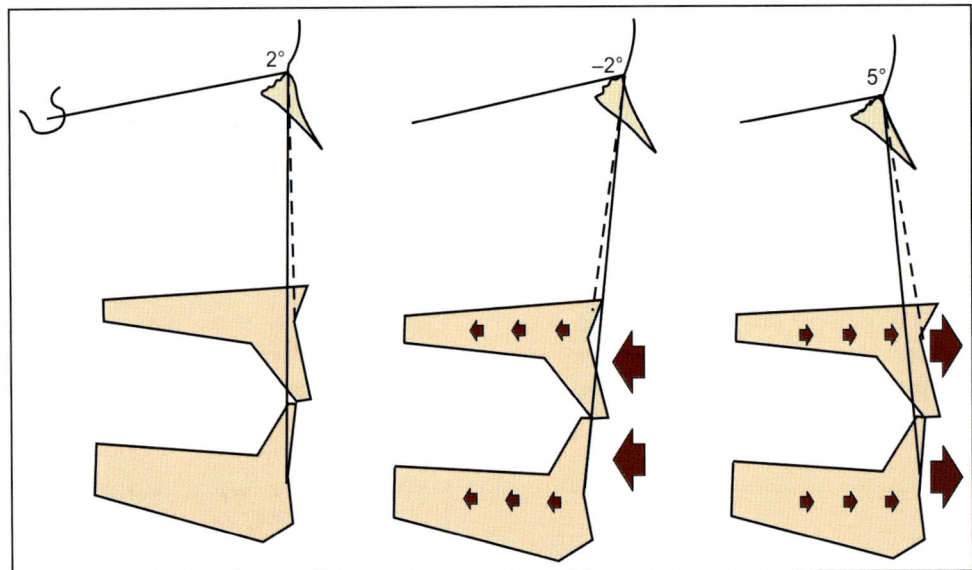

Fig. 9.29: Effect of short and long cranial bases on ANB angle

- A-B plane angle
- Mandibular plane angle
- Y-axis

Dental Parameters

- Cant of occlusal plane
- Interincisal angle
- Incisor–occlusal plane angle
- Incisor–mandibular plane angle
- Upper incisor to A-Pog line

Facial angle: It is the angle formed by the intersection of N-Pog plane and FH plane. It signifies the antero-posterior positioning of the mandible to the upper face

- *Normal value:* The average value of facial angle is 87.8° while the range is 82–95°.

- *Increased facial angle:* It is seen in class III malocclusion
- *Decreased facial angle:* It is seen in class II malocclusion

Angle of Convexity

It is formed by the intersection of a line from nasion to point A and a line from point A to pogonion. It helps in determining convexity or concavity of the skeletal profile.

Mean value: The average value of angle of convexity is "0" while the range is −8.5 to 10°.

- *Positive angle or increased angle:* If it is more than nomal value, it is referred as positive or increased angle of convexity. It indicates prominent maxillary base relative to mandible.
- *Negative angle:* If the angle is below its normal value. It indicates of prognathic profile.

Beta Angle

The beta angle is a new measurement for assessing the skeletal discrepancy between the maxilla and the mandible in the sagittal plane. It uses three skeletal landmarks—point A, point B and the apparent axis of the condyle-C

Lines used are:
- Line connecting the center of the condyle C with B point—C-B line
- Line connecting A and B points
- Lines from point A perpendicular to C-B line.
  The beta angle is measured as the angle between the last perpendicular line and the A-B line.

Normal values:
- Class I skeletal pattern—27° and 35°
- Class II skeletal—less than 27°
- Class III skeletal pattern—greater than 35°

Advantages:
- It does not depend on the cranial landmarks and only single parameter is measured.
- It can be used in serial cephalograms for comparisons in the changes of the sagittal relationship of the jaws either by growth or orthodontic or orthognathic intervention.

Disadvantage: It does not the position of the jaw bases to the skull.

BJORK-JARABAK ANALYSIS

This polygon is very useful to predict growth patterns both from a qualitative and quantitative point of view, i.e. direction and amount. It also contributes to a better definition of the facial type. When evaluating a young patient who requires orthodontic, orthopedic or a combination of both treatments, it is imperative for the clinician to know as accurately as possible what the patient's growth pattern is.

His observations are based on a study of approximately 300 children aged 12 and a similar number of soldiers whose ages ranged from 21 to 23 in whom almost 90 measurements were determined.

Tracing of the Polygon

Planes:
- S-Na—anterior cranial base
- S-Ar—posterior cranial base
- Ar-Go—ramus height
- Go-Me—mandibular body length
- Na-Me—anterior facial height
- S-Go—posterior facial height
- Go-Na—it divides the gonial angle into two halves, a upper and an inferior one.

Angles of polygon:
- Saddle angle—Na-S-Ar
- Articulare angle—S-Ar-Go
- Gonial angle—Ar-Go-Me
- Upper gonial angle—Ar-Go-Na
- Lower gonial angle—Na-Go-Me

Saddle Angle

It is formed by the union of the anterior cranial base with the posterior cranial base. This point is located in the intersection of the radiographic inferior contour of the spheno-occipital bones and the posterior border of the neck of the condyle. It represents the TMJ because it is located where the condyle comes out of the glenoid cavity.

Normal value—122°.

A high angle indicates a more horizontal S-Ar line while a lower angle indicates that the line is more vertical. This variation also results in a different location of the glenoid cavity thus influencing the mandible position anteroposteriorly.

If the angle is lower than the normal, there will be a downwards and slightly backward displacement of the joint cavity resulting in a more forward implantation of the mandible.

If the angle is more open than the normal, during growth, the articular fossa will be located more downward and backward causing a more distal placement of the mandible.

Although the saddle angle cannot be modified by an orthodontic treatment, it is a structural factor that should be taken into account in growth forecast, because mandibular projection might result in different angulations. In general, open angles are frequent in dolichofacial subjects, while closed angles are usually seen in brachyfacial and mesofacial subjects.

Articular Angle

It is formed by the posterior cranial base and the tangent to the posterior border of the mandibular ramus.

Normal value—143°

A lower angle tends to favor mandibular prognathism whereas high angle will favor retrognathism.

This angle should not only be taken into account in growth forecast, but also in the study of the patient's facial type and, therefore, in the treatment planning. This is one of the two polygon angles that can be modified by treatment.

Gonial Angle

- It is formed by the tangents to the posterior border of the mandibular ramus and inferior border of the body of the mandible.
- Normal value—130°
- The *upper gonial angle* is formed by the tangent to the posterior border of the ramus and by a line traced between the gonial angle and nasion.
- The *lower gonial angle* is formed by the union of the Go-Na line with the tangent to the inferior border of the corpus, the angle is called Na-Go-Me.
- The norm for the upper gonial angle—52 to 55°.
- The norm for lower gonial angle—70 to 75°.
- The total gonial angle describes the shape of the mandible.
- It determines the direction of the growth of the lower half of the face.
- Low angle characterizes a square mandible, subtle antegonial notch, high mandibular arch, brachyfacial type and orthognathic profile.
- The lower gonial angle describes the slant of the mandibular body. A high angle indicates a downward inclination and a tendency for an open bite.
- A closed lower gonial angle denotes a horizontal mandibular body and a tendency for an overbite.
- Open gonial angles suggest a dolichofacial jaw, a low mandibular dental arch, marked antegonial notch, convex profile and open facial axis.
- The norm for the sum is 396 ±6°. A lower combined value suggests anterior growth of the symphysis; a high angle predicts vertical growth and limited chin advancement.

SUPERIMPOSITION

Superimpositions are used to retrospectively study changes in jaw and tooth positions brought about through orthodontic treatment and growth. To study maxillary changes, pre-treatment and post-treatment cephalograms are superimposed on the lingual curvature of the palate. The mandibular composite is registered on the internal cortical outline of the symphysis with best fit on the mandibular canal to assess mandibular tooth movement as well as incremental growth of the lower jaw. Superimposition of the cephalometric records on sella enables the evaluation of overall growth and treatment changes.

This technique is also used in orthognathic surgery cases to confirm growth cessation in the craniofacial region by superimposing two sequential cephalograms taken within a 6 to 12 months interval. The lack of bony changes affirms that no further growth has taken place in that time interval.

Recent Advances in Diagnosis

- Digital photography
- Digital radiographs
- Digiceph and digigraphs
- Denofacial planner
- Vistadent—for surgical VTO
- Dentoptix

BIBLIOGRAPHY

1. Jacobson A. Radiographic Cephalometry: From Basics to Videoimaging, Chicago, 1995, Quintessence.
2. Jacobson A. "Wits" appraisal of jaw disharmony. Am J Orthod 1975;67:125–38.
3. Steiner CC. Th use of cephalometric as an aid to planning and assessing orthodontic treatment. Am J Orthod 1960;46:721–35.
4. Tweed CH. The diagnostic facial triangle in the control of treatment objectives. Am J Orthod 1969; 55: 651.
5. Tweed CH. The Frankfort-mandibular incisor angle (FMIA) in orthodontic diagnosis, treatment planning and prognosis. Angle Orthod 1954;24:121–9.

PREVIOUS YEAR'S UNIVERSITY QUESTIONS

Essay

1. Define cephalometric. Describe the cephalostat and write in detail about Steiner's analysis.
2. Write advantages and disadvantages of cephalometrics. Discuss in detail about Tweed's diagnostic triangle.
3. Write various soft tissue and hard tissue landmarks, planes and angles.

Short Questions

1. Steiner's analysis.
2. ANB angle.
3. Wits analysis
4. Tweed's analysis

MCQs

1. *Types of cephalograms are:*
   a. Lateral cephalogram
   b. Frontal cephalogram
   c. Occlusal cephalogram
   d. Both a and b **(Ans: d)**

2. *Lateral cephalogram provides:*
   a. A lateral view of skull
   b. An anteroposterior view of the skull

c. Both a and b

d. None of the above   **(Ans: a)**

3. *Frontal cephalogram provides:*
   a. An anteroposterior view of the skull
   b. A lateral view of skull
   c. Both a and b
   d. None of the above   **(Ans: a)**

4. *The distance between the X-ray source and the mid-sagittal plane of the patient in cephalometric radiograph should be:*
   a. 5 feet
   b. 6 feet
   c. 7 feet
   d. 8 feet   **(Ans: a)**

5. *Cephalometric tracing in orthodontics is made on:*
   a. The frosted surface of acetate tracing sheet
   b. The plane paper
   c. The white paper
   d. None of the above   **(Ans: a)**

6. *Which of the following is hard tissue landmark in cephalometrics:*
   a. Condylion
   b. Posterior nasal spine
   c. Gonion
   d. All of the above   **(Ans: d)**

7. *Basion in cephalometrics refers to:*
   a. Lowest point on the anterior margin of the foramen magnum in the midline
   b. Lowest point on the posterior margin of the foramen magnum in the midline
   c. Highest point on the anterior margin of the foramen magnum in the midline
   d. Highest point on the posterior margin of the foramen magnum in the midline
   (Ans: a)

8. *Condylion in cephalometrics refers to:*
   a. Superior most point of the head of the condyle of the mandible.
   b. Inferior most point of the head of the condyle of the mandible.
   c. Superior most point of the neck of the condyle of the mandible.
   d. Inferior most point of the neck of the condyle of the mandible.   **(Ans: a)**

9. *Se in cephalometrics refers to:*
   a. Mid-entrance point of sella turcica
   b. Midpoint of sella turcica

c. Mid-inferior point of sella turcica

d. None of the above   **(Ans: a)**

10. *ptm in cephalometrics refers to:*
    a. Intersection of the inferior border of the foramen rotundum with the posterior wall of the pterygomaxillary fissure
    b. Intersection of the superior border of the foramen rotundum with the posterior wall of the pterygomaxillary fissure
    c. Intersection of the anterior border of the foramen rotundum with the posterior wall of the pterygomaxillary fissure
    d. Intersection of the posterior border of the foramen rotundum with the posterior wall of the pterygomaxillary fissure   **(Ans: a)**

11. *FH plane is also called:*
    a. Frankfort horizontal plane
    b. Frankfort vertical plane
    c. Frankfort oblique plane
    d. All of the above   **(Ans: a)**

12. *E-plane is also called:*
    a. Esthetic plane
    b. External plane
    c. Both a and b
    d. None of the above   **(Ans: a)**

13. *Normal facial angle is about:*
    a. 82–95°
    b. 70–82°
    c. 95–110°
    d. 120–130°   **(Ans: a)**

14. *Increased facial angle indicates:*
    a. Skeletal Class III malocclusion
    b. Skeletal Class II malocclusion
    c. Skeletal Class I malocclusion
    d. All of the above   **(Ans: a)**

15. *Decreased facial angle indicates*
    a. Skeletal Class III malocclusion
    b. Skeletal Class II malocclusion
    c. Skeletal Class I malocclusion
    d. All of the above   **(Ans: b)**

16. *Facial angle signifies:*
    a. Anteroposterior positioning of the mandible to the upper face
    b. Anteroposterior positioning of the maxilla to the upper face
    c. Maxillomandibular relationship
    d. All of the above   **(Ans: d)**

17. *Angle of convexity in cephalometric analysis helps in:*
    a. Determining convexity of the skeletal profile
    b. Determining concavity of the skeletal profile
    c. Both a and b
    d. None of the above **(Ans: d)**

18. *The average value of the angle of convexity is*
    a. 8.5–10°
    b. 3.5–5.5°
    c. 0.0–3.0°
    d. 3.8–5.9° **(Ans: a)**

19. *Y-axis in Down's cephalometric analysis helps in:*
    a. Diagnosing horizontal pattern
    b. Assessing vertical growth pattern
    c. Both a and b
    d. None of the above **(Ans: c)**

20. *Decreased mandibular plane angle in Steiner's cephalometric analysis indicates:*
    a. Vertical growth pattern
    b. Horizontal growth pattern
    c. Both a and b
    d. None of the above **(Ans: b)**

21. *Upper incisor to NA angle is formed by:*
    a. The long axis of upper central incisors and the line joining nasion to point A
    b. The long axis of upper lateral incisors and the line joining nasion to point B
    c. The long axis of lower central incisors and the line joining nasion to point A
    d. The long axis of lower lateral incisors and the line joining nasion to point A **(Ans: a)**

22. *The normal angle of upper incisor to NA angle is*
    a. 20°
    b. 25°
    c. 22°
    d. 18° **(Ans: c)**

23. *IMPA in Tweed's cephalometric analysis stands for:*
    a. Frankfort mandibular plane angle
    b. Incisor mandibular plane angle
    c. Frankfort mandibular incisor plane angle
    d. All of the above **(Ans: b)**

24. *Decreased FMIA in Tweed's triangle indicates:*
    a. Lower incisor proclination
    b. Lower incisor rotation
    c. Lower incisor retroclination
    d. Upper incisor proclination **(Ans: c)**

25. *Who described Wits appraisal:*
    a. Jacobson
    b. Rakosi
    c. Rickett
    d. Down **(Ans: a)**

26. *If the point BO is ahead than the point AO in Wit's appraisal, it denotes:*
    a. Skeletal Class II jaw dysplasia
    b. Skeletal Class III disharmonies
    c. Skeletal Class I jaw dysplasia
    d. All of the above **(Ans: b)**

27. *Wits analysis was developed in:*
    a. University of New York
    b. University of Bristol
    c. University of Witwatersrand
    d. None of the above **(Ans: c)**

28. *Wits analysis was developed primarily to study the:*
    a. Inter-relationship of maxilla and mandible anteroposteriorly
    b. Relationship of maxilla to the anterior cranial base
    c. Relationship of mandible to the posterior cranial base
    d. None of the above **(Ans: a)**

29. *Who discovered the X-ray:*
    a. Roentgen
    b. Herbert Hofrath
    c. Pacini
    d. Rickett's **(Ans: a)**

30. *In which year, Roentgen discovered X-ray:*
    a. 1931
    b. 1890
    c. 1895
    d. 1995 **(Ans: c)**

9.3 STUDY MODEL AND MODEL ANALYSIS

Chapter Outline

- Introduction
- Carey's analysis
- Ashley Howe's analysis
- Pont's analysis
- Linder Harth index
- Korkhaus analysis

- Bolton's analysis
- Mixed dentition analysis
- Kesling diagnostic setup
- Huckaba radiographic analysis
- Occlusogram

INTRODUCTION

The study models are the accurate plaster reproductions of the teeth, alveolar process and their surrounding soft tissues.

They are essential diagnostic records, which allow examination of teeth and the occlusion from all directions.

They aid in diagnosis, treatment planning and fabrication of selected appliances, as well as in patient education and monitoring the progress of the orthodontic treatment.

USES

Orthodontic study models serve a number of purposes.

Diagnostic purpose: With the help of study models, the occlusion from all aspects can be easily inspected. They are helpful in carrying out the model analysis. They help in assessing the nature and severity of malocclusion.

Patient and parent education purpose: They are useful in explaining the treatment plan to the patient and/or parents and motivating the patient for orthodontic treatment.

Record purpose: It is one of the most important pre-treatment records. They are useful in comparing the pre-treatment and post-treatment.

Laboratory purpose: Fabrication of removable orthodontic appliances on the models. They are useful in the repairing of removable orthodontic appliances. Direct banding and bonding procedure can be done on the cast.

Referral purpose: Study models are useful to transfer records in case the patients are to be treated by another clinician orthodontist.

Requirements to do Model Analysis (Fig. 9.30)

- Well prepared study models
- Vernier calipers
- Divider
- Ruler
- 0.003" soft brass wire

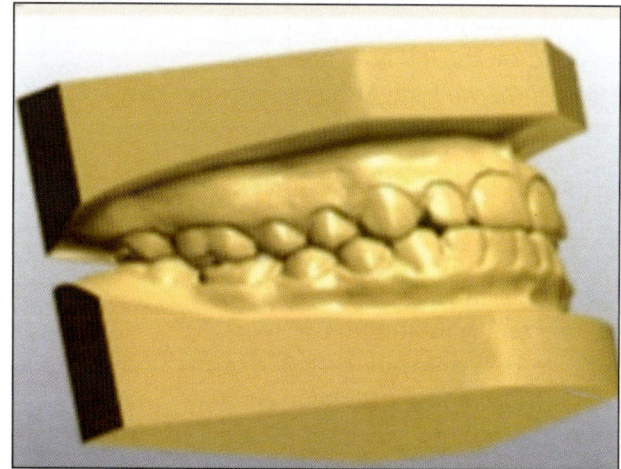
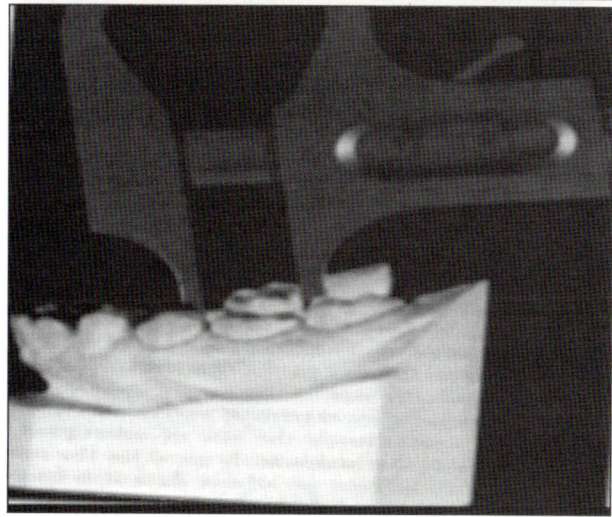

Fig. 9.30: Vernier calipers

Model Analysis

The model analysis used to assess the need of arch expansion:

- Pont's analysis
- Linder Harth analysis
- Korkhaus analysis

Analysis used to assess the need of extraction:

- Arch perimeter analysis
- Carey's model analysis

CAREY'S ANALYSIS

It is used to assess the need of extraction in mandibular arch only.

Procedure

- Determination of arch length in Carey's analysis is done using 0.012 inch soft round brass wire
- In case of proclined anterior teeth, the brass wire is passed on the cingulum of anteriors.
- In case of retroclined anteriors, the brass wire is passed on the labial to anterior.
- In case of well aligned anterior, the wire is passed on the incisal edge.

Inference

In Carey's analysis, if the discrepancy is 2.5 mm or less, it indicates a non-extraction case where in minimal tooth material excess. It is a boderline case where it requires reproximation only.

- If the discrepancy is 2.5–5 mm, it indicates a extraction of 2nd premolar.
- If the discrepancy is more than 5 mm, it indicates a extraction of 1st premolar (Fig. 9.31).

ASHLEY HOWE'S ANALYSIS

Ashley Howe believed that crowding results due to a deficiency in arch width rather than that of the arch

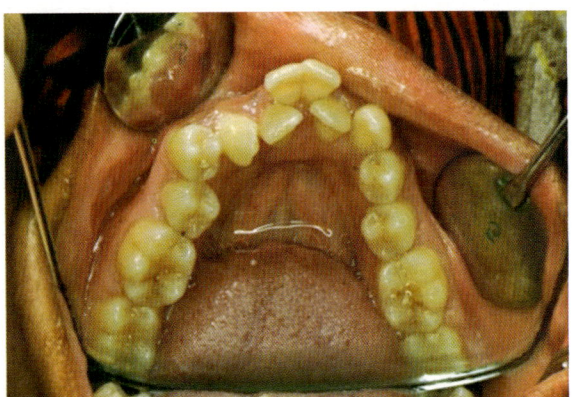

Fig. 9.31: Severity of crowding

length. He established a relationship between total widths of the 12 teeth anterior to the second molars to the width of the dental arch in the first premolar region.

Procedure

- **Determination of total tooth material (TTM):** The mesiodistal width of all the teeth mesial to the second permanent molar is measured with the help of bow divider and all the values are summed up. This value is called **total tooth material.**
- **Determination of premolar dimension (PMD):** It is determined from the tip of buccal cusp of left first permanent premolar to the right first permanent premolar in the same arch.
- **Determination of premolar basal arch width (PMBAW):** It is measured from left canine fossa to the right canine fossa. If the canine fossa is not clearly noticed, the measurements are made from a point that is 8 mm apical the crest of the interdental papilla distal to the canine.

$$PMBAW\% = \frac{PMBAW \times 100}{TTM}$$

Inference

- Expansion of an arch is possible, if PMBAW is greater than PMD.
- Expansion is not possible, if PMBAW is less than PMD
  - If the ratio is between 34 and 44%, it indicates borderline case.
  - If the ratio is 44% or more, it indicates non-extraction case.
  - If the ratio is less than 37%, it indicates extraction case.

Arch Perimeter Analysis

It is similar to the Carey's analysis but it is used to assess the need of extraction in maxillary arch.

PONT'S ANALYSIS

Pont in 1909 proposed this analysis.

Procedure (Fig. 9.32)

- It is determined the sum of incisor in Pont's analysis by measuring mesial distal width of four maxillary incisors and values are summed up (SI).
- The premolar value is measured by placing the tip end of divider at distal pit of 1st premolar of right side and another at the distal pit of left side of 1st premolar (MPV).

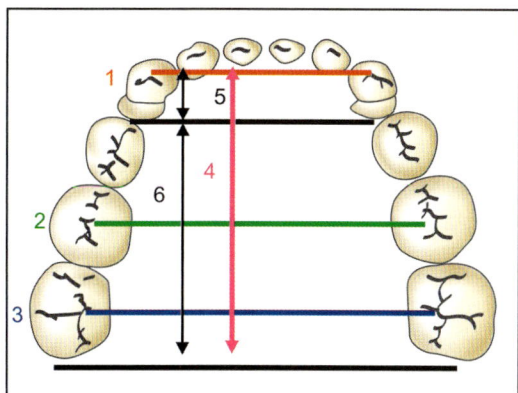

Fig. 9.32: Maxillary and mandibular dental width measurements. 1. Intercanine distance. 2. Interpremolar distance. 3. First intermolar distance. 4. Dental arch total length. 5. Anterior segment length. 6. Posterior segment length

- The measured molar value (MMV) is determined by placing the divider at the mesial pit of right side 1st molar to the mesial pit of left side 1st molar.
- The calculated premolar value (CPV) is determined by using the following formula

$$CPV = \frac{\text{Sum of incisors (SI)} \times 100}{80}$$

The calculated molar value (CMV) is determined by the formula which is mentioned below

$$CMV = \frac{SI \times 100}{64}$$

How much expansion needed in premolar region is determined by the formula as CPV–MPV?

How much expansion needed in molar region is determined by the formula as CMV–MMV?

The only difference between Pont's analysis and Linder Harth model analysis is 85 instead of 80 as in Pont's analysis.

- It helps in determining whether the dental arch is narrow or wide.
- It gives inference the need for lateral arch expansion.
- It gives as how much expansion is possible in premolar and molar regions.

Drawback of Pont's Analysis

- Maxillary laterals are the teeth most commonly missing from the oral cavity.
- Maxillary laterals may undergo morphogenetic alteration like 'peg'-shaped lateral.
- This analysis is derived solely from the casts of the French population.
- It does not take skeletal malrelationship by using the Pont's indexs into consideration.

- Pont's index does not account for the relationship of the teeth to the supporting bone, or the difficulties in increasing the mandibular dimensions.
- It should always be remembered that the patient's original mandibular and maxillary arch form should be considered as the ultimate guide for arch width rather than the values arrived at by using the Pont's index.

LINDER HARTH INDEX

Linder Harth proposed an analysis, which is very similar to Pont's analysis. However, he made a variation in the formula to determine the calculated premolar and molar values.

The calculated premolar value is determined using the formula:

$$\frac{SI \times 100}{85}$$

The calculated molar value is determined using the formula:

$$\frac{SI \times 100}{64}$$

Where SI = sum of mesiodistal width of incisors

KORKHAUS ANALYSIS

This analysis makes use of the Linder Harth's formula to determine the ideal arch width in the premolar and molar regions. An additional measurement is made from the midpoint of the interpremolar line to a point in between the two maxillary incisors. According to Korkhaus, for a given width of upper incisors, a specific value of the distance between the midpoint of interpremolar line to the point between the two maxillary incisors should exist. In case of proclined upper anteriors, an increase in this measurement is seen while a decrease in this value denotes retroclined upper anteriors.

For the values noted the mandibular value (LI) should be equal to the maxillary value (Lu) in millimeters minus 2 mm.

BOLTON'S ANALYSIS

According to Bolton, there exists a ratio between the mesiodistal width of maxillary and mandibular teeth. Malocclusion occurs when there is disparity between the mesiodistal dimensions of maxillary and mandibular teeth. Figure 9.33 and Tables 9.1 and 9.2.

Procedure

- *Sum of mandibular 12 teeth:* The mesiodistal width of all the teeth mesial to the mandibular second permanent molars is measured and summed up.

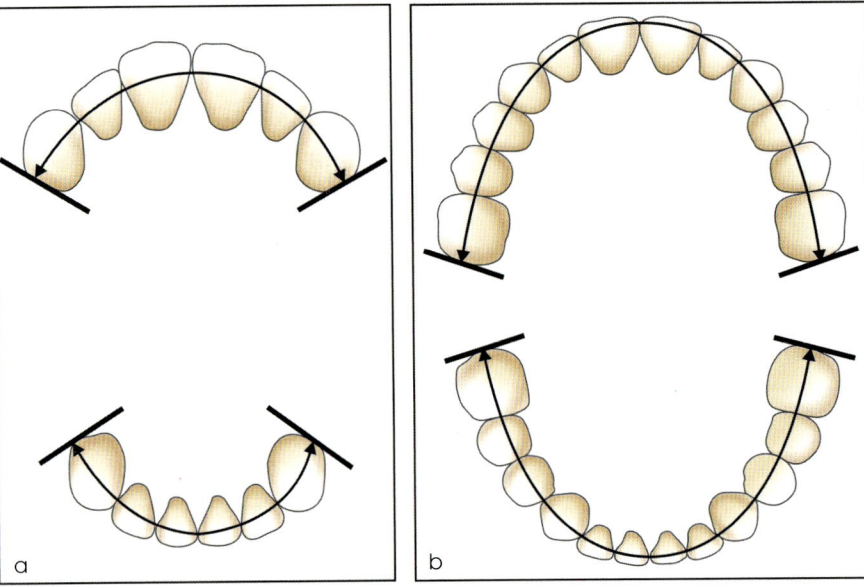

Fig. 9.33: (a) Anterior Bolton analysis; (b) Full arch Bolton analysis

Table 9.1: Bolton's chart: Overall ratio					
Max 12	Man 12	Max 12	Man 12	Max 12	Man 12
85	77.6	94	85.8	103	94
86	78.5	95	86.7	104	95
87	79.4	96	87.6	105	95.9
88	80.3	97	88.6	106	96.8
89	81.3	98	89.5	107	97.8
90	82.1	99	90.4	108	98.6
91	83.1	100	91.3	109	99.5
92	84	101	92.2	110	100.4
93	84.9	102	93.1		

Table 9.2: Bolton's chart: Anterior ratio					
Max 6	Man 6	Max 6	Man 6	Max 6	Man 6
40	30.9	45.5	35.1	50.5	39
40.5	31.3	46	35.5	51	39.4
41	31.7	46.5	35.9	51.5	39.8
41.5	32	47	36.3	52	40.1
42	32.4	47.5	36.7	52.5	40.5
42.5	32.8	48	37.1	53	40.9
43	33.2	48.5	37.4	53.5	41.3
43.5	33.6	49	37.8	54	41.7
44	34	49.5	38.2	54.5	42.1
44.5	34.4	50	38.6	55	42.5
45	34.7				

- *Sum of maxillary 12 teeth:* The mesiodistal width of all the teeth mesial to the maxillary second permanent molars is measured and summed up.
- *Sum of mandibular 6 anterior teeth:* The mesiodistal width of all the anterior teeth is measured and summed up.

- *Sum of maxillary 6 anterior teeth:* The mesiodistal width of all the anterior teeth is measured and summed up.

Determination of Overall Ratio

The sum of mesiodistal width of the mandibular teeth should be 91.3% of the mesiodistal width of maxillary anterior.

The overall ratio is determined by the formula

$$\text{Overall ratio} = \frac{\text{Sum of mandibular 12}}{\text{Sum of maxillary 12}} \times 100$$

Inference

If the ratio is less than 91.3%, then it indicates maxillary tooth material excess. Amount of maxillary tooth excess is determined by the formula,

$$\text{Sum of maxillary 12} = \frac{\text{Sum of mandibular 12}}{91.3} \times 100$$

If the ratio is more than 91.3%, then it indicates mandibular tooth material excess.

Amount of mandibular excess is determined by the formula,

$$\text{Sum of mandibular 12} = \frac{\text{Sum of maxillary 12}}{100} \times 100$$

Determination of Anterior Ratio

The sum of mesiodistal width of mandibular anteriors should be 77.2% of the mesiodistal width of maxillary anteriors.

The anterior ratio is obtained by the formula,

$$\text{Anterior ratio} = \frac{\text{Sum of mandible } 6}{\text{Sum of maxillary } 6} \times 100$$

Inference

If the ratio is less than 77.2%, then the maxillary anterior tooth material is excessive. If it is greater than 77.2%, then the mandibular anterior tooth material is excessive.

The amount of mandibular tooth material excess is calculated by using the formula: Mandibular anterior tooth material excess =

$$\text{Sum of mandibular } 6 - \frac{\text{Sum of max. } 6 \times 77.2}{100}$$

The amount of maxillary tooth material excess is calculated by using the formula: Maxillary anterior tooth material excess=

$$\text{Sum of maxillary } 6 - \frac{\text{Sum of max. } 6 \times 100}{77.2}$$

Drawbacks of the Analysis

- This study was done on a specific population and the ratios obtained need not be applicable to other population groups.
- Bolton analysis does not take into account the sexual dimorphism in the maxillary canine widths.

Bolton advocated the reduction of tooth material in the anterior region, if the anterior ratio shows an excess of tooth material. He prefers to do proximal stripping on the upper arch, if the upper anterior tooth material is excess and extraction of a lower incisor, if necessary, to reduce tooth material in the lower arch.

MIXED DENTITION ANALYSIS

It is an analysis to study the relationships of tooth size and available space during the mixed dentition. It is used to evaluate the amount of space available for the unerupted permanent canines and premolars.

Estimation of the size of the unerupted teeth can be carried out using three basic approaches:

- Measurement of the teeth on radiograph
- Estimation from proportionality table
- A combined approach of collecting data from radiograph and prediction tables.

Non-Radiographic

- Moyer's analysis
- Tanaka Johnston analysis
- Ballard and Wyile analysis

- Radiographic
- Huckaba analysis
- Nance analysis
- Combination of radiograph and prediction chart
- Hixon and Old Father
- Staley Kerber

Indications

- Premature loss of permanent canine.
- Rotation or blocking of lateral incisor because of lack of space.
- Ectopic eruption of permanent 1st molars.
- Distal terminal planner

Aramentarium

- Dental cast
- Boley's gauge
- Probability chart

Procedure

- The mesiodistal width of mandibular incisors is measured with Boley's gauge and summed.
- Place one tip of Boley's gauge in midline and the other on the distal surface of mandibular lateral incisor. This point is marked and repeated on the other side.
- The second mark will be on the deciduous canine.
- The distance from the mesial surface of mandibular first molars to the marked point is the space available for the eruption of mandibular canine and premolars.
- Based on the width of lower incisors, the width of the canine and premolars are predicted.
- Greater space available—spacing
- Lesser space available—crowding
- In case of upper canine and premolar width prediction, a different probability chart is employed.

Advantages

- No radiographs needed
- Can be used inside the patients mouth.
- Does not require sophisticated clinical judgment.
- It has minimal systemic error.
- Allows for sexual dimorphisms with equal accuracy.
- Used for both arches
- Not time consuming

Disadvantages

- Does not take into account the natural increase in arch perimeter that occurs in the transitional period.

- Does not account for tipping of mandibular incisor either lingually or facially.
- Maxillary tooth size is predicted by mandibular teeth.

Moyer's Mixed Dentition Analysis

- This is done only in study models. In this analysis, the size of the unerupted permanent cuspids and premolars are predicted.
- It is done with the knowledge of certain erupted permanent teeth.
- The lower incisor mesiodistal widths are measured and added to predict the sizes of unerupted teeth from the Table 9.3.

Tanaka and Johnston

It is suggested by **Tanaka and Johnston in 1974.** The width of unerupted canine and premolars is predicted. It is based on the sum of width of lower incisor.

Procedure

- Measure the total arch length.
- The mesiodistal width of lower incisor is measured and summed up.
- Upper canine and premolar width prediction—divide the value by 2 and add 11 mm to it.
- Lower canine and premolar width prediction—divide the value by 2 and add 10.5 mm to it.
- Space available = Total arch length – sum of lower incisors + 2 (calculated width of canine and premolar)

Advantages

- Radiograph is not required.
- Reasonably good accuracy.
- Simple and practical.

KESLING DIAGNOSTIC SETUP

HD Kesling introduced the diagnostic set up which is made from an extra set of trimmed study models. This helps the clinician in treatment planning as it simulates various tooth movements, which are to be carried out in the patient. The individual teeth along with their alveolar process are sectioned off from the model using a saw and replaced back in the desired final position.

The procedure is as follows:
- Dental cast is related to FMIA.
- Constant FMIA = 65° and find ideal position of mandibular incisors mesiodistally.
- Align both the lower central and lateral incisors on the lower cast at FMIA = 65°.

- Mandibular incisors are placed at right angles to mandibular plane.
- Canines are the next teeth to be positioned.
- First and second premolars are then set on the model.
- If the remaining space on each side is adequate to receive the permanent first molars, then extraction is not required.
- If space is inadequate and amounts is more than that can be gained by uprighting the permanent second molars, then some teeth must be removed usually the first premolar.
- When the mandibular set up is completed, the maxillary teeth are cut from their base and repositioned, then articulated to the mandibular set up.

Uses of Diagnostic Setup

- Aids in treatment planning as it helps to visualize tooth size arch length discrepancies and determine whether extraction is required or not.
- The effect of extraction and tooth movement following it on occlusion can be visualized.
- It acts as a tool as the improvements in tooth positions can be shown to the patient.

HUCKABA RADIOGRAPHIC ANALYSIS

This method relies on intraoral radiograph to predict the size of unerupted tooth using a formula. This makes use of a study cast and radiograph.

Procedure

- True size of the erupted deciduous molar is measured in the model.
- Radiographic width of the erupted deciduous molar is measured with the help of intraoral radiograph.
- Radiographic size of the unerupted premolar is measured using the intraoral radiograph.
- True width of the unerupted premolar is calculated using the formula

$$\frac{\text{Actual width of primary molar}(X1)}{\text{Apparent width of primary molar}(X2)} = \frac{\text{Actual width of unerupted premolar}(Y1)}{\text{Apparent width of unerupted premolar}(Y2)} \quad \text{or}$$

$$Y1 = \frac{X1 \times Y2}{X2}$$

Disadvantages

- Radiographic measurement are prone to distortion
- Difficult to measure rotated tooth in radiograph.
- Cumbersome procedure

Table 9.3 Probability chart for predicting the sizes of unerupted cuspid and bicuspids (Moyer 1988)

A. Mandibular bicuspids and cuspids

Males

21/12 (%)	19.5	20	20.5	21	21.5	22	22.5	23	23.5	24	24.5	25	25.5
95	21.6	21.8	22.0	22.2	22.4	22.6	22.8	23.0	23.2	23.5	23.7	23.9	24.2
85	20.8	21.0	21.2	21.4	21.6	21.9	22.1	22.3	22.5	22.7	23.0	23.2	23.4
75	20.4	20.6	20.8	21.0	21.2	21.4	21.6	21.9	22.1	22.3	22.5	22.8	23.0
65	20.0	20.2	20.4	20.6	20.9	21.1	21.3	21.5	21.8	22.0	22.2	22.4	22.7
50	19.5	19.7	20.0	20.2	20.4	20.6	20.9	21.1	21.3	21.5	21.7	22.0	22.2
35	19.0	19.3	19.5	19.7	20.0	20.2	20.4	20.7	20.9	21.1	21.3	21.5	21.7
25	18.7	18.9	19.1	19.4	19.6	19.8	20.1	20.3	20.5	20.7	21.0	21.2	21.4
15	18.2	18.5	18.7	18.9	19.2	19.4	19.6	19.9	20.1	20.3	20.5	20.7	20.9
5	17.5	17.7	18.0	18.2	18.5	18.7	18.9	19.2	19.4	19.6	19.8	20.0	20.2

Females

95	20.8	21.0	21.2	21.5	21.7	22.0	22.2	22.5	22.7	23.0	23.3	23.6	23.9
85	20.0	20.3	20.5	20.7	21.0	21.2	21.5	21.8	22.0	22.3	22.6	22.8	23.1
75	19.6	19.8	20.1	20.3	20.6	20.8	21.1	21.3	21.6	21.9	22.1	22.4	22.7
65	19.2	19.5	19.7	20.0	20.2	20.5	20.7	21.0	21.3	21.5	21.8	22.1	22.3
50	18.7	19.0	19.2	19.5	19.8	20.0	20.3	20.5	20.8	21.1	21.3	21.6	21.8
35	18.2	18.5	18.8	19.0	19.3	19.6	19.8	20.1	20.3	20.6	20.9	21.1	21.4
25	17.9	18.1	18.4	18.7	19.0	19.0	19.5	19.7	20.0	20.3	20.5	20.8	21.0
15	17.4	17.7	18.0	18.3	18.5	18.8	19.1	19.3	19.6	19.8	20.1	20.3	20.6
5	16.7	17.0	17.2	17.5	17.8	18.1	18.3	18.6	18.9	19.1	19.3	19.6	19.8

B. Maxillary bicuspids and cuspids

Males

21/12 (%)	19.5	20	20.5	21	21.5	22	22.5	23	23.5	24	24.5	25	25.5
95	21.2	21.4	21.6	22.9	22.1	22.3	22.6	23.8	23.1	23.4	23.6	23.9	24.1
85	20.6	20.9	21.1	21.3	21.6	21.8	22.1	22.3	22.6	22.8	23.1	23.3	23.6
75	20.3	20.5	20.8	21.0	21.3	21.5	21.8	22.0	22.3	22.5	22.8	23.0	23.3
65	20.0	20.3	20.5	20.8	21.0	21.3	21.5	21.8	22.0	22.3	22.5	22.8	23.0
50	19.7	19.9	20.2	20.4	20.7	20.9	21.2	21.5	21.7	22.0	22.2	22.5	22.7
35	19.3	19.6	19.9	20.1	20.4	20.6	20.9	21.1	21.4	21.6	21.9	22.1	22.4
25	19.1	19.3	19.6	19.9	20.1	20.4	20.6	20.9	21.1	21.4	21.6	21.9	22.1
15	18.8	19.0	19.3	19.6	19.8	20.1	20.3	20.6	20.8	21.1	21.3	21.6	21.8
5	18.2	18.5	18.8	19.0	19.3	19.6	19.8	20.1	20.3	20.6	20.8	21.0	21.3

Females

95	24.1	21.6	21.7	21.8	21.9	22.0	22.2	22.3	22.5	22.6	22.8	22.9	23.1
85	20.8	20.9	21.0	21.1	21.3	21.4	21.5	21.7	21.8	22.0	22.1	22.3	22.4
75	20.4	20.5	20.6	20.8	20.9	21.0	21.2	21.3	21.5	21.6	21.8	21.9	22.1
65	20.1	20.2	20.3	20.5	20.6	20.7	20.9	21.0	21.2	21.3	21.4	21.6	21.7
50	19.6	19.8	19.9	20.1	20.2	20.3	20.5	20.6	20.8	20.9	21.0	21.2	21.3
35	19.2	19.4	19.5	19.7	19.8	19.9	20.1	20.2	20.4	20.5	20.6	20.8	20.9
25	18.9	19.1	19.2	19.4	19.5	19.6	19.8	19.9	20.1	20.2	20.3	20.5	20.6
15	18.5	18.7	18.8	19.0	19.1	19.3	19.4	19.6	19.7	19.8	20.0	20.1	20.2
5	17.8	18.0	18.2	18.3	18.5	18.6	18.8	18.9	19.1	19.2	19.3	19.4	19.5

Recent Advances

- Digital study model
- Occlusogram
- Ortho CAD

OCCLUSOGRAM

It is developed by **Burston in 1961.** Occlusograms are actual sized photographs of the occlusal surfaces of the dental casts. The tracing of these occlusograms allow the orthodontist to simulate treatment in the occlusal view. These actual sized images of the occlusal views of the dental casts can be a valuable aid in determining arch form and widths, solution to arch length discrepancies (crowding or spacing), anchorage requirements in each quadrant for extraction cases, the presence and extent of skeletal asymmetrics and the presence and extent of tooth mass discrepancies, occlusograms can also be used as an aid in archwire construction.

DIGITAL STUDY MODEL

Refer Chapter 29.

BIBLIOGRAPHY

1. Bolton WA. Disharmony in tooth size and its relationship to the analysis and treatment of malocclusion. Angle Orthod 1958;28:113.
2. Bolton WA. The clinical application of a tooth-size analysis. Am J Orthod 1962;48:504–29.
3. Moyers E, Handbook of Orthodontics, 4th ed., Year Book Medical Publishers, Inc., 1988.
4. Huckaba GW. Arch size analysis and tooth size prediction. Dent Clinic North Am July 1964;431
5. Rakosi, Joanes, Graber. Orthodontic Diagnosis. In:Color Atlas of Dental Medicine, 1st ed., Thieme, 1993.
6. Tanaka, Johnston. The prediction of size of unerupted canines and premolars. Jam Dent Asso 1974;88:798.

PREVIOUS YEAR'S UNIVERSITY QUESTIONS

Essay

1. Enumerate various mixed dentition analyes and write in detail about Tanaka and Johnston mixed dentition analysis.

Short Questions

1. Pont's index
2. Study models
3. Bolton's ratio

4. Arch perimeter analysis
5. Uses of study model
6. Kesling diagnostic setup
7. Occlusogram

MCQs

1. *Analysis used to assess the need of extraction:*
   a. Arch perimeter analysis
   b. Carey's model analysis
   c. Both a and b
   d. Bolton's model analysis   **(Ans: c)**

2. *Which is the model analysis used to assess the need of arch expansion?*
   a. Pont's analysis
   b. Linder Harth analysis
   c. Korkhaus analysis
   d. All of the above   **(Ans: d)**

3. *Which model analysis is used to assess the tooth material excess?*
   a. Korkhaus analysis
   b. Carey's analysis
   c. Bolton's analysis
   d. All of the above   **(Ans: c)**

4. *Which model analysis is used to assess both the need of extraction as well as the expansion?*
   a. Ashley Howe's analysis
   b. Pont's analysis
   c. Linder Harth analysis
   d. All of the above   **(Ans: a)**

5. *CPV in Pont's analysis stands for:*
   a. Computer premolar value
   b. Calculated premolar value
   c. Calculated 1st premolar value
   d. Calculated 2nd molar value   **(Ans: b)**

9.4 SKELETAL MATURITY INDICATORS

Chapter Outline

- Introduction
- Maturity indicators
- Anatomy of hand-wrist
- Methods to assess skeletal maturity
- Cervical vertebrae as indicators of skeletal maturity
- Teeth mineralization as skeletal maturity indicator

INTRODUCTION

The maturational status of the patient has a strong bearing on orthodontic diagnosis, treatment planning, outcome of the treatment and post-treatment stability.

Chronological age, appearance of secondary sexual characteristics, growth charts, dental development and skeletal maturation are often used for growth prediction in clinical orthodontic practice.

The growth maturation occurs at different times in different individuals. The stage of skeletal maturation of an individual is essential for formulating diagnosis and treatment planning as this may affect the final prognosis of the orthodontic treatment. The basis for skeletal age assessment by radiographs is that during growth every bone goes through a series of changes that is studied by radiograph. Different ossification centers appear and mature at different times. The order, rate, time of appearance and progress of ossification in the various ossification centers occur in a predictable sequence.

Ideal Requirements

The anatomical site for the determination of skeletal status should have ideal requirements:

- It should be accurate.
- It should be valid over time and across age groups.
- It should be easily accessible.
- It should need minimum radiation.
- The stages of maturity should be well defined and easily identifiable.
- It requires minimum armamentarium.

Hand-Wrist Radiographs Predictable

It is made up of numerous small bones. These bones show a predictable and scheduled pattern of appearance, ossification and union from birth to maturity. Hence this region is one of the most suited to study growth.

Indications of Hand and Wrist X-rays

- In patients who exhibit a marked discrepancy between chronological age and dental or skeletal age.
- To assess the skeletal age in a patient whose normal growth is affected by endocrinological disturbances, infections, nutritional imbalances or trauma conditions.
- To predict the timing and variation of pubertal growth spurt.
- It helps to know cessation of active growth for taking the right decision to treat orthognathic surgical procedures.
- It helps as research tool.

Disadvantages

- It is complex in nature to study.
- It needs separate X-ray and additional radiation exposure to patients.
- Hand-wrist site is far away from the jaw which is the site of orthodontic correction.

Six types of skeletal development have been recognized:
- **1st group:** Average children.
- **2nd group:** Children who are tall in their childhood only because they have matured faster than average; they will not be particularly tall adults.
- **3rd group:** Children who not only mature early, but are also genetically tall. The children are taller than average from early childhood and will be tall adults.
- **4th group:** Children who are small because they mature late, but will eventually be of average stature.
- **5th group:** Children who are both late in developing and genetically short in stature.
- **6th group:** Indefinite group who start puberty either much earlier or much later than usual.

MATURITY INDICATORS

The key to successful treatment is to start at the right age. The age can be expressed in number of ways:
- Neural age

- Mental age
- Physiological age and biochemical age
- Chronological age
- Sexual/pubertal age
- Dental age
- Age determination using growth charts
- Skeletal/anatomical/radiological age

Neural Age

The neural age helps us to understand that the patient is mentally developed to understand the need for treatment and to what extent would he/she be able to cooperate and follow proper instructions.

Mental Age

The mental age is thus an index of maturation of the mind and like radiological age, increases at a rate that depends on many intrinsic and environmental factors.

A convenient way of classifying intelligence test performance is by the use of the concept of the intelligence quotient (IQ) which is the mental age expressed as a percentage of the chronological age. Thus, a child with a mental age of 12 years and a chronological age of 10 would have an IQ of 120.

The ability to draw a human figure is often used to assess development and the items the child include in the drawing can be scored and rated in terms of mental age. There is good correlation between assessments made at 5 and 11 years of age. Another method of estimating mental development is simply to use as the standard capacity of the child to read.

Physiological and Biochemical Age

A series of physiological and biochemical changes occur during growth which can be correlated to skeletal and chronological age.

Many physiological and biochemical changes during growth show a sex difference in timing, for they are more closely related to other indices of maturation than to chronological age. Thus, girls show a spurt in systolic blood pressure which occurs earlier than the corresponding spurt in the male and the resting mouth temperature which falls by 0.5 to 1°C from infancy to maturity, reaches its adult value earlier in girls. The erythrocyte count and blood value of boys diverge away from the figures for girls at the time of the adolescent spurt.

In the plasma, inorganic phosphate shows a steady fall from the high levels of childhood to reach adult figures by the ages of 15 in girls and 17 in boys.

The alkaline phosphatase raises significantly in parallel with growth velocity between the ages of 8–12 in girls and 10–14 in boys and thereafter it falls rapidly to adult levels.

More promising index of maturity is the ratio of creatine to creatinine in the urine, this ratio is thought to fall progressively with age after about the age of 14 and half years, probably under hormonal influences. Girls maturing early have a lower ratio than those of the same chronological age maturing late and a measurement of this ratio might be made to afford information regarding maturity, if considered along with skeletal and other data obtained at the same time.

Chronological Age

It is defined as age measured by years lived since birth. It is considered as a poor indicator of maturity as it provides little validity for identifying the stages of development progression through adolescence to adulthood. It may help to categorize the individual as early, average or late mature.

This enables an orthodontist to determine and predict the rate and magnitude of facial growth and help decide the time duration and method of treatment.

Sexual/Pubertal Age

There is a great deal of individual variation but puberty and the adolescent growth spurt occurs on an average in early second decade of life. It is generally seen 2 years earlier in girls than in boys. The stage of development of secondary sexual characteristics provides a physiologic calendar of adolescence that correlates with the individual's physical growth status.

The stages of sexual development in boys are more difficult to specifically define than in girls. Puberty begins later and extends over a longer period of about 5 years in boys as compared to 3½ years in girls.

Girls

If the menarche has occurred, peak height velocity (PHV) has been attained and the growth rate is decelerating.

If the menarche has not occurred, the growth rate may be decreasing but has certainly not yet reached the level of the end of the pubertal growth spurt (20 mm per year).

Boys

- If a boy has a prepubertal voice, it is most probable that the peak height velocity has not yet been reached.

- If the voice change has begun, the boy is in the pubertal spurt.
- If a boy has a male voice, the growth rate has begun to decelerate.
- No boy will reach the end of the pubertal spurt without having a male voice.

Dental Age

Dental age can be correlated to skeletal and chronological age but there is some controversy existing as eruption time table can be altered due to general and local factors.

Methods to Determine Dental Age

Eruption time table: Chronological age can be correlated to the eruption time table of primary and secondary teeth. Radiological appearances of developing jaws and teeth are taken into account. Radiological development of root of lower canine is considered to be an accurate method to correlate dental age to skeletal age.

Age Determination using Growth Chart

Growth charts involve the height, weight and chronological age of the child. There is variation seen in boys and girls. It is used to understand growth pattern in terms of deviations from the usual pattern and to express variability quantitatively. It can be done on individual basis or growth can be compared using standard growth charts. The importance is to determine whether growth is normal/abnormal or the child is in early/late developmental phase.

Growth charts can be used to follow the child over a time to evaluate, whether there is unexpected change in growth pattern hence the pattern, timing, variability, velocity and predictability of growth can be determined.

It can determine the peak height velocity which is the circumpubertal (the apex of the pubertal growth spurt), i.e. maximum period at which rate of increase in height is the highest.

Height and weight measurements are one of the powerful tools in growth assessment but become impractical in clinical orthodontics, as it requires longitudinal data which is seldom available and needs time and repeated observations. This method can be accurately correlated with pubertal and skeletal age.

Skeletal Age

Skeletal/radiological/anatomical age is considered to be the most reliable age for assessment of growth for orthodontic purposes. It is closely related to the growth of an individual. The stages of growth can be accurately determined using methods based on the skeletal maturation indicators and these can be used by the orthodontist to decide the type of treatment and determine the prognosis of a particular case.

Anatomical Regions

Anatomical regions suitable for skeletal maturational assessment should have ideally:
- Region should be small to restrict radiation exposure and expense.
- Should have many ossification centers which ossify at separate times and which can be standardized.
- Region should be easily accessible

Regions Normally used for Age Assessment

a. *Head and neck:* Skull cervical vertebrae
b. *Upper limb:* Shoulder joint—scapula, elbow, hand, wrist and fingers
c. *Lower limb:* Femur, hip joint, knee, ankle, foot— tarsals, metatarsals, phalanges.
d. Hand-wrist radiographs

ANATOMY OF HAND-WRIST (Figs 9.34 and 9.35)

It consists of the following four groups of bones:
- Distal ends of long bones of forearm
- Carpals
- Metacarpals
- Phalanges

Distal ends of long bones of forearm: It is formed by the distal ends of radius and ulna, which are the long bones of the forearm. In the anatomical position with

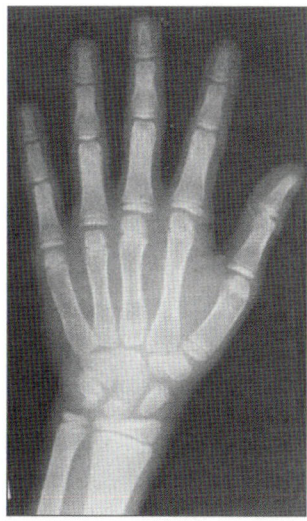

Fig. 9.34: Anatomy of hand-wrist

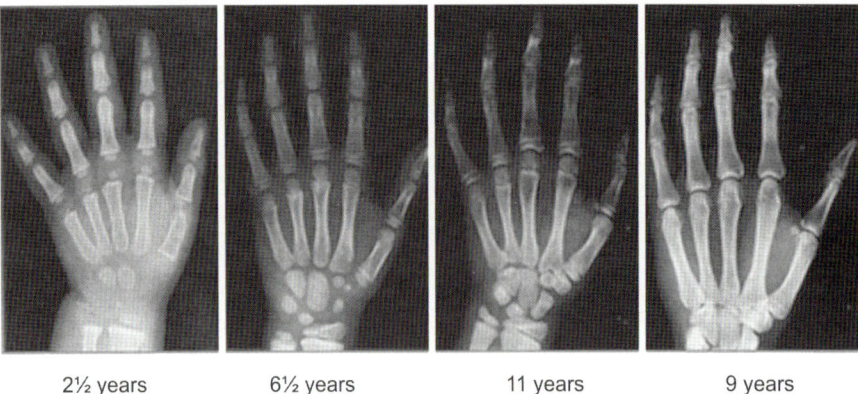

| 2½ years | 6½ years | 11 years | 9 years |

Fig. 9.35: Hand–wrist X-ray during growing period at different age levels

the palm facing upwards or front, the ulna is on the medial aspect (towards finger) while the radius is on the distal aspect (towards thumb). The method is rarely used nowadays and is of more interest for theoretical purpose than for its clinical applicability.

Carpals: They consist of eight small, irregularly shaped bones, arranged in two rows:
1. *Proximal row:* The bones of the proximal row are scaphoid, lunate, triquetral and pisiform.
2. *Distal row* of bones includes trapezium, trapezoid, capitates and hamate.

Metacarpals: These are the 5 miniature long bones forming the skeletal framework of the palm of the human hand. They are numbered 1 to 5 from the thumb to the little finger. All the metacarpals ossify from one primary ossifying center located in their shafts and a secondary center on their distal end; except the first metacarpal where it appears at the proximal end.

Phalanges: They are small bones that form the fingers. There are three phalanges in each finger. The thumb has only two phalanges. The bones of phalanges are referred to as the proximal, middle (absent in thumb) and distal phalanges. The phalanges have been considered to ossify in three stages (Fig. 9.36a to f):
- *Stage 1:* The epiphysis and diaphysis are equal.
- *Stage 2:* The epiphysis caps the diaphysis by surrounding it like a cap.
- *Stage 3:* Fusion occurs between the epiphysis and diaphysis.

The sequence of the four ossifications stages progresses through epiphyseal widening on selected phalanges, the ossification of the adductor sesamoid of the thumb, the capping of selected epiphysis over their diaphysis and the fusion of selected epiphyses and diaphysis.

Widening of the epiphysis to its diaphysis is a progressive process. The epiphysis first appears as a small center of ossification centrally located in the diaphysis. When it has developed laterally to the width of the diaphysis, it is considered applicable as a skeletal maturational indicator in this system.

Capping occurs in the transition between initial widening and fusion of the epiphysis and diaphysis. It is the stage in which the rounded lateral margins of the epiphysis begin to flatten and point towards the diaphysis, with an acute angle on the side facing the diaphysis. The time of first appearance of the capping is applicable as a skeletal maturational indicator.

Fusion between the epiphysis and diaphysis follows capping. It also begins centrally and progresses laterally, until the two formerly separate bones become one. The time of completion of this fusion with a smooth continuity of the surface at the junction area, is applicable as an SMI.

Ossification of the adductor sesamoid of the thumb first appears as a small relatively round center of ossification medial to the junction of epiphysis and diaphysis to the proximal phalanx. It then becomes progressively larger and denser. It is the first observation of the existence of this bone that is considered applicable as an SMI.

METHODS TO ASSESS SKELETAL MATURITY

A number of methods have been described to assess skeletal maturity. The followings are the most commonly used methods:
- Greulich and Pyle method
- Singer's method of assessment
- Fishman's skeletal maturity indicators
- Bjork, Grave and Brown method
- Maturation assessment by Hagg and Taranger

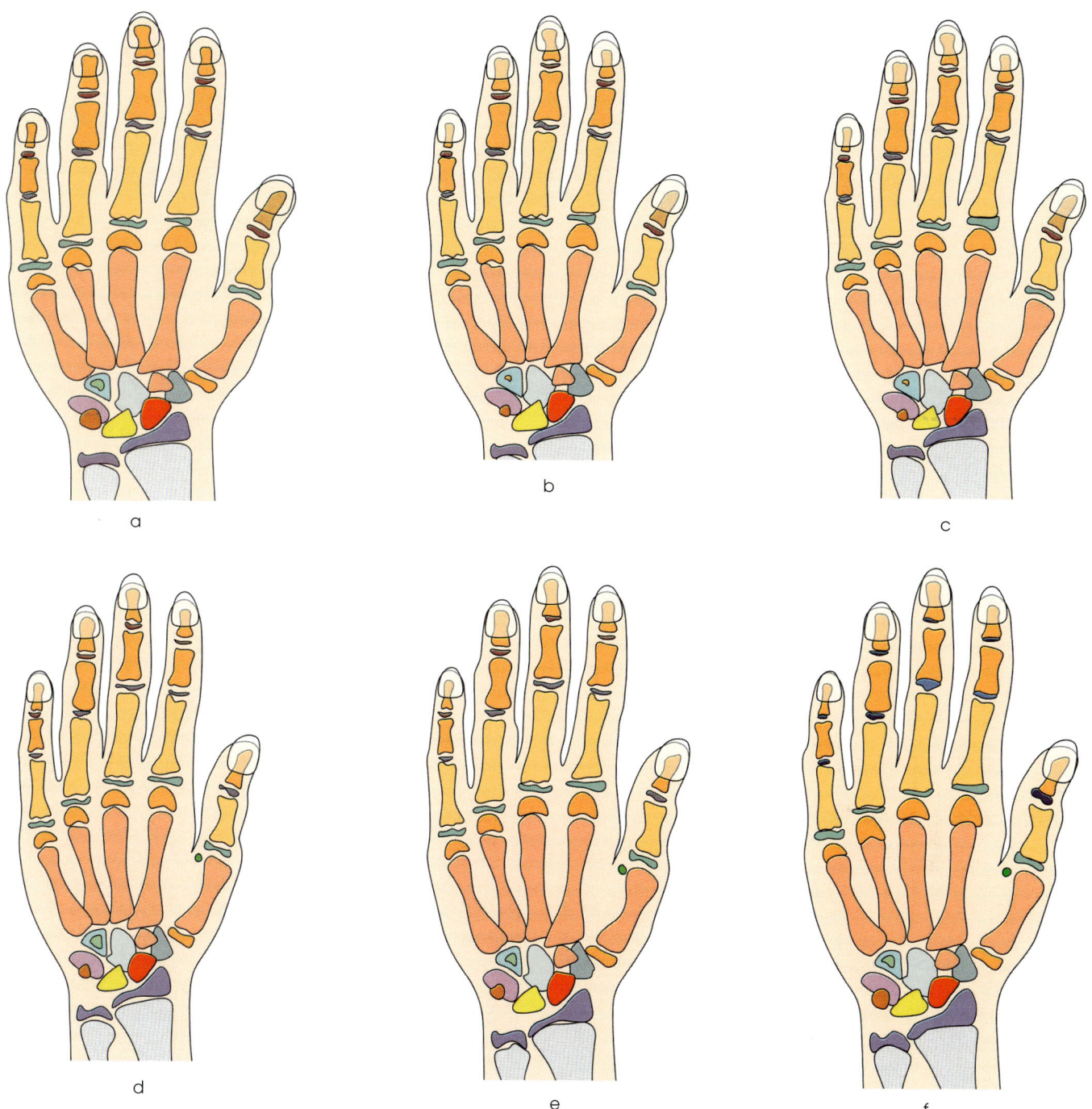

Fig. 9.36: Six stages of hand-wrist development: (a) Stage I: Early; (b) Stage II: Prepubertal; (c) Stage III: Pubertal onset; (d) Stage IV: Pubertal; (e) Stage V: Pubertal deceleration; (f) Stage VI: Growth completion

Greulich and Pyle Method

They published an atlas containing ideal photographs of hand-wrist radiographs of children of different chronological ages. Separate sets of photographs exist for male and female patients. The patient's radiograph is matched on an overall basis with one of the photographs in the atlas.

Singer's Method of Assessment

Julian Singer in 1980 proposed a system of hand-wrist radiograph assessment which helps the clinician to rapidly determine the maturational status of the adolescent patient.

Six stages of hand-wrist development are described (Table 9.4 and Fig. 9.36a to f).

Table 9.4: Six stages of hand-wrist development	
Stage	*Characteristic*
Early	This stage is characterized by absence of the pisiform, absence of hook of the hamate and epiphysis of proximal phalanx of second finger being narrower than its diaphysis
Pre-pubertal	This stage is characterized by initial ossification of hook of the hamate, initial ossification of pisiform and proximal phalanx of second finger being equal to its epiphysis
Pubertal onset	This stage is characterized by beginning of calcification of ulnar sesamoid, increased width of epiphysis of proximal phalanx of the second finger and increased calcification of hook of hamate and pisiform
Pubertal	Characterized by calcification of the sesamoid and capping of the diaphysis of the middle phalanx of third finger by its epiphysis.
Pubertal deceleration	This stage is characterized by calcified ulnar sesamoid, fusion of epiphysis of distal phalanx of third finger with its shafts and epiphysis of radius and ulna not fully fused with respective shafts
Growth completion	No remaining sites seen

Table 9.5 Fishman's skeletal maturity indicators	
SMI 1	Proximal phalanx of the third finger shows equal widths of epiphysis and diaphysis
SMI 2	Width of the epiphysis is equal to that of diaphysis in the middle phalanx of the third finger
SMI 3	Width of the epiphysis is equal to that of diaphysis in the middle phalanx of the fifth finger
SMI 4	Appearance of the adductor seasmoid of the thumb
SMI 5	Capping of epiphysis seen in the distal phalanx of the third finger
SMI 6	Capping of epiphysis seen in the middle phalanx of the third finger
SMI 7	Capping of epiphysis in the middle phalanx of the fifth finger
SMI 8	Fusion of epiphysis and diaphysis in the proximal phalanx of third finger
SMI 9	Fusion of epiphysis and diaphysis in the proximal phalanx of third finger
SMI 10	Fusion of epiphysis and diaphysis in the middle phalanx of third finger
SMI 11	Fusion of epiphysis and diaphysis seen in the radius

Fishman's Skeletal Maturity Indicators

Leonord S Fishman in 1982 made use of four anatomical sites located on the thumb (adductor sesamoid), third finger, fifth finger and radius. Elevan discrete adolescent skeletal maturity indicators (SMIs) were proposed which covered the entire period of adolescent development (Table 9.5). The Fishman's system of interpretation uses four stages of bone maturation which include:

- **MP_3:** The middle phalanx of the third finger, the epiphysis equal in width to diaphysis.
- **S stage:** Appearance of adductor sesamoid of the thumb.
- **MP_{3cap}:** The middle phalanx of the third finger, the epiphysis caps its diaphysis.
- **DP_{3u} and MP_{3u}:** The distal phalanx and the middle phalanx of the third finger, complete fusion of epiphysis.

Maturation Assessment by Hagg and Taranger

They investigated in 1982 a prospective longitudinal study in 212 Swedish children with the data comprised of standing height, tooth emergence, pubertal development and hand–wrist radiographs. It is analyzed by taking annual radiographs between the ages of 6 and 18 years.

Joint of the first finger (S) and certain specified stages of three epiphyseal bones: The middle and distal phalanges of the third finger (MP3 and DP3) and the distal epiphysis of the radius (R).

MP3-F: The epiphysis is as wide as the metaphysis. This stage is attained before the onset of pubertal growth spurt which indicates that more than 80% of the pubertal growth remaining.

MP3-FG: The epiphysis is as wide as metaphysis and there is distinct medial and/or lateral border of the epiphysis forming a line of demarcation at right angles to the distal border. This stage indicates the accelerating slope of the pubertal growth spurt is attained 1 year before or after peak height.

MP3-G: The sides of epiphysis have thickened and also cap their metaphysis, forming a sharp edge distally at one or both sides. This stage is attained at about peak height of pubertal growth spurt.

MP3-H: This stage is characterized by the beginning of fusion of the epiphysis and metaphysis. This stage is indicated by the decelerating slope of the peak height velocity but before end of growth spurt.

MP3-I: This stage is characterized by the completion of fusion of the epiphysis and metaphysis. This is attained at the end of growth spurt in all subjects except a few girls (Fig. 9.37).

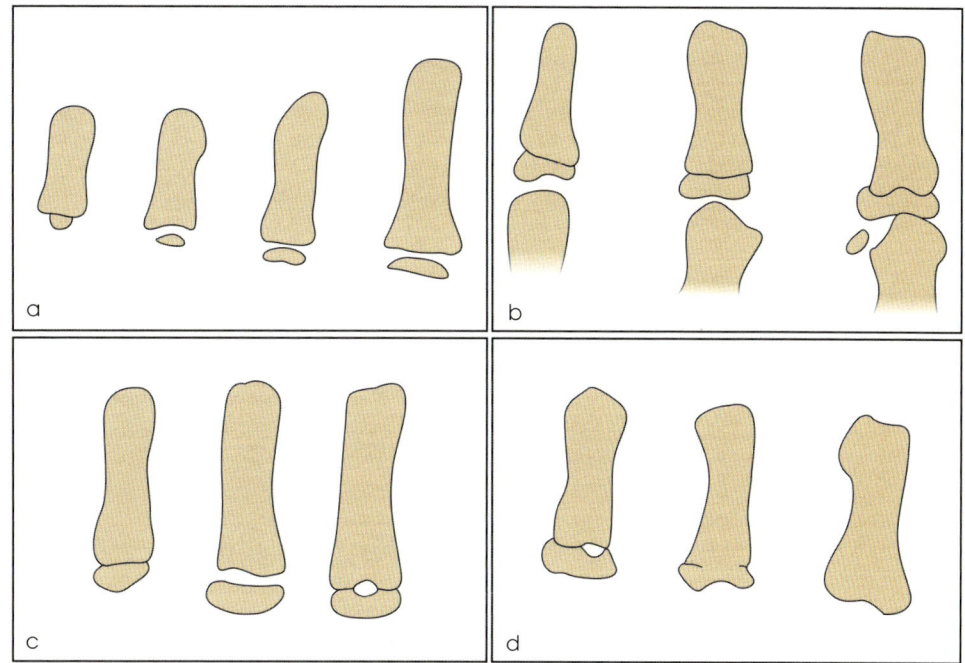

Fig. 9.37: Radiographic identification of skeletal mautrity indicators: (a) Epiphysis equal in width to diaphysis; (b) Appearance of adductor sesamoid of the thumb; (c) Capping of epiphysis; (d) Fusion of epiphysis

Third Finger Distal Phalanx

DP3-I: Fusion of the epiphysis and metaphysis is completed. It indicates the decelerating period of the pubertal growth spurt.

Radius

R-1: Fusion of epiphysis and metaphysis on radius has begun. This stage is attained 1 year before or at the end of growth spurt by about 80% of the girls and 90% of the boys.

R-IJ: Fusion is almost complete except for a small gap still remaining at one or both the margins.

R-J: This is characterized by complete fusion of the epiphysis and metaphysis.

Maturation Assessment by Hagg and Taranger and the KR (Kansal and Rajagopal) Modified MP3 Method

Kansal and Rajagopal modified MP3 indicators further and compared to the cervical vertebrae maturation indices (CVMI) as described by Hassel and Farman.

For the purpose of easy understanding, the parameters studied by Hagg and Taranger are mentioned in blue, additional features observed by Kansal and Rajagopal in pink and Hassel and Farmen in red.

Bjork, Grave and Brown Method (Table 9.6)

They divided skeletal development into nine stages. Each of these stages represents a level of skeletal

maturity. Later in the year 1978, Schopf gave the appropriate chronological age for each of the stages. Skeletal age is assessed by matching the characteristics of patient's radiograph with any of these stages (Fig. 9.38).

CERVICAL VERTEBRAE AS INDICATORS OF SKELETAL MATURITY

A new system of skeletal maturation assessment using the cervical vertebrae was first developed by Hassel and Farman. One of the main advantages of this method is that cervical vertebral maturation can be assessed on lateral cephalogram which is used regularly in orthodontic diagnosis obviates the need for an additional radiograph (Table 9.7).

He developed a method of skeletal maturation assessment in which there are six stages of development using the morphologic characteristics of the cervical (C2, C3 and C4) vertebrae such as:

- Shape of the vertebral bodies
- Height of the vertebral bodies
- Concavity of the lower border of the cervical bodies. The changes in the shape of cervical vertebral bodies of C3 and C4 at each level of skeletal development are assessed.
- At first wedge-shaped, then changed to rectangular, next to square-shaped.

Certain levels of bone development are associated with change in the shape of cervical vertebrae. By this

Table 9.6: Bjork, Grave and Brown method

Stage	Male (years)	Female (years)	Characteristics
1	10.6	8.1	The epiphysis and diaphysis of the proximal phalanx of index finger are equal
2	12	8.1	The epiphysis and diaphysis of the middle phalanx of the middle finger are equal
3	12.6	9.6	Three areas of ossification: a. The hamular process of the hamate exhibits ossifications b. Ossification of pisiform c. The epiphysis and diaphysis of radius are equal
4	13	10.6	This stage marks the beginning of the pubertal growth spurt. It is characterized by a. Initial mineralization of the ulnar seasamoid of the thumb b. Increased ossification of the gamular process of the hamate bone
5	14	11	This stage heralds the peak of the pubertal growth spurt. Capping of diaphysis by the epiphysis is seen in: a. Middle phalanx of the third finger b. Proximal phalanx of the thumb c. Radius
6	15	13	This stage signifies the end of the pubertal growth spurt. It is characterized by union between epiphysis and diaphysis of the distal phalanx of the middle finger
7	15.9	13.3	Union of epiphysis and diaphysis of the proximal phalanx of the little finger occurs
8	15.9	13.9	This stage shows fusion between the epiphysis and diaphysis of the middle phalanx of the middle finger
9	18.5	16	This is the last stage and it signifies the end of skeletal growth. It is characterized by fusion of epiphysis and diaphysis of the radius

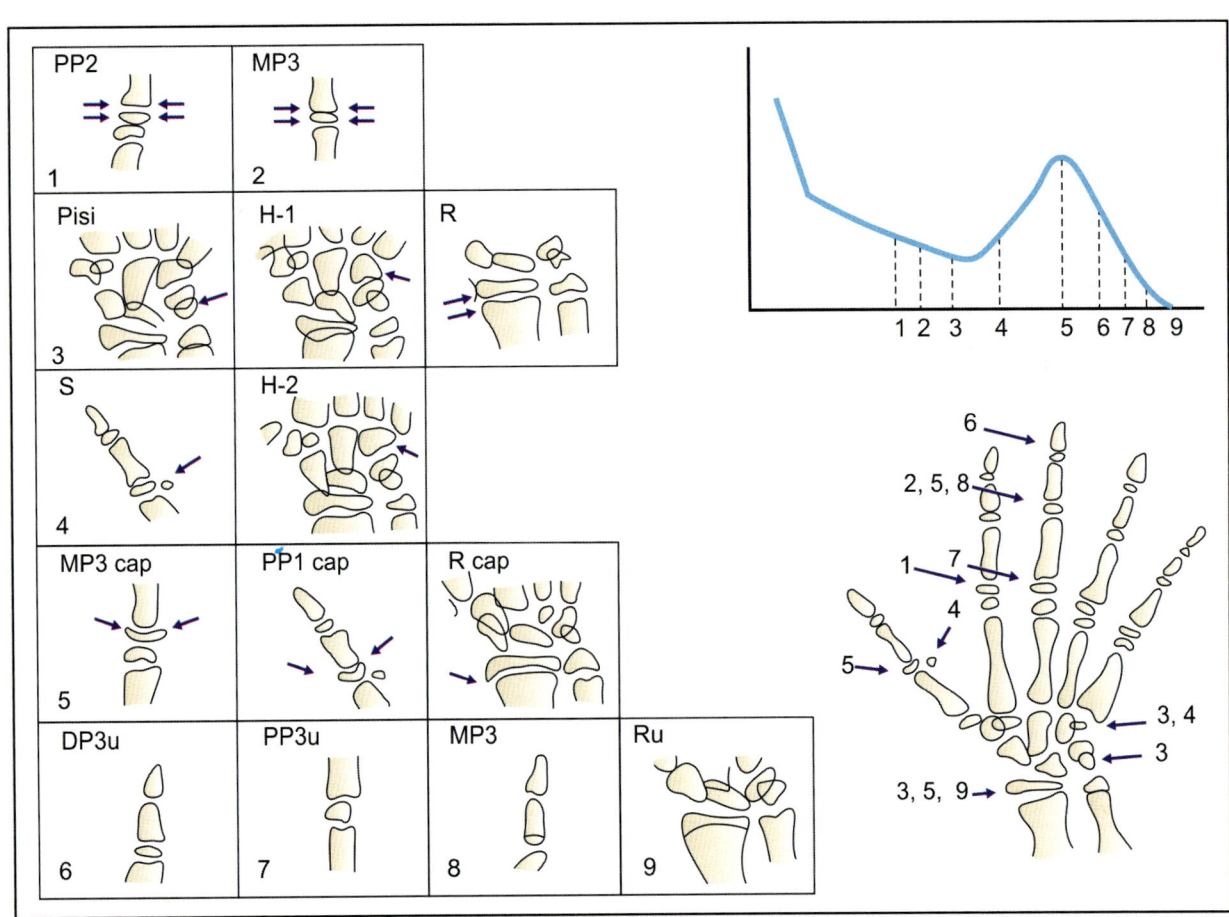

Fig. 9.38: Nine stages represents skeletal maturity

Table 9.7: Stages of cervical vertebrae maturation

Stage	Name	Changes in vertebrae
Stage 1	Initiation	Marks the beginning of adolescent growth. Cervical vertebral bodies and C2, C3 and C4 are wedge shaped with their superior borders tapering posteroanteriorly. Their inferior borders are flat 80–90% of pubertal growth is remaining
Stage 2	Acceleration	Acceleration of growth occurs. Concavities are developing on the lower borders of C2 and C3. Lower border of C4 vertebral body is flat. C3 and C4 assume rectangular shape. 65–85% of pubertal growth remains
Stage 3	Transition	Growth is accelerated to reach peak height velocity. Distinct concavity seen in lower borders of C2 and C3. Concavity is developing in the lower borders of C2, C3 and C4. They are more rectangular in shape. 25–65% pubertal growth is remaining
Stage 4	Deceleration	Deceleration of adolescent growth spurt begins. Distinct concavities seen at the lower borders of all three vertebrae—C2, C3 and C4. C3 and C4 are more square in shape.10–15% pubertal growth remaining
Stage 5	Maturation	Cervical vertebrae attain maturity. Concavities at lower borders of C2, C3 and C4 become more accentuated. C3 and C4 are more square in shape. 5–10% pubertal growth remaining
Stage 6	Completion	Adolescent growth is nearly complete. More accentuated concavities are seen at lower borders of C2, C3 and C4. Shape of C3 and C4 is square with greater vertical dimension than width. Pubertal growth is complete with no more growth potential remaining.

observation, Hassel and Farman proposed 6 stages of cervical vertebrae maturation (Fig. 9.39).

TEETH MINERALIZATION AS SKELETAL MATURITY INDICATOR

The stages of calcification of the left mandibular canine could be used as a first level diagnostic tool to estimate the timing of the pubertal growth spurt. Relationships between the stages of tooth mieralization of the mandibular canine appear to correlate better with ossification stages than the other teeth.

The teeth are rated according to the technique described by Demirjian's stages of dental calcification, where the development of the tooth is divided into 8 defined stages identified by the letters A to H. The E to H stages are taken to study for skeletal maturation (Fig. 9.40).

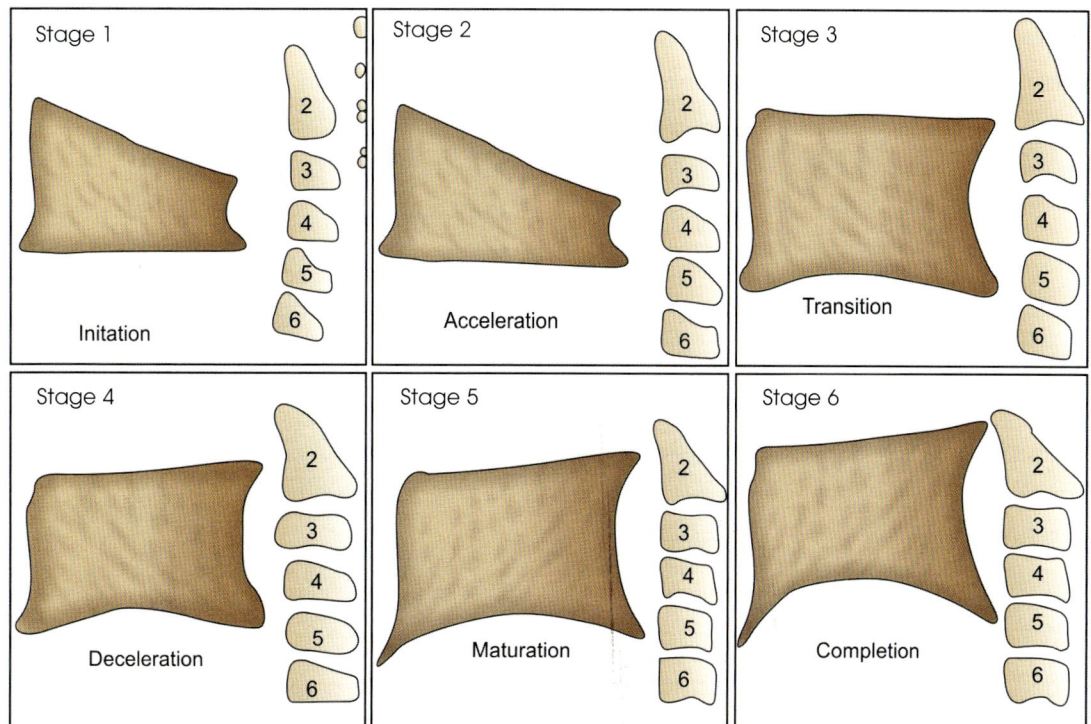

Fig. 9.39: Stages of cervical vertebrae maturation

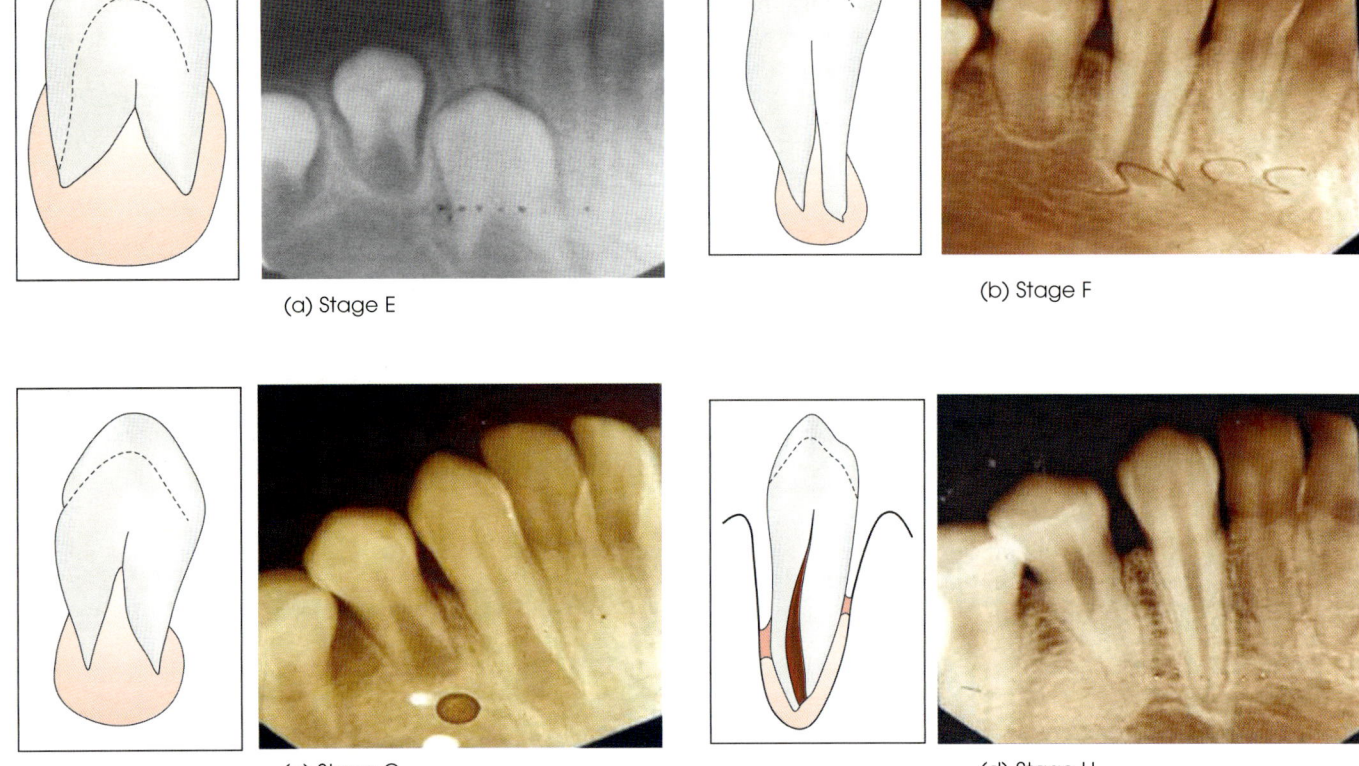

Fig. 9.40: Demirjian's stages of mandibular canine calcification: (a) Stage E: The walls of the pulp chamber form straight lines whose continuity is broken by the presence of the pulp horn. The root length is less than the crown height; (b) Stage F: The walls of the pulp chamber now form a more or less isosceles triangle. The apex ends in a funnel shape. The root length is equal to or greater than the crown height; (c) Stage G: The walls of the root canal are now parallel and their apical end is still is partially open; (d) Stage H: The apical end of the root canal is completely closed. The periodontal membrane has a uniform width around the root and the apex

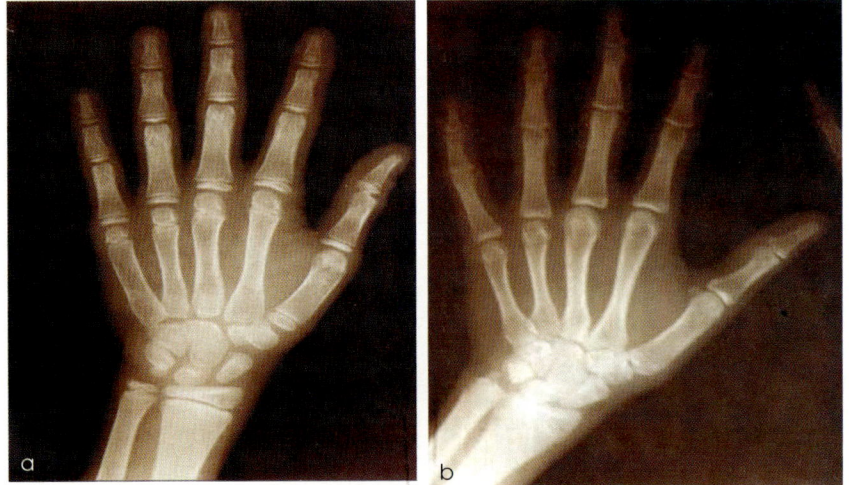

Fig. 9.41: (a) Stage G is coincident with capping; (b) Stage H is coincident with fusion

Stage E: The walls of the pulp chamber form straight lines whose continuity is broken by the presence of the pulp horn. The root length is less than the crown height.

Stage F: The walls of the pulp chamber now form a more or less isosceles triangle. The apex ends in a funnel shaped. The root length is equal to or greater than the crown height.

Stage G: The walls of the root canal are now parallel and their apical end is still partially open.

Stage H: The apical end of the root canal is completely closed. The periodontal membrane has a uniform width around the root and the apex.

Stages E and F are coincident with the epiphyseal widening in the third finger—proximal, middle phalanx and middle phalanx of the fifth finger.

Stage G is coincident with the ossification of adductor sesamoid, capping of third finger—middle phalanx, distal phalanx and fifth finger middle phalanx indicating its association with accelerative phase of growth (Fig. 9.41a).

Stage H is coincident with fusion of proximal, middle, distal phalanx of third finger and fusion of radius indicating its association with decelerative phase of growth (Fig. 9.41b).

BIBLIOGRAPHY

1. Demirjian, Buschang, Tanguay, and Patters: Interrelationship among measures of somatic, skeletal, dental and sexual maturity. Am J Orthod 1985; vol 433–438.
2. Fishman LS. Radiographic evaluation of skeletal maturity. Angle Orthod 1982; 52:88–112.
3. Grave KC, Brown T. Skeletal ossification and adolescent growth spurt. Am J Orthod 1976; 69:611–9.
4. Hassel and Farman: Skeletal maturation evaluation. Am J Orthod 1955;58–66.

PREVIOUS YEAR'S UNIVERSITY QUESTIONS
Essay
1. Describe the anatomy of hand–wrist X-ray
2. Discuss Demirjian's stages of mandibular canine calcification with suitable illustrations.

Short Questions
1. Fishman's skeletal maturity indicators
2. Cervical vertebrae
3. Carpal bones
4. Sesamoid

MCQs
1. *The following are biologic indicators of maturity, except:*
   a. Dental age
   b. Chronological age
   c. Skeletal age
   d. Sexual age   **(Ans: b)**

2. *All the following are ideal requirements of a maturity indicator, except:*
   a. Radiation exposure should be minimal
   b. Criteria should be different for boys and girls
   c. The stages of maturity should be well defined and easily identifiable
   d. It should be cost-effective   **(Ans: b)**

3. *Skeletal age for assessing biologic maturity is useful:*
   a. In childhood
   b. For adolescence only
   c. Throughout the postnatal growth period
   d. From birth to early adolescence   **(Ans: c)**

4. *Hand-wrist region consists of a total of:*
   a. 51 bones
   b. 29 bones
   c. 27 bones
   d. 13 bones   **(Ans: b)**

5. *The long bones of hand-wrist region are:*
   a. Trapezium and trapezoid
   b. Capitates and hamate
   c. Radius and ulna
   d. All of the above   **(Ans: c)**

6. *The skeleton of hand-wrist region is made up of the following groups of bones, except:*
   a. Distal ends of radius and ulna
   b. Carpals and metacarpals
   c. Phalanges
   d. Proximal ends of radius and ulna   **(Ans: d)**

7. *Carpal bones are arranged in:*
   a. Two rows: left and right
   b. Two rows: proximal and distal
   c. Three rows: left, right and center
   d. None of the above   **(Ans: b)**

8. *Proximal row of carpal bones is made of:*
   a. Scaphoid, lunate
   b. Trapezium and trapezoid
   c. Triquetrum and pisiform
   d. Both a and c   **(Ans: d)**

9. *The distal row of carpal bones is made of:*
   a. Trapezium and trapezoid
   b. Capitates and hamate
   c. Pisiform and hamular process
   d. Both a and b   **(Ans: d)**

10. *The phalanges are the small bones that form the skeleton of the fingers and there are a total of:*
   a. 15 phalanges
   b. 14 phalanges

c. 5 phalanges

d. 10 phalanges **(Ans: b)**

11. *Each digit of the hand has how many phalanges?*
    a. 3 phalanges except thumb which has 2 phalanges
    b. 3 phalanges except thumb which has 1 phalanges
    c. All digits have 3 phalanges each
    d. All digits have 2 phalanges each except thumb which has 3 phalanges **(Ans: a)**

12. *Sesamoid bone is a:*
    a. Long bone of hand
    b. One of carpal bone
    c. Small modular bone
    d. One of metacarpal bone **(Ans: c)**

13. *Which is the recent method of skeletal maturity of indicator gaining popularity?*
    a. Hand-wrist radiographs
    b. Cervical vertebrae assessment on lateral cephalogram
    c. Pelvic radiographs
    d. All of the above **(Ans: b)**

14. *Following are the methods to assess skeletal age using hand-wrist radiographs, except:*
    a. Grave and Brown method
    b. Greenwich and Pyle method
    c. Lamparski method
    d. Ringer's method **(Ans: c)**

15. *Growth modification procedures are best carried out in which stage of singer's method?*

a. Stage 1(early)

b. Stage 3 (pubertal onset)

c. Stage 4 (pubertal onset)

d. Stage 2 (prepubertal) **(Ans: d)**

16. *Who first developed a method for skeletal maturity assessment using cervical vertebrae?*
    a. Hassel and Farman
    b. Lamparski
    c. San Roman
    d. Tarranger **(Ans: a)**

17. *Hassel and Farman cervical vertebrae maturation method has how many stages of development?*
    a. 9
    b. 6
    c. 11
    d. 5 **(Ans: b)**

18. *In Hassel and Farman method, the cervical vertebrae studied are:*
    a. C1, C2 and C3
    b. C2, C3 and C4
    c. C3, C4 and C5
    d. C2 and C3 **(Ans: b)**

19. *In Hassel and Farman method, which of the following morphologic characteristics of the cervical vertebrae are taken into account for assessing skeletal maturity?*
    a. Shape of the vertebral bodies
    b. Height of vertebral bodies
    c. Concavity, if the lower border of the cervical bodies
    d. All of the above **(Ans: d)**

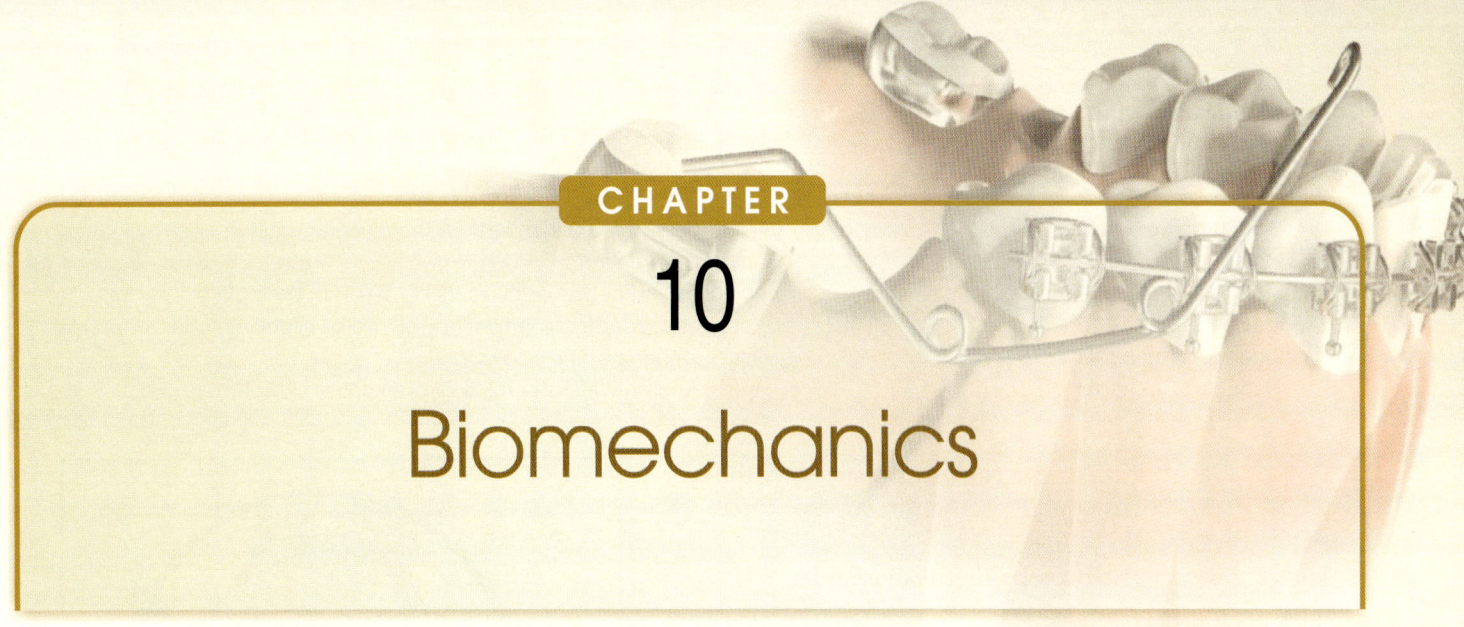

10.1 MECHANICS OF TOOTH MOVEMENT

Chapter Outline

- Introduction
- Mechanics
- Center of resistance
- Couple

- Center of rotation
- Moment to force ratio
- Different types of tooth movement
- Forces according to their duration

INTRODUCTION

An understanding and proper application of the biomechanical principles enables efficient tooth movement in the shortest possible duration and with minimal tissue damage.

Newton's First Law

Everybody continues in its state of rest or uniform motion in a straight line, unless it is compelled to change the state by forces impressed upon it, and teeth are no exception.

MECHANICS

Mechanics is defined as that branch of engineering science that describes the effect of force on a body. A clear understanding of the theories of mechanics has potential applications in three areas:

1. Precise application of forces
2. A better understanding of clinical and histological response to various magnitudes of forces
3. Improving the design of orthodontic forces
    The response of a tooth to an applied force can be at three levels:
1. Clinical

2. Cellular
3. Stress-strain activity within the investing tissues
    For a better understanding of mechanics, the following terminologies should be known:
- Force
- Center of resistance
- Moment
- Couple
- Center of rotation

Force

Force is a load or external influence applied to a body that changes or tends to change the position of the body. Force types are:
- Compression (squeezing together)
- Tension (stretch a body)
- Shear force (lateral shifting of body)
    Force is measured in 'grams' or 'ounces'.

Center of Resistance (Table 10.1)

- Center of resistance is defined as the point in the object at which the resistance to movement is at maximum.

Table 10.1: Center of resistance for different structures	
Single rooted tooth	1/3rd to 1/4th the distance from the alveolar crest to apex
Molars	Apical to furcation
Maxillary dentition	Apical to and between the roots of 1–2 mm premolars
Maxilla	Posterosuperior to zygomaxillary suture or slightly inferior to orbitale
Intrusion of upper anterior	Distal to the lateral incisor roots
Mandibular dentition	Apical and between the roots of premolars

- If a force is applied to the center of resistance, the whole body moves equally in the direction of force applied.

The center of resistance of a tooth is variable.

It depends on:

- Root morphology
- Number of roots
- Level of alveolar bone support
- Root length

Factors which can change the position of the center of resistance are the root length and alveolar bone height. Longer the root the center of resistance will be placed more apically. Likewise, if the alveolar crest is higher, the center of resistance will be placed more coronally.

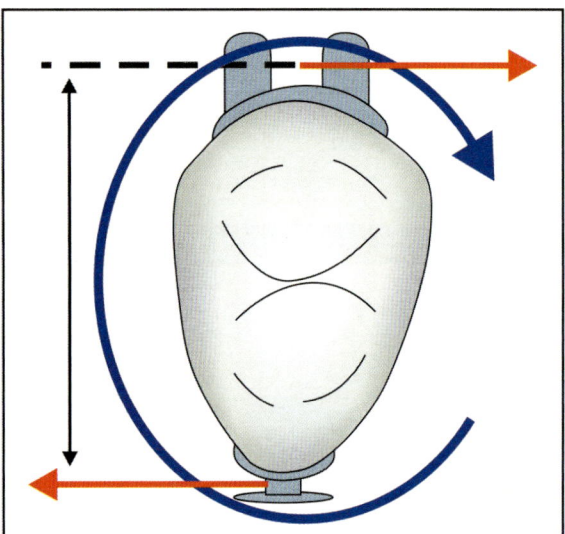

Fig. 10.1: Couple

Couple (Fig. 10.1)

Couple is two forces which are equal in magnitude but opposite in direction. Application of two forces in this manner produces pure moment, because the bodily movements get cancelled as the forces are acting in opposite direction. Rotation can be achieved by applying a couple.

If the two forces of the couple act on opposite side of the center of resistance, their effect is additive. However, if they are on the same side of the center of resistance, their effect is subtractive.

Center of Rotation (Fig. 10.2 and Table 10.2)

Center of rotation can be varied by applying a force and couple. Center of rotation differ for each tooth movement. Center of rotation is any point around which rotation occur when the tooth is being moved

MOMENT TO FORCE RATIO (Fig. 10.3)

Moment

Moment is defined as the tendency or measure of a tendency to produce movement around a particular axis. Moment is force acting at a distance. It is calculated by the formula:

$$\text{Moment} = f \times d$$

- Where 'f' is the magnitude of force.

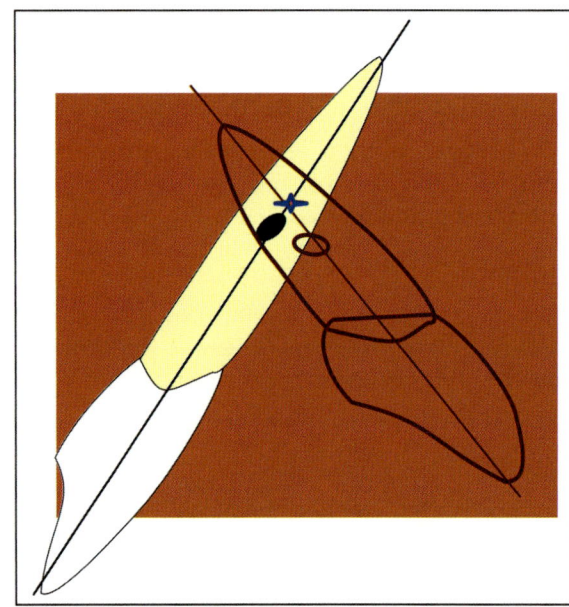

Fig. 10.2: Center of rotation

- 'd' is the perpendicular distance between the point of force application and center of resistance.
- The unit of moment is 'grams millimeter'.
- When an orthodontic force is applied, a moment is created when line of force does not pass through the center of resistance.

Table 10.2: Type of tooth movement and center of rotation

Tooth movement	Center of rotation
Uncontrolled tipping	Between center of resistance and apex
Controlled tipping	At the root apex
Bodily tooth movement	At infinity
Root movement	At incisal edge
Rotation	No net force acts at crest

Table 10.3: Tooth movement and moment to force ratio

Tooth movement	Moment to force ratio
Uncontrolled tipping	0:1 to 5:1
Controlled tipping	7:1
Translation	10:1
Root movement	12:1

- When a moment is created, the force tends to move the object plus it tends to rotate the object through the center of resistance.
- By altering the moment to force ratio, the desired tooth movement can be achieved.

The relationship between the applied force system and the type of tooth movement can be explained by moment to force ratio. M/F ratio determines the center of rotation and thereby the type of tooth movement also (Table 10.3).

DIFFERENT TYPES OF TOOTH MOVEMENT

Tipping (Table 10.4)

Tipping, in practice, is the easiest type of tooth movement. When a single force is applied to a bracket

Table 10.4: Optimum orthodontic force for different types of tooth movement

Tipping	60
Bodily movement	75–120
Root uprighting	50–100
Rotation	35–60
Extrusion	35–60
Intrusion	10–20

on a round wire, the tooth tips about its center of rotation, located in the middle of the root, close to its center of resistance.

Controlled and Uncontrolled Tipping

Uncontrolled tipping: In this situation, when force is applied the crown moves in one direction and root moves in the opposite direction. Here, center of rotation lies near to center of resistance. This is referred as uncontrolled tipping (Fig. 10.4).

Controlled tipping: In this situation, crown moves in the direction of force but the root position remains the same or gets minimally displaced. Here, center of rotation lies at apex of the root (Fig. 10.5).

Translation: In this situation, tooth moves bodily, e.g. both crown and root portion of tooth moves bodily in the direction of force. Here, center of rotation lies at infinity. All the points in the tooth move by same distance in the same direction in translation (Fig. 10.6).

Root movement: In this situation, root moves in the direction of force but the crown position remains the

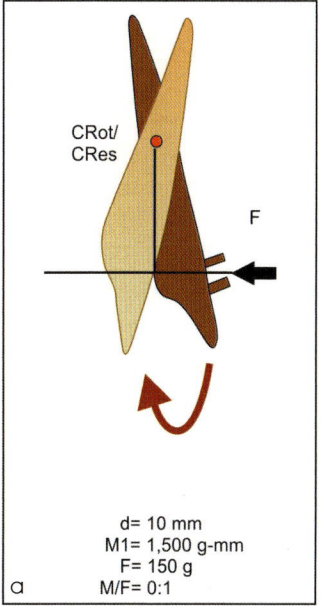
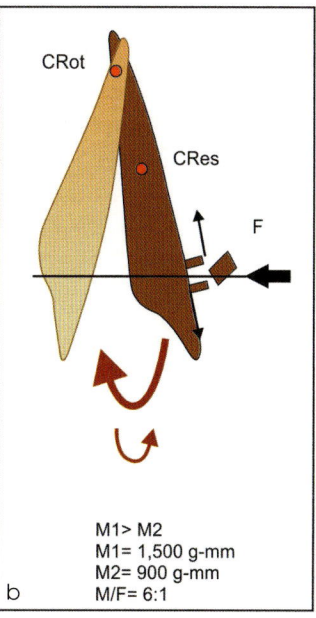
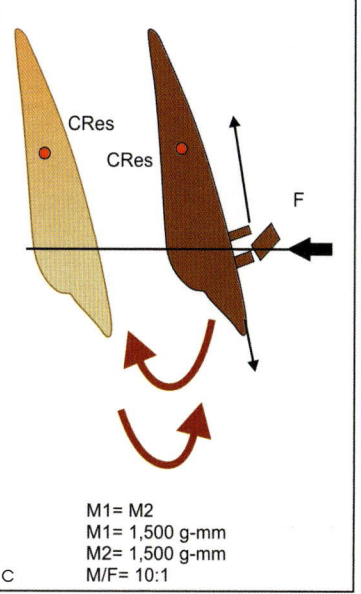
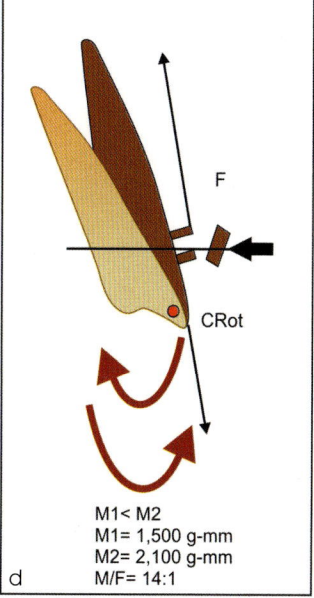

Fig. 10.3: M/F ratio

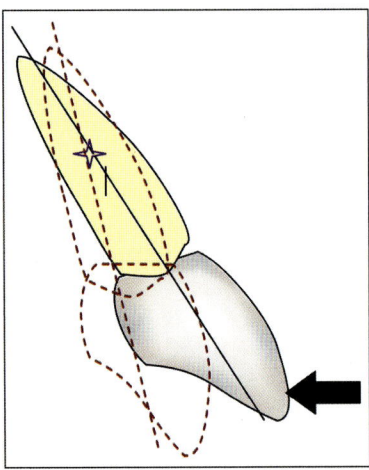

Fig. 10.4: Uncontrolled tipping

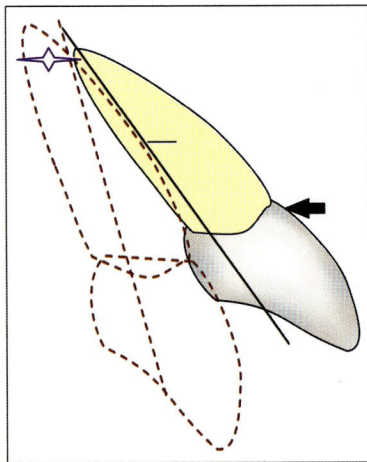

Fig. 10.5: Controlled tipping

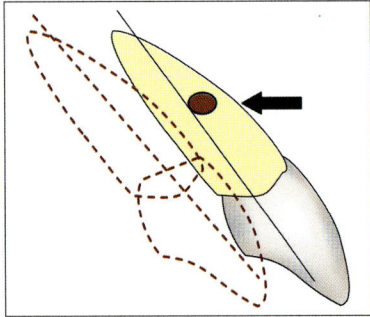

Fig. 10.6: Translation

same or gets minimally displaced. Here, center of rotation lies at incisal edge of the crown (Fig. 10.7).

Intrusion: Intrusion is the bodily displacement of a tooth along axis in an apical direction. It requires least amount of forces and is most sensitive (Fig. 10.8 and Table 10.4).

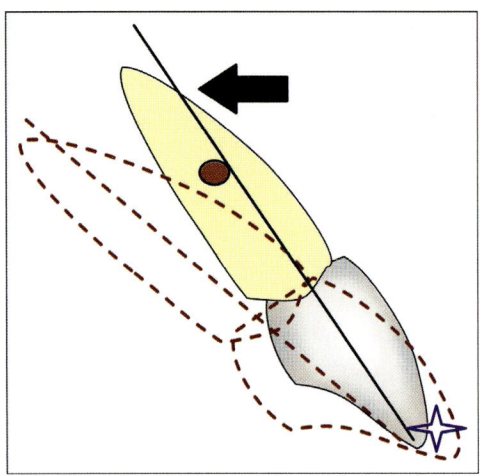

Fig. 10.7: Root movement

Extrusion: Extrusion is the bodily displacement of a tooth along its long axis in an occlusal direction (Fig. 10.8 and Table 10.4).

Uprighting

The axial inclination of teeth is such that the crowns of these teeth will be tipped abnormally in mesiodistal direction and the roots tipped in the opposite direction. Tipping of these roots back to get an acceptable mesiodistal orientation is termed uprighting.

Forces According to their Duration (Fig. 10.9)

Continuous Forces

A continuous force can be obtained by using wires with low load/deflection rate and high working range. In the leveling phase, where there is considerable variation in level between teeth, it is advantageous to use these wires to control anchorage and maintain longer intervals between appointments.

Continuous force depreciates slowly, but it never diminishes to zero within two activation periods (clinically, this period is usually 1 month); thus, constant and controlled tooth movement results. For example, the force applied by nickel titanium (NiTi) open coil springs is a continuous force.

Interrupted Forces

Interrupted forces are reduced to zero shortly after they have been applied. If the initial force is relatively light, the tooth will move a small amount by direct resorption and then will remain in that position until the appliance is reactivated.

After the application of interrupted forces, the surrounding tissues undergo a repair process until the second activation takes place. The best example of an

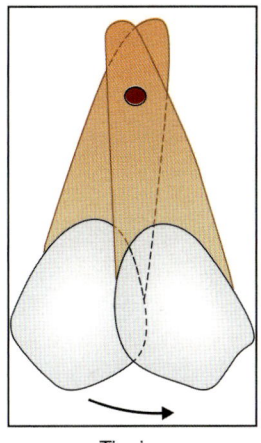
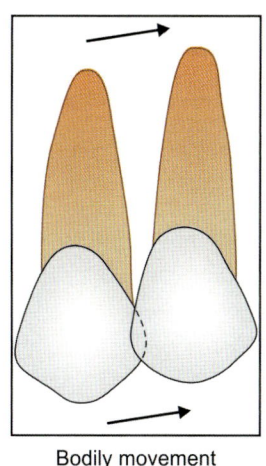
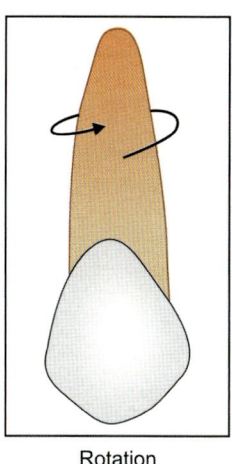
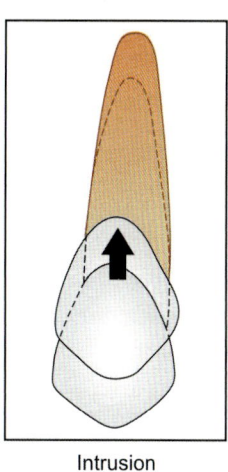
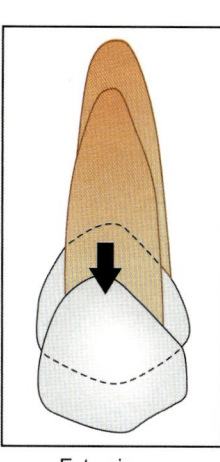

| Tipping | Bodily movement | Rotation | Intrusion | Extrusion |

Fig. 10.8: Different types of tooth movement

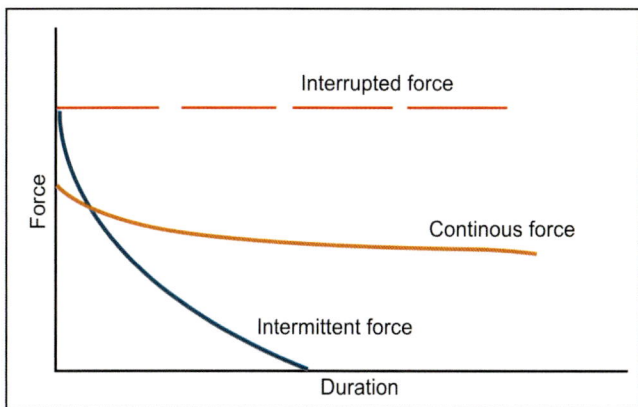

Fig. 10.9: Forces according to their duration

active element that applies interrupted force is the rapid expansion screw.

Intermittent Forces

During intermittent force application, the force is reduced to zero when the patient removes the appliance. When it is placed back into the mouth, it continues from its previous level, reducing slowly. Intermittent forces are applied by extraoral appliances.

BIBLIOGRAPHY

1. Textbook of Orthodontics by Sridhar Premkumar.
2. Textbook of Orthodontics by SI Bhalajhi.

PREVIOUS YEAR'S UNIVERSITY QUESTIONS

Essay

1. Discuss different types of tooth movement and its center of rotation.
2. What is the optimum orthodontic force for different types of tooth movement?

Short Questions

1. Intermittent force
2. Center of rotation
3. Center of resistance
4. Couple of force

MCQs

1. *The center of resistance for maxilla is about:*
   a. 5–10 mm inferior to the orbitale
   b. Between roots of maxillary molars
   c. The center of maxillary arch
   d. 1–2 mm apical to furcation of maxillary molar
      (Ans: a)

2. *A force couple brings about:*
   a. A bodily tooth movement
   b. Pure rotation
   c. Tipping movement
   d. Intrusion of tooth   **(Ans: b)**

3. *Movement of tooth around mesiodistal axis is called:*
   a. Tipping
   b. Torquing
   c. Rotation
   d. Translation   **(Ans: a)**

4. *During uncontrolled tipping, stresses in the periodontal ligament are:*
   a. Uniformly disturbed all around the tooth
   b. Concentrated near apex
   c. Concentrated near cervical areas
   d. Not uniform and are concentrated near apex and cervical area   **(Ans: d)**

10.2 BIOLOGY OF TOOTH MOVEMENT

Chapter Outline

- Introduction
- Biological control of tooth movement
- Theories of tooth movement
- Phases of tooth movement

- Biochemical control of tooth movement
- Interventions for accelerating orthodontic tooth movement
- Root resorption

INTRODUCTION

Aulius Cornelius Celsus advocated that the teeth can be moved by finger pressure. The modern era in dentistry began in 1728 with the publications of the first comprehensive book on dentistry by Fauchard who described a procedure of **"Instant orthodontics"** whereby he aligned ectopically erupted incisors by bending the alveolar bone. A century and a half later in 1888, **Farrar** tried to explain that the teeth move either the orthodontic forces bend the alveolar bone or they resorb it. The bone resorption idea of Farrar was proven by Sandstedt in 1904. In 1932, **Schwarz** concluded that an optimal force in smaller in magnitude than that capable of occluding PDL capillaries, occlusion of these blood vessels, he reasoned, would lead to necrosis of surrounding tissues, which is harmful and slow down the velocity of tooth movement. This opinion was suggested by **Reitan** in 1971.

Oppenheim in 1911 was the first person to study the tissue changes in the bone incident to orthodontic tooth movement. Orthodontic treatment is based on the principle that if prolonged pressure is applied to a tooth, the tooth movement will occur as the bone around the tooth remodels. Bone is selectively removed in some areas and added in other. In essence, the tooth moves through the bone carrying its attachment apparatus with it as the socket of the tooth migrates (Fig. 10.10)

BIOLOGIC CONTROL OF TOOTH MOVEMENT

Orthodontic tooth movement is a complex and wonderful process as one calcified structure (tooth) moves over another calcified structure (bone). The final event which is responsible for this movement is remodeling. To initiate remodeling, the orthodontic force which is mechanical energy should be converted into a biological signal. This process of conversion of energy is called **transduction**. It is based on how these signals are elicited to induce tooth movement, various theories of tooth movement have been put forward.

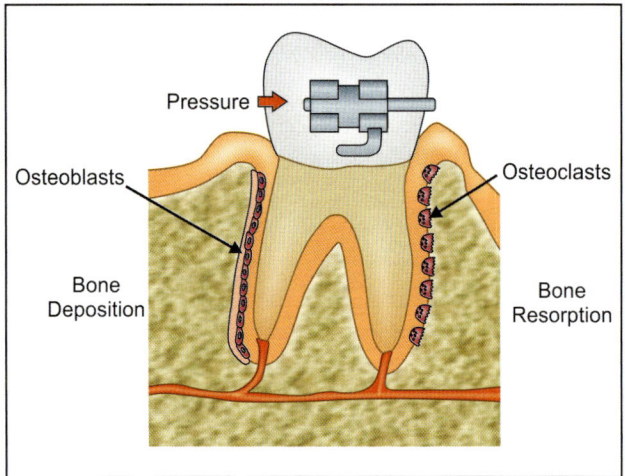

Fig. 10.10: Tooth movement

Definition: The optimum orthodontic force is one that produces maximum tooth movement in the desired direction with minimum damage to the supporting tooth tissues and without any discomfort to the patient.

The orthodontic force should not occlude the blood vessels in the periodontal ligament. Ideally, it should be less than the capillary pulse pressure. According to Schwarz and Oppenheim, the optimum orthodontic force should be in the range of 20–26 gm/cm² of root surface. Schwarz further stated that optimum orthodontic force for tooth movement as 15–20 mmHg of vascular pressure.

THEORIES OF TOOTH MOVEMENT

- Mechanochemical hypothesis (Flowchart 10.1)
- Pressure tension theory/classic theory
- Piezoelectric theory/bone-bending piezoelectric theory
- Blood flow theory/fluid dynamic theory

Two possible control elements, biologic electricity and pressure tension in the periodontal ligament that affects blood flow are contrasted in two major theories of orthodontic tooth movement.

Piezoelectric Theory

It relates tooth movement at least in part to changes in bone metabolism controlled by the electric signals that are produced when alveolar bone flexes and bends.

Pressure Tension Theory

Schwarz proposed the pressure tension theory in 1932. The view of tooth movement shows three stages:

1. Alterations in blood flow associated with pressure within PDL.
2. The formation and/or release of chemical messengers.
3. Activation of cells.

It relates tooth movement to cellular changes produced by chemical messengers, traditionally thought to be generated by alterations in blood flow through PDL.

The two theories are neither incompatible nor mutually exclusive from a contemporary perspective; it appears that both mechanisms may play a part in the biologic control of tooth movement.

According to this theory, whenever a tooth is subjected to an orthodontic force, it results in areas of pressure and tension. The area of the periodontium in the direction of tooth movement is under pressure while the area of periodontium opposite to the tooth movement is under tension. The areas of pressure show bone resorption while the areas of tension show bone deposition (Fig. 10.11).

The histological changes occurring during tooth movement vary according to the magnitude and duration of the force applied. The histological changes occurring during tooth movement can be described under the following headings (Fig. 10.12):

* Changes following application of mild orthodontic forces (Table 10.5)
* Changes following application of excessive orthodontic forces

Flowchart 10.1: Mechanochemical hypothesis

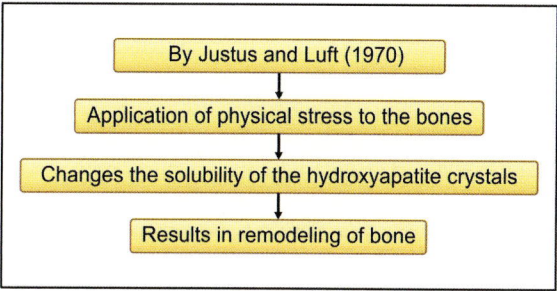

Changes following Application of Mild Orthodontic Forces

Changes on pressure side (Table 10.5): The periodontal ligament gets slightly compressed on the pressure side. As the mild forces are not sufficient to occlude the blood vessels of the periodontal ligament, vessels may dilate and there will be recruitment of osteoclasts to that area of periodontal ligament. The osteoclasts will cause resorption of the alveolar bone immediately adjacent to the periodontal ligament. This kind of resorption where the periosteal bone from the inner wall of the socket is resorbed, is called frontal resorption or direct resorption (Fig. 10.13).

Changes on tension side: An area of tension is created in the supporting structure of the tooth, opposite to the direction of force. The periodontal ligament is stretched in this area and vascularity is increased. Increased vascularity leads to mobilization of osteoblasts and fibroblasts in those areas. The osteoblasts lay down a layer of osteoid bone immediately adjacent to the lamina dura.

To summarize:

* Hyperemia within the periodontal ligament, dilatation of the blood vessels.
* Increased number of osteoclasts and osteoblasts.
* Lamina dura resorbed from the area next to periodontal ligament on pressure side—frontal or direct bone resorption.
* Deposition of osteoid bone on the tension side which calcifies subsequently.
* Tooth movement occurs due to bone resorption and deposition.
* No root resorption.

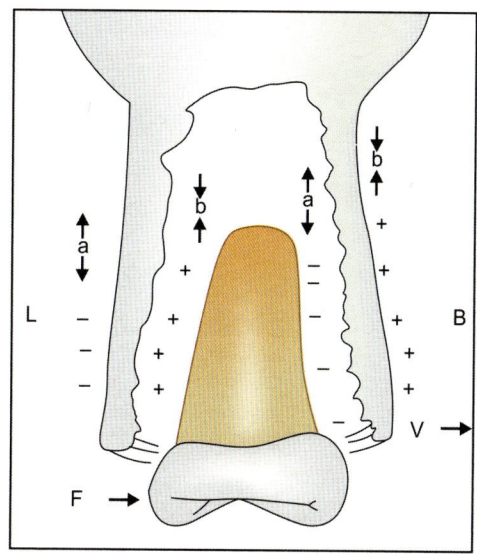

Fig 10.11: Pressure/tension area

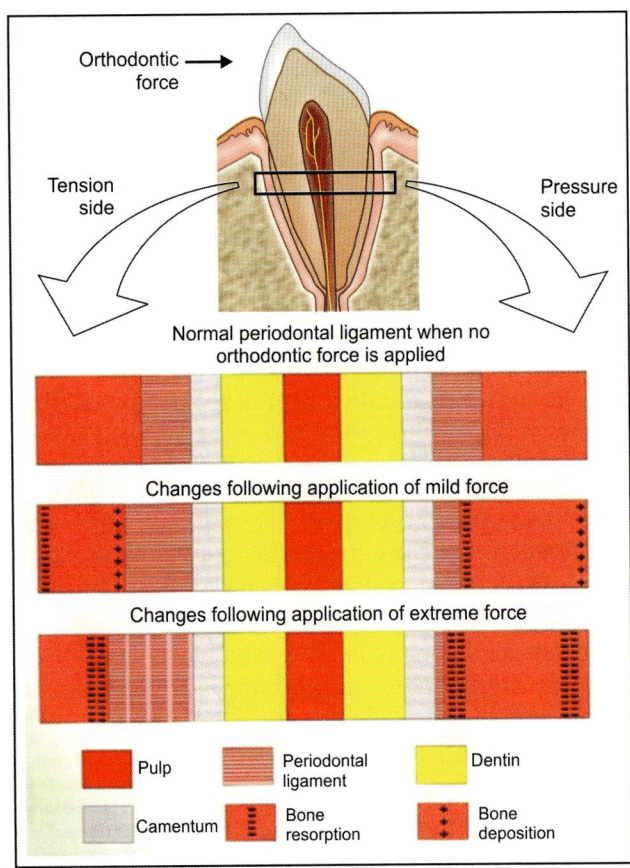

Fig. 10.12: Histological changes during tooth movement

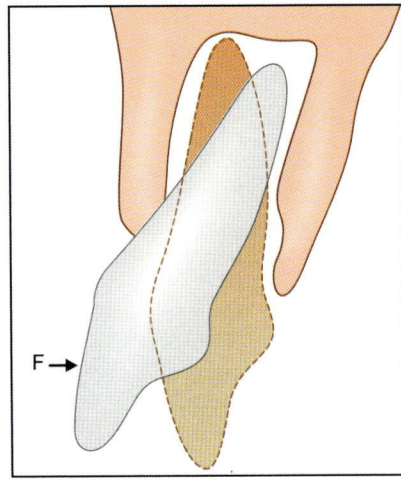

Fig. 10.13: Frontal resorption

Changes following Application of Excessive Orthodontic Forces (Table 10.5)

Changes on pressure side: On applying excessive forces, the periodontal ligament on the pressure side is extremely compressed causing contact between the tooth and the alveolar bone. This leads to occlusion of blood vessels in that area. As a result, the periodontal

ligament in these areas gets deprived of nutritional supply and begins to show regressive changes with cell-free areas called hyalinization (Fig. 10.14). Due to ischemia and hyalinization, there is no recruitment of osteoclasts in the pressure side. No resorption occurs on the periosteal surface of the socket and thus tooth does not move for a period of time. Nonvitality and ankylosis of the tooth are other possible consequences of extreme orthodontic force.

Changes on tension side: The periodontal ligament is overstretched leading to tearing of blood vessels and ischemia. When excessive force is applied, there is an increased osteoclastic activity as compared to osteoblastic activity and thus the tooth may become loosened in its socket.

Thus, if the force applied is severely excessive and prolonged, the periodontal ligament in the area of pressure will be deprived of its blood supply and there

Table 10.5 Physiologic response to sustained pressure against a tooth

Light pressure	Heavy pressure	Event
< 1 sec	< 1 sec	PDL fluid incompressible, alveolar bone bends, piezoelectric signal generated
1–2 sec	1–2 sec	PDL fluid expressed, tooth moves within PDL space
3–5 sec		Blood vessels within PDL partially compressed on pressure side, dilated on tension side; PDL fibres and cells mechanically distorted
Minutes		Blood flow altered, oxygen tension begins to change; prostaglandins and cytokines released.
Hours		Metabolic changes affect the cellular activity
– 4 hrs		Cellular differentiation begins within PDL
– 2 days		Tooth movement begins- remodeling of bony socket
	3–5 sec	Occluded blood vessels within PDL on pressure side
	Minutes	Blood flow cut off to compressed PDL area
	Hours	Cell death in compressed area
	3–5 days	Cell differentiation in adjacent narrow & undermining resorption begins
	7–14 days	Tooth movement occurs

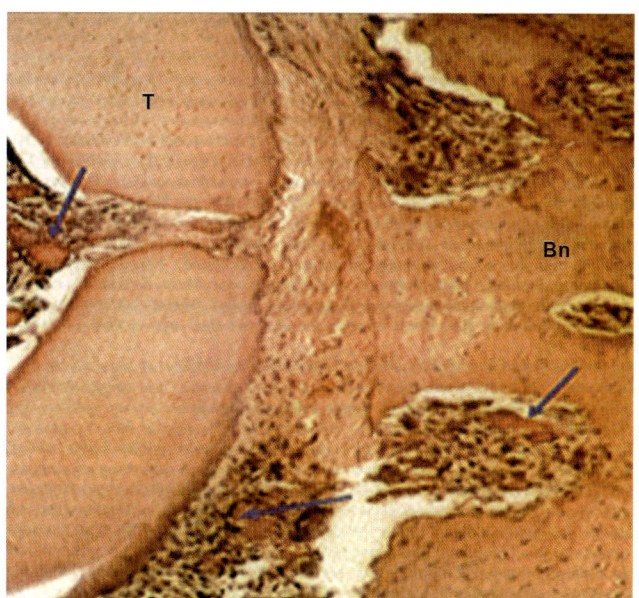

Fig. 10.14: Microscopic features of hyalinization

may be necrosis of the ligament, with massive undermining resorption (Fig. 10.15) and possibly resorption of the root surface of the tooth. Application of very heavy orthodontic forces causes pain, loosening of the tooth in its socket and healing may occur by ankylosis of the tooth to the alveolar bone.

To summarize:

- Compression of periodontal ligament and occlusion of blood vessels in the areas of pressure and ischemia.
- Formation of wide zones of hyalinization and extended lag period.
- No frontal resorption and no immediate tooth movement.
- Increased endosteal vascularity and endosteal resorption of the socket wall under the hyalinized area-undermining resorption

- Eventually tooth moves as a result of this undermining resorption.
- Relatively rapid tooth movement will bone deposition in the areas of tension.
- Grossly excessive forces may cause root resorption, loosening, nonvitality and ankylosis of the tooth.

Bone-bending Piezoelectric Theory

There are different types of electric signals generated:
1. Piezoelectricity
2. Streaming potential
3. Bioelectric potential

Piezoelectric effect was described by Fukada and Yasuda in 1957. When orthodontic force is applied to teeth, it causes deformation or bending of the alveolar bone, the bone which is deformed by stress becomes electrically charged and exhibits a phenomenon called piezoelectricity (Fig. 10.16).

When a force is applied to tooth, the distorted adjacent alveolar bone forms areas of concavity and convexity. Bone deposition occurs in the areas of concavity, which is negatively charged. Areas of concavity become positively charged and bone resorption occurs (Flowchart 10.2).

The possible sources of piezoelectricity in alveolar bone are:

- Hydroxyapatite crystals
- Collagen fibers
- Collagen–hydroxyapatite interface
- Mucopolysaccharide of ground substance

Piezoelectricity is characterized by two unique properties: Quick decay rate and reverse piezoelectricity.

Quick decay rate: When a force is applied, piezoelectric signal is created in response that quickly dies away to zero even though the force is maintained.

There is production of an equivalent signal opposite in direction, when the force is released.

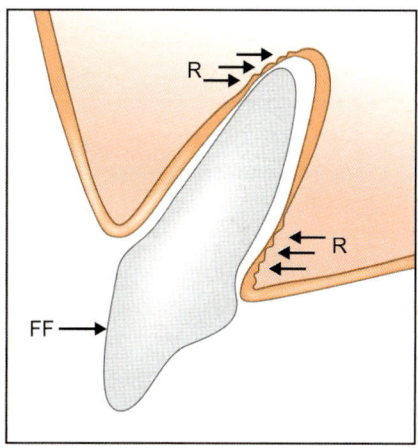

Fig.10.15: Undermining resorption

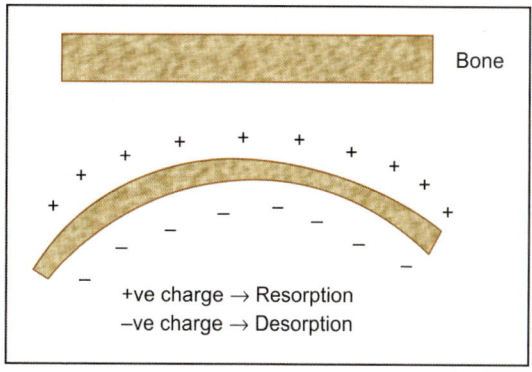

Fig. 10.16: Bone bending

Flowchart 10.2: Depicts changes after force application

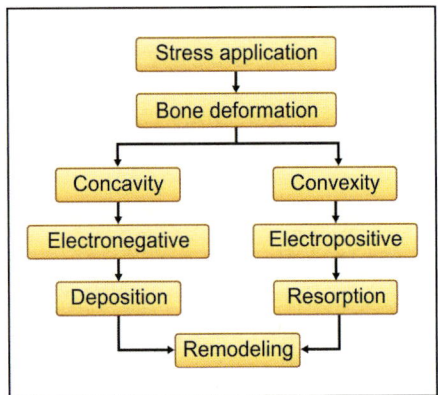

Flowchart 10.3: Changes after piezoelectricity

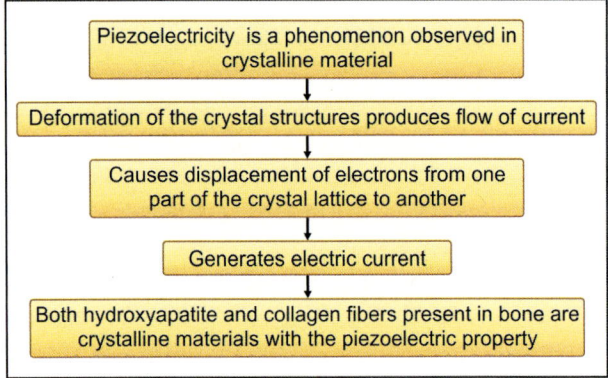

Flowchart 10.4: Reverse piezoelectricity

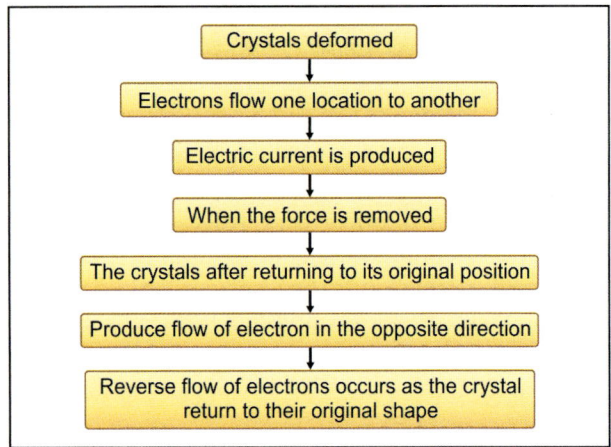

Both these characteristics are explained by the migration of electrons within the crystal lattice as it is distorted by pressure. When the crystal structure is deformed, electrons migrate from one location to another and electric charge is observed. As long as the force is maintained, the crystal structure is stable and no further electric events are observed. When the force is released, however, the crystal returns to its original shape and a reverse flow of electrons is seen. With this arrangement, rhythmic activity would produce a constant interplay of electric signals, whereas occasional application and release of force would produce only occasional electric signals.

Ions in the fluids that bathe living bone interacting with the complex electric field generated when the bone bends causing temperature changes as well as electric signals. As a result, both convection and conduction currents can be deleted in the extracellular fluids and the currents are affected by the nature of the fluids. The small voltages that are observed, are called streaming potential.

Endogenous electric signals can be observed in bone that is not stressed. These are called the bioelectric potentials.

Today, it is proven fact that adding exogenous electric signals can modify cellular activity. The effects presumably are felt at cell membranes. The external electric signals, probably affect cell membrane receptors, membrane permeability or both. It has also been proved that when low voltage direct current is applied to the alveolar bone, it modifies the bioelectric potential and increase the rate of tooth movement. Also, a pulsed electromagnetic field increased the rate of tooth movement, apparently by shortening the initial lag phase before tooth movement begins.

Not only is bone mineral, a crystal structure with piezoelectric properties, but the collagen itself is piezoelectric and the other possible sources of electric current are hydroxyapatite, collagen–hydroxyapatite interface and mucopolysaccharide fraction of ground substance (Flowchart 10.3).

Reverse piezoelectricity (Flowchart 10.4).

Blood Flow Theory/Fluid Dynamic Theory

The fluid dynamic theory is also called the blood flow theory as proposed by Bien.

According to this theory, tooth movement occurs as a result of alterations in fluid dynamics in the periodontal ligament. The periodontal ligament occupies the periodontal space which is confined between the tooth and alveolar socket. The periodontal space contains a fluid system made up of interstitial fluid, cellular elements, blood vessels and viscous ground substance in addition to periodontal fibers. It is a confined space and the passage of fluid in and out of the space is limited.

The contents of periodontal ligament thus create a unique hydrodynamic condition resembling a hydraulic mechanism and a shock absorber. When the force is removed, the fluid is replenished by diffusion from capillary walls and recirculation of the interstitial fluid. When the force applied is of short duration such as mastication, the fluid in the periodontal space is replenished as soon as the force is removed. But when a force of greater magnitude and duration is applied such as during orthodontic tooth movement, the interstitial fluid in the periodontal space gets squeezed out and moves towards the apex and cervical margins and results in decreased tooth movement. This is called the "squeeze film effect" by Bein.

When an orthodontic force is applied, it results in compression of the periodontal ligament. Blood vessels of the periodontal ligament get trapped between the principal fibers and these results in their stenosis. The vessel above the stenos is then balloons resulting in formation of an "aneurysm". These aneurysms are minute flexible walled sacs of fluid (Flowchart 10.5).

Bien suggested that there is an alteration in the chemical environment at the site of vascular stenosis due to decreased oxygen level in the compressed areas as compared to the tension side. The formation of these aneurysms and vascular stenosis causes blood gases to escape into the interstitial fluid thereby creating a favorable local environment for resorption.

PHASES OF TOOTH MOVEMENT (Fig. 10.17)

Burstone categorized three distinct stages of tooth movement as initial phase, lag phase and post-lag phase.

Initial phase: The initial phase of tooth movement is immediately following the application of force onto the tooth. The phase is characterized by a sudden displacement of the tooth within its socket. The movement of the tooth into the periodontal space and the bending of the alveolar bone probably cause it. The extent of movement achieved is nearly same for both light and heavy forces.

Lag phase: The lag phase is characterized by very little or no tooth movement. The lag phase is longer, if heavy

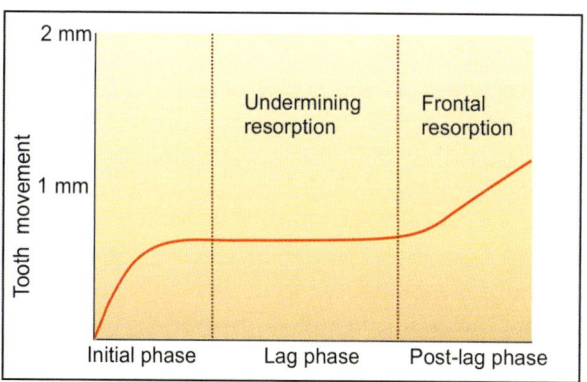

Fig. 10.17: Phase of tooth movement

forces are applied. This stage usually lasts from one to three weeks though Reitan has reported hyalinization period up to 40 days. As the area of hyalinization created is large and the resorption is rearward. Shorter duration of the lag phase is noticed for lighter forces. There is very little, if any area of hyalinization and frontal resorption is noticed.

Post-lag phase: There occurs a mechanical displacement of the tooth associated with cellular activity of resorption and deposition. This may be any type of movement and may be rapid or slow. It occurs spontaneously at the conclusion of the hyalinization period.

Interrupted lag phase: Not included in previous classification, but the concept that little or no movement occurs during the hyalinization period or lag phase appears subject to some qualifications. Movement can occur following reactivation of spring force before undermining resorption has eliminated the hyalinized areas resulting from the previous activation. This might be termed as an interrupted lag phase.

BIOCHEMICAL CONTROL OF TOOTH MOVEMENT

Cells respond to signals from other cells and to changes in the environment.

Extracellular signal can be:
- *Endocrine:* Endocrine organs release hormones, usually carried by blood to the distant target cells.
- *Paracrine signaling;* The cell is close to the target cell and the compound that is released (local mediator) affects only the group of cells adjacent to it.
- Autocrine signaling cells respond to substance that they themselves release.

Some hormones bind to receptors within the cells; others bind to cell surface receptors.

- *Intracellular receptors:* Steroids, retinoic acid and thyroxines, being hydrophobic, enter the cell and

Flowchart 10.5: Blood flow theory

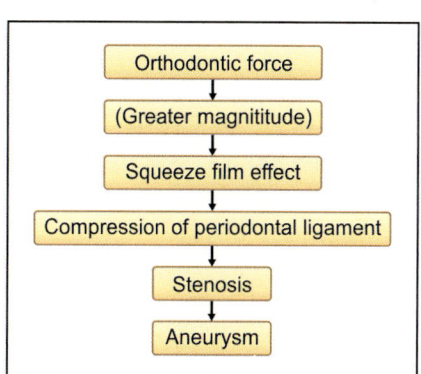

bind to specific receptors in the cytosol or nucleus and act on nuclear DNA to alter transcription of specific gene.

- *Cell surface receptors:* Peptide and protein hormones, prostaglandins, amino acids epinephrine and other water-soluble signaling molecules called ligands act as 1st messengers and bind to cell surface receptors proteins and thereby activate enzymes that generate an increase or decrease in the concentration of intracellular signaling compounds termed 2nd messenger (these include compounds such as adenosine 3', 5' monophosphate).

Surface receptors may open or close certain gated ion channels in the plasma membrane and in turn may allow the influx of certain ions into the cell. Ca^{2+} has been shown to act as 2nd messengers. Certain prostaglandins have also been shown to act as local mediators during paracrine signaling (Fig. 10.18 and Flowchart 10.6).

Tissue trauma stimulates prostaglandin release. Their concentration tends to increase even following the gentle manipulation of tissues. Ischemia has been shown to trigger prostaglandin synthesis. Epinephrine, angiotensin, prolactin and histamine have also been shown to increase prostaglandin synthesis.

The biochemical control of orthodontic tooth movement is a complex and as yet not completely understood phenomenon.

Effect of Drugs/Medications on Tooth Movement

- Orthodontic tooth movement enhancers:
  - Vitamin D administration enhances tooth movement.
  - Direct injection of prostaglandin into the PDL has shown to increase the rate of tooth movement (painful).
- Orthodontic tooth movement:
  - Bisphosphonates (used for treatment of osteoporosis, e.g. alendronate).
  - Prostaglandin inhibitors (e.g. indomethacin used for arthritis treatment).

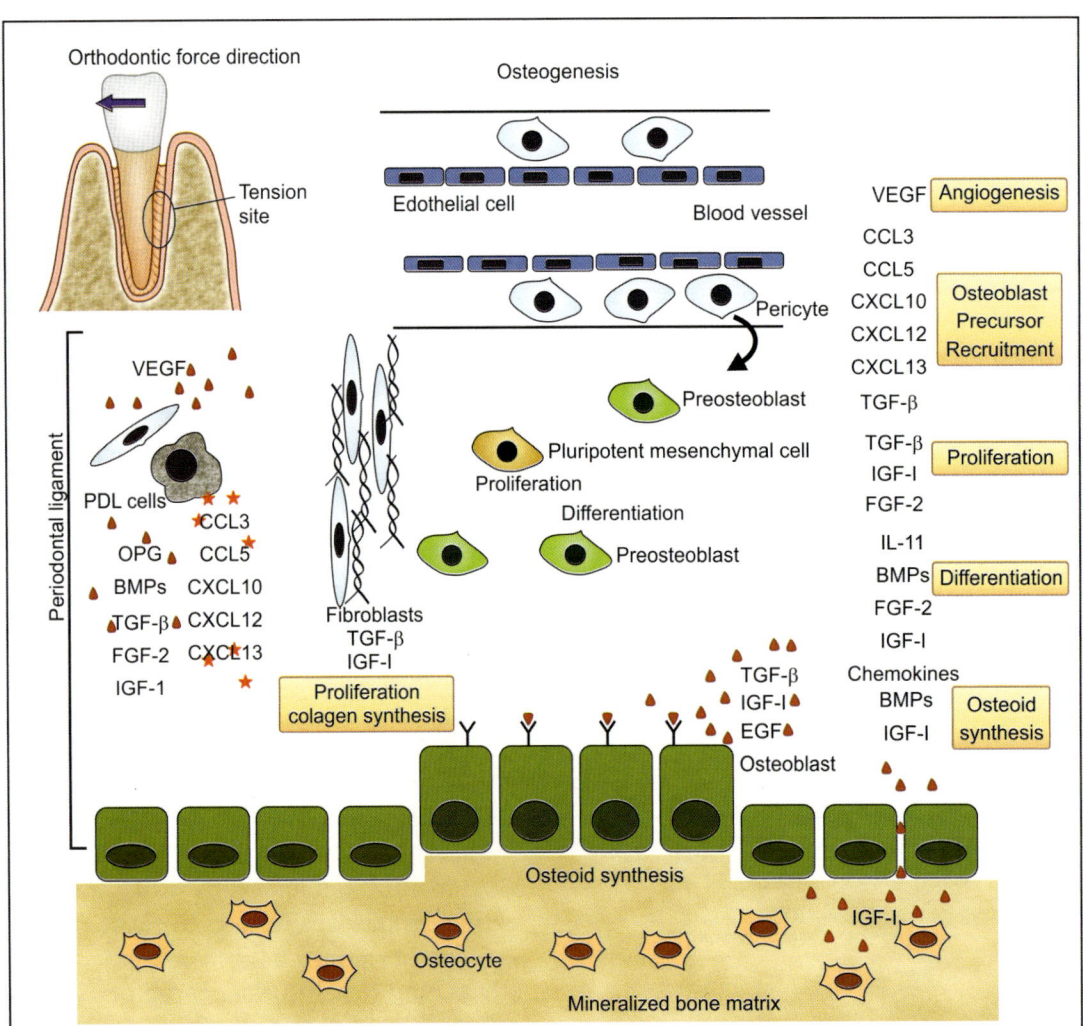

Fig. 10.18: Biochemical control of tooth movement

Flowchart 10.6: Summary of changes in intracellular level

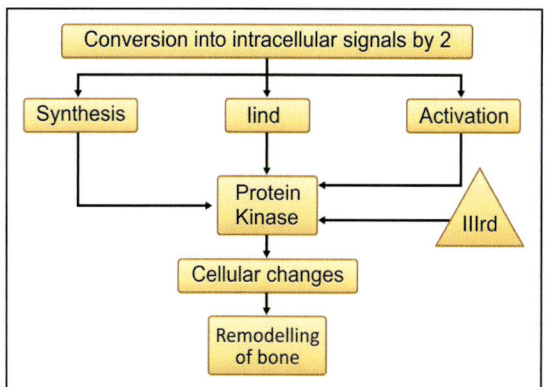

Flowchart 10.6: Summary of changes in intracellular level

Deleterious effects of orthodontic forces are listed in Table 10.6.

INTERVENTIONS FOR ACCELERATING ORTHODONTIC TOOTH MOVEMENT

Currently, fixed orthodontic treatment requires a long duration of about 2–3 years, which is a great concern and poses high risks of caries, external root resorption, and decreased patient compliance. There are two basic ways to reduce the treatment duration:

- One approach is by making the treatment mechanics more efficient.
- Another approach involves interventions to increase the velocity of orthodontic tooth movement by enhancing the bone remodeling.

Different Methods to Accelerate Tooth Movement

More efficient mechanics:
- Low friction mechanics
- Self-ligating brackets
- Preformed robotic archwires
- Microimplants

Enhance bone remodeling
- Biochemical
- Parathyroid hormone
- Parathyroid hormone
- Osteocalcin
- Dihydroxyvitamin D_3 $(1,25\text{-}(OH)_2D_3)$

Table 10.6: Deleterious effects of orthodontic forces	
Effects on the pulp	• Modest and transient inflammatory response within the pulp, at least at the beginning of tooth movement with no long-term significance • A large enough abrupt movement of the root apex could severe the blood vessels as they enter • According to some studies endodontically treated teeth are slightly more prone to root resorption during orthodontics than are teeth with normal vitality.

Effects on root structure	• Root remodeling is a constant feature of orthodontic tooth movement, but permanent loss of root structure would occur only if repair did not the initially resorbed cementum
	• Above average resorption can be anticipated, if the teeth have:
	  – Conical roots with pointed apices
	  – Distorted root form
	  – History of trauma
	  – Root apices in contact with cortical bone
	  – Excessive force during orthodontic treatment, particularly if heavy continuous forces are used.

Effects on alveolar bone height	• Excessive loss of crestal bone height is almost never seen as a complication of orthodontic tooth movement • Almost never exceeds 1 mm, greatest changes at extraction sites
Mobility	• Radiographically, it can be observed that the periodontal ligament space widens during orthodontic tooth movement • Heavier the orthodontic force—greater the amount of undermine resorbing expected—greater the mobility. • If a tooth becomes extremely mobile during orthodontic treatment, all forces should be discontinuied until the mobility decreases to moderate levels
Pain related to orthodontic treatment	• Pain of any type involves a great deal of individual variation. • Pain is related to the development of ischemic areas in the periodontal ligament. Hence, lighter forces because more pain. • If light forces are used, the amount of pain experienced by patients can be decreases by having the engaged in repeated chewing during the first 8 hours after the orthodontic appliance is activated

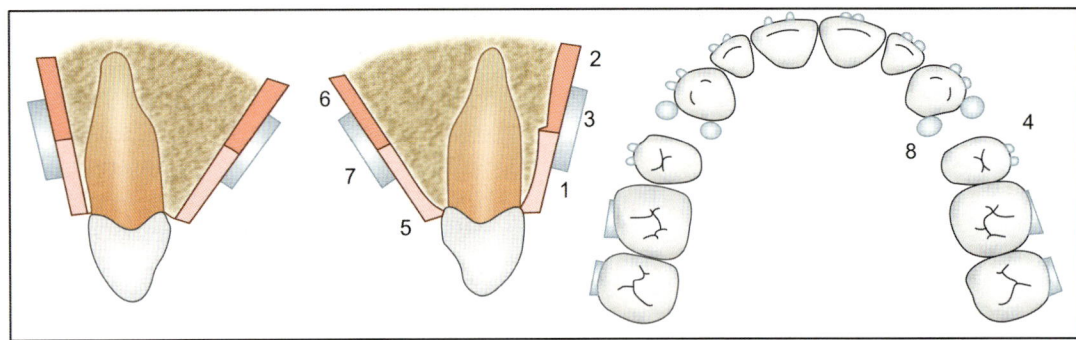

Fig. 10.19: Low level laser therapy

Physical stimulation:
- Micropulse and cyclic vibration
- Low level laser therapy
- Low intensity pulsed ultrasound

Surgical approach:
- Corticotomy
- Periodontally assisted osteogenic orthodontics
- Piezocision assisted orthodontics

Low-level laser therapy: Low-level laser therapy was performed through a laser device from which the laser was emitted to the desired mucosa areas. Low-level laser therapy is safe regarding periodontal and root health and it is unable to accelerate orthodontic tooth movement (Fig. 10.19).

Corticotomy: Corticotomy is performed by making small perforations on the alveolar bones along the way by which the tooth would be moved (Fig. 10.20).

Electrical current: Electrical current was delivered to the mucosa of canines through a fixed electrical appliance assembly (20 mA, 5 hours per day) on canines (Fig. 10.21a and b).

Pulsed electromagnetic fields: Pulsed electromagnetic fields are produced by an integrated circuit embedded in a removable denture (0.5 mT and 1 Hz, 8 hours per day overnight).

Dentoalveolar Distraction vs Periodontal Distraction

- Dentoalveolar distraction was performed by making monocortical perforations on alveolar bones around canines, followed by distracting canines using distractors.
- Periodontal distraction was performed by making vertical grooves on the mesial side of the first premolar extraction sockets followed by the same distracting technique (Fig. 10.22).
- The distractor was composed of an anterior segment fixed on the canine, a posterior segment fixed on the first molar, and a connecting sliding rod.

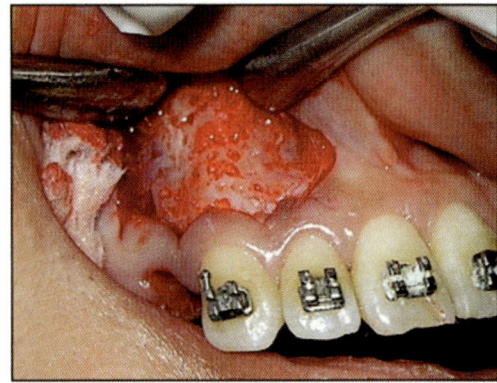

Fig. 10.20: Flap design with cortical perforations extended to the apex of the canine

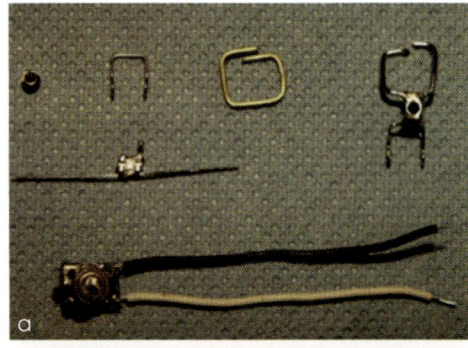

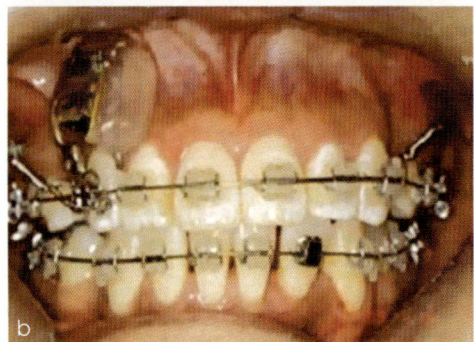

Fig. 10.21: Electric current on canines

- Canine distraction (0.5 mm/d) was achieved by sliding the anterior segment toward the posterior segment (Fig. 10.23).

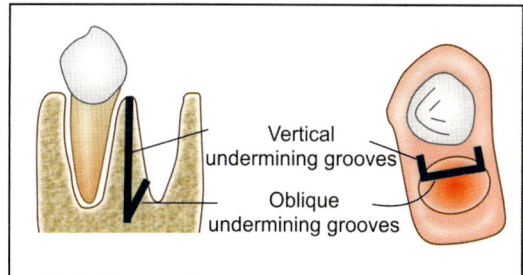

Fig. 10.22: Technique for periodontal distraction (PD)

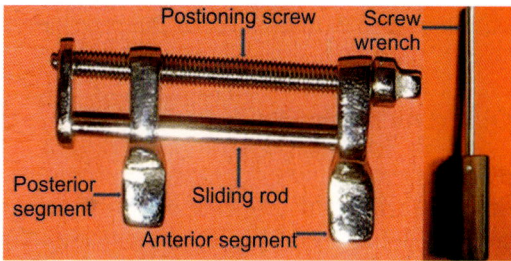

Fig. 10.23: Canine distraction

Recent Advances

- Gene therapy
- Vibrations
- Biomodulators

To conclude:

- Among these interventions, corticotomy, dento-alveolar distraction and periodontal distraction have strong clinical evidence.
- Low-level laser therapy is safe but unable to accelerate orthodontic tooth movement; corticotomy is safe and able to accelerate orthodontic tooth movement.
- Current evidence does not reveal whether electrical current and pulsed electromagnetic fields are effective in accelerating orthodontic tooth movement; dentoalveolar or periodontal distraction is promising in accelerating orthodontic tooth movement but lacks convincing evidence.

ROOT RESORPTION

Root resorption is a common sequela of orthodontic treatment. It is an inflammatory process leading to an ischemic necrosis in a localized area of periodontal ligament when the orthodontic force is applied.

Risk Factors of Root Resorption after Orthodontic Treatment

Certain risk factors are associated with the onset and progression of root resorption like:

1. Duration of treatment
2. Magnitude of force applied
3. Direction of tooth movement
4. Method of force application whether intermittent or continuous
5. Type of orthodontic tooth movement

Patient-related risk factors are:

1. The individual susceptibility on a genetic basis
2. Some systemic diseases
3. Abnormal root morphology
4. Dental trauma
5. Previous orthodontic treatment

The prevention of root resorption during orthodontic treatment may be done by controlling risk factors. The periodic radiographic examination during the treatment is necessary to detect the occurrence of root damages and thus plan the further treatment. Root resorption is considered as clinically important when 1–2 mm (one-fourth) of the root length is lost. Severe root resorption during orthodontic treatment (>5 mm) occurs rarely.

Types of Root Resorption

It is of three types:

1. *Microresorption* is confined to cementum. It is localized, superficial and gets repaired.
2. *Progressive root resorption* appears at the site of continuous and heavy forces; it may involve entire apex.
3. *Idiopathic root resorption* is seen even before the start of orthodontic treatment. It gets aggravated by the orthodontic treatment.

Degrees of Severity of Root Resorption

There are three degrees of severity of root resorption:

1. Cementum or surface resorption, occurring together with remodeling, when only outer cementum layer is resorbed, which regenerates or remodels later. This process is similar to trabecular bone remodeling.
2. Dentin resorption with repair (deep resorption), when cementum and outer dentin layer are resorbed; resorption is irreversible because only cementum regenerates. Tooth root form after this resorption and remodeling may stay the same or altered.
3. Surrounding apical root tissue is fully resorbed and root shortening is observed. Apical tissues under cementum are lost, root tissues do not regenerate. Repair of outer surface occurs in the cementum layer.

Degree of Root Resorption and Root Resorption Index

1. *Grade I:* Irregular root contour

2. *Grade II:* Apical root resorption is less than 2 mm.
3. *Grade III:* Apical root resorption is from 2 mm to one-third of the initial root length.
4. *Grade IV:* Apical root resorption is more than one-third of the initial root length of root resorption.

Risk Factors for Root Resorption

These factors can be divided into biological, mechanical and combined factors.

Biological Factors

a. *Genetics*
b. *Systemic factor:* Allergic patients are susceptible to increased risk of root resorption. Lack of estrogens induces quick orthodontic tooth movement and calcitonin inhibits activity of odontoclasts.
c. *Impacted third molars:* It may cause the root resorption of second molar. Maxillary impacted canines can induce the root resorption of the incisors and first premolars.
d. *Tooth structure:* Levander and Malmgren divided the root forms to:
   • Normal
   • Short
   • Blunt dilacerated
   • Pipette shaped
   Most authors have shown that roots with abnormal shape have a higher susceptibility to root resorption. According to Sinclaire, normal and blunt tooth roots resorb the least. Pipette-shaped roots are the most susceptible to root resorption. Short roots have a greater risk for root resorption than average length roots.
e. *Chronological age:* Periodontal membrane becomes narrower and less vascularized, aplastic, alveolar bone becomes denser, less vascularized and aplastic and cementum becomes wider with age. Through these changes, adults show higher susceptibility to root resorption. When a patient is older than 11 years, risk for root resorption increases due to closure of apical foramen.
f. *Dental change:* Rosenberg has stated that teeth with incomplete root formation undergo less root resorption than those with completely formed roots. The teeth that are treated orthodontically lose averagely 0.5 mm of the root length. Longer roots are more likely to be resorbed than shorter ones because longer roots need stronger forces to be moved and the actual displacement of root apex is greater during tipping or torqueing movements. Endontically treated tooth subjected to orthodontic

forces is more prone for root resorption. Dental trauma may lead to root resorption without orthodontic treatment.

BIBLIOGRAPHY

1. Bassett CAL. Beneficial effects of electromagnetic fields. J Cell Biochem 1993; 51:387–93.
2. Melsen B. Biologic reaction of alveolar bone to orthodontic tooth movement. Angle Orthod 1999;6992): 151–8
3. Melsen B. Tissue reaction to orthodontic tooth movement: a new paradigm. Eur J Orthod 2001;23(6):671–81.
4. Zengo AN, Pawluk RJ, Basset CAL. Stress induced bioelectric potentials in the alveolar complex: Am J Orthod 1973; 64:17.

PREVIOUS YEAR'S UNIVERSITY QUESTIONS

Essay

1. Enumerate different theories of tooth movement. Discuss in detail about pressure tension theory.
2. Discuss tissue changes during orthodontic tooth movement.

Short Questions

1. Optimum orthodontic force
2. Phases of tooth movement
3. Types of tooth movement
4. Undermining resorption
5. Root resorption

MCQs

1. *Which of the below is not a theory of tooth eruption:*
   a. Blood eruption theory
   b. Root growth theory
   c. Blood flow theory
   d. Hammock ligament therapy **(Ans: c)**

2. *Hammock ligament theory was proposed by:*
   a. Bien
   b. Sicher
   c. Oppenheim
   d. Schwarz **(Ans: b)**

3. *Which theory is most accepted among tooth eruption theories?*
   a. Blood pressure theory
   b. Root growth
   c. Hammock ligament
   d. Periodontal ligament traction **(Ans: d)**

4. *Physiological tooth movement includes:*
   a. Pre-eruptive tooth movement
   b. Eruptive tooth movement

c. Posteruptive tooth movement

d. All of the above   **(Ans: d)**

5. *Posteruptive tooth movement is a compensatory movement for:*
   a. Proximal wears only
   b. Occlusal wears only
   c. Both a and b
   d. None of the above   **(Ans: c)**

6. *Frontal or direct resorption occurs:*
   a. As a result of mild orthodontic forces
   b. Occurs on the pressure side of tooth movement
   c. Does not cause resorption of root
   d. All of the above   **(Ans: d)**

7. *When a force is applied to tooth:*
   a. Areas of pressure are created
   b. Areas of tension are created
   c. Bone resorption and deposition occur
   d. All of the above   **(Ans: d)**

8. *Tooth movement occurs due to:*
   a. Osteoblastic activity only
   b. Osteoclastic activity only
   c. Both a and b
   d. None of the above   **(Ans: c)**

9. *Frontal resorption occurs as a result of:*
   a. Mild orthodontic forces
   b. Excessive orthodontic forces
   c. Compression on pressure side of tooth movement
   d. All of the above   **(Ans: a)**

10. *Periodontal ligament deprives of nutritional supply and showing regressive changes with:*
    a. Direct resorption
    b. Frontal resorption
    c. Hyalinization
    d. Undermining resorption   **(Ans: c)**

11. *Undermining or rearward resorption occurs as a result of:*
    a. Changes following mild forces
    b. Changes following moderate forces
    c. Changes following extreme forces
    d. None of the above   **(Ans: c)**

10.3 ANCHORAGE

Chapter Outline

- Definitions
- Classification
- Sources of anchorage
- Anchorage loss
- Anchorage planning
- Tweed's classification of anchorage preparation
- Temporary anchorage device (TAD)

DEFINITIONS

1. Anchorage is defined as the nature and degree of resistance to displacement offered by an anatomic unit for the purpose of effecting tooth movement **(Graber).**
2. Anchorage is the site of delivery from which a force is exerted **(White and Gardiner).**
3. **Louis Ottofy** (1923): Defined it as "the base against which orthodontic force or reaction of orthodontic force is applied".
4. **Nanda:** The amount of movement of posterior teeth (molar and premolar) to close the extraction space in order to achieve selected treatment goals.
5. **According to Proffit:** It is the resistance to unwanted tooth movement.

Classification

According to Moyer

Manner of force application
- Simple anchorage
- Stationary anchorage
- Reciprocal anchorage
- Jaws involved
- Intramaxillay anchorage
- Intermaxillary anchorage

Site of anchorage
- Intraoral
- Extraoral
- Cervical
- Occipital
- Parietal

Number of anchorage units
- Single or primary anchorage
- Compound anchorage
- Multiple or reinforced anchorage

According to Ottofy

Anchorage (intraoral) can be classified according to manner of force application as:
A. Simple
B. Stationary
C. Reciprocal

According to White and Gardiner

- Simple
- Stationary
- Reciprocal
- Reinforced
- Intermaxillary
- Extraoral

The force used to move teeth is derived from certain anatomic areas, which acts as anchors. Poor anchorage management can result in a non-ideal occlusion, over-retraction or under-retraction of the incisors and poor facial esthetics. Anchorage devices can be classified according to the tissues providing resistance to unwanted tooth movement. The anchor unit should incorporate as many teeth as possible, so that the force threshold needed to initiate tooth movement is not exceeded.

Newton's third law: For every action, there is an equal and opposite reaction. The resistance that the anchorage areas offer to these unwanted tooth movements is called *sources of anchorage.*

The anchorage potential of teeth depends on a number of factors such as:
- Root form
- Root size
- Number of roots
- Root length
- Root inclination
- Root form

It depends largely on its root form. The cross-section of roots can be of three types:

1. *Round:* Bicuspids, palatal root of maxillary molars
2. *Flat:* Mandibular incisors, molars and the buccal roots of maxillary molars.
3. *Triangular:* Canine, maxillary central and lateral incisors

Size and number of roots: Multirooted teeth with large roots have a greater ability to withstand stress than single-rooted teeth.

Root length: In physiologic conditions, the root length indicates the depth to which the tooth is embedded in bone. The longer the root, the deeper it is embedded in bone and the greater is its resistance to displacement.

Inclination of tooth: The axial inclination of a tooth is important in assessing its value as a source of anchorage.

A greater resistance to displacement is offered when the force exerted to move teeth is opposite to that of their axial inclination.

Ankylosed: Ankylosed teeth are directly fixed to the alveolar bone and hence lack a periodontal ligament. Orthodontic movement of such teeth is not possible and they can, therefore, serve as excellent anchors whenever possible.

Intercuspation: Good intercuspation leads to greater anchorage potential. Interlocking of the cusps prevents the mesial drift of the teeth.

Contact points: Teeth with tight and broad contact provide greater anchorage.

Mesial drift: Resistance value is least in downward and forward directions. Maxillary posterior teeth drift more readily by mesial migration.

ANCHORAGE LOSS

It is defined as the undesirable movement of anchor tooth in excess to that of planned treatment.

Reasons for anchorage loss:
- Excessive force
- Impingement of roots of incisors or anterior teeth to the labial cortical plate
- Improper anchorage preparation
- Improper treatment planning
- Resistance between archwire and brackets

Anchorage loss in all three planes of space:
- Sagittal plane:
  - Mesial movement of molars
  - Proclination of anterior

- Vertical plane:
  - Extrusion of molars
  - Bite deepening due to anterior extrusion
- Transverse plane:
  - Buccal flaring due to over expanded arch form and unintentional lingual root torque
  - Lingual dumping molars

Methods to prevent anchorage loss:
- Use of mini-screws
- Use of stabilizing appliances like transpalatal arch, Nance palatal arch and lingual arch
- Use of light forces
- Extraoral anchorage using headgears
- Utilizing muscular force

Simple Anchorage

It is defined as dental anchorage in which the manner and application of force is such that it tends to change the axial inclination of the tooth or teeth that form the anchorage unit in the plane of space in which the force is being applied. Thus, the resistance of the anchorage unit to tipping is utilized to move another tooth or teeth. Simple anchorage is obtained by engaging with the appliance a greater number of teeth than are to be moved within the same dental arch. Thus, the resistance offered by the anchorage unit is greater than that offered by the tooth or teeth being moved, e.g. when a palatally placed premolar is pushed bucally with the teeth in the dental arch as the anchor units (Fig. 10.24).

Stationary Anchorage

It is defined as dental anchorage in which the manner and application of force tends to displace the anchorage unit bodily in plane of space in which the force is being applied.

The anchorage provided by a tooth resisting bodily movement is considerably greater than one resisting tipping force (Fig. 10.25).

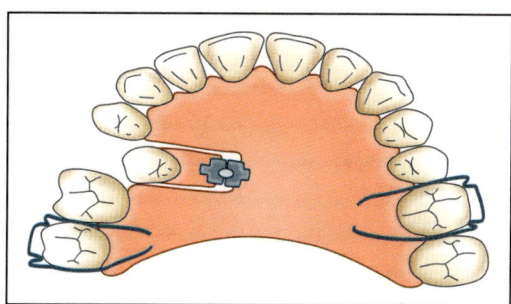

Fig. 10.24: Simple anchorage

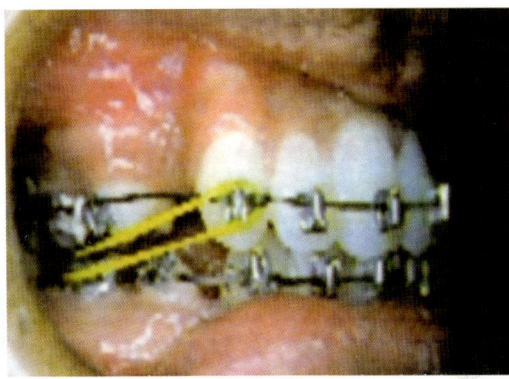

Fig. 10.25: Stationary anchorage

Reciprocal Anchorage

The term refers to the resistance offered by two malposed units when the dissipation of equal and opposite forces tends to move each unit towards a more normal occlusion. Here two teeth or two groups of teeth of equal anchorage value are made to move in opposite directions (Fig. 10.26a and b).

A frequently used form of reciprocal anchorage is known as intermaxillary traction. The forces used to move the whole or part of one dental arch in one direction are anchored by equal forces by moving the opposite arch in opposite direction, thus, correcting discrepancies in both the dental arches.

Closure of a midline diastema is done by moving the two central incisors towards each other, the use of crossbite elastics and dental arch expansion.

Intraoral Anchorage

- Anchorage in which all the resistance units are situated within the oral cavity is termed intraoral anchorage.
- The teeth to be moved and the anatomic areas that offer anchorage are all within the oral cavity.
- Various intraoral anatomic units that may be employed are the teeth, palate and lingual alveolar bone of mandible.

Extraoral Anchorage

- Certain extraoral areas can be utilized as sources of anchorage to bring about orthodontic or orthopedic changes.
- They are mainly used when adequate resistance cannot be obtained from intraoral sources for the purpose of anchorage.
- The extraoral sources of anchorage include the cranium, the back of the neck and the facial bones.
- Anchorage in which the resistance units are situated outside the oral cavity is termed extraoral anchorage.

Cranium (Occipital or Parietal Anchorage)

Extraoral anchorage can be obtained by using headgears that device anchorage from the occipital or parietal region of the cranium. These devices are used along with a face bow to restrict maxillary growth or to move the dentition or maxillary bone distally.

- *Cervical headgear:* Anchorage from cervical region (Fig. 10.27).
- *Occipital headgear:* Anchorage from occipital bone (Fig. 10.28).
- *High pull headgear:* Anchorage from parietal and occipital bones.
- *Chin cup:* Anchorage from chin region.
- *Facemask or reverse pull headgear:* Anchorage from frontal bone and chin.
- *Combination headgear:* Anchorage from occipital as well as cervical region (Fig. 10.29).

Cortical Anchorage

The cortical bone is more resistant to resorption than the medullary bone. The cortical anchorage concept

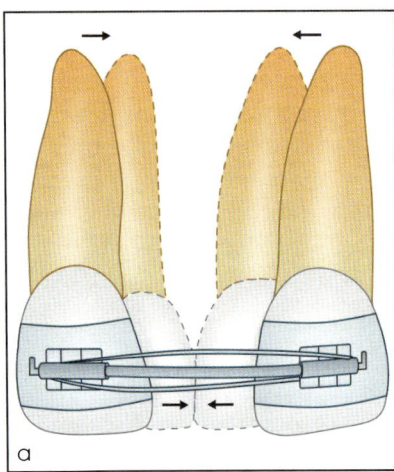

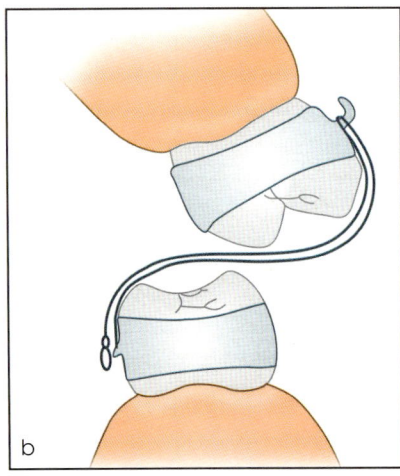

Fig. 10.26: Reciprocal anchorage

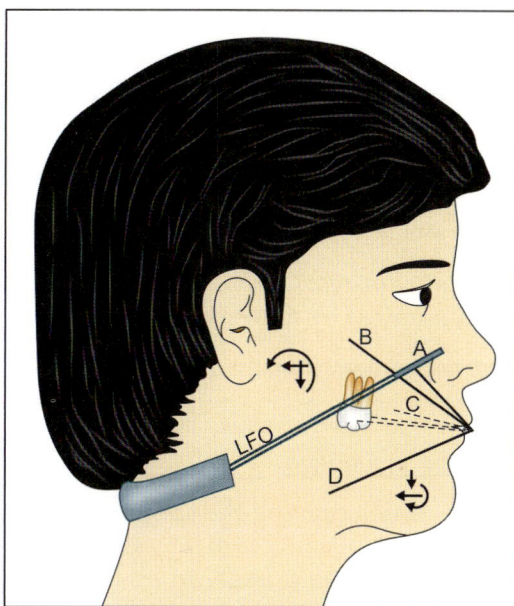

Fig. 10.27: Cervical anchorage

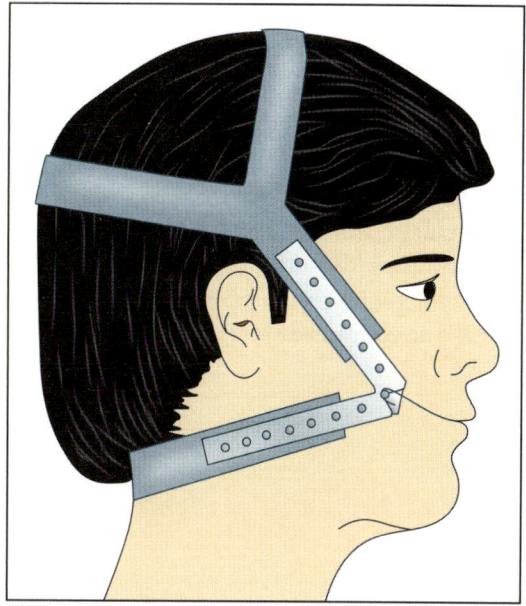

Fig. 10.29: Combination anchorage

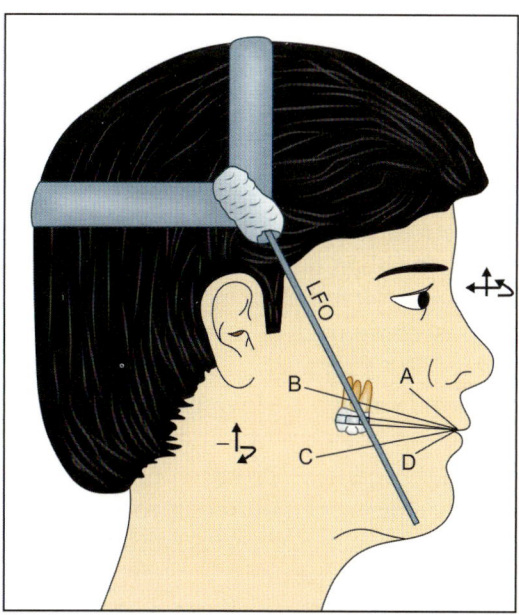

Fig. 10.28: Occipital anchorage

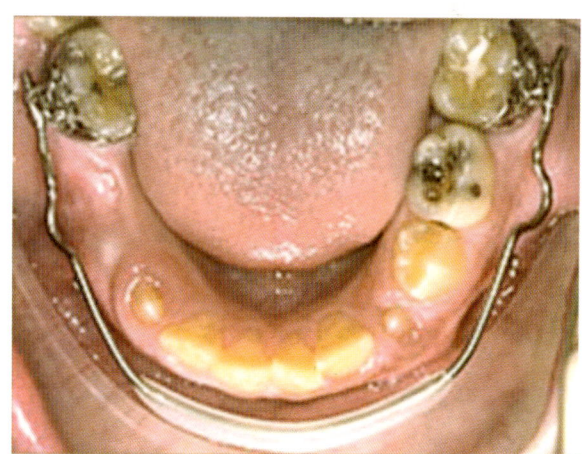

Fig. 10.30: Mascular anchorage

makes use of this. The torqueing of the roots of buccal teeth outwards against the cortical plate serve as a way to inhibit their mesial movement.

It depends upon:
- Radicular position with respect to cortical bone.
- Alveolar border narrowing in edentulous space.

It increases with age due to decrease of blood circulation.

Muscular Anchorage

It depends upon:
- Lips and cheek strength
- Habits such as lips, cheek, tongue thrust
- Mandibular elevating muscular strength
- Cusps integrity
- Presence or absence of antagonist teeth

Muscular anchorage makes use of forces generated by muscles to aid in the movement of teeth. In certain cases, the perioral musculature is employed as resistance units (Fig. 10.30).

Intramaxillary Anchorage

When all the units offering resistance are situated within the same jaw the anchorage is described as intramaxillary. In this type of anchorage, the teeth to be moved and the anchorage units are all situated either entirely in the maxillary or the mandibular arches.

Intermaxillary Anchorage

Anchorage in which the resistance units situated in one jaw is used to affect tooth movement in the opposing jaw is called intermaxillary anchorage.

- It is also termed as **Baker's anchorage.** It was introduced in 1893.
- Class II elastic traction applied between the lower molar and upper anterior (Fig. 10.31).
- Class III elastic traction applied between the upper molar and lower anterior (Fig. 10.32).

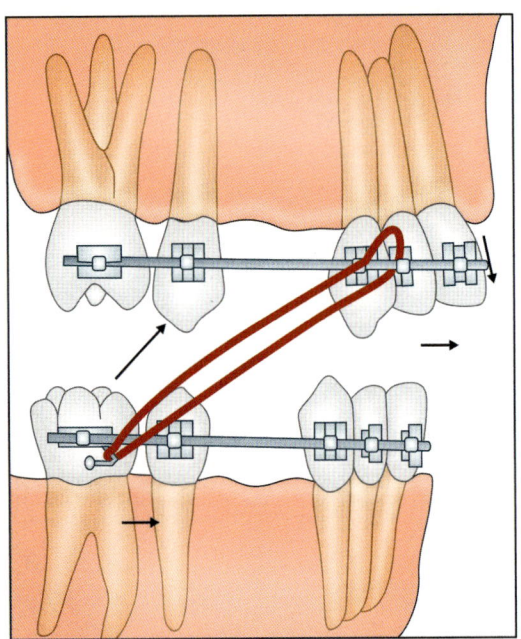

Fig. 10.31: Class II intermaxillary elastics

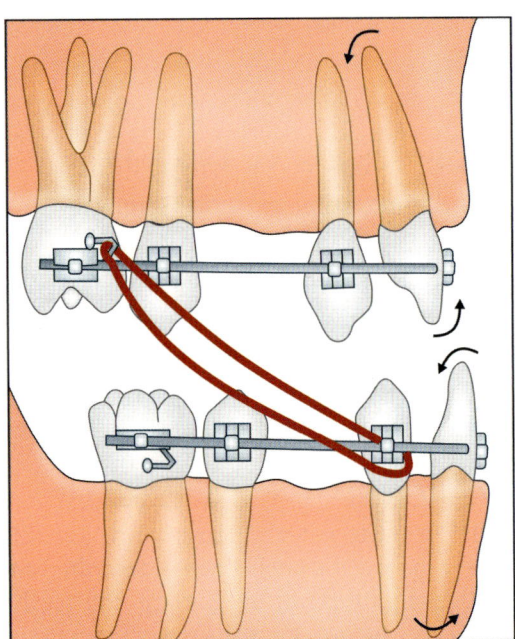

Fig. 10.32: Class III intermaxillary elastics

Maximum anchorage

- No more than 25% of extraction space should be lost by forward movement of anchor teeth.
- 75% or more of the extraction space is needed for the retraction of the anterior.
- In maximum anchorage cases, the mesial movement of posteriors is not advised.

Moderate anchorage: 25–50% of extraction space closure is permitted by movement of anchor teeth.

Minimum anchorage: More than half of extraction space closure is permitted.

ANCHORAGE PLANNING

At the time of determining the space requirement to resolve the malocclusion in a given case, it is essential to plan for space that is likely to be lost due to the invariable movement of the anchor teeth. The anchorage requirement depends on:

- *The number of teeth to be moved:* The greater the number of teeth being moved the greater is the anchorage demand. Moving teeth in segments as in retracting the canine separately rather than retracting the complete anterior segment together will decrease the load on the anchor teeth.
- *The type of teeth to be moved:* Teeth with large flat roots and/or more than one root exert more load on the anchor teeth. Hence, it is more difficult to move a canine as compared to an incisor or a molar as compared to a premolar.
- *Type of tooth movement:* Moving teeth bodily requires more force as compared to tipping the same teeth.
- *Periodontal condition:* Teeth with decreased bone support or periodontally compromised teeth are easier to move as compared to healthy teeth attached to a strong periodontium.
- *Duration of tooth movement:* Prolonged treatment time places more strain on the anchor teeth. Short-term treatment might bring about negligible amount of change in the anchor teeth whereas the same teeth might not be able to withstand the same forces adequately if the treatment becomes prolonged.

TWEED'S CLASSIFICATION OF ANCHORAGE PREPARATION

Tweed is credited with refining the edge-wise appliance and it is important to understand that at the time headgears were used in practically each and every case. Also the forces used to bring about tooth movement were very high as compared to what we use today.

Tweed classified anchorage preparation so as the anchor molars would not move into the extraction and sufficient space would be available to bring about the retraction of the anterior teeth.

First degree or minimal anchorage preparation is reserved for cases where the facial esthetics are good with an ANB angle equal to or less than 0 to 4°. The total discrepancy should be less than or equal to 10 mm.

The anchorage preparation consisted of inclining the terminal molars which are angulated such that the direction of pull of the intermaxillary elastic force during function will not exceed 90° when related to the long axis of these teeth.

Second degree or moderate anchorage preparation is usually required in cases where the ANB angle exceeds 4.5° with a Class II profile (retrognathic mandible).

Tweed recommended the banding of mandibular second molars in all such case with the terminal molars so angulated that their distal marginal ridge is at gum level. With such an anchorage preparation, the direction of pull from the Class II elastics would be greater than 90° during function. Such a pull will further depress than elongate the terminal molars.

Third degree or total anchorage is reserved for cases with an ANB angle of more than or equal to 5° and the total discrepancy was 14–20 mm.

The anchorage preparation is such that all the molars and premolars are tipped distally with the distal marginal ridge of the second molar being located below the gum level.

Such anchorage preparation is usually not required nowadays.

TEMPORARY ANCHORAGE DEVICE (TAD)

A TAD is a device that is placed into bone in order to enhance orthodontic anchorage. They either support

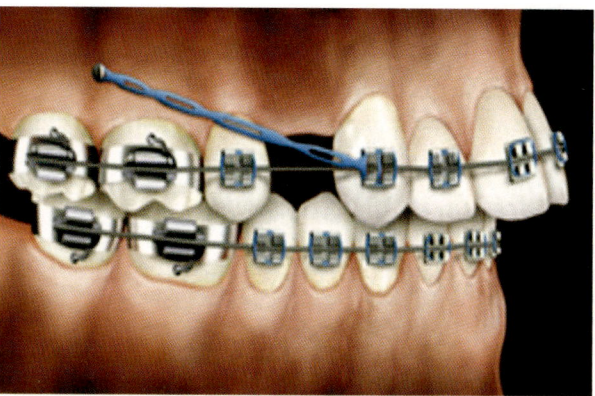

Fig. 10.33: Temporary anchorage device

the anchorage teeth or act by themselves as anchorage element/unit. They are temporary and are subsequently removed after use. They can be located on the bone surface (transosteal), under the periosteum (sub-periosteal), or inside the bone (endosteal) and can be fixed to bone either mechanically (cortically stabilized) or biologically (osseointegration) (Fig. 10.33).

Currently available skeletal anchorage devices can be classified either as biocompatible or biological. Ankylosed teeth are biological anchorage units.

It can be further subclassified based on Flowchart 10.7.

- Nature of mechanical retention in the bone (modification of surgical fixation methods), such as fixation wires, fixation screws in combination with mini-plates and mini-screws.
- Biological osseointegration such as endosseous prosthetic implants.

Since orthodontic patients do not usually display edentulous alveolar bony ridges for the insertion of an implant, special implants for orthodontic anchorage purposes were developed for the retromolar and palatal areas.

Flowchart 10.7: TAD—classification

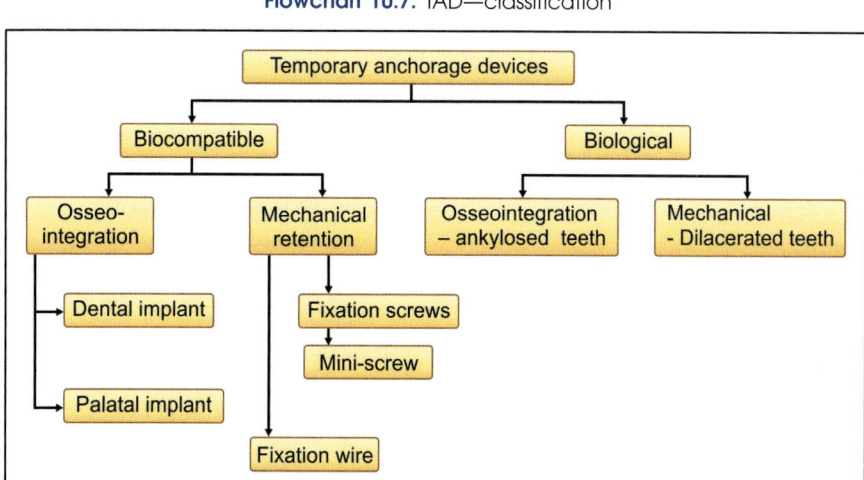

BIBLIOGRAPHY

1. Block MS, Hoffman DR. A new device for absolute anchorage for orthodontics. Am J Orthod 1995;107:251–8.
2. Gould E. Mechanical principles in extraoral anchorage. Am J Orthod 1957;17:319–33.
3. Melsen B, Bosch C. Different approaches to anchorage: a survey and an evaluation. Angle Orthod 1997;67:23–30.

PREVIOUS YEAR'S UNIVERSITY QUESTIONS

Essay

1. Classify anchorage. Write in detail about extra oral anchorage.
2. Define anchorage. What are the governing factors to value the anchorage?

Short Questions

1. TAD
2. Tweed classification of anchorage preparation
3. Methods to prevent anchorage loss
4. Cortical anchorage

MCQs

1. *Definition of anchorage is given by:*
   a. Graber
   b. White and Gardner
   c. Both a and b
   d. None **(Ans: c)**

2. *Extraoral sources of anchorage are:*
   a. Cranial bones
   b. Facial bones
   c. Basal jaw bones
   d. Both a and b **(Ans: d)**

3. *The following is an example of intramaxillary anchorage:*
   a. Class I elastics
   b. Class II elastics
   c. Class III elastics
   d. Box elastics **(Ans: a)**

4. *Cross-elastic is an example of:*
   a. Reciprocal anchorage
   b. Intermaxillary anchorage
   c. Stationary anchorage
   d. Both a and b **(Ans: d)**

5. *Bilateral symmetrical expansion is a type of:*
   a. Reciprocal anchorage
   b. Intermaxillary anchorage
   c. Stationary anchorage
   d. Simple anchorage **(Ans: a)**

6. *Correction of midline diastema is an example of:*
   a. Reciprocal anchorage
   b. Intermaxillary anchorage
   c. Stationary anchorage
   d. Simple anchorage **(Ans: a)**

7. *Transpalatal arch is:*
   a. Reinforced anchorage
   b. Reciprocal anchorage
   c. Compound anchorage
   d. Stationary anchorage **(Ans: a)**

8. *Which type of anchorage is not critical:*
   a. Maximum anchorage
   b. Minimum anchorage
   c. Moderate anchorage
   d. None of the above **(Ans: b)**

9. *More the number of the teeth to be moved:*
   a. Less the anchorage needed
   b. Greater is the demand of anchorage
   c. Not related to anchorage
   d. None of the above **(Ans: b)**

10. *'Anchorage is the site of delivery from which force is exerted' was defined by:*
    a. Graber
    b. White and Gardiner
    c. Newton
    d. Robert J Nicoli **(Ans: b)**

11. *Extraoral sources of anchorage include:*
    a. Cranium
    b. Back of the neck
    c. Facial bone
    d. All of the above **(Ans: d)**

12. *Anchorage from cranium is obtained by:*
    a. Occipital bone
    b. Parietal bone
    c. Frontal bone
    d. All of the above **(Ans: d)**

13. *Lip bumper to distalize molars is an example of:*
    a. Extraoral anchorage
    b. Intraoral anchorage
    c. Intramaxillary anchorage
    d. Muscular anchorage **(Ans: d)**

14. *Reinforced anchorage uses:*
    a. Extraoral sources
    b. Intraoral sources
    c. Combination of a and b
    d. None of the above **(Ans: c)**

15. *Modification of anterior inclined plane is*
    a. Baller's appliance
    b. Sved appliance
    c. Activator
    d. All of the above **(Ans: c)**

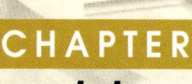

Preventive Orthodontics

Chapter Outline	
• Space maintenance	• Classification of space maintainers
• Preventive measures undertaken	• Types of space maintainer
• Space maintainers	

SPACE MAINTENANCE

Most orthodontic problems begin during the period of time when the development of the dental arch and occlusion proceeds from the primary to permanent dentition.

Unfortunately, many patients do not see the orthodontic specialist during this time, because the general dentist is the one who cares for the dental needs of the vast majority of growing children, it is imperative that they should be able to recognize growth problems as they occur. This will allow them to either actively intervene or immediately refer these patients to the orthodontist.

The stages of occlusal development are classified as follows:
- 1st stage: 3—primary dentition
- 2nd stage: 6—eruption of first permanent molars
- 3rd stage: 6–9—exchange of the incisors
- 4th stage: 9–12—eruption of the cuspids and bicuspids
- 5th stage: 12—eruption of the second molars

Unfortunately, a smooth transition through these stages is often disrupted by the premature loss of teeth. Tooth decay, trauma from a fall, or some other accidental injury is just some of the common reasons teeth are lost early. When this occurs, pediatric space management is the key to preventing a serious malocclusion in the permanent dentition. In the posterior quadrants, the early loss of primary teeth often results in a reduction of arch length. This change can directly affect the normal eruption of the adult teeth. If space loss has not already occurred, rapid intervention with a space-maintaining appliance is of utmost importance. In the anterior region, space maintenance is important to maintain normal speech, function, and esthetics.

Adults

Proper space management is important for the adult patient in a variety of situations. During active restorative treatment, there is often a need for an interim appliance to maintain space. For example, an interim space maintainer is often used in young patients who, because of an accident, rampant caries, or hereditary partial anodontia, are missing either anterior or posterior teeth. Other indications for an interim space maintainer seen in the general practice on a daily basis are:
- To maintain space.
- To re-establish occlusion.
- To replace visible missing teeth while definitive restorative procedures are being accomplished.
- To serve while the patient is undergoing periodontal or other prolonged treatment.
- When healing is progressing after an extraction or a traumatic injury.
- To maintain function while accomplishing minor tooth movement.

Definitions

Graber (1966) has defined as the action taken to preserve the integrity of what appears to be a normal occlusion at a specific time.

Proffit and Ackerman (1980) have defined as prevention of potential interference with occlusal development.

PREVENTIVE MEASURES UNDERTAKEN

- Caries control
- Parent counseling
- Space maintenance
- Exfoliation of deciduous teeth
- Abnormal frenal attachment
- Treatment of locked permanent first molar
- Abnormal oral musculature and related habits.

Caries Control

Caries involving the deciduous teeth especially the proximal caries is the main cause of development of a malocclusion. In case of proximal decay, the adjacent tooth tends to tilt into the proximally decayed area resulting in the loss of arch length, thereby resulting lesser space for the succedaneous tooth to erupt in the right position.

Parental Counseling

It may be divided into:
- Prenatal counseling
- Postnatal counseling

Postnatal Counseling

It is associated with the clinical examination of the child at:
a. Six months to one year
b. Two years of age
c. Three years of age
d. Five to six years of age

Six months to one year of age:
- Teething problems
- Bottle milk is recommended until first deciduous tooth erupts in the oral cavity.
- Child should be initiated to drinking from a glass by one year of age

Two years of age:
- Bottle feeding should be withdrawn completely by 18–24 months of age. This would decrease the bottle caries development.
- Bushing the teeth

Three years of age:
- Clinical examination—generally the full complement of deciduous dentition should have erupted by now.
- The occlusion, molar and canine relationship should be checked. Any presence of discrepancies like crossbite, supernumerary, missing teeth, etc. should be checked.
- Oral habits such as thumb sucking, lip sucking, oral breathing should be considered. Parents should be aware of these habits development.

Five to six years of age:
- Parents are informed about the exfoliation of deciduous teeth till 12–13 years.
- Space maintainers in case of premature loss of deciduous teeth.

SPACE MAINTAINERS

Early loss of primary molar often allows the adult first molar to tip and move mesially. The basic unilateral space maintainer is used for holding molar position.

Space maintainers are defined as the appliances that prevent the loss of arch length and which in turn guide the permanent teeth into a correct position in the dental arch.

Factors to be Considered for Space Maintenance

- Time elapsed since loss of tooth
- Dental age of the patient
- Amount of bone covering the developing succedaneous tooth bud
- Stage of root formation
- Congenitally missing tooth
- Eruption of permanent tooth in the opposite arch
- Oral musculature and habits

Indications of Space Maintainers

- When the forces acting upon the tooth are unbalanced and space analysis indicates a possible space inadequacy for the succedaneous.
- When a malocclusion exists that would aggravate the reduction of existing space.
- Maximum closure within the first 6 months after extraction. Therefore, it is best to insert an appliance as soon as possible after extraction.
- Delayed eruption of permanent tooth.

Contraindications for Space Maintainers

- When there is no alveolar bone overlying the crown of erupting tooth and there is sufficient space for its eruption.

- When permanent succeeding tooth is congenitally absent and space closure is desired.
- When the space left is in excess of the mesiodistal dimensions required for the eruption and space loss is not expected.

Ideal Requirements of Space Maintainer

- Should maintain the desired mesiodistal dimension of the space
- Should not interfere with physiological vertical eruption of the opposite teeth
- Should not interfere with eruption of permanent teeth.
- It should be simple in fabrication
- It should be strong enough to withstand the normal functional force

CLASSIFICATION OF SPACE MAINTAINERS

There are different methods of classifying space maintainers. They may be unilateral or bilateral.

According to hitchcock:
- Removable or fixed or semifixed
- With bands or without bands
- Functional or nonfunctional
- Active or passive
- Combinations of above

According to Raymond Thurow:
- Removable
- Complete arch-lingual arch

According to Hinrichson:
1. *Fixed space maintainers*
   a. *Class I*
      - Non-functional types
        1. Bar type
        2. Loop type
      - Functional type
        1. Pontic type
        2. Lingual arch type
   b. *Class II:* Cantilever type (distal shoe, band and loop)
2. *Removable space maintainer:* Acrylic partial dentures

TYPES OF SPACE MAINTAINERS

Removable Space Maintainers

They are the space maintainers which can be removed and reinserted into the oral cavity by the patient. They can be classified as functional and non-functional.
- *Functional:* Removable partial dentures that incorporate teeth to aid in mastication, speech and esthetics (Fig. 11.1).

- *Non-functional:* They have only an acrylic extension over the edentulous area to prevent space closure and over eruption of opposite teeth (Fig. 11.2).

Acrylic partial dentures: It is used in patients with multiple losses of teeth.

Full or complete dentures: They are used in cases of rampant caries when most of the primary teeth may require extraction. Due to improved preventive measures, they are quite rare in children nowadays.

Removable distal shoe space maintainer: It is devised by Starkey. This is indicated in premature loss of primary second molar before the eruption of permanent first molar. This is an immediate acrylic partial denture with an acrylic distal shoe extension. The acrylic extension is placed in the alveolus to guide the first permanent molar into position. This extension is grinded away when once the first molars cut into oral cavity.

Fixed Space Maintainer

There are two types:
- Bonded space maintainer
- Banded space maintainers

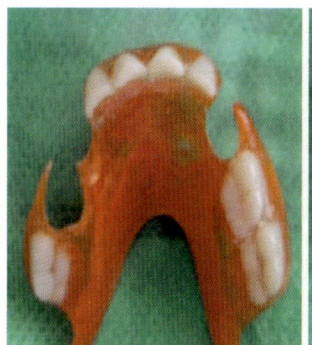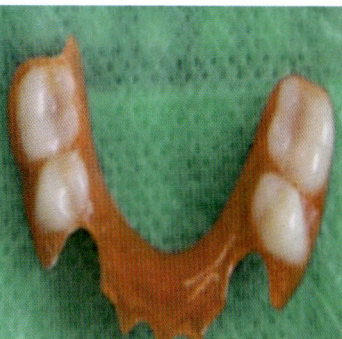

Fig. 11.1: Functional removable space maintainers

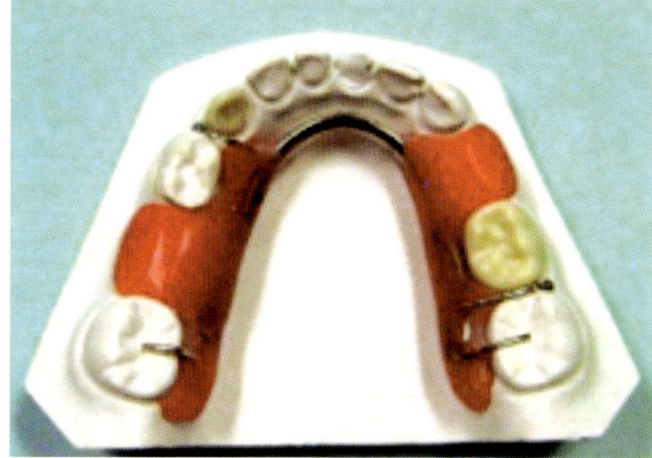

Fig. 11.2: Non-functional removable space maintainer

Band and Loop

Band and loop space maintainers used in dentistry. It is a passive fixed non-functional type. It is a unilateral fixed appliance indicated for space maintenance in the posterior segments when single tooth is lost. It can be used individually on both sides (Fig. 11.3).

Mayne space maintainer: This is a modification of band and loop where instead of a loop there is only lingual guiding wire with no wire on buccal side.

Crown and Loop Appliance

It is similar in all aspects to band and loop except that a stainless steel crown is used for the abutment teeth. Two methods can be used:
1. The loop can be directly attached to crown by soldering.
2. It can also be welded or soldered to a band which is adopted over the crown.

Lingual Arch Space Maintainer

The lingual arch space maintainer is the most effective appliance for space maintenance and minor tooth movement in the lower anterior in case of minor imbrications (Fig. 11.4).

Lingual Arch with Stops

When a primary cuspid is lost prematurely, the anterior can shift into its position. This causes a loss of arch length in that area. This can be prevented with the use of a lingual arch with stops. In the design shown here, loops have also been added to the archwire. These loops allow the doctor to adjust the length of the archwire to gain a small amount of arch length (Fig. 11.5).

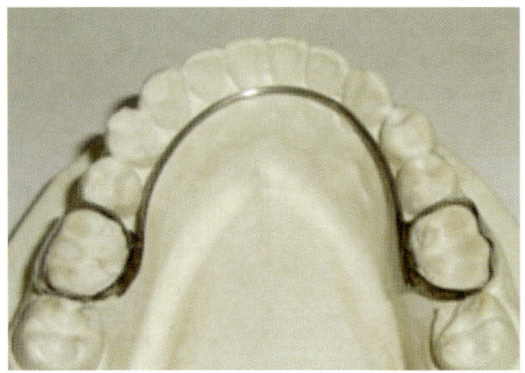

Fig. 11.4: Lingual arch space maintainer

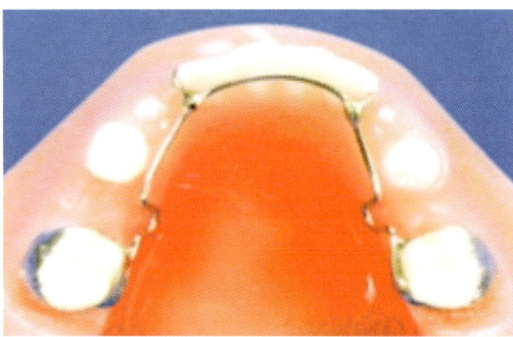

Fig. 11.5: Lingual arch with stops

Nance Holding Arch

This can be considered as a maxillary counterpart of lower lingual arch. The palatal portion approximates an acrylic button that the palatal tissue which provides resistance to the anterior movement of posterior teeth. They are constructed using 0.036 inch diameter hard stainless steel wire. Both the lower lingual arch and upper Nance holding arch can be used to reinforce the anchorage. It is indicated in case of bilateral loss of deciduous molars. It can be combined with a habit breaking appliance (Fig. 11.6).

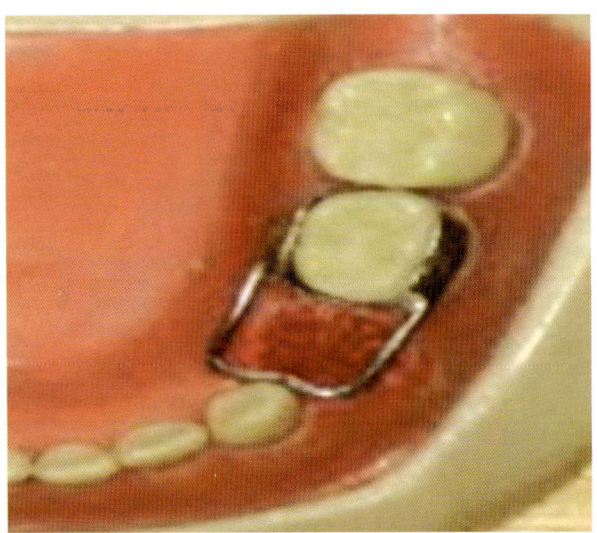

Fig. 11.3: Band and loop space maintainer

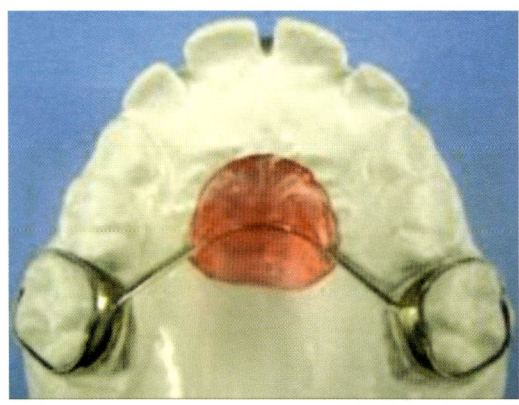

Fig. 11.6: Nance holding arch

Transpalatal Arch (Goshgarian Arch)

Transpalatal arch (TPA) has been recommended for stabilization of maxillary first permanent molars when the primary molars require extraction. It was introduced by Robert A Goshgarian of Illinois in 1972. It consists of 0.036 inch or 0.040 inch stainless steel round wire which is bent to the palatal contour and extends towards the palatal surface of the bands placed on the first permanent molar of one side to the other. It is indicated in the cases where unilateral loss of space is seen when one side of the arch is intact and several primary teeth on the other side are missing.

Transpalatal with Omega Loop

By adding a mid-palatal Omega loop to the standard transpalatal design, this appliance not only acts as an anchor, but when carefully activated can be used to rotate, torque, distallize or intrude the molars (Fig. 11.7).

Distal Shoe Space Maintainer

It was developed by Willets in 1932. It is also called Willet's appliance and eruption guided appliance. Popularly used distal shoe appliance is crown or band bar appliance described by Roche in 1942. Thus the appliance which is used in practice now is Roche's distal shoe or its modification using crown and band appliances with distal intragingival extension. The main difference between the two appliances is gingival extension. The Roche variety had a 'V' shaped gingival extension while the Willet's one had a bar type. Early loss or removal of the second primary molar prior to the eruption of the first permanent molar is the prime indication (Fig. 11.8a and b).

Limitations

- Overextension causes injury to the permanent tooth bud, i.e. second premolar.

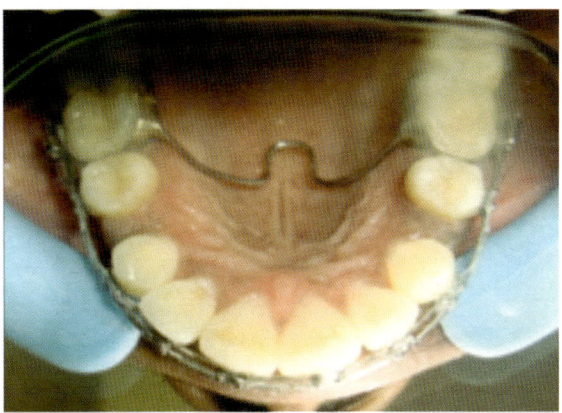

Fig. 11.7: Transpalatal with omega loop

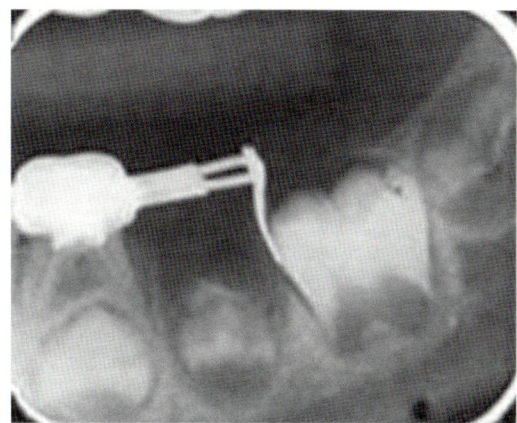

a

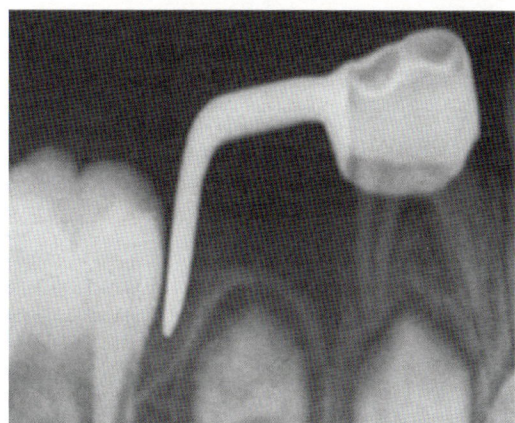

b

Fig. 11.8: (a) Roche distal shoe space maintainer; (b) Willet's appliance

- If underextended, it may allow the molar to tip into the space or over the band.
- Prevents complete epithelialization of extraction socket.

To be effective, the guide plane must extend into the alveolar process so that it contacts the permanent first molar approximately 1 mm below the mesial marginal ridge, at or before its emergence from the bone.

Band and Bar Type

The abutment teeth on either side of the extraction space are banded and connected to each other by a bar. Alternatively stainless steel crown can be placed on abutments and is called crown and bar space maintainer.

Preformed Posterior Space Maintainer

A new posterior space maintainer consists of solid steel foil pad bases, one anterior and one posterior. Stainless steel tubing of 9 mm long and an internal diameter of 1–2 mm soldered to posterior wire. The wire length is measured intraorally and cuts off the excess.

The appliance is adjusted according to the mesiodistal dimension of the extraction space. The wire is inserted into tube and crimped in place. The appliance is ready for direct bonding. It can be inserted in both upper and lower arch (Fig. 11.9a and b).

Advantages

- No bands or impression are necessary
- It can be completed in one appointment
- It can be used for posterior spaces of any length
- It permits the normal eruption of teeth
- It can be used in partially erupted where bands may not
- It can be bonded either buccally or lingually

Glass Fiber-reinforced Composite Resin (GFRCR) as a Space Maintainer

In order to determine the length of GFRCR required, the distance between the mesiobuccal line angle of the primary canine and distobuccal line angle of the second primary molar is measured using a digital vernier caliper. After administration of adequate anesthesia, isolation is done using a rubber dam and suction. Both the abutment teeth (primary canine and second primary molar) are cleaned with pumice slurry and then etched with 35% orthophosphoric acid for 40 seconds. The teeth are rinsed, air-dried, and wetted with an adhesive that is as light-cured for 20 seconds.

This application is repeated 2–3 times to prevent contraction gap formation. A thin layer of flowable composite is applied to the buccal surfaces of the abutment tooth without light-curing it. The cut length of GFRCR is placed on this flowable composite, extending from the buccal aspect of primary second molar to buccal aspect of primary canine. The ends of the fiber are adapted to the teeth surfaces with a plastic filling instrument. Preliminary curing is done individually at each end of the fiber framework for 40 seconds, during which the other end is protected from the light source.

An additional layer of flowable composite is applied over the area where the fiber abutted the tooth surface and this is light-cured for 40 seconds. A similar procedure is repeated on the lingual aspect of the abutment teeth. Any uncovered fiber is further covered with flowable composite. The space maintainer is checked for gingival clearance and occlusal interference. Finishing is done using composite finishing burs. Finally, as per the manufacturer's instructions, bonding agent is applied over the fiber frame and light-cured at multiple points for the purpose of reactivation (Fig. 11.10).

Buccal Bar

Two bands and a buccal bar are used for maintaining space where a long span prohibits the use of a basic space maintainer and allow you to regain a small amount of lost space (Fig. 11.11).

Occlusal Bar

This two-band space maintainer with an occlusal bar is designed top prevent supereruption of the opposing

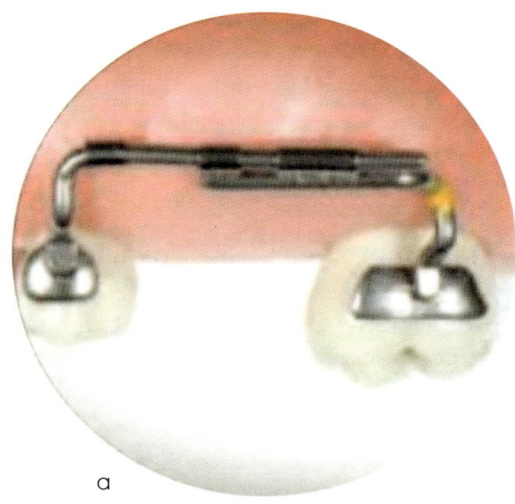

a

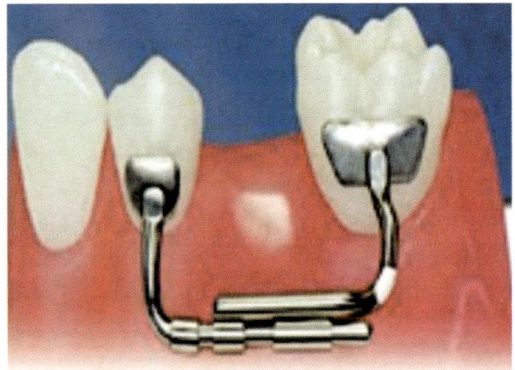

b

Fig. 11.9: (a) EZ space maintainer in upper arch; (b) EZ space maintainer in lower arch

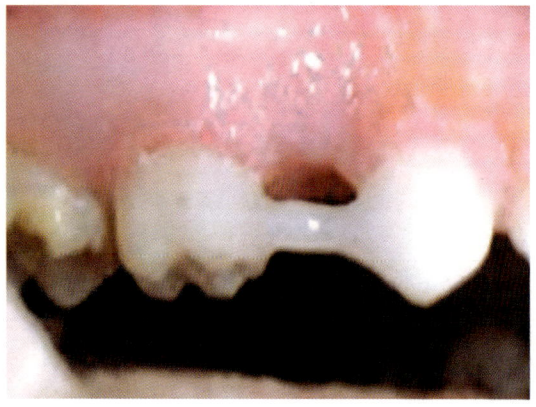

Fig. 11.10: Bonded space maintainer

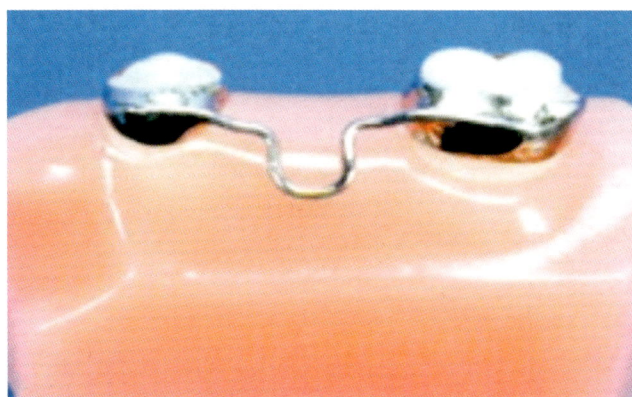

Fig. 11.11: Buccal bar

teeth. This cleansable design allows patients to easily maintain their oral hygiene.

Occlusal Pad

This two-band space maintainer has an acrylic pad over the edentulous region. It is designed with an occlusal surface of the pad in function with the opposing teeth and the tissue side cleared away to eliminate any interference with the normal eruption of the succedaneous teeth.

This appliance can act as a food trap. This can be controlled easily with the use of an oral irrigator (Fig. 11.12).

Crown and Loop

A crown may be used in conjunction with a space maintainer. As with the other unilateral space maintainers, an occlusal rest on the adjacent tooth will prevent unwanted mesial tipping of the molar.

Crown and Loop with Rest

When your treatment plan requires that a crown and loop space maintainer be used for an extended period of time, it is suggested that the appliance include the

rest on the abutment tooth to prevent unwanted mesial movement and tipping.

Essix

The Essix retainer is a popular retainer for the extremely appearance conscious patient. It is fabricated by thermoforming a thin sheet of Essix material over the entire arch. Essix material is made of a clear acrylic that is tough, stain and abrasive resistant and has the light-reflecting properties to make the teeth appear brilliant when the retainer is in place. The appliance covers the buccal, labial, and lingual surfaces and extends onto the gingival tissue.

Wilson 3D Lingual Arch

The Wilson 3D system has special attachment to the bands that permit the lingual arch to be removed in a vertical direction. The adjustment loops in the wire (referred to as "activators") make this lingual arch much more than just an arch length space-maintaining device. The activator is a diamond-shaped loop that is easily adjusted with a flat-on-round light wire plier. Proper adjustment of the activator loops can provide a number of different movements such as: anterior-posterior arch length increase, buccal expansion, distal molar movement, molar torque or tip, and molar rotation (Fig. 11.13).

Groper Fixed Anterior Bridge (Fig. 11.14)

Esthetics and strength are the key advantages to this popular design.

This design is often used when the abutment teeth are partially compromised, or when superior strength of the overall appliance is desired.

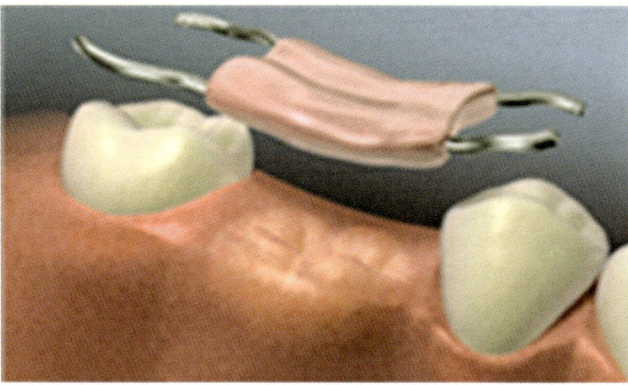

Fig. 11.12: Occlusal pad

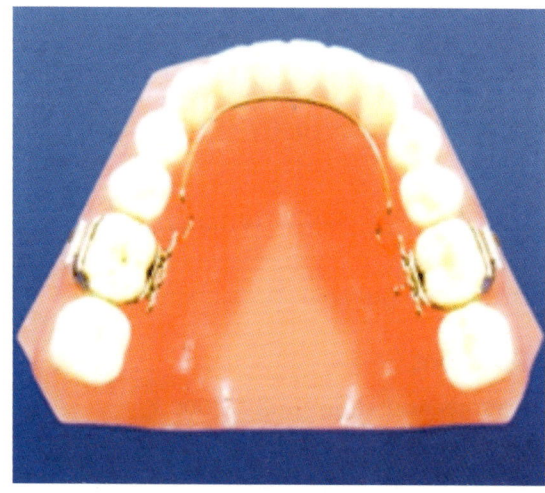

Fig. 11.13: Wilson 3D lingual arch

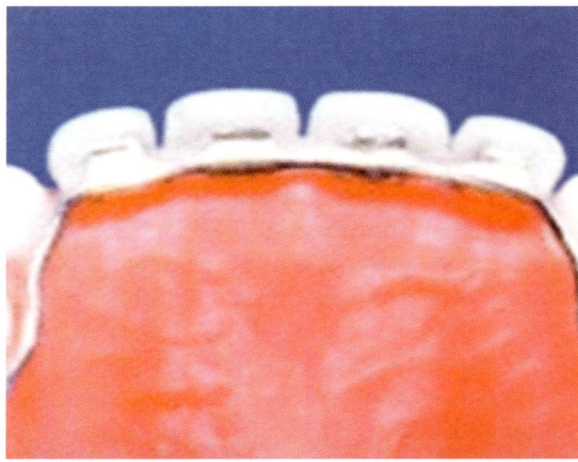

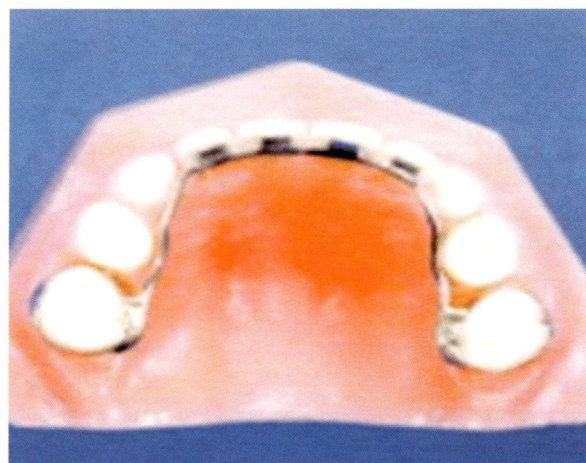

Fig. 11.14: Groper fixed anterior bridge—with crowns

This is particularly useful for patients who tend to be tough on their appliances.

BIBLIOGRAPHY

1. Ackerman JL, Proffit WR. Preventive and interceptive orthontics: A strong theory proves weak in practice. Angle Orthod 1980; 50:75–86.
2. Dewel BF. Serial extraction, its limitations and contra-indications in orthodontic treatment. Am J Orthod 1967; 53:904–21.

PREVIOUS YEAR'S UNIVERSITY QUESTIONS

Essay

1. Classify space maintainer. Write in detail about distal shoe appliance.
2. Discuss the removable space maintainer.

Short Questions

1. Indications and contraindications
2. Glass fiber-reinforced composite resin as a space maintainer
3. Nance holding arch
4. TPA
5. Parent's counseling

MCQs

1. *Preventive orthodontics is undertaken:*
a. Before development of a malocclusion
b. After the malocclusion has already manifested
c. After eruption of 3rd molars
d. All of the above   **(Ans: a)**

2. *If the child is bottle fed, the mother is advised to use:*
a. Physiologic nipple
b. Conventional nipple
c. Artificial nipple
d. All of the above   **(Ans: a)**

3. *Physiologic nipple permits:*
a. Sucking of milk resembling normal functional activity
b. Easy passage of milk into child's oral cavity
c. Dental caries prevention
d. All of the above   **(Ans: a)**

4. *Classical example of natural space maintainer is:*
a. Deciduous dentition
b. Deciduous molar
c. Permanent molars
d. Permanent dentition   **(Ans: a)**

5. *Enamel pearls may cause:*
a. Occlusal interference
b. Premature contact
c. Both a and b
d. None of the above   **(Ans: c)**

6. *Example of a removable space maintainer:*
a. Acrylic partial denture
b. Full or complete denture
c. Removable distal shoe space maintainer
d. All of the above   **(Ans: d)**

7. *Crown and bar space maintainer is a modification of:*
a. Crown and loop
b. Bar and loop
c. Band and loop
d. Band and bar   **(Ans: d)**

8. *According to Hinrichsen, a distal shoe appliance comes under:*
a. Class I fixed space maintainer.
b. Class II fixed space maintainer
c. Class III fixed space maintainer
d. Class IV fixed space maintainer   **(Ans: b)**

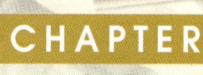

Interceptive Orthodontics

Chapter Outline

- Introduction
- Serial extraction
- Space regainers
- Muscle exercises

INTRODUCTION

Interceptive orthodontics involves the early treatment of occlusal disturbances to eliminate or simplify their future management. Such intervention is usually undertaken during the mixed dentition stage of development. The number of situations encountered are listed during various stages of the developing dentition that may benefit from interceptive treatment.

Unlike preventive orthodontic procedures, interceptive orthodontics is undertaken at a time when the malocclusion has already developed or is developing. It basically refers to measures undertaken to prevent a potential malocclusion from progressing into a more severe one. Some of the procedures carried out in preventive orthodontics but the timings are different.

The interceptive treatment may benefit a number of the clinical situations outlined below.

Early mixed dentition:
- Digit sucking habit
- Delayed eruption
- Supernumerary tooth
- Early loss of deciduous teeth
- Anterior crossbite
- Posterior crossbite
- Severe crowding
- Increased overjet

Late mixed dentition:
- Ectopic maxillary canines
- Infraocclusion
- Hypodontia
- Traumatic overbite
- Increased overjet

Early permanent dentition:
- Impacted teeth
- Crowding

Interceptive orthodontic procedures:
- Serial extraction
- Space regaining
- Control of abnormal habits
- Correction of developing crossbite
- Diastema closure
- Removal of premature contacts
- Interception of skeletal malrelationship
- Removal of soft tissue or bony barrier to eruption of teeth

SERIAL EXTRACTION

Serial extraction is an interceptive orthodontic procedure undertaken in the early mixed dentition period that involves planned removal of certain primary and permanent teeth in a programmed sequence, so as to relieve crowding in the arches and to guide the remaining erupting permanent teeth into more favorable position.

Definition

Tweed defined serial extraction as the planned and sequential removal of the primary and permanent teeth to intercept and reduce dental crowding problems.

Historical Perspective

Robert Bunon in early 1743 was the first to advise the extraction of primary teeth to achieve a better alignment of permanent teeth.

The term serial extraction was first coined by Kjellgren in 1929. However, it was Nance who popularized the procedure in 1940s in England and he is considered as the *father of serial extraction technique*.

Indications

- Premature exfoliation of deciduous canine especially in the lower arch.
- Lingual eruption of lower lateral incisors (Fig. 12.1).
- Severe arch length—tooth material discrepancy of 10 mm or more in the arch.
- Midline shift due to displacement of lateral incisors following premature loss of unilateral deciduous canine.
- Proclination of permanent upper and lower incisors associated with crowding.
- Absence of developmental/physiologic spacing in the deciduous dentition.
- Abnormal root resorption pattern of deciduous canines. Radiological examination reveals a crescent pattern of resorption on the mesial side of the primary canine roots.

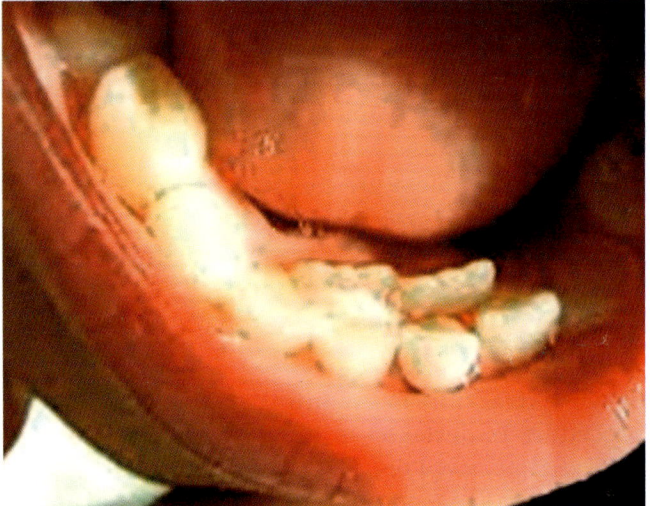

Fig. 12.1: Typical case of serial extraction

Contraindications

- Congenitally missing teeth
- Presence of deep bite or open bite
- In cleft palate and cleft lip cases
- When there is collapsed arch
- Presence of midline diastema and spacing
- Class II and class III malocclusion with skeletal abnormalities
- Anodontia/oligodontia
- Class I malocclusion with minimal space deficiency
- Unerupted malformed teeth, e.g. dilacerations
- Mild disproportion between arch length and tooth material.

Procedure

No single extraction sequence applies to all patients. Some of the commonly used methods are described here.

- Dewel's method
- Nance method
- Tweed's method
- Grewe's method

Dewel's Method (1978) (Extraction of CD4)

Step-1: In this step, the deciduous canines are extracted at around 8–9 years to create space for the alignment of the incisors.

Step-2: In this step, deciduous first molars are extracted when first premolars reach half of the root length as seen in intraoral radiographs.

This is done at 12 months after the extraction of deciduous canines. The objective of deciduous first molar extraction is to accelerate the eruption of first premolars. This ensures that the first premolars emerge into the oral cavity before the eruption of permanent canines.

Step-3: In this step, first premolars are extracted as they are emerging into the oral cavity and when the permanent canines have developed beyond half of the root length. Extraction of first premolars facilitates proper eruption and alignment of permanent canines (Box 12.1).

However, the establishment of proper intercuspation usually requires orthodontic mechanotherapy of minimal duration.

Tweed's Method (1966) (Extraction of D4C)

This method involves the extraction of the deciduous first molars at 8 years of age. This is followed by the extraction of the first premolars and the deciduous canines simultaneously (Fig. 12.2).

Box 12.1: Summary of Dewel method

Steps	Tooth extracted	Purpose
Step-1	Extraction of deciduous canine	To facilitate alignment of incisors
Step-2	Extraction of deciduous first molar	To facilitate the eruption of first premolars before the eruption of permanent canines
Step-3	Extraction of first premolars	To facilitate the eruption of permanent canines

Nance Method

Nance method is the modification of Tweed's method which involves the extraction of the deciduous first molars followed by the extraction of the first premolars and the deciduous canines.

Grewe's Method

It is based on the planning of extraction sequence for different clinical conditions.

Class I malocclusion with premature loss of a mandibular deciduous canine: This will lead to midline shift, when the arch length discrepancy is 5–10 mm/arch, then the remaining deciduous canine should be extracted next, if the first premolar have their roots more than half formed. If the roots of the first premolars are not developed more than half, then extractions of the deciduous first molar is delayed. The first premolars should be extracted as they emerge.

Class I malocclusion with severe mandibular anterior crowding: Deciduous canines are extracted, when there is arch length deficiency and more than 5 mm per quadrant. The deciduous first molars are extracted next on completion of at least half of the premolar root formation and the extraction of first premolars follow as they erupt into the oral cavity.

Class I malocclusion where minimal mandibular anterior crowding (6–10 mm arch deficiency): The deciduous first molars are extracted when the roots of the premolars are more than half formed (Fig. 12.3).

SPACE REGAINING

If a primary molar is lost early and space maintainers are not used, reduction in arch length by mesial movement of 1st permanent molar can be expected. Space lost can be regained by distal movement of first molar. Estimation of space lost can be done by mixed dentition analysis. The space can be regained up to 3 mm. Space regaining procedures are preferably undertaken prior to eruption of 2nd permanent molar.

SPACE REGAINERS

- Modified Hawley's appliance
- *Sling shot appliance:* Two hooks on buccal and lingual side of molar to be incorporated in the acrylic plate to hold the elastic. The elastic is stretched at the mesial aspect of molar to ditalize it.

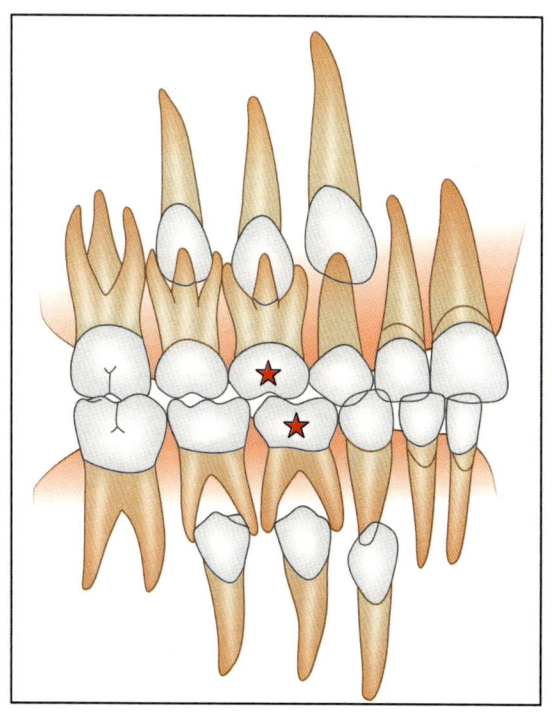
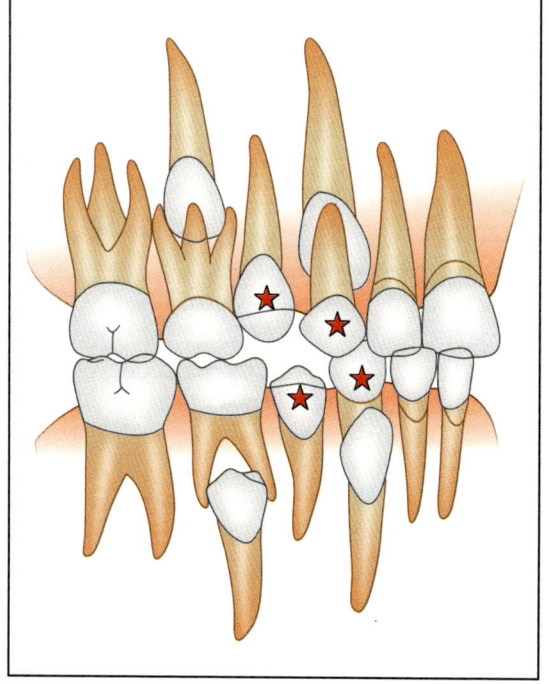

Fig. 12.2: Tweed's method

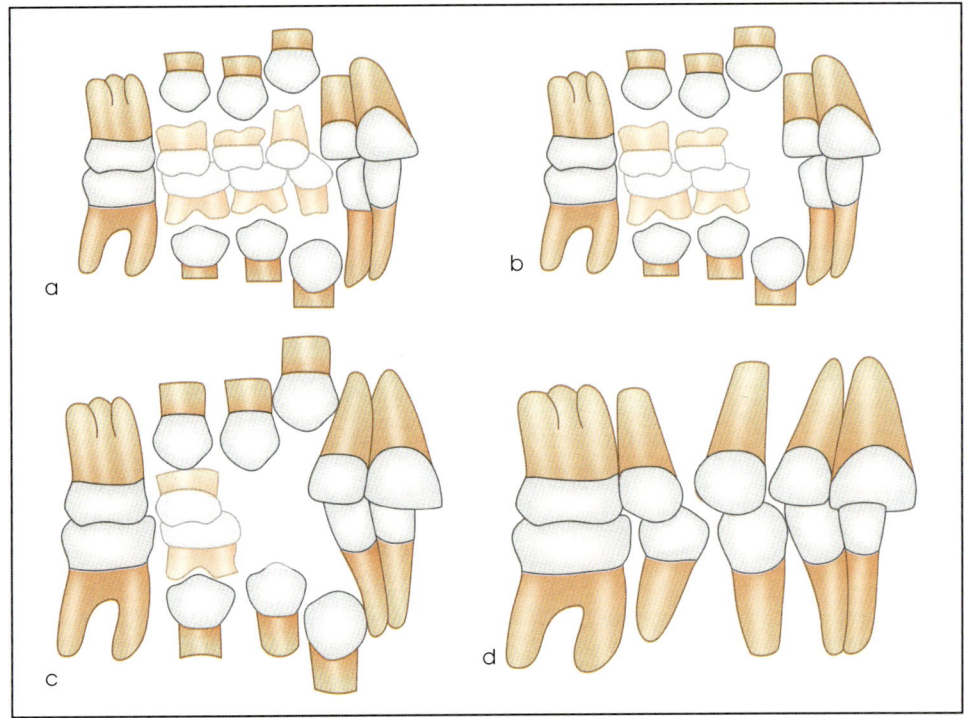

Fig. 12.3: Grewe's method

- Modified Humphery appliance
- Removable or fixed lingual arch with springs
- Expansion screw regainer
- Recurved helical spring regainer
- Knee spring regainer
- Clasp rings
- Modified bonded space regainer
- Gerber space regainer
- Open coil space regainer

Modified Bonded Space Regainer

Modified space regainer/maintainer are a simple appliance that can be placed chairside in single visit. A composite dimple is bonded on the buccal side of permanent first molar and with the help of an explorer; a tunnel is burrowed into the mesial of the dimple. This creates a composite tunnel that is open only on the mesial. A piece of .016″ NiTi wire then bonded on the buccal side of primary molar and extended beyond the dimple. After the composite has set on both teeth, with the help of bird beak plier, direct the free end of wire into the tunnel made in the dimple of first molar. This will give a form of activated loop NiTi wire. A small amount of bonding material is placed in the opening of tunnel to make the attachment more permanent.

Over the time, the loop returns to its original shape due to the memory properties of NiTi wire, at the same time distalizing and uprighting the first molar. Once the active correction is completed, the wire segment is left in place as a passive space maintainer, until the eruption of second premolar (Fig. 12.4).

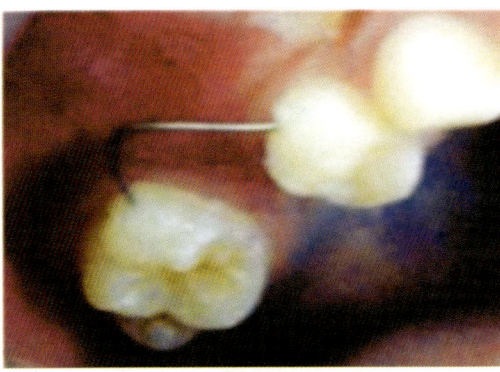

Before

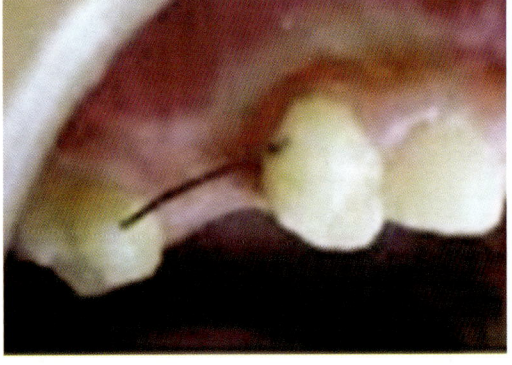

After

Fig. 12.4: NiTi sface regainer

Gerber Space Regainer

It consists of U-shaped hollow tubing in which U-shaped rod is inserted. Tube is soldered on the mesial aspect of molar to be moved distally, base of rod contacting tooth mesial to edentulous area. Open coil springs are placed around free ends of rod and inserted into tubing assembly. Forces generated by compressd coil spring moves molar distally.

Open Coil Space Regainer

The buccal and lingual tubes are soldered to the adapted permanent first molar. The tubes should be parallel to one another in all planes. 0.7 mm stainlessl steel wire is bent to U shape which fits passively in both the buccal and lingual tubes. At the junction of the straight and curved part of the wire, both buccally and lingually, a stop is prepared by soldering. Then cut enough spaced open coil spring so as to extend from the stop to a point about 2 mm distal to the anterior limit of the tube on the molar band. The coil spring is slipped on the wire. The wire is then put in the tubes and the band with the wire and compressed spring is cemented on the molar. The compressed spring become passive and exert reciprocal pressure mesially to the premolar and distally to the permanent molar (Fig. 12.5).

Hawley's Appliance with Split Acrylic Dumb-Bell Spring

Hawley's appliance on the mandibular arch is constructed with a split acrylic dumb-bell spring. It is used to regain up to 2 mm of lost space by tipping one of the permanent first molars distally. It is an effective and comfortable appliance during treatment.

Dumb-bell spring allows easy adjustments to add distalizing force to the lower molar and the limit of

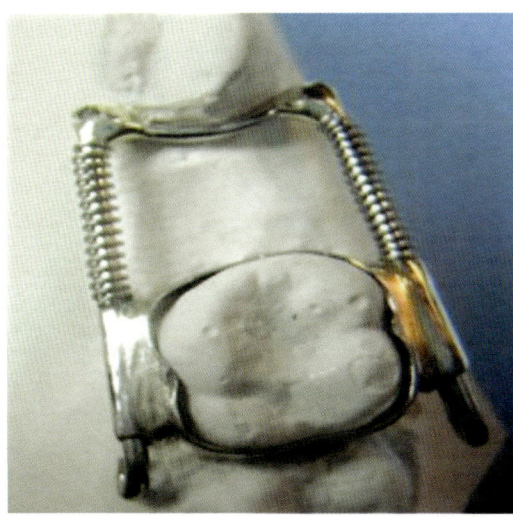

Fig. 12.5: Open coil space regainer

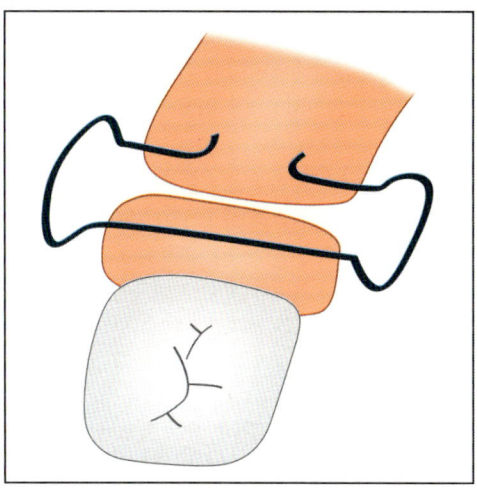

Fig. 12.6: Split acrylic dumb-bell spring

possible spring opening is at least 3 mm which is beyond the necessity of the usual movement of this tooth. The spring should be adjusted twice a month, creating an increment of opening in the split acrylic area of 0.5 mm at a time (Fig. 12.6).

MUSCLE EXERCISES

Exercises for the Lips

A number of exercises have been advocated for the lips and circumoral musculature in patients with hypotonic lips and short upper lips.

- Stretching of the upper lip to maintain lip seal is an important therapeutic measure in patients having short hypotonic lips. To aid in the stretching, the patient is asked to hold a piece of paper between the lips.

- Patient can be asked to stretch the upper lip inferiorly towards the chin.

- Holding and pumping of water back and forth behind the lips.

- Lip massaging.

- Button pull exercise
  a. A button of one and half inch is taken and a thread passed through the button hole. Patient is asked to place the button behind the lips and pull the thread, while restricting it from being pulled out by using lip pressure.
  b. *Tug of war exercise:* This involves use of two buttons, with one kept behind the lips while the other button is held by another person to pull the thread.
  c. Playing a reed musical instrument produces fine lip tonicity.

Exercise for Tongue

- *Barnet's tongue positioning exercises:*
  a. Identify the incisal papilla as the spot behind front teeth.
  b. Practice touching spot with the tongue tip
  c. Swallow with lips and teeth closed and tongue tip touching the incisal papilla
  d. Have patient practice this with lips apart.
- Andrew recommends practice of swallow correctly 20 times before meals with water in the mouth and mirror in hand. Each practice is followed by relaxation of muscles until the swallowing progress smoothly. Use of sugarless mint held against roof of the mouth stimulates saliva and makes it necessary to swallow.
- *Single elastic swallow of Gardiner:* Using orthodontic elastic band of 1/4" or 5/16" placed on the tip of the tongue plus speech exercises—'D', 't'.
- *Double elastic swallow:* Place 1 elastic each at tip and middle of tongue contact with tip and mid-part of palate. Lips open with buccal teeth together. Speech exercises—'C', 'h', 'g'.
- *Peanuts and elastic band:* Patient chews peanuts but not to swallow it. The chewed peanuts are placed in the middle of the tongue. Place the elastic at tip of tongue. Instruct the practice of swallow. Then, speech exercises—'C', 'g', 'k'.

BIBLIOGRAPHY

1. Ackerman JL Proffit WR. Preventive and interceptive orthodontics: Strong theory work in practice. Angle Orthod 1980; 50:75–86.
2. Dewel BF. Serial extraction: its limitations and contra-indications in orthodontic treatment. Am J Orthod 1967;53:904–21.
3. Norton A, Wickwire Na, Gellin ME. Space management in mixed dentition. J Dent Child 1975;42:0112–8.

PREVIOUS YEAR'S UNIVERSITY QUESTIONS

Essay

1. Define serial extraction. Write about Nance method.
2. List out the various space regainers. Write a note on Gerber space regainer.

Short Questions

1. Exercise for lips
2. Hawley's appliance with split acrylic dumb-bell spring
3. Indications and contraindications
4. Open coil space regainer

MCQs

1. *The term serial extraction was first used by:*
   a. Kjellgren
   b. Nance
   c. Dewey
   d. Raymond C Thurrow   **(Ans: a)**

2. *Planned and progressive extraction is related to:*
   a. Wilkinson's extraction
   b. Serial extraction
   c. Therapeutic extraction
   d. Any of the above   **(Ans: b)**

3. *The first tooth to be extracted in Tweed's method:*
   a. Deciduous first molar
   b. Deciduous second molar
   c. Deciduous canine
   d. Permanent first premolar   **(Ans: a)**

4. *Best time to correct anterior crossbite:*
   a. 6 years
   b. 7 years
   c. First time it is seen
   d. After eruption of all anterior   **(Ans: c)**

5. *Functional anterior crossbite is seen in:*
   a. Class I malocclusion
   b. Class II malocclusion
   c. Class III malocclusion
   d. Pseudo Class III malocclusion **(Ans-D)**

6. *Button pull exercise is done for:*
   a. Lips
   b. Tongue
   c. Cheeks
   d. Teeth   **(Ans: a)**

7. *Tug of war exercise is a good exercise for:*
   a. Masseter muscle
   b. Buccinator muscle
   c. Tongue
   d. Lips **(Ans: d)**

8. *One elastic swallow exercise is for:*
   a. To prevent tongue thrusting
   b. To prevent lip biting
   c. To prevent bruxism
   d. To correct improper positioning of tongue
      (Ans: d)

9. *Hold pull exercise is helpful in:*
   a. Preventing tongue thrusting

b. Proper positioning of tongue

c. Stretching the lingual frenum

d. Lip seal   **(Ans: c)**

10. *One relastic swallow and two elastic swallow are exercises for:*

a. Lips

b. Tongue

c. Cheeks

d. Preventing bruxism   **(Ans: b)**

11. *Father of serial extraction is*

a. Kjellgren

b. Tweed

c. Nance

d. Dewel   **(Ans: c)**

Surgical Orthodontics

Chapter Outline

- Canine impaction
- Two-stage Interalveolar corticotomy
- Circumferential supracrestal fibrotomy

- Frenectomy
- Orthognathic surgery
- Distraction osteogenesis

INTRODUCTION

They can be used as an adjunct or in conjunction with orthodontic treatment. Some surgical procedures are carried out before orthondontic treatment, and some during orthodontic therapy. These surgical procedures are usually carried out:

- To eliminate the existing etiologic factor, e.g. labial frenectomy for abnormal frenal attachment, surgical exposure and removal of impacted teeth.
- As a part of treatment, e.g. therapeutic extractions and serial extraction
- Stabilize the orthodontic treatment results and prevent relapse; e.g. supracrestal fibrotomy
- To correct severe skeletal discrepancies; e.g. orthognathic surgeries.

Surgical orthodontics is divided into minor surgical and major surgical procedures.

Minor Surgical Procedure

- Canine/incisor impaction
- Supracrystal fibrotomy
- Frenectomy
- Two-stage interalveolar corticotomy
- Therapeutic extraction
- Supernumerary extraction
- Removal of soft tissue and bony barrier to enable eruption of teeth
- Canine retraction by distraction osteogenesis

CANINE IMPACTION

The permanent canines play a pivotal role in achieving an esthetic smile, functional occlusion and also in establishing the arch form. They are the most dimensionally stable teeth in the oral cavity because they are the longest, with good labiolingual thickness and effective anchorage in the alveolar process. However, the incidence of an impacted canine is high which can be due to various reasons. A thorough clinical examination and radiographic evaluation is required to evaluate whether the impacted canine is in favorable or unfavorable position for guiding into the oral cavity.

The maxillary canine is the most commonly impacted tooth. The prevalence of maxillary canine impaction is 1–2% with a female: male ratio of 2:1. 85% of impaction is palatal while the remainder 15% occurs buccally.

Normal Development of Maxillary Canine

The maxillary canine begins its development high in the maxilla at the age of 4–5 months. The tooth has a long path of eruption, passing along the distal root surface of the lateral incisor, buccal to the deciduous canine and its final position reaches at 11–12 years. The canine should be palpable high in the buccal sulcus by the age of 10 years.

Etiology of Canine Impaction

- *The genetic theory:* It states that genetic factors may be important in determining crypt position or the direction of eruption.
- *The guidance theory:* It suggests that the distal root surface of the maxillary lateral incisor is important in guiding the maxillary canine into the arch. When the lateral incisor is small or absent there is a predisposition to canine impaction.
- *Crowding:* It is the most common cause of buccal canine impaction.

The canine impaction is caused by primary and secondary causes.

Primary causes:
- Rate of root resorption of deciduous teeth
- Trauma to the deciduous tooth bud
- Lack of availability of space in the arch
- Disturbances in tooth eruption sequences
- Rotation of tooth buds
- Premature of root closure
- Canine eruption into the cleft palate area

Secondary causes:
- Abnormal muscle pressure
- Febrile diseases
- Endocrine disturbances
- Vitamin D deficiency

It is imperative to assess whether the impacted canine is in favorable position or unfavorable position for management. If it is an unfavorable position, the treatment plan will depend on:
1. Whether it is symptomatic or
2. Whether it is associated with pathology or
3. Whether it is non-symptomatic without pathology

No.1 and 2 situations require surgical extraction and no.3 requires observation to assess, if orthodontic/prosthodontic management is required.

If the tooth is in a favorable position, then the following treatment plan can be considered.
- Surgical exposure and spontaneous eruption
- Surgical exposure and orthodontic traction.

Clinical and Radiographic Signs of Impaction

Clinical signs of impaction include:
- Failure to palpate the canine buccally by 10 years of age
- Immobility of the deciduous canine
- A palatal bulge indicating the presence of the underlying canine.

- Inadequate space within the dental arch for canine eruption.
- Increased mobility or non-vitality of the maxillary central and lateral incisors.

Radiographic signs include:
- A palatal canine position demonstrated using the parallax technique
- The canine overlapping the lateral or central incisor root
- The long axis of the canine angled more than 25° to the vertical plane.

Radiographic Assessment of Canine Position

This is commonly accomplished using the vertical (dental panoramic tomogram; DPT; and upper anterior occlusal radiograph) or horizontal (two periapical taken at different angles) parallax techniques. A palatally positioned canine will move in the same direction as the tube shift between the radiographs.

The buccal canine will move in the opposite direction of the tube shift. A canine in the line of the arch will remain static between tube shifts. A lateral cephalogram can also be used to assess vertical and anteroposterior position. Factors to consider when assessing canine position and the prognosis for alignment include the vertical position, horizontal position and angulation.

Management of Palatally Displaced Canines

There are several options for the management of palatally impacted canines.
- Extraction of the deciduous canine
- No treatment
- Orthodontic alignment
- Surgical removal
- Autotransplantation

Extraction of the deciduous canine in patients aged between 10 and 13 years, where the permanent canine is palatal, may help to normalize its eruptive path particularly if there is adequate space within the arch. If there is crowding, the chances of normalization are reduced. If there is no sign of radiographic improvement after 12 months, it is unlikely to occur and other options should be considered.

No treatment is indicated when the patient is poorly motivated. They should be warned about the potential risk of resorption of the adjacent incisor roots and cystic change within the canine follicle. Annual radiographic review is advised to check for complications.

Orthodontic alignment following surgical exposure is indicated in well-motivated patients where the canine has a favorable position (Fig. 13.1). Alignment is most commonly accomplished using fixed appliances with traction applied via chain (Fig. 13.2) or ligature or elastic thread (Fig. 13.3) and magnets (Fig. 13.4) bonded to the crown of the canine at the time of surgical exposure or to a bracket directly attached to its surface. Space must be available within the arch to accommodate the impacted tooth. This can be gained by redistributing space already present, the use of headgear to distalize

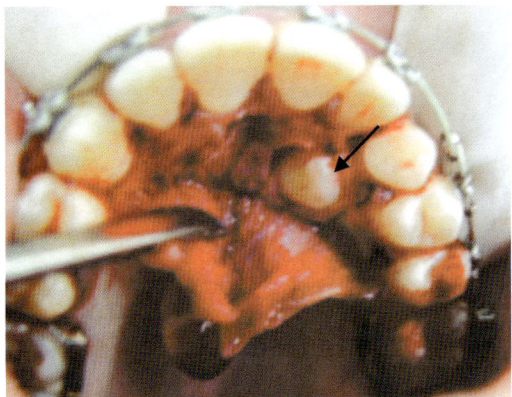

Fig. 13.1: Surgical exposure of palatally impacted canine

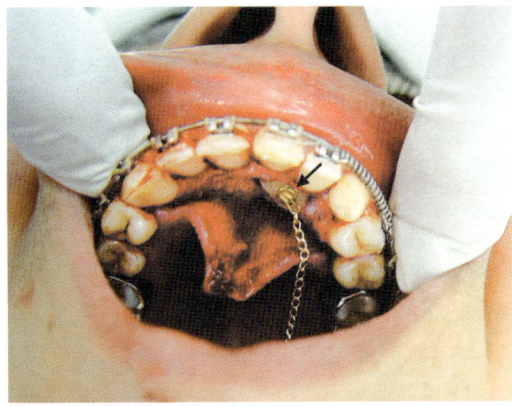

Fig. 13.2: After surgical exposure, orthodontic traction by chain

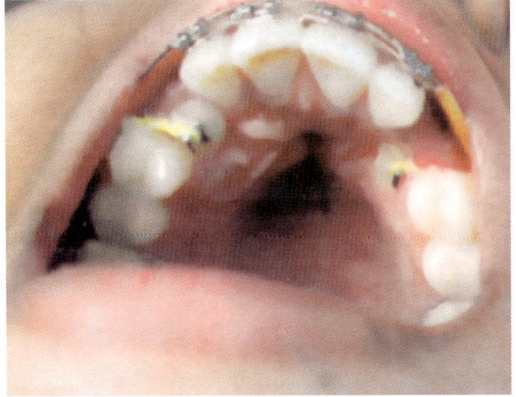

Fig. 13.3: Palatally impacted canine treated with fixed appliance using elastic thread

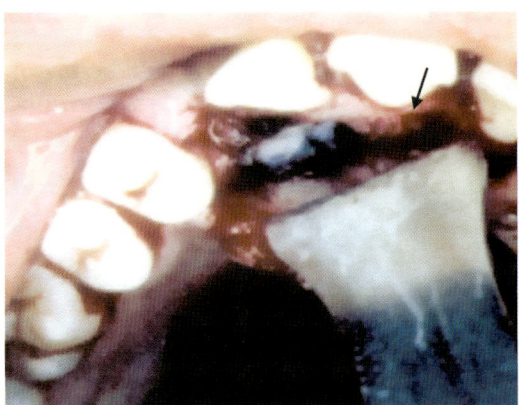

Fig. 13.4: Using magnets in correcting palatally impacted canine

the buccal segments or by extractions. Treatment may take between 2 and 2.5 years.

Surgical removal should be considered when the canine is in a very unfavorable position, in poorly motivated patients in whom orthodontic treatment is contraindicated and in cases of severe crowding. In the latter case, the first premolar can be substituted as a canine.

Buccally Displaced Maxillary Canines and Incisors

The most common cause is severe crowding where the canine gets deflected buccally. The canine will erupt in the majorities of cases, if the crowding is relieved. If the impacted canine is unfavorable position, it should be removed surgically, if it causes any problems.

The treatment methods for favorable impacted canines consist of two aspects. They are the:
- Surgical procedures
- Methods of attachment

Surgical Procedures

Surgical exposure is described to make a tunnel for eruption to occur. It is stated that injury to the soft tissue is less when compared with the completed exposure of the crown of canine. If the canine impaction is not in the favorable position, the extraction is the only choice (Fig. 13.5).

The open eruption technique: This is the exposure of the entire labial aspect of the anatomic crown with total excision of all keratinized tissue (window approach). It is reported to result in significant loss of periodontal attachment, recession, gingival inflammation, lack of keratinized gingiva and reduced sulcus depth.

The apically repositioned flap is a modification aimed at improving the periodontal outcome by raising a full flap taken from the crest of the ridge and relocating it higher upon the crown of the newly

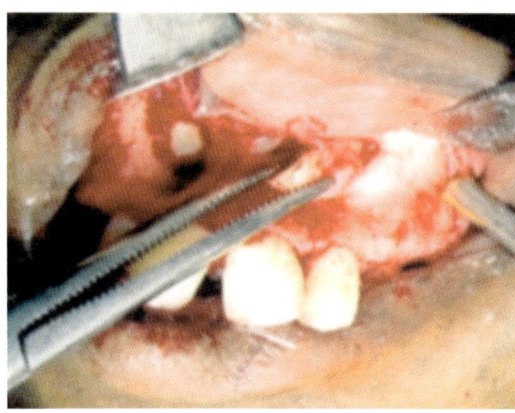

Fig. 13.5: Extraction of unfavorable canine impaction

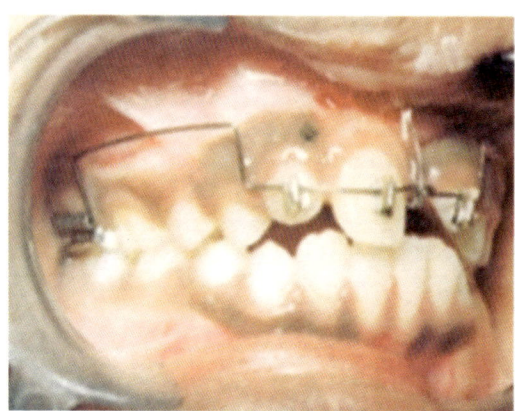

Fig. 13.6: Incisor impaction and 2 × 4 appliance with utility arch design

exposed. The method is a recognized and accepted procedure in periodontics.

The closed eruption technique: For labially impacted canine, a surgical flap is raised from the attached gingiva at the crest of the ridge with suitable releasing cuts and elevated as high as to expose the unerupted canine. An attachment is then bonded to the tooth and the flap is fully sutured back to the former place. The twisted stainless steel ligature wire that has been placed on the attachment is then drawn inferiorly and through the sutured edges of the replaced flap.

Method of Attachment

Many auxiliary attachments can be fixed on the exposed impacted canines by which the orthodontic forces can be applied. They are cast gold canine caps, gold chain (Fig. 13.7a) or threaded pin drilled into the tooth tip. The orthodontic brackets can be directly bonded to the impacted tooth and extruded by ligature wire, (Fig. 13.7b), elastic thread and elastic chains (Fig. 13.8). Magnets are also used. U-flex eruption device with flexible base curved to fit incisal edge of upper incisor has also been used. Sectional Fixed appliance can be given for incisor impaction (2 × 4 appliances with utility arch design) (Fig. 13.6).

Incisor Impaction

The Easy-Way-Coil (EWC) system—consisting of a stainless steel coil spring, an orthodontic attachment, and a stainless steel ligature wire—was introduced in 2008 as an alternative means of applying a continuous eruptive force to an impacted tooth. Although it is easily inserted and activated, like similar techniques, it is designed for use with a base archwire. The palatal anchorage is effective alternative to a rigid, full-arch orthodontic wire or a Nance holding arch, improving force control while minimizing side effects on the

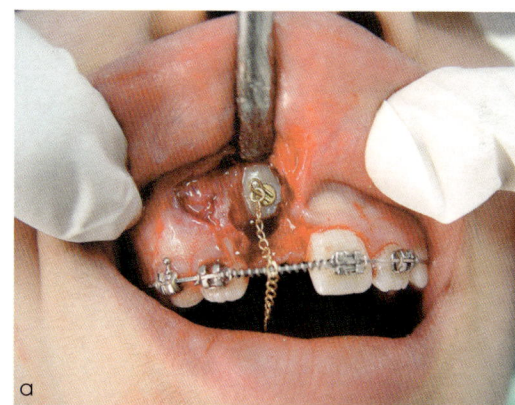

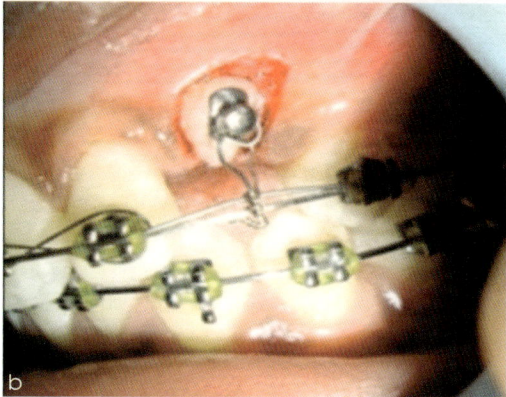

Fig. 13.7: Surgical exposure of incisor impaction: (a) Orthodontic traction by gold chain; (b) Traction by ligature

adjacent teeth. Overall treatment time can be significantly reduced because the impaction is corrected independently in an initial phase.

TWO-STAGE INTERALVEOLAR CORTICOTOMY

The orthodontic correction of adult malocclusion with interalveolar corticotomy as described by Kole is an effective method to carry out dento-osseous movements by heavy orthodontic forces to bring out rapid tooth

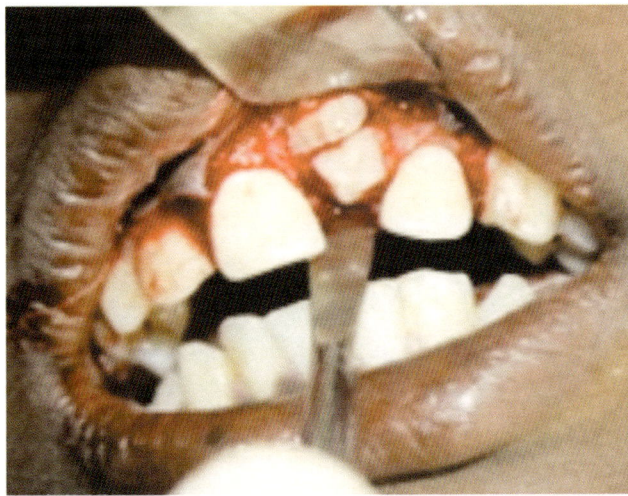

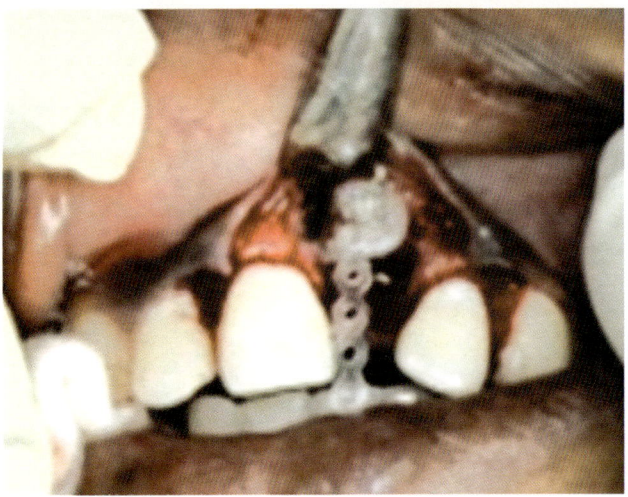

Fig. 13.8: Incisor impaction surgically exposed and supernumerary tooth seen

- After preoperative evaluation of the patient, the surgery is performed in two stages with an interval of two weeks between the stages.
- After achieving good local anesthesia, a full thickness mucoperiosteal flap is raised from the first molar to the opposite side first molar.
- Next, the longitudinal bone cuts are marked between the roots of the teeth to be moved with the help of a fine rose head bur. These markings are made radially and are approximately located between the roots of the teeth to be moved onto the mesial and distal sides.
- These bony cuts are connected with a fine tapering fissure bur till the cuts reached the corticocancellous junction to an approximate depth of 2 mm.
  The longitudinal parallel cuts made along the roots are widened depending upon the diastema.
- Since the cuts are extended only to the cortico-cancellous junction, damage to the roots is minimized.
- The vertical cuts are connected at the apical area 4–5 mm above the apices of the teeth with a horizontal cortical cut which reached the cancellous portion to the depth of 2 mm.
- The flap is sutured.
- After two weeks, the patient is scheduled for the next stage of treatment on the labial side. The procedure is repeated the same way as it is done on the palatal side (Fig. 13.10).

Orthodontic Treatment

The orthodontic treatment is started with fixed appliance at the commencement of fourth week after the second stage.

Fixed appliance and orthopedic elastics are used to compress the weakened bone. Class I and Class II elastics are used to close the residual space distal to canines simultaneously to retract the proclined anterior (Fig. 13.11).

movement and to improve the stability of the results achieved. It is mainly in Angle Class II division 1 with severe proclination and large spacing of upper anterior. It should be assessed radiologically, if there is sufficient inter-radicular distance of more than 2 mm (Fig. 13.9).

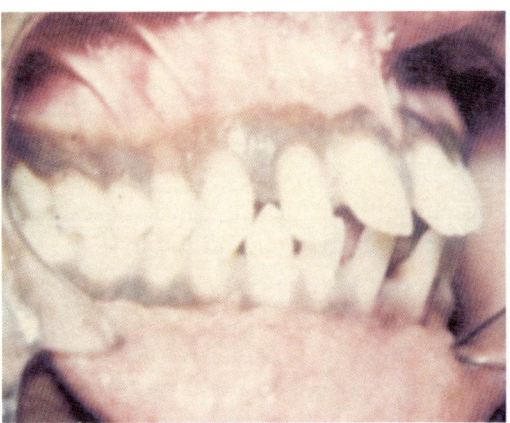
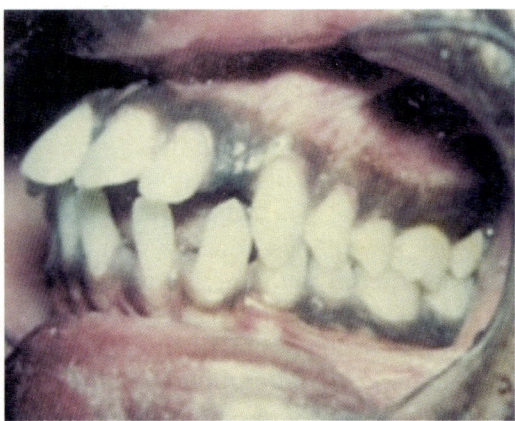

Fig.13.9: Ideal case for corticotomy

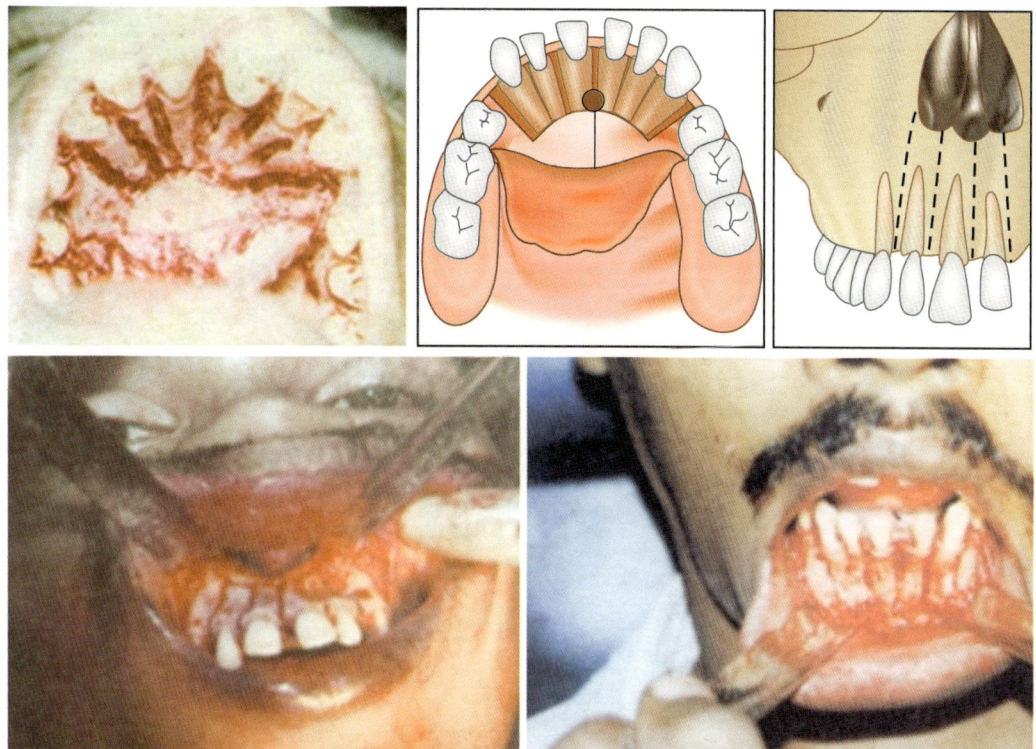

Fig. 13.10: Interalveolar corticotomy

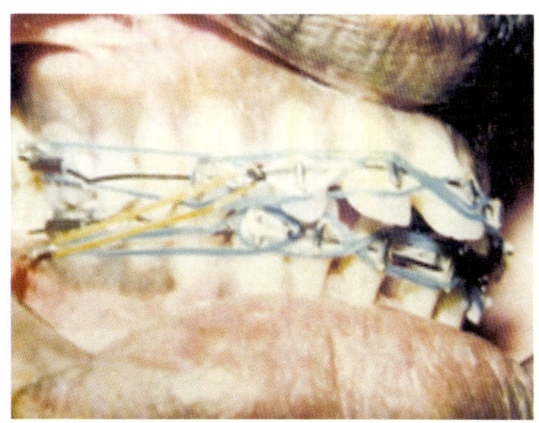

Fig. 13.11: Orthodontic fixed appliances with orthopedic force

Advantages

The two-stage interalveolar corticotomy followed by fixed appliance gives manifold advantages.

- The duration of the active orthodontic treatment is only 6 to 9 months. This is considerably shorter time taken than cases treated by orthodontic means alone.
- The patient's satisfaction and comfort with this combined procedure are highly encouraging.
- It is both simple and safe for the patient.
- No complication such as non-vitality, necrosis of bone and damage to the periodontal ligaments are observed.

- It obviates the need for root paralleling springs.
- There is no relapse.
- This procedure is advantageous even in adults where there is periodontal involvement.

Hence, this procedure can be adjunct to orthodontic treatment where there is difficult clinical situation.

If the midline diastema is severe more than 5 mm, the corticotomy can be one of the treatment modalities (Fig. 13.12).

CIRCUMFERENTIAL SUPRACRESTAL FIBROTOMY (CSF)

It is also known as pericision. It is undertaken as an adjunctive retention procedure after the correction of severe rotations. The transseptal and alveolar crestal group of gingival fibers are responsible for relapse tendencies after correction of rotations. These fibers that were stretched during derotation have the tendency to recoil back predisposing to relapse. This group of fibers do not readily readapt and reorganize to the new tooth position and may take around 36 weeks following correction of rotations, hence cause relapse.

Pericision involves surgical sectioning of these supracrestal fibers and allowed to heal while the teeth are held in the proper stable position; thus the tendency for relapse is greatly reduced. Reattachment of these fibers at a new relaxed position on the root surface stabilizes the tooth in its new position (Fig. 13.13).

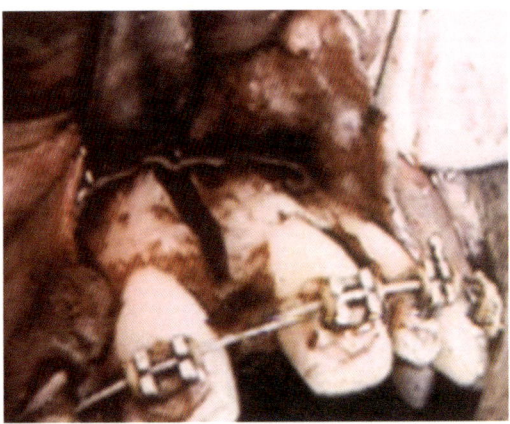

Fig. 13.12: Correction of midline diastema by corticotomy and fixed appliance

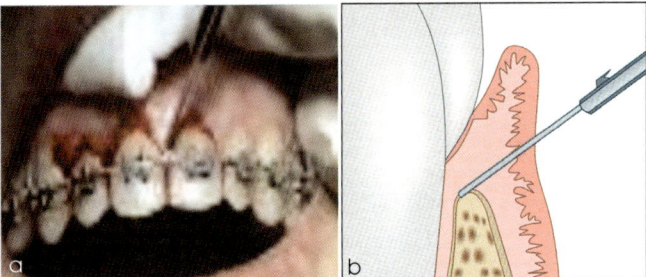

Fig. 13.13: Supracrestal fiberotomy

Edard's Technique

Under local anesthesia, a no 11 knife or a sharp narrow scalpel is passed through the gingival sulcus up to 2 mm apical to the alveolar crest. Cuts are made interproximally on each side of a rotated tooth and along the labial or lingual gingival margin.

Alternatively, an incision can be made in the center of each gingival papilla separating it from below the margin 1–2 mm below the height of the bone buccally and lingually. This is called "vertically papillary fibrotomy".

- This procedure is done only at the end of the finishing phase of orthodontic treatment.
- Retainers must be given immediately after debonding of the active appliance.

FRENECTOMY

One of the causes for midline diastema is abnormal labial frenum which prevents approximation of midline diastema. Clinically, it is confirmed by blanch test. When the upper lip is moved towards right or left, the gingiva blanches. This is called positive blanch test.

Frenectomy is a surgical procedure performed to excise the frenum and remove the deeply embedded fibrous tissue. Frenectomy should not be attempted before the eruption of permanent lateral incisors and canines.

Controversy exists regarding the timing of the frenectomy during orthodontic procedures. According to some authors, frenectomy should be performed prior to close the midline diastema by orthodontic appliances. However, some others advocate that frenectomy should be performed after space closure. This is to reduce the scar tissue formation that can prevent closure of the midline space. It can be done either before or after appliance therapy has approximated the central incisors.

Procedures (Figs 13.15 to 13.18)

- The whole length of the frenum and the mucosa should be totally excised and all fibrous tissue should be cleared to bone level but the periosteum is left intact.
- Any palatally attached fibrous tissue should be removed completely so as to release the frenum from the palatal attachment and is left attached to the lip at its anterior end only (Fig. 13.14).
- Fibrous tissue attached to the intermaxillary suture area between the two central incisors should also be removed.
- To prevent the reattachment of the fibrous tissue, it is advised to undermine the mucosa of the lip.

V-shaped radiographic appearance of the intrerproximal bone between the maxillary central incisors is a diagnostic sign for high frenal attachment as the caused for diastema (Fig. 13.19).

REMOVABLE OF SOFT TISSUE AND BONY BARRIER TO ENABLE ERUPTION OF TEETH

Removable soft tissue and bony barrier is a surgical interceptive orthodontic procedure, which involves excision of the soft tissue and removable of bone, covering the crown of the unerupted tooth and to create the space so that the tooth can erupt without any

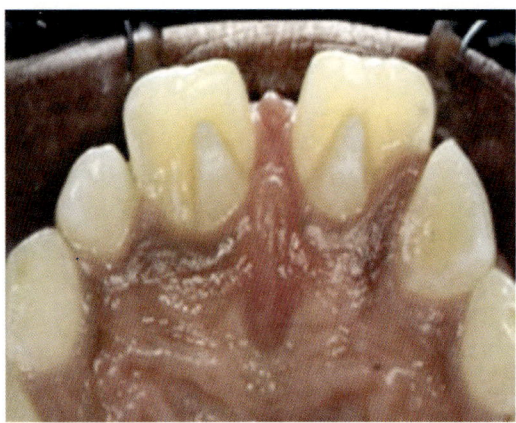

Fig. 13.14: Frenal attachment extended on palatal side

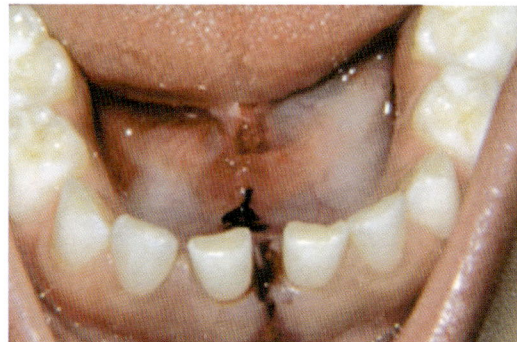

Fig. 13.15: Lower frenectomy

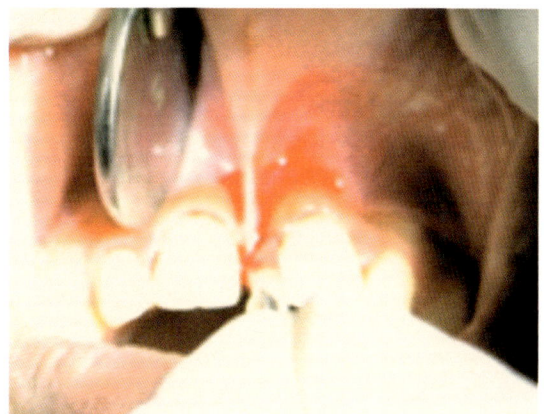

Fig. 13.16: Upper frenectomy—high frenal attachment

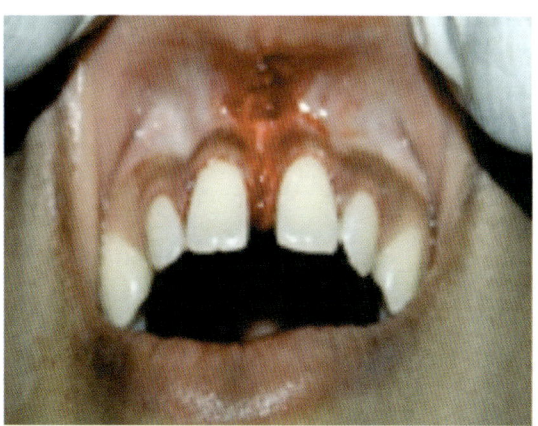

Fig. 13.17: Upper frenectomy—done surgically

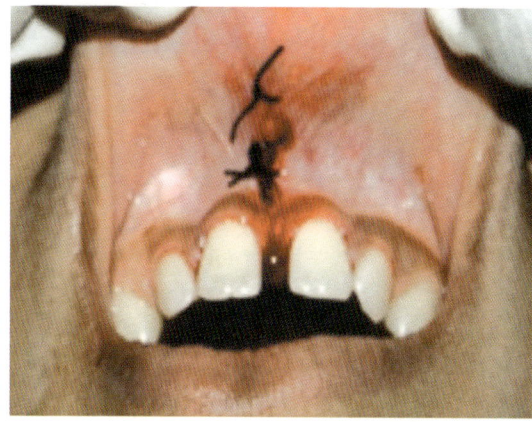

Fig. 13.18: Upper frenectomy: After surgery, the flap was sutured

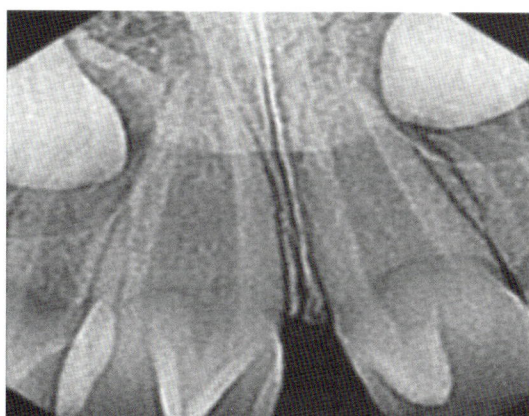

Fig. 13.19: V-shaped radiographic appearance

hindrance. The extent of soft tissue and bone removal should be such that the greatest diameter of the crown of the tooth should be able to easily emerge. The surgical wound is given a cement dressing for a period of two weeks.

ORTHOGNATHIC SURGERY

Orthognathic surgery is the surgical correction of skeletal anomalies or malformations involving the mandible or maxilla. The objective of orthognathic surgery is the correction of wide range of minor and major facial and jaw irregularities and benefits include an improved ability to chew, speak, breath and appearance.

Note: The envelop of discrepancy, showing the amount of change in all three planes of space that could be produced by orthodontic tooth movement alone (inner circle); orthodontic tooth movement combined with growth modification in a growing child, myofunctional appliances (middle circle); and orthognathic surgery (outer circle).

Severe skeletal dentofacial deformities cannot be corrected by orthodontic treatment alone. It requires surgery along with orthodontic treatment. The limits of orthodontic treatment can be determined somewhat by the "envelop of discrepancy" (Fig. 13.20).

Orthognathic surgery includes diagnosis, treatment planning and execution of the treatment by combining orthodontics and oral and maxillofacial surgery to correct the musculoskeletal, dentofacial and soft tissue deformities of the jaw and associated structures. The

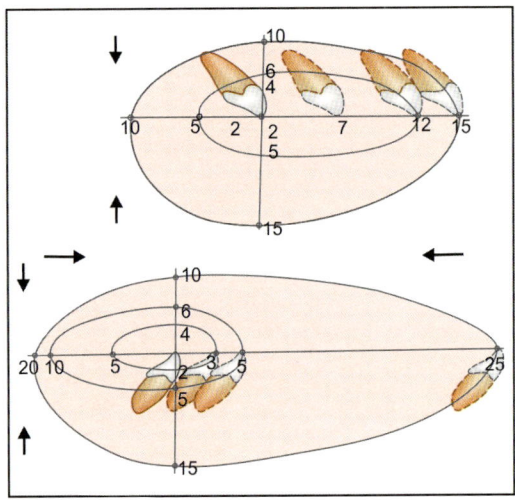

Fig. 13.20: Envelop of discrepancy

ideal time for orthognathic surgery is when the growth potential is completely over.

The various types of severe skeletal dentofacial deformities are:

- *Mandibular excess:* Mandibular prognathism
- *Mandible deficiency:* Mandibular retrognathism
- *Maxilla excess:* Vertical maxillary excess
- *Maxilla deficiency:* Vertical maxillary deficiency
- Combination:
  - Bimaxillary protrusion
  - Naso-maxillary hypoplasia associated with prognathic maxilla
  - Naso-maxillary hypoplasia associated with cleft lip and palate
- *Facial asymmetry:* Asymmetric prognathism of mandible

Asymmetrical Mandibular Prognathism

With Anterior Open Bite

Clinical features:

1. Facial asymmetry
2. Deviation of the chin to one side
3. Midline of the mandible is shifted
4. High gonial angle
5. Eccentric bilateral mandibular protrusion
6. Anterior open bite

Without Anterior Open Bite

Clinical features:

1. Facial asymmetry
2. Deviation of the chin
3. Midline shift
4. High gonial angle
5. No anterior open bite

Nasomaxillary Hypoplasia with Cleft Lip and Palate

Facial features:

1. Severe midface hypoplasia
2. Distorted upper lip
3. Asymmetry of the face
4. Pseudomandibular prognathism

Dental features:

1. Angle's Class III molar relation
2. Crowding of maxillary teeth
3. Anterior crossbite
4. Constricted maxillary arch

Nasomaxillary Hypoplasia with Prognathic Mandible

Features:

1. Angle's Class III molar relation
2. Anterior and posterior crossbites
3. Maxillary incisors tend to be protruded in relation to the hypoplastic maxilla
4. Mandibular posterior teeth tend to lean outward

Unilateral Condylar Hyperplasia

It is of two types:

1. Hemimandibular elongation
2. Hemimandibular hyperplasia

1. **Hemimandibular elongation**

Clinical features:

a. Horizontal displacement of the mandible and chin to the affected side.
b. Occlusal cant is seen.
c. Lateral open bite on the unaffected side.
d. Secondary overeruption of the maxillary teeth in the affected side to maintain functional occlusion.
e. The occlusal plane slopes upwards to the unaffected side.
f. In severe cases, lateral open bite is seen in the affected side.
g. OPG and PA view shows elongation of the condylar neck with increased ramal height and may show condylar head enlargement.

2. **Hemimandibular hyperplasia:** It is characterized by three-dimensional enlargement of the one side of the mandible that includes condylar head, neck, ramus and the body of the mandible.

Clinical features:

a. One side of the face may be enlarged.
b. Horizontal displacement of the mandible and the chin to the affected side.
c. Occlusal cant is seen.

d. Open bite is seen in the affected side.

e. Over eruption of the maxillary teeth on the affected side.

f. Mandibular plane steeps upwards to the unaffected side.

Radiographic features:

a. Deforming enlargement of the condyle

b. Elongation of the condylar neck

c. Elongation of the ascending ramus

d. Typical bowing at the inferior border of the mandible

e. The angle is rounded off

f. Increased height of the body of the mandible
  • Unilateral condylar hypoplasia
  • Hemifacial hypertrophy

Facial Esthetic Analysis

The entire face is divided into three equal parts:
• *Upper third:* Hairline to glabella
• *Middle third*: Glabella to subnasale
• *Lower third:* Subnasale to soft tissue menton

Frontal View Analysis

Larry Wolford and Field recommended the evaluation of 14 anatomic relationship in the frontal view analysis

Examination of the Patient

The patient is asked to sit upright with:
• The interpupillary line parallel to the floor
• The plane of the ears parallel to the floor
• Frankfort horizontal plane, i.e. a line from the tragus of the ear to the infraorbital rim should be parallel.

The patient should be examined with the teeth in the centric position with the lips relaxed

Anatomic Relationships

The forehead, eyes, orbits and nose are evaluated for symmetry, size and deformity.

To find out the symmetry of the face:
• The perpendicular line is drawn from both right and left canthus and it coincides with alar of the nose. The intercanthal distance is 31+3 mm.
• The perpendicular line is drawn from both right and left papillary and it coincides with commissure of the oral cavity. The interpupillary distance is 65 +3 mm.
• The intercanthal distance, alar base width and palpebral fissures width should be equal
• The width of the nasal dorsum is one-third of the intercanthal distance and nasal lobule is two-thirds of the intercanthal distance.

• A line through the medial canthus and a perpendicular to the papillary line should fall on the alar base.
• The upper lip length is measured from subnasale to the upper tooth to the lip stomion:
  – It is 22 +2 mm in males
  – It is 20 +2 mm for females
• A normal upper tooth to the lip relationship is 1 to 4 mm of the incisal edge at rest.
• The facial midline, nasal midline, lip midline, dental midline and chin midline all should fall in one straight line.
• Lip incompetence, if present, should be measured from the upper lip stomion to the lower lip stomion with lips in repose.
• During smile, the vermilion of the upper lip should be in the cervical third of the upper tooth with not more than 1 or 2 mm of gingival exposed
• The distance between glabella to the subnasale and subnasale to the menton is 1:1.
• The length of the upper lip should be one-third of the lower third of face.
• The lower eyelid should be at the level or slightly above the most inferior aspect of the iris.

Facial contour angle: It is the angle formed between the upper facial contour and the upward extension of the lower facial contour. Normal value is –8° to –11°.

Nasolabial angle: It is the angle formed at the subnasale by a line drawn tangent to the base of the nose with the line drawn from the upper lip to subbnasale.

Normal value = 100° to 110° in males

110° to 120° in females

Lip position: The upper lip should protrude ahead of the lower facial contour plane by 3.5 mm and lower lip should be at 2.2 mm.

Lower lip, chin throat angle: The angle between the line drawn from the lower lip to pogonion and a line drawn tangent to the soft tissue contour below the body of the mandible:
• Normal value = 110 + 8°
• Greater values show recessive chin
• Lower values show excessive chin

Chin to throat length: The distance between the angle of the throat and soft tissue menton:
• Normal value is 51 +6 mm
• Greater value shows mandibular prognathism with concave face, acute lower lip, chin throat angle.

Cephalometrics for Orthognathic Surgery

The first step in the diagnosis of the orthognathic surgical patient is to determine the nature of the dental and skeletal defects. A number of cephalometric assessments are commonly used for orthodontic case analysis. These analyses are primarily designed to harmonize position of the teeth with the existing skeletal pattern. Patients who require orthognathic surgery usually have facial bones as well as tooth positions that must be modified by combined orthodontic and surgical procedures. For this reason, a specialized cephalometric appraisal system, called cephalometrics for orthognahic surgery (COGS) was developed at the University of Connecticut.

The chosen landmarks and measurements can be altered by various surgical procedures; the comprehensive appraisal includes all of the facial bones and a cranial base reference; rectilinear measurements can be readily transferred to a study cast for mock surgery.

The 10 Measurement Analyses

Skeletal Assessment

1. SNA
2. SNB
3. ANB
4. Posterior face height/anterior face height (Jarabak ratio):
   - Normal—65°
   - N-ANS—40 mm
   - ANS-Me—2 mm
   - S-PNS—32 mm
   - PNS-MP—55 mm

   The vertical components N-NAS and ANS-ME help us to diagnose anterior upper and lower facial height problems.

   S-PNS and PNS-ME help to diagnose the posterior upper and lower facial height problems. Any deviation from the normal values suggests a vertical maxillary excess or deficiency.
5. Anterior facial height:
   - SN/MP = 31.3°
   - Greater than 32°—skeletal open bite
   - Less than 32°—skeletal deep bite
6. Witt's appraisal:
   - Perpendicular line is dropped from point-A and B on the occlusal plane
   - In females—0 mm
   - In males—1 to 2 mm

- When it is +8 mm or more—skeletal Class II
- When it is –12 mm or more—skeletal Class III
7. Chin angle:
   - The angle is formed between the nasion and pogonion line to the true horizontal line.
   - Normal—87.5°
   - It is used for chin prominence or deficiency

Soft Tissue Assessment

Nasolabial angle:
- It is the angle formed by a tangent to the columella of the nose and the upper lip tangent
- Normal+ 193 +5°
- If there is 90° or less—maxilla to be repositioned posteriorly.
- If there is 114° or more—maxilla to be repositioned anteriorly.

Dental Assessment

IMPA and perpendicular to SN plane:
- IMPA is the angle formed by a line passing through the axis of the lower incisor to the mandibular plane:
  - Normal value is 90+5°
  - Lesser value—mandibular incisor protrusion
- Perpendicular to SN plane is the angle formed by the line passing through the tip of the upper incisor to SN plane:
  - Normal value—104 + 5°
  - Greater than 110°—upper incisor protrusion
  - Less than 110°—upper incisor retrusion

Interincisal angle: It is the angle formed by a line passing through the incisal edge and apex of the root of maxillary and mandibular incisors.
- Normal value—132°
- Greater than 132°—upper and lower incisor retrusion
- Less than 132°—upper and lower incisor protrusion

Presurgical Orthodontics

For orthognathic surgery to be carried out, certain orthodontic treatment procedures should be done prior to the surgery. The mechnotherapy and treatment objectives are the opposite of the normal orthodontic treatment plan in presurgical orthodontics. These include:
- Align the teeth with inclination and angulation
- To relieve arch crowding
- To close spaces
- To correct derotations
- To eliminate gross dental interferences

Osteotomy Procedures

The various osteotomy procedures for the correction of dentofacial deformities are given below:

Mandibular body osteotomy:
- Anterior body osteotomy
- Posterior body osteotomy
- Mid-symphysis osteotomy

Segmental subapical mandibular surgeries:
- Anterior subapical mandibular osteotomy
- Posterior subapical mandibular osteotomy
- Total subapical mandibular osteotomy

Genioplasty—horizontal osteotomy in the chin region
- Augmentation genioplasty
- Reduction genioplasty
- Straightening genioplasty

Mandibular ramus osteotomy
- Subcondylar ramus osteotomy
  - Extraoral subcondylar ramus osteotomy
  - Intraoral subcondylar ramus osteotomy
  - Arching ramus osteotomy
  - Intraoral modified sagittal split osteotomy

Maxillary osteotomy procedures: Intraoral

Segmental maxillary osteotomy procedures
- Single tooth dentoosseous osteotomy
- Interdental osteotomies
- Anterior maxillary osteotomy
- Posterior maxillary osteotomy

Usage of midface osteotomies
- LeFort I
  - Low midface hypoplasia
  - Retromaxilla
  - Cleft patients
- LeFort II
  - Nasomaxillary hypoplasia
  - Cleft patients
  - Binders syndrome
- Bimaxillary procedures—for both jaws

Correction of Mandibular Abnormalities

Mandibular Excess

Mandibular excess was one of the first dentofacial deformities treated by a combination of orthodontics and surgery.

Excess growth can occur in anteroposterior direction (sagittal) or vertical dimension. Mandibular excess frequently results in Angle's Class III malocclusion with reverse overjet. The following are some of the commonly used surgical techniques to treat patients with mandibular excess.

1. *Vertical ramus osteotomy:* Transoral vertical ramus osteotomy was popularized by Caldwell and Letterman in the early 1950s, where lateral aspect of ramus was exposed through a submandibular incision. Intraoral incision is used in recent times. The technique can be utilized for mandibular setback.

In this technique, the ramus is sectioned in a vertical fashion and the entire body and anterior ramus section of the mandible are moved posteriorly. The proximal segment containing condyle is overlapped on the posteriorly positioned anterior portion of the ramus; the jaw is then stabilized during healing phase.

2. *Bilateral sagittal split osteotomy (BSSO) with mandibular setback:* BSSO technique has become one of the most popular methods for treatment of both mandibular deficiency and mandibular excess. This technique can be used to either advance or retrude the mandible. Class III patients with mandibular excess are treated by BSSO with mandibular setback.

BSSO was first described by trainer and Obswegerer and later modified by Dalpont, Hunsuch and Epker. The technique involves the splitting of the ramus and posterior body of the mandible in a sagittal fashion, which allows either advancement or setback of the mandible. This type of splitting produces large area of bony overlap that provides flexibility necessary to move the mandible in several directions. The significant bony overlap also allows for adequate bone healing and improved postoperative stability (Fig. 13.21).

3. *Manbibular subapical osteotomy:* When the reverse overjet relationship is isolated to the anterior dentoalveolar area of the mandible, a subapical osteotomy technique can be used for correction of mandibular dental prognathism. In this technique, bone

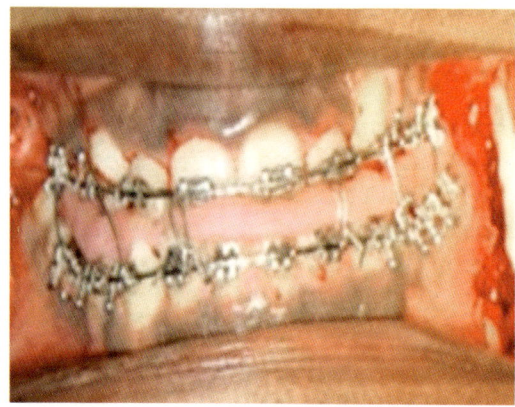
Fig. 13.21: Intraoral operative bilateral sagittal split osteotomy

is removed in the area of an extraction site of a bicuspid or molar tooth, and the anterior dentoalveolar segment of the mandible is moved to more posterior position.

Mandibular Deficiency

Patients with mandibular deficiency typically show retried position of the chin (as viewed from profile aspect) and Angle's Class II malocclusion with an increased overjet. The following techniques are used for the advancement of the mandible.

1. **BSSO with mandibular advancement:** BSSO technique as described earlier is the most popular technique for mandibular advancement. After splitting of the jaw, anterior segment of the mandible is advanced and stabilized into its new position.

2. **Mandibular total subapical osteotomy:** Total subapical osteotomy may be adequate in a patient with Class II malocclusion. Dentoalveolar segment of mandible is moved anteriorly allowing correction of Class II malocclusion without increasing chin prominence.

3. **Vertical 'L' or 'C' osteotomy:** When extreme mandibular advancement of greater than 10–15 mm is necessary, a vertical 'L' or 'C' osteotomy is preferred. The technique combines the sagittal split with a vertical ramus osteotomy. Iliac crest bone grafts may be filled in the osteotomy defect.

Correction of Maxillary Abnormalities

Le Fort I osteotomy (total maxillary osteotomy) are currently the most common procedures performed to correct the anteroposterior, transverse and vertical abnormalities of the maxilla. After total surgical separation, the maxilla can be moved and repositioned in all three planes of space. Maxilla can be moved in upward, downward or forward direction after Le Fort I osteotomy.

Maxillary Excess

Maxillary excess can occur in transverse, anteroposterior and vertical dimensions.

Maxillary excess in anteroposterior dimension:

1. *Anterior maxillary subapical setback:* This technique is used when skeletal Class II malocclusion is caused by a maxillary excess limited to the anteroposterior dimension with no vertical increase of the maxilla. Patient typically exhibits midface protrusion. Maxillary excess in the anterior region can effectively be treated with surgical retraction of the maxillary anterior segment by utilizing the maxillary first premolar extraction space.

2. *LeFort I osteotomy with maxillary setback:* LeFort I osteotomy (total maxillary osteotomy) is the most common procedure to correct maxillary abnormalities. After total separation, maxilla can be moved and repositioned in all three planes of space.

Vertical maxillary excess: Vertical maxillary excess may result in excessive lower facial height, incompetent lips, excessive vertical display of incisors and gingival or skeletal anterior open bite. Posterior portion of maxilla shows excessive downward growth. Thus, when molar teeth are in occlusion of this anatomic abnormality, the anterior teeth are left without contact.

1. *LeFort I osteotomy with maxillary impaction:* It is done when the excess is present in anterior as well as posterior segment. Bone removed at osteotomy site to permit superior repositioning of the maxilla.

2. *Segmental maxillary osteotomy:* A maxillary excess which is mostly in posterior region causing anterior open bite can be treated by bilateral posterior segmental maxillary osteotomies. Maxillary first premolar is removed and maxilla is sectioned into posterior and anterior dentoalveolar segment. Excess bone is cut at the osteotomy sites and segments are moved superiorly and posterior to allow even contact between all the teeth.

Maxillary Deficiency

Patients with maxillary deficiency may exhibit retruded upper lip, inadequate tooth exposure, prominent chin and Class III malocclusion. Maxillary deficiency can occur in anteroposterior, vertical and transverse dimensions.

- LeFort I osteotomy with advancement of maxilla is done to correct anteroposterior maxillary deficiency (Figs 13.22 and 13.23).
- Maxillary bone can be segmented to allow for transverse expansion when maxilla is constricted.

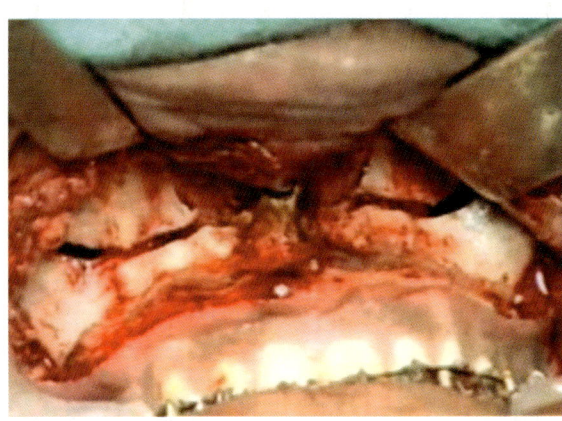

Fig. 13.22: LeFort I osteotomy

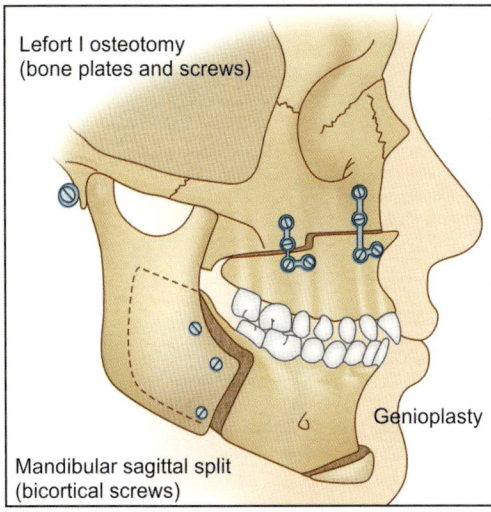

Fig. 13.23: Treatment for maxillary deficiency and skeletal Class III

- In case of vertical maxillary deficiency, elongation of lower 3rd of face can be achieved by inferior positioning of maxilla with bone grafts using a LeFort I osteotomy.

Post-surgical orthodontics: After a period of healing, final alignment and positioning of teeth and closure of any extraction space is accomplished by orthodontic tooth movement. The final setting of occlusion occurs rapidly within 6–10 months. Retention after surgical orthodontic management is similar to routine orthodontic management.

Surgical Assisted Rapid Palatal Expansion

A transverse deficiency of the maxilla in adult patients can be treated with surgically assisted rapid maxillary expansion. This procedure involves the techniques of orthodontic palatal widening with a modification of the LeFort I osteotomy.

A cut is made along the lateral surface of the maxilla, which is similar to the LeFort I cut in this area. Then a vertical cut is made in the anteronasal spine above the apices of central incisors to open/split the midpalatal suture. Activation of the maxillary expansion appliance is now begun. When the maxilla reaches its desired width, the expansion appliance is stabilized for 3 months in a retention phase.

Selection of Orthodontic Appliance

Straight wire appliance is only used as it aids in tooth movement and stabilize them during stresses, during surgery and during intermaxillary fixation. Begg appliance is not used. Ceramic or tooth-colored brackets are also not used as it is susceptible for breakage and discoloration.

Modifications
1. At the area of osteotomy, it is mandatory to tip the tooth for root divergence.
2. Sometimes deliberate switching of the orthodontic brackets of the right and left canines and premolars should be done for root divergence.

Rhinoplasty
- Cosmetic surgery of the nose focused on the contour of the nasal dorsum, the shape of the nasal tip and the width of the alar base.
- Particularly effective when nose is deviated to one side, has a prominent dorsal hump, or has a bulbous or distorted tip.
- Usually, follows LeFort I osteotomy which compromises the appearance of nose.

Chin augmentation or reduction
- Most frequently used adjunct to orthodontics.
- Improves the stability of the lower incisors as well as enhancing facial appearance, tightens the suprahyoid musculature and produces desirable changes in chin-neck contour.
- Reduction of the chin with osteotomy can be a possibility to camouflage a skeletal Class III problem (Fig. 13.24).

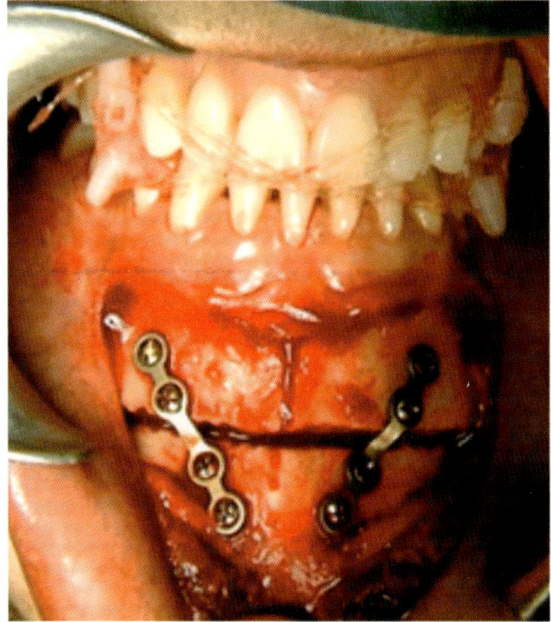

Fig. 13.24: Genioplasty

DISTRACTION OSTEOGENESIS

Distraction osteogenesis (DO) is the biologic process of new bone formation between bone segments gradually separated by incremental traction. Recently, distraction osteogenesis has been extensively applied

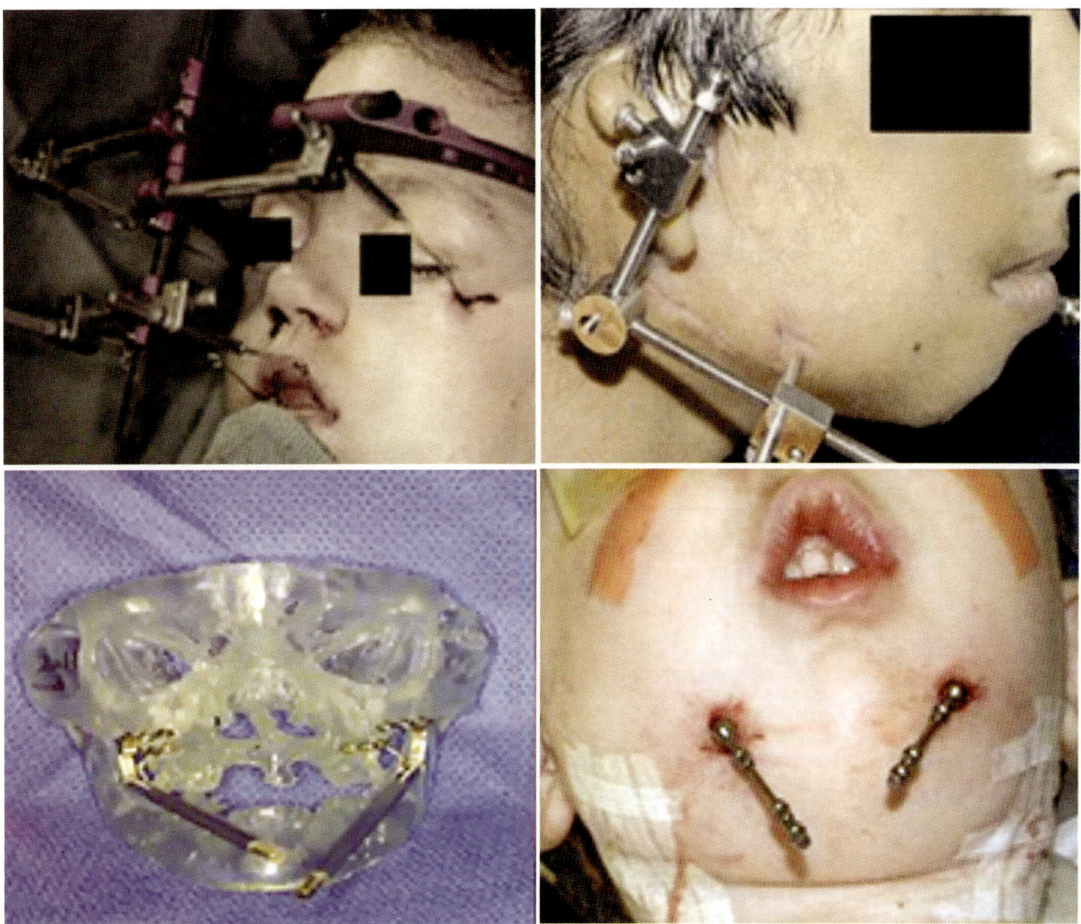

Fig. 13.25: Surgical procedure for distraction osteogenesis

to the craniofacial complex and is becoming a viable treatment option in the correction of craniofacial deformities.

This process begins when a distraction force is applied to the healing callus that joins the divided bone segments, and continues as long as the tissue is stretched. Importantly, a distraction force applied to bone also creates tension in the surrounding soft tissues, initiating a sequence of adaptive changes termed distraction histogenesis. It should be emphasized that under the influence of tensional stresses produced by gradual distraction, active histogenesis occurs in different tissues, including skin, fascia, muscle, tendon, cartilage, blood vessels and peripheral nerves (Fig. 13.25).

Difference between orthognathic surgery and distraction osteogenesis is shown in Fig. 13.26.

Basic Principles of Distraction Osteogenesis

- Preservation of blood supply
- Close apposition of cut bone surfaces to allow early bridge formation
- Gradual distraction at regular rhythm.

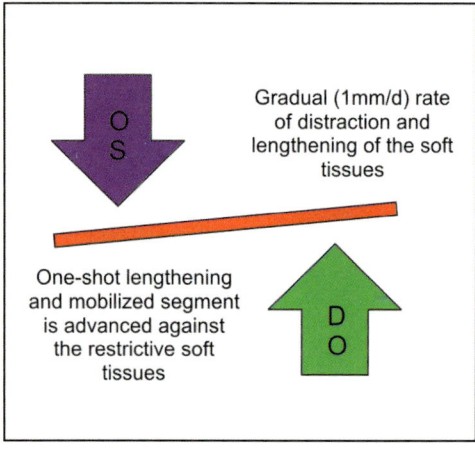

O S

Gradual (1mm/d) rate of distraction and lengthening of the soft tissues

One-shot lengthening and mobilized segment is advanced against the restrictive soft tissues

D O

Fig. 13.26: Difference between surgery and distraction osteogenesis

Rate of distraction: Number of millimeters per day at which the bone surfaces are stretched. The rate of 1 mm a day is considered optimal.

Rhythm of distraction: Number of distractions per day usually in equally divided increments to total the rate. The rhythm may vary from one cycle per day of 1 mm to 0.25 mm four times per day or 0.5 mm twice daily.

Classification of Distraction Device

The distraction device is a semirigid fixator that connects the proximal and distal segments of the mandible.

1. *Based on site*
   - Mandibular
   - Midface or maxillary
   - Alveolar
   - Transport (reconstruction of neomandible/ neocondyle)
   - Rigid external distractor (RED)
2. *Based on use*

   External distractor:
   - Unidirectional (activated in one plane of space)
   - Bidirectional (activated in two plane of space)
   - Multiplanar (activated in three plane of space)
   - Rigid external distraction (RED) system

   Internal distractor:
   - Mandibular intraoral distractor
   - Modular internal distractor (MID)
   - Tooth-borne distractor, e.g. rapid canine distractor, alveolar distractor
3. *Based on direction*
   - Horizontal
   - Oblique
   - Vertical

Large Maxillomandibular Advancement Possible

- Can be done at any age. There have been reports of rapid, early mandibular distraction to prevent tracheotomy in a newborn with micrognathia that was causing severe airway obstruction.
- Minimized need for orthognathic surgery, hence reduce complication
- Minimized relapse because of histogenesis during distraction
- Shorter hospital stay
- No bone graft required
- New bone formed in distraction osteogenesis is more native and permit orthodontic tooth movement

Disadvantages

- Lack of precision
- Poor three-dimensional control, but current distractor are constantly modified for desired results
- In some cases, multiple daily outpatient visit required
- Pain due to manipulation of healing corticotomy daily

- Difficult access for orthodontist during distraction osteogenesis
- Difficult plaque control
- Damage to TMJ due to incorrect vector orientation
- Cutaneous scarring resulting from transcutaneous fixation pins

Classification of Treatment Modalities with DO

DO in the field of craniofacial reconstruction is applicable for the following six treatment techniques:

1. To lengthen the mandible
2. To advance the maxilla/midface or monobloc advancement
3. Bone segment transportation
4. Trifocal distraction treatment as in case of symphyseal defect
5. Distraction for alveolar augmentation
6. Distraction implantology

Indications

Distraction osteogenesis is indicated in all cases of mandibular shortening or maxillary hypoplasia where orthognathic surgery is not first choice. Various acquired and congenital condition in which distraction osteogenesis is indicated are given below.

Congenital Deformities

- Pierre-Robin syndrome
- Severe retrognathic syndrome, e.g. Treacher Collins and Goldenhar syndrome
- Non-syndromic congenital micrognathia
- Severely constricted mandible/maxilla
- Craniofacial microsomia unilateral/bilateral
- Midfacial hypoplasia
- Obstructive sleep apnea (OSA)
- Facial asymmetry

Acquired Conditions

- Post-traumatic growth disturbances of mandible, e.g. temporomandibular joint ankylosis
- Non-union fractures
- Atrophy of edentulous segments
- Oncologic mandibular osseous defects

Others

- Rapid canine distraction for rapid distalization of canine to reduce orthodontic treatment time.
- Distraction for ankylosed teeth to create optimum height of alveolar bone.

Diagnostic Database

- Study models
- Photographs
- Llateral head and PA cephalograms
- Orthopantomograms
- Computed tomography scans

Management of a case with craniofacial deformities with distraction osteogenesis involves a team approach among the surgeons and orthodontists. Orthodontist plays a crucial role in diagnosis and treatment planning. This would involve a thorough clinical examination of the face and structures. A diagnostic data base is created with the aid of study models, photographs, lateral head and PA cephalograms, orthopantomograms, computed tomography scans. In addition to treatment planning, the data base is also useful for evaluation of treatment result.

Mandibular Distraction Devices

1. *External unidirectional distraction (McCarthy, 1992)* (Fig. 13.27): The distractor consists of single calibrated rod with two clamps which hold two 2 mm half pins that are placed on either side of the osteotomy.

- Approx. 20–24 mm of bone stock is necessary to place this device.
- Disadvantages of this type of distractor include:
  - Scarring due to pins
  - Difficulty predicting the direction in which the distraction would proceed
  - Inability to change the direction of distraction once the process has started

2. *Eternal bidirectional distraction* (Fig. 13.28)

- Provides an additional degree of freedom over unidirectional device

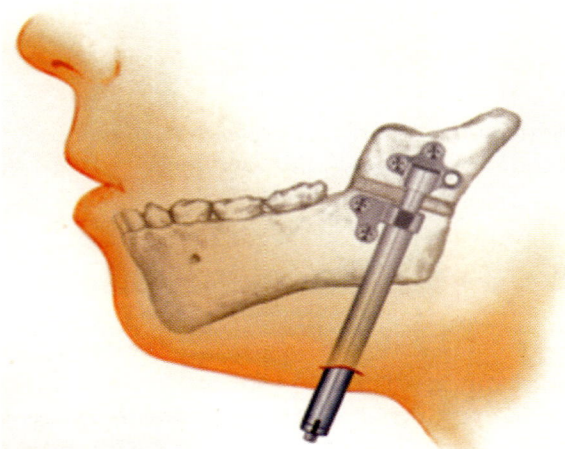

Fig. 13.27: External unidirectional distraction

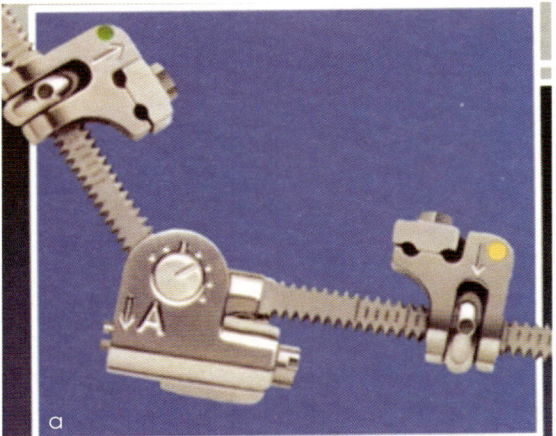

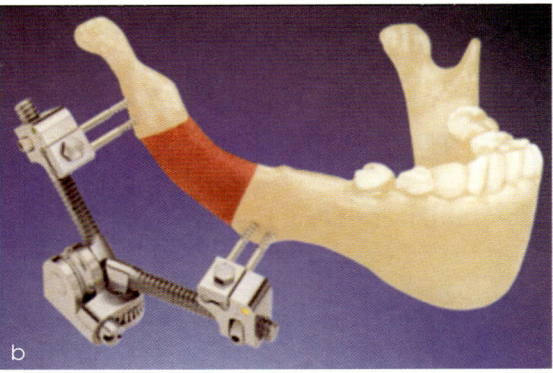

Fig. 13.28a and b: External bidirectional distraction

- Bidirectional distraction is necessary for correction of the two step occlusal plane and ramus deficiency.

3. *Multiplanar distraction* (Fig. 13.29)

- The device consists of a central housing with two worm gears in different planes.
- Two arms extend from the housing with pin clamps at either ends.
- Each quarter turn results in an expansion of 0.25 mm.
- Each arm is 20 mm in length for a total linear expansion of 40 mm.
- Two activation screws enable changes in transverse and vertical angulation.

4. *Internal distraction* (Fig. 13.30)

- Due to the criticism of the external distractors, internal distractors were developed to eliminate the problems of facial scarring, pin tract infections and high visibility.
- McCarthy (1995) introduced an intraoral distraction appliance tested on the canine model.
- Vasquez and Diner developed two internal distractors—one for lengthening of mandibular body and other for ramus.

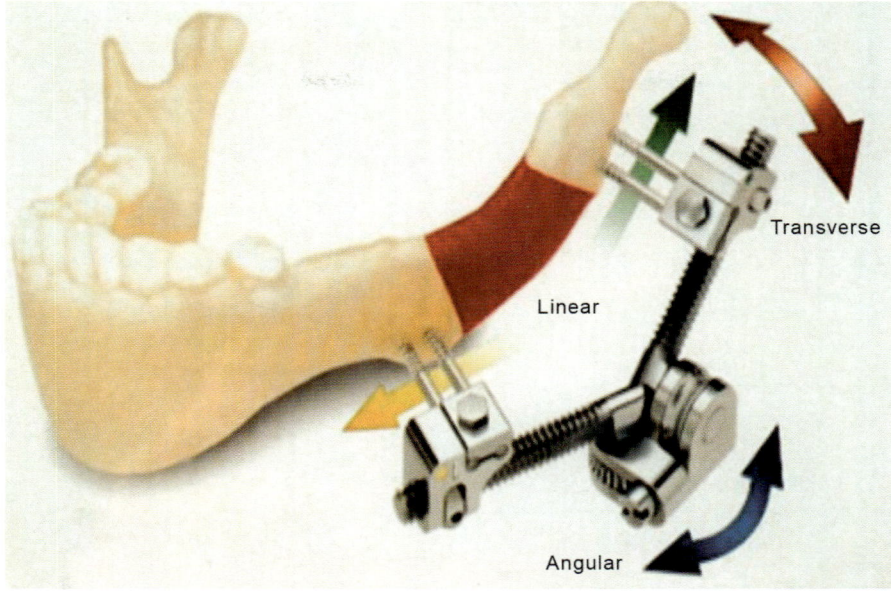

Fig. 13.29: Multiplanar distraction

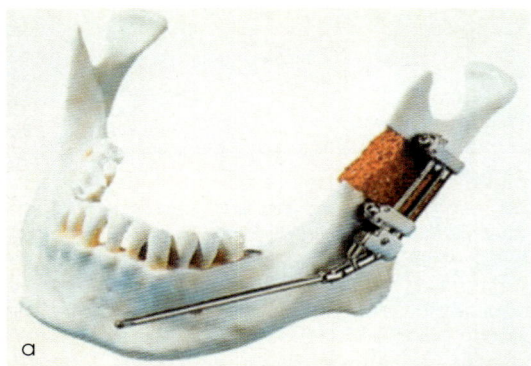

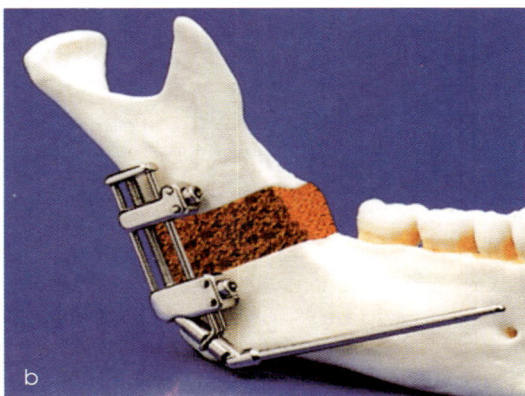

Fig. 13.30a and b: Internal distraction

5. ***Tooth-borne appliances*** (Fig. 13.31)
- Razdolsky (1997) introduced a completely tooth-borne IO distractor capable of linear changes.
- Current technique starts by fitting preformed SS crowns to one tooth on either side of the anticipated osteotomy site.

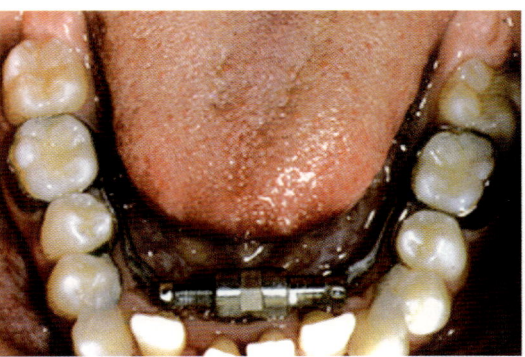

Fig. 13.31: Tooth-borne appliance

- A rubber base impression is then taken and an IO distractor is fabricated in the laboratory

Vertical Device Placement (Fig. 13.32)
- Vertical device placement results in an increase in the vertical dimension of the mandibular ramus.
- During activation, a change occurs in appliance orientation that appears to be caused by the nonlinear molding effect of the neuromusculature on the regenerate as it is formed. The mandible autorotates in a counterclockwise direction and the lower incisors take a more advanced position.
- A posterior open bite may occur on the side that has undergone vertical distraction in the ramus.
- Bilateral vertical lengthening of the ramus results in counterclockwise uprighting of the mandibular symphysis. When combined with the sagittal advancement of the mandibular body, the increased prominence of the lower third of the face is evident.

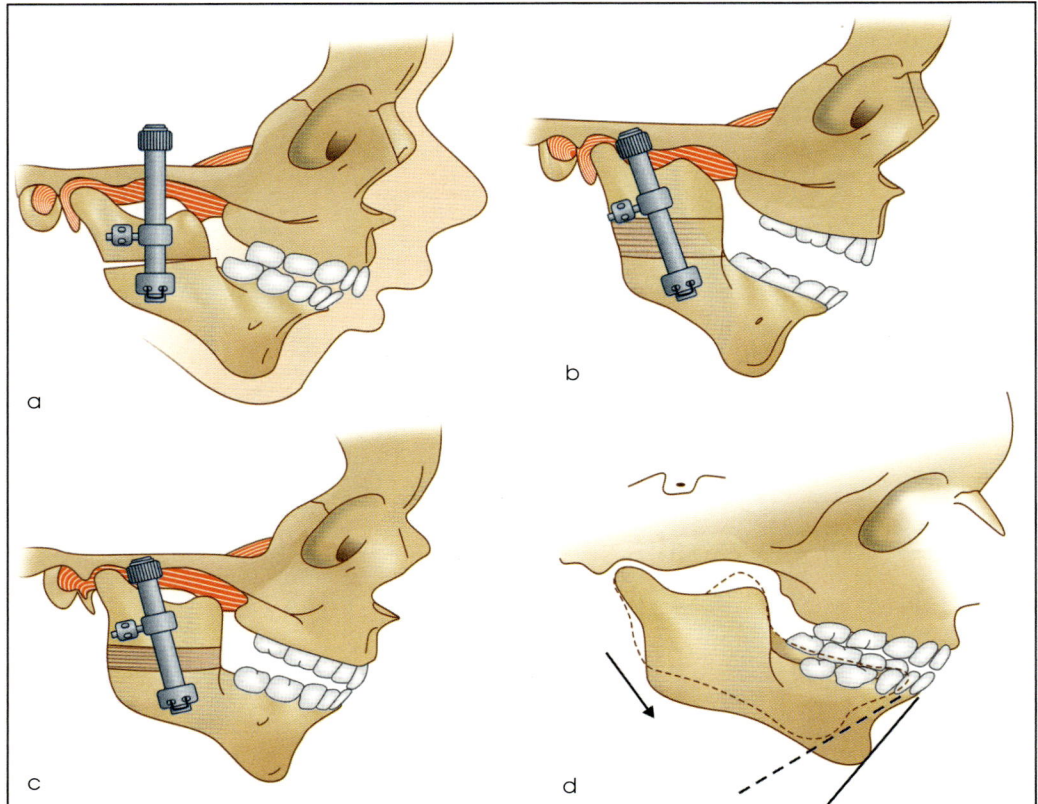

Fig. 13.32: Vertical device placement: (a) The device placed vertically in the mandibular ramus before activation; (b) Activation of the device results in an increase in the vertical height of the ramus. Note the separation between the maxillary and mandibular dentition before closure of the mandible; (c) The authors believe the change in appliance orientation is caused by the nonlinear molding effect of the neuromusculature on their generate as it is formed. As the mandible autorotates in a counterclockwise direction, the lower incisors take a more advanced position, and a posterior open bite may present itself on the side that has been lengthened vertically; (d) Note that bilateral vertical lengthening of the ramus is associated with counterclockwise uprighting of the symphysis. This, along with sagittal advancement of the mandibular body, contributes to the perception of increased prominence of the lower third of the face

- The unilateral vertical ramal lengthening is usually associated with transverse correction of the chin position and the cant correction of the mandibular occlusal plane.

In most of the unilateral cases, the pins/device have been inserted along a predominantly vertical vector with a more oblique position of the device in the bilateral cases in which sagittal thrust of the body and chin is also desired (oblique vector).

Horizontal Device Placement (Fig. 13.33)

- The most efficient approach for achieving sagittal projection of the mandibular body and symphysis is by placement of the distraction device in a horizontal position in relation to the mandibular body.
- There is a tendency in horizontal distraction of the mandibular body to rotate in a clockwise direction, resulting in an open bite. The suprahyoid musculature, in balance with the muscles of mastication and the distraction device itself, has a role in this occurrence.
- It is reported that here is an improvement in the patency of the oropharyngeal airway and tongue position subsequent to mandibular sagittal advancement. Neonatal mandibular distraction has been performed when life-threatening airway problems exist.

A horizontal vector is used in bilateral cases in which only anterior mandibular projection is required.

Multidirectional Device Placement (Fig.13.34)

The introduction of a multidirectional device provides more control in achieving:
1. The fundamental vertical elongation of the ramus,
2. Horizontal elongation (body) and recreation of the mandibular angle with control over the incisor vertical bite relationships (open bite, closed bite), and
3. Transverse widening or increase in the bigonial distance.

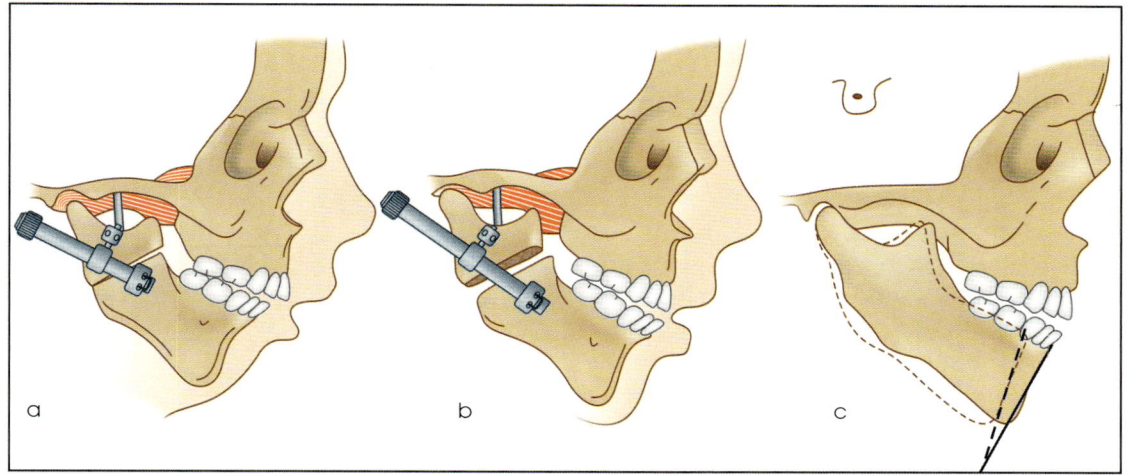

Fig. 13.33: Horizontal device placement: (a, b) Horizontal device placement results in an increase in the anteroposterior dimension of the mandibular body with increased sagittal projection of the symphysis; (c) There is a tendency in horizontal distraction for the body to rotate in a clockwise direction, sometimes resulting in open bite. The pull of the suprahyoid musculature may have a role in this occurrence. There has been a reported improvement in patency of the oropharyngeal airway and tongue position subsequent to mandibular sagittal advancement

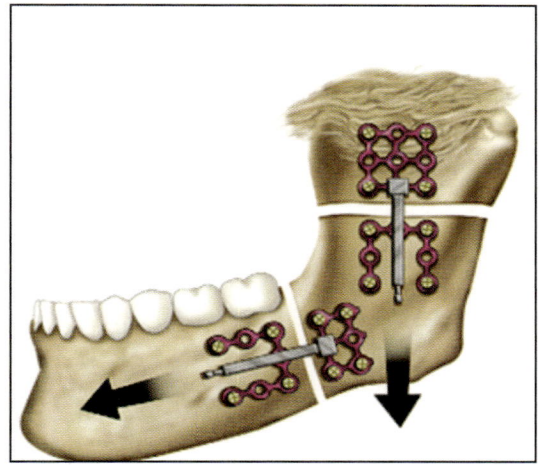

Fig. 13.34: Placement of distractor

4. Intraoral devices, offering the decided advantage of avoiding an external cutaneous scar, will find more application in the bilateral deficiencies (micrognathia) in which there is sufficient bone stock for device placement and when a horizontal vector is optimal.
5. In the cases of unilateral distraction with severe ramal deficiency and the need for a vertical vector, the extraoral device is still preferred.

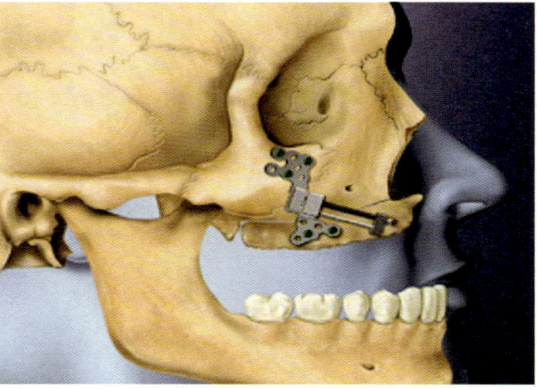

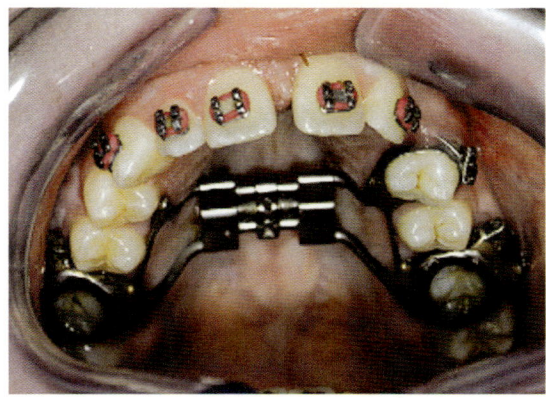

Fig. 13.35: Tooth-borne distractor

Buccal Bone-Borne Versus Tooth-Borne Appliances (Fig.13.35)

Either a tooth-borne or bone-borne appliance may be used to widen the mandible. The tooth-borne osteodistractor tends to widen more superiorly than at the inferior border of the mandible. Generally, the tooth-borne appliance has not been tolerated as well as the bone-borne distractor, because of tongue impingement and oral hygiene. Nevertheless, good results have been achieved with both appliances.

Orthodontic Treatment Protocol

- Predistraction orthodontics
- Orthodontics during distraction and consolidation phase
- Post-distraction orthodontics
- Retention

Maxillary and mandibular dental arches are prepared for distraction osteogenesis by leveling and alignment, decompensation, and correction of curve of Spee. The teeth should be moved to the ideal positions relative to the basal bone so that an ideal maxillo-mandibular relationship is not compromised by existing dental compensations. Standard predistraction orthodontic protocol includes appropriate transverse arch width coordination of both maxillary and mandibular arches followed by passive rectangular archwires with the hooks for engaging interarch elastics during and after distraction. Predistraction preparation should consider root divergence of the tooth with a fixed orthodontic appliance at the osteotomy site. This is to facilitate the osteotomy and to ensure adequate alveolar bone on the both sides for periodontal health.

Orthodontics during Distraction and Consolidation Phase (Figs 13.36 and 13.37)

Four influences that are presumed to affect the observed vector are:

1. The unique biomechanical characteristics of the selected distraction device,
2. Orientation of the distraction device to the mandibular anatomy,

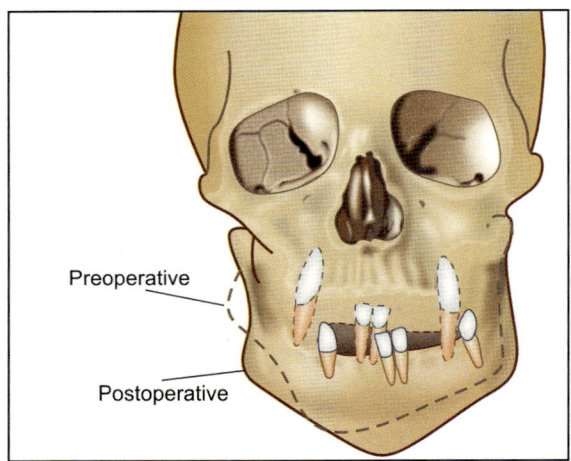

Fig. 13.36: Difference between pre- and post-operative

Note: In predistraction planning, the orthodontist evaluates and determines the desired vector based on a skeletal appraisal. However; the clinically observed vector often varies from the planned vector.

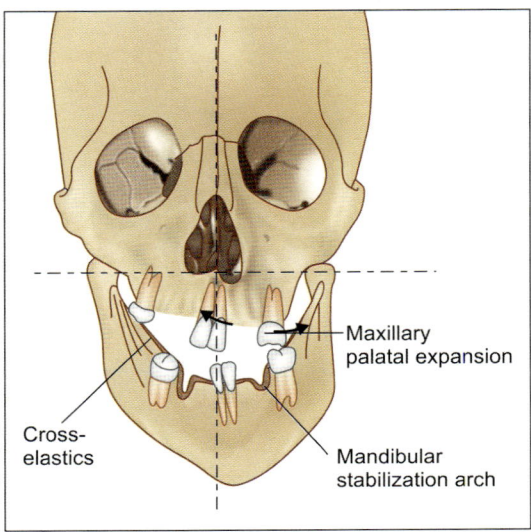

Fig. 13.37: Reduction of anterior open bite

Note: Intermaxillary elastics may be helpful in the reduction of an anterior openbite and may be used transversely to correct crossbite or lateral shift of the mandible during active distraction. In this illustration, the mandible has shifted toward the contralateral side resulting in posterior crossbite. The ipsilateral side shows openbite.

Cross-elastics combined with a mandibular lingual stabilization arch are used to correct the crossbite.

3. Neuromuscular influence, and
4. Externally exerted forces.

During distraction and consolidation phase, orthodontics' management aimed to direct the tooth-bearing segment to their post-distraction positions. In mandibular distraction, interarch elastics during this phase influence the vector and are useful in remodeling of regenerated bone and close the open bite. Unilateral mandibular distraction (hemifacial microsomia) can lead to posterior open bite on distraction side and crossbite on normal side. Expansion of maxillary arch along with use of interarch elastics can be used to correct developing transverse and vertical discrepancies. Occlusal bite-block can be used during the consolidation and post-consolidation phase to supraerupt posterior dentition to correct the cant and open bite.

For the maxillary and midfacial distraction, force should be directed through the center of resistance (CR) of maxilla. If force is directed below the center of resistance, an open bite is the result. Light vertical elastics from the maxillary arch to the lower arch would help in controlling clockwise rotation of the mandible and open bite.

Over Correction

- The amount of over correction is influenced by the amount of expected post-distraction growth remaining in the craniofacial skeleton. A young child with much growth ahead would be overcorrected more than a child who is close to the completion of growth.

- The process of distraction does not measurably alter the growth rate of the affected mandible after completion of the procedure. The expanded mandibular ramus in a very young child will need considerable post-distraction growth to achieve full adult dimensions. With the expectation that the post-distraction growth will be syndromic and inadequate to keep up with the normal side, there is a need for greater overcorrection of the ramus in a very young child.
- After completion of activation, the device is maintained in position for approximately 8 weeks (consolidation phase). The device is not removed until there is radiographic evidence of a cortical outline or mineralization of their generated portion of the mandible.
- The device is removed in the office as an outpatient procedure.

Methods of occlusal plane management include the use of:

1. An occlusal acrylic wafer that is reduced one tooth at a time to allow for serial eruption of the maxillary posterior dentition.

2. An functional appliance with lingual shields to provide lateral control of mandibular position. Included in this appliance is a bite plane that is adjusted one tooth at a time for passive eruption of the maxillary teeth.

3. Occlusal acrylic build ups that are reduced one tooth at a time to allow for serial eruption of the maxillary teeth (Fig. 13.38).

In the unilateral distraction cases, the orthodontist is often confronted with a posterior open bite on the distracted side and a crossbite on the contralateral side. The crossbite resulting from mandibular shift across the midsagittal plane may be corrected by a combination of transpalatal arches, lingual arches, intermaxillary cross elastics, and a palatal expansion devices (Fig. 13.38a). The open bite may be managed with gradual adjustment of a bite plate worn on either the mandibular or maxillary dentition (Fig. 13.38b). The bite plate is relieved, one tooth at a time, under the occlusal surface of the maxillary posterior teeth. This results in gradual eruption of the teeth down to the level of the corrected mandibular occlusal plane (Fig. 13.38c and d).

Post-distraction Orthodontics

Post-distraction orthodontics should be initiated after the consolidation phase which is aimed at finishing and settling the occlusion. Essix type retainers may not be

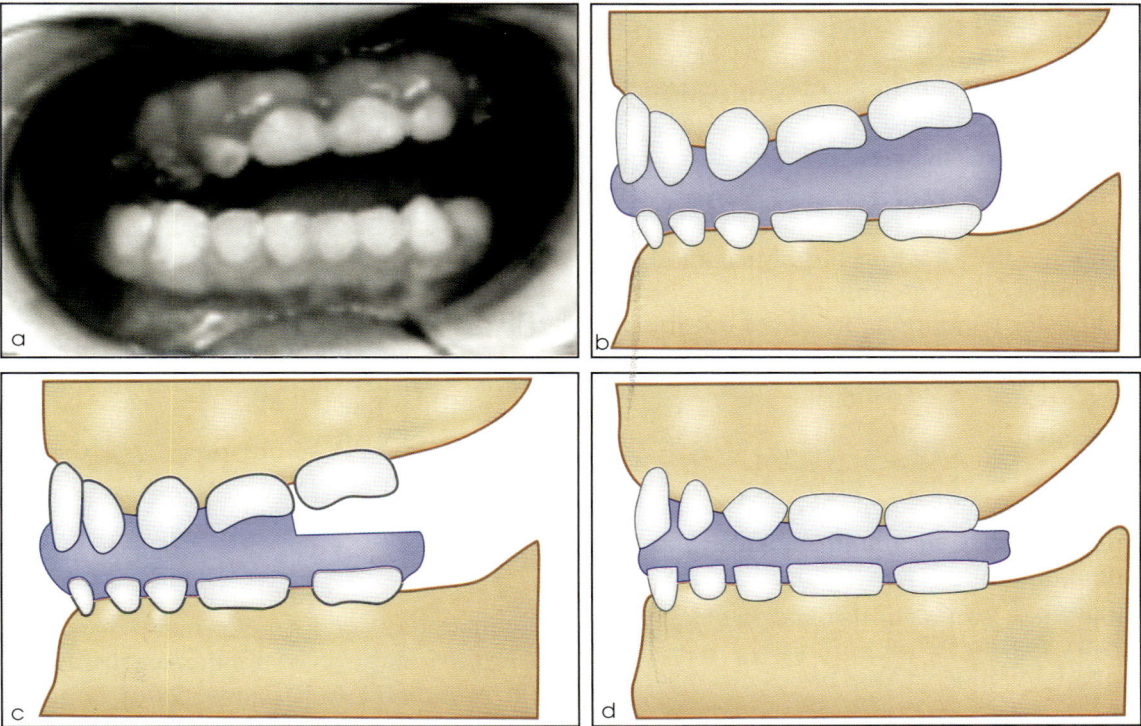

Fig. 13.38: Occlusal acrylic reduction

sufficiently rigid to maintain the increased transverse dimension. If an Essix retainer is required for patient esthetics and compliance, it should only be used during the day and a Hawley retainer used for evening and night-time wear. Fixed lower canine-to-canine wire will adequately maintain the canine width and anterior alignment, but cannot be expected to aid in maintaining any posterior expansion. Consequently, a Hawley retainer with integral lingual support wire is a good form of mandibular retention.

BIBLIOGRAPHY

1. Larry J Peterson. Principles of oral and Maxillofacial Surgery, 2 ed., Lippincott.
2. Epker BN, Stell JP, Fish Le. Dentofacial deformities: integrated orthodontic and surgical correction, 2 ed., St Louis: Mosby, 1998.
3. McNeill RW; Proffit WR and White RP. Cephalometric prediction for orthodontic surgry. Angle Orthod 42:154 April 1972
4. Proffit WR, Epker BN. In: Bell et al (editors), surgical correction of dentofacial deformities, Philadelphia: Saunders, 1980.
5. Kaplan RG. Supracrestal fiberotomy. J Am Dent Assoc 1977; 95(6):1127–32.
6. Kyu-Rhim Chung, Moon-Young Oh, Su-Jin KO. Corticotomy-Assisted Orthodontics. J Clin Orthod 2001; 35 (5):331–339.

PREVIOUS YEAR'S UNIVERSITY QUESTIONS

Essay

1. Describe the different orthognathic surgeries for Class II skeletal conditions.
2. Classify distraction osteogenesis.

Short Questions

1. Corticotomy
2. Pericision
3. Frenectomy
4. BSSO
5. Genioplasty
6. Decompensation

MCQs

1. *The common impacted tooth next to third molar is:*
   a. Maxillary lateral incisors
   b. Maxillary canine
   c. Maxillary premolars
   d. Mandibular canine **(Ans: b)**

2. *Before surgical exposure, the impacted tooth is localized by:*
   a. Two radiographs taken at different angulations (SLOB) technique
   b. More than 1 radiograph technique
   c. Both a and b
   d. None of the above **(Ans: c)**

3. *Decompensation refers to:*
   a. Repositioning the teeth properly over the dental bone
   b. Alignment of crowded teeth
   c. Repositioning the teeth properly over the skeletal bone without consideration of bite relationship to the opposing arch
   d. All of the above **(Ans: c)**

4. *BSSO stands for:*
   a. Biomechanical surgical septal osteotomy
   b. Bimaxillary sagittal split osteotomy
   c. Bilateral sagittal split osteotomy
   d. None of the above **(Ans: c)**

5. *Following is the most popular method for treating both mandibular deficiency and excess:*
   a. LeFort I osteotomy
   b. Vertical ramus osteotomy
   c. BSSO
   d. Mandibular subapical osteotomy **(Ans: c)**

6. *Who popularized the transoral vertical osteotomy:*
   a. Obswequer
   b. Caldwell and letterman in 1950
   c. Trainer
   d. Httnsuck **(Ans: b)**

7. *Who first described the BSSO orthognathic surgical procedure:*
   a. Letterman
   b. Obswequer
   c. Caldwell
   d. Dalpont **(Ans: b)**

8. *Cosmetic surgeries include the following, except:*
   a. Rhinoplasty
   b. Genioplasty
   c. Vertical osteotomy
   d. Molar augmentation **(Ans: c)**

9. *Distraction osteogenesis includes:*
   a. Cutting osteotomy to separate the segments of bone
   b. Application of traction appliances
   c. Incremental separation of bone segments to facilitate bone formation
   d. All of the above **(Ans: d)**

10. *Distraction osteogenesis can be used in:*
    a. Maxilla only
    b. Mandible only
    c. Maxilla and mandible
    d. TMJ   **(Ans: c)**

11. *Presurgical orthodontics is aimed at:*
    a. Done before orthognathic surgery
    b. Correcting the dental compensation that has occurred in response to skeletal deformity
    c. Done after orthognathic surgical procedure
    d. Both a and b   **(Ans: d)**

Abnormal Pressure Habits and their Management

Chapter Outline

- Definitions of habits
- Classification of oral habits
- Development of habit (theories)
- Tongue thrusting habit
- Thumb/finger sucking habit

- Abnormal swallowing habit
- Mouth breathing habit
- Lip habits
- Postural habit
- Bruxism

DEFINITIONS OF HABITS

William James in 1972, an eminent psychologist, stated that it is acquired habit from a psychological point of view and is nothing but a new pathway of discharge formed in the brain by which certain incoming currents tend to escape.

Johnson (1938): A habit is an inclination or attitude for some action acquired by frequent repetition and showing itself in increased facility to performance and reduced power of resistance.

Maslow in 1949: A habit is a formed reaction that is resistant to change, whether useful or harmful, depending on the degree to which it interferes with the child's physical, emotional and social functions

Moyer: Habits are learned patterns of muscular contractions, which are complex in nature.

Stedman: Habit is an act, behavioral response, practice or custom established in one's repertoire by frequent repetitions of the same act.

Habit is an automatic response to a situation acquired normally as the result of repetition and learning strictly applicable only to motor responses. At each repetition, the act becomes less conscious and can lead onto unconscious habit.

Dorland: Fixed or constant practice established by frequent repetition.

Buttersworth: Frequent or constant practice or acquired tendency which has been fixed by frequent repetition.

Harry in 1971 stated that orthodontically habit is manifested as self implicated trauma or force which affects the shape, size, position and posture of the tongue, jaws and lips.

Finn (1972): A habit is an act which is socially unacceptable.

CLASSIFICATION OF ORAL HABITS

Different authors have proposed various systems of classifying oral habits. These systems of classification are based upon the fact which they consider most important in the development, etiology and correction of these habits.

1. **William James** (1923) has classified oral habits as:
   - *Useful:* It includes habits of normal functions such as correct tongue position, proper respiration and deglutition and normal use of the lips in speaking.
   - *Harmful:* It includes all that exert perverted stresses against the teeth and dental arches as well as those habits such as open mouth habit, lip biting, lip sucking and thumb sucking.
2. **Morris and Bohanna** (1969)
   - Non-pressure habit

- Pressure habit
  - *Sucking habit:* Lip, thumb sucking, tongue thrusting
  - *Biting habit:* Nail biting, needle, thread holding
  - *Posturing habit:* Pillow, hand rest
  - *Miscellaneous:* Bruxism, cheek biting
3. **Tandon**
   - *Obsessive* (deep rooted):
     - Intentional or meaningful
     - Masochistic or self-inflicting injurious habit
   - *Non-obsessive* (empty learned):
     - Empty or unintentional: Abnormal pillowing, chin propping
     - Functional: Tongue thrusting
4. **ET Klein** (1952) classified abnormal pressure habits into intrinsic and extrinsic.
   a. *Intrinsic pressure habits*:
      - Thumb sucking
      - Finger sucking
      - Tongue sucking
      - Lip sucking
      - Cheek sucking
      - Nail biting
      - Lip biting
      - Tongue biting
      - Tongue thrusting
      - Macroglossia
      - Incorrect swallowing
      - Mouth breathing
   b. *Extrinsic pressure habits*:
      - Chin propping
      - Face leaning on hand
      - Abnormal pillowing positions leaning on forearm or hand.

   Habitually sleeping on the right side of the face may cause the nose to turn leftward or vice versa, a deviated septum may also result from this sleeping habit.
5. **A broader system of classification based on the nature of habit by Kingsley** (1958).

   Functional oral habits: Mouth breathing

   Muscular habits: Tongue thrusting, lip and cheek biting.

   Combined muscular action (involvement of oral and other muscles):
   a. Finger sucking,
   b. Thumb sucking, and
   c. Dummy sucking.

   Postural habits: Chin propping, face leaning on hand, abnormal pillowing, habitually sleeping on one side (left/right side of the face).

Self-mutilating habits or masochistic: Peeling of gingival with finger nail, lip and cheek biting and bruxism.
6. **TM Graber (1988) classification:** Described earlier.
7. **Sim and Finn's classification:**
   a. *Non-compulsive oral acts:* Habits that are easily dropped out from the child behavior pattern as he or she matures. It shows more consistent behavior and an increased level of maturity and responsibility. Children appear to undergo continuing behavior modification which permits them to release certain undesirable habit patterns and form new and more socially acceptable ones.
   b. *Compulsive habits:* It is a habit that has acquired fixation in the child to the extent that he or she reverts to the practice of this habit whenever his security is threatened by events which occur around the child. He tends to suffer from an increased anxiety when attempts are made to correct the habit. They have deep-seated emotional need and is possibly the only safety valve when emotional pressures become too much to cope with.

Some of the other common classifications of habits are as follows:
1. *Habits can be classified according to the cause of the habit:*
   - *Physiologic habits:* Those require for normal physiologic functioning, e.g. nasal breathing, sucking during infancy.
   - *Pathologic habits:* Those that are pursued due to pathologic reasons, e.g. mouth breathing due to deviated nasal septum (DNS)/enlarge adenoids.
2. *Classification based on the origin of the habit:*
   - *Retained habits:* Those that are carried over from childhood into adulthood.
   - *Cultivated habits:* Those that are cultivated during socioactive life of an individual.
3. *Classification based on the patient awareness to the habit:*
   - *Unconscious habits:* They are sustained by unconscious behavior. Simple attenuation of sensory feedback mechanism aid in cessation.
   - *Conscious habits:* Involve choice or need, making treatment more difficult and complex.

DEVELOPMENT OF HABIT

Many theories, which reason out the development of habit, are:
1. Psychoanalytic theory of Sigmund Freud
2. Behavior learning theory.

Psychoanalytic Theory

According to this theory, the oral habits are the product of pleasure; the child derives from stimulating the oral erogenous zone. The pleasure derived may be sexual or escape from a painful situation as in the case of infant who sucks when he is hungry. Freud suggested that orally in the infant is related to progenitor organization and that sexual activity is not yet separated from the taking of nourishment.

Psychoanalytical theory states that if there is either frustration or over indulgence of oral needs during infancy, later behavior will show some form of impairment.

Thumb sucking may be the only manifestation of insecurity maladjustment/deep-seated internal conflicts.

Behavior Learning Theory—Palermo (1956)

Supporters of this theory believed that the habit is a learned behavior and confirm to the laws of learning theory.

Learning theorists say that it is the foundation of behavioral pattern. A conditioned reflex is a reflex response to a stimulus that previously elicited little or no response, acquired by repeated pairing the stimulus with another stimulus that normally does produce the response. This is an example of associative learning where the organism learns about the relation of one stimulus to another.

Conditioning and stimulus generalization can initiate a habit, which if continuously repeated reinforced, will become a learned pattern.

Benjamin's Theory (1962)

He suggested that thumb sucking manifests from the rooting/placing reflex seen in all mammalian infants. Rooting reflex is the movement of infant's head and tongue towards an object touching the cheek. The object is usually the mother's breast while feeding, but may also be a finger or a pacifier. The rooting reflex usually disappears around 7–8 months of age.

Oral Gratification Theory: Sheldon (1932)

If the child is not satisfied with sucking during the feeding period, it will persist as a symptom of an emotional conflict/disturbance in the form of digit sucking.

Oral Drive Theory: Sears and Wise (1982)

This theory suggests that the strength of oral drive depends on how long a child continues to feed by sucking. In other words, prolongation of nursing strengthens the oral drive in the child and thus NNS is the result of prolongation of nursing and not the frustration of weaning.

This theory agrees with Freud's theory that sucking increases the erotogenesis of the mouth.

Eric Johnson and Brent Larsson (1993)

Origin of NNS is a combination of psychoanalytical and learning theories.

TONGUE THRUSTING HABIT

Definition

Boucher (1963) defined tongue thrust as thrusting or tongue between the anterior teeth especially in the initial stage of swallowing. It is often combined with resting position also between the teeth that can inhibit normal eruption and so produce an open bite.

Proffit (1990) defined tongue thrust swallowing as the placement of the tongue tip forward between the incisors during swallowing.

Norton and Gellin (1978): Condition in which the tongue protrudes between anterior and posterior teeth during swallowing with ot without affecting tooth position.

Tulley (1969): It is forward movement of the tongue tip between the teeth to meet the lower lip during deglutition and sounds of speech so that the tongue becomes interdental.

Classification

Backlund (1963)
- Anterior tongue thrust: Forceful anterior thrust
- Posterior tongue thrust: Lateral thrusting in case of missing teeth.

Pickett (1966)
- Adaptive tongue thrust: Tongue adapts to an open bite caused by missing teeth/thumb sucking. Transitory tongue is put forward only for a short period. Forceful and rapid.
- Habitual: Due to postural problem, a habit or presence of open bite.

Moyers classified tongue thrusting into three types:
1. The simple tongue thrust swallow
2. The complex tongue thrust swallow
3. Retained infantile swallow: Persistence of infantile swallow even after permanent teeth appear
1. *Simple tongue thrust:* Swallow usually is associated with a history of digital sucking, even though the

sucking habit may no longer be practiced, since it is necessary for the tongue to thrust forward into the open bite to maintain an anterior oral seal with the lips during the swallow. There is an increase in tongue thrust swallowing seen with both pacifiers sucking and digital sucking (Fig. 14.1).

It typically displays contractions of the lips, mentalis muscle and mandibular elevators and the teeth are in occlusion as the tongue protrudes into an openbite. There is a normal teeth-together swallow, but a tongue thrust is present to seal the open bite.

2. *Complex tongue thrust:* It is defined as a tongue thrust with a teeth apart swallow. Patients with complex tongue thrust combine with contractions of the lip, facial and mentalis muscles, lack of contraction of the mandibular elevators. It is more diffuse and difficult to define than that is seen with a simple tongue thrust. Examination of the dental casts typically reveals a poor occlusal fit and instability of intercuspation because the intercuspal position is not repeatedly reinforced during the swallow. Since persistent teeth-apart swallows do not stabilize the occlusion, the patients with this type of thrust usually demonstrate occlusal interferences in the retruded position.

James Braner and Holt:

Type I: Nondeforming tongue thrust

Type II: Deforming tongue thrust
- Subgroup 1: Anterior open bite
- Subgroup 2: Anterior proclination
- Subgroup 3: Posterior crossbite.

Type III: Deforming lateral tongue thrust
- Subgroup 1: Posterior open bite
- Subgroup 2: Posterior crossbite
- Subgroup 3: Deep overbite.

Type IV: Deforming anterior and lateral tongue thrust
- Subgroup 1: Anterior and posterior open bite

- Subgroup 2: Proclination of anterior teeth
- Subgroup 3: Posterior crossbite.

Etiology of Tongue Thrusting

1. This kind of thrust is associated with chronic nasal—respiratory distress, mouth breathing, tonsillitis or pharyngitis. When the tonsils are inflamed, the root of the tongue may encroach on the enlarged facial pillars. To avoid this encroachment, the mandible reflex drops separating the teeth and providing more room for the tongue to be thrust forward during swallowing to more comfortable position.

2. **Thumb sucking:** Moyers writes that tongue thrust often accompanies or is a residuum of thumb sucking.

3. **Open spaces during mixed dentition:** When a child loses deciduous teeth especially a canine or an incisor, the tongue frequently protrudes into the space at rest and during speech and swallowing activities.

4. Macroglossia (Fig. 14.2) and microglossia

5. **Sleeping habits:** When some patients sleep on their back on a low pillow, open mouth results. The tongue rests on the mandibular arch and moves forward against the teeth during swallowing.

6. **Abnormal tongue posture:** In Class III, the tongue lies below the plane of occlusion. In Class II, short mandible and steep mandibular plane angle may position the tongue forward. Two types of variation from normal tongue posture are seen.

   a. *Retracted tongue/cocked tongue:* The tongue tip is withdrawn from all anterior. Posterior open bite occurs because the tongue spreads laterally as it is present in edentulous patients. The tongue loses its positional sense with the removal of teeth and periodontal ligaments and 10% of all children have this posture.

   b. *Protracted tongue:* There are two types:
      i. *Endogenous:* Retention of infantile swallowing always present between the incisors. It also

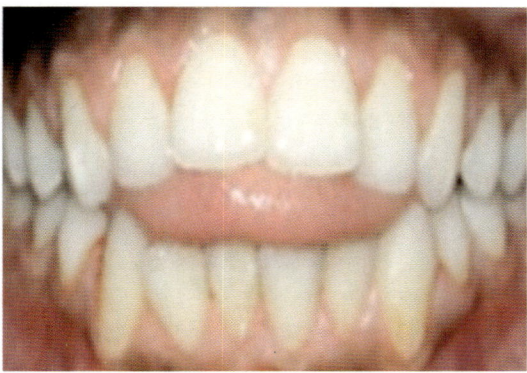

Fig. 14.1: Simple tongue thrust

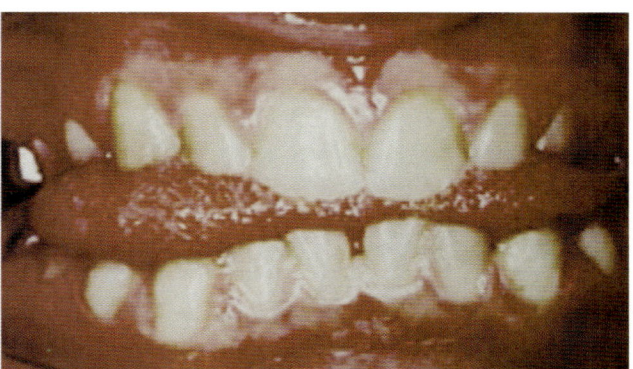

Fig. 14.2: Macroglossia

causes excessive vertical anterior face height or the skeletal pattern which predisposes to the tongue protraction. Surgical correction of every skeletal dysplasia is the only treatment.

ii. *Acquired:* It is transitory adaptation to enlarged tonsils. Dramatic change is seen in the tongue and mandibular posture.

Treatment of Tongue Thrust Habit

- Myofunctional therapy
- Speech therapy
- Mechanotherapy

Myofunctional Therapy

Garliner: Guidance of correct posture of tongue during swallowing by various exercises

- Placement of tongue tip in rugae area for 5 minutes.
- Orthodontic elastics and sugarless fruit drops
- 2S, 4S exercises
  - Identification of spot
  - Salivating
  - Squeezing in spot
  - Swallowing
- Other exercises
  - Whistling
  - Reciting from 60 to 90
  - Yawning
- *Lip exercise:* Tug of war and button pull exercise
- *Lip massage:* Lower lip over upper massage
- *Subconscious therapy:*
  - Time—special time for reminding
  - Subliminal therapy: Placing reminder sign in sight during meal
  - Autosuggestion: 6 times swallow before sleeping

Speech Therapy

- Training of correct position of tongue
- Articulation of speech
- Repetition of words with "S" sound

Mechanotherapy

Purpose
- Reeducation of tongue position
- Maintaining tongue in the confines of dentition
- Maintaining the interocclusal distance: Prevention of overeruption and narrowing of maxillary buccal segment
- Preorthodontic trainer for myofunctional training (Fig. 14.3):

– It aids in correct positioning of tongue with the help of tongue tags.
– Tongue guard

Appliance Therapy

- Hawley's appliance with palatal crib (Fig. 14.4)
- Oral screen and vestibular screen
- Modified Thurow appliance—skeletal open bite correction—AJODO 2005 (Fig. 14.5)
- Dillingham habit breaking appliance (Fig. 14.6)

Since the tongue thrust decreases with age, treatment must be based on age:

- *3–11 years:* Normal occurrence is not to be concerned and reassure parents. If child is under 7 years, there is no need to be concerned since speech sound that elicits a lisp is not matured until 7–8 years of age.
- *Conservative approach:* Demonstrate the correct swallowing pattern or procedure and observe the child.
- *11 years or older:* Tongue thrust is not a normal pattern.

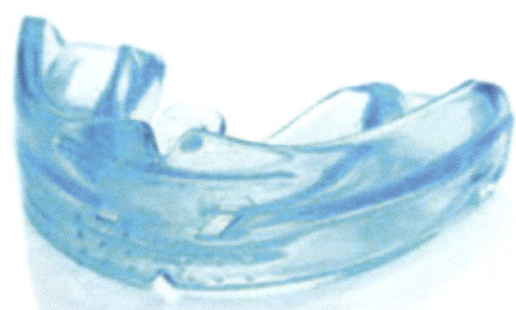

Fig. 14.3: Preorthodontic trainer

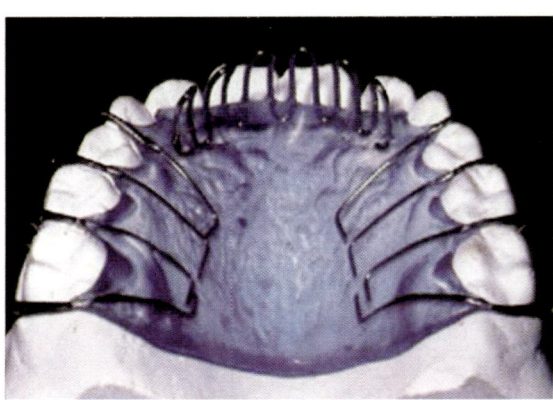

Fig. 14.4: Hawley's appliance with palatal crib

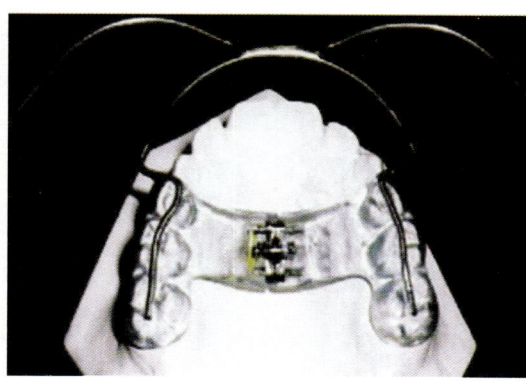

Fig. 14.5: Modified Thurow appliance

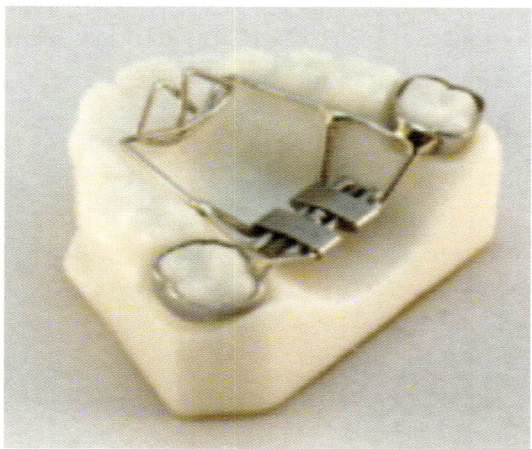

Fig. 14.6: Dillingham habit breaking appliance

Management of Simple Tongue Thrust

Three phases (Moyers):
- Conscious learning of new reflex—cognitive approach
- Transferring to subconscious level—reflexive approach
- Reinforcement of new reflex.

Cognitive approach: Myofunctional approach: Advantages of postponing tongue therapy until treatment of malocclusion is begun include:
- Correction of malocclusion results in disappearance of habit.
- It gives maximum opportunity for transition to mature adult swallow.
- Therapy is most effective when carried out with orthodontic treatment.
- Muscle exercises

Reflective approach: When new swallowing pattern has been learned at a conscious level, it is necessary to transfer it to the subconscious level. At the second appointment, the patient should be able to swallow correctly at will.

Neuromuscular facilitation: Subcortical method of affecting swallowing act. Sensory input is correlated with motor activities on a subconscious level.

Reinforcement of new reflex: This is achieved by means of mechanical restraints which may be removable or fixed. Cribs or rakes are valuable in breaking the habit. Oral screen also may be used.

Treatment of Complex Tongue Thrust
- Treat the occlusion first
- When orthodontic treatment is in its retentive stages, careful occlusal equilibration is completed.
- The muscle training is begun similar to simple tongue thrust with minor modifications.

THUMB/FINGER SUCKING HABIT

Definition of Thumb Sucking

Gellin (1978): It is defined as displacement of thumb or one or more fingers in varying depths into the mouth.

Moyers: Repeated and forceful sucking of thumb with associated strong buccal and lip contractions.

The habit of sucking the thumb for oral gratification, it is normal in infants and young children as a pleasure-seeking or comforting device, especially when the child is hungry or tired.

The habit reaches its peak when the child is between 18 and 20 months of age and it normally disappears when the child develops and matures. Thumb sucking beyond 4 to 6 years of age may lead to malocclusion of the teeth and deformation of the bony tissue of the thumb. Excessive thumb sucking especially in older children may be indicative of some emotional problem (Fig. 14.7).

All digital sucking habits should be studied for their psychological implications for they may be related to hunger, satisfying of the sucking instinct, insecurity or even desire to attract attention (Tables 14.1 and 14.2).

Classification of Thumb Sucking

Thumb sucking is classified into 5 types:

1. Cook (1958)

α-**group:** Pushed palate in a vertical direction and displayed only little buccal wall contractions

β-**group:** Registered strong buccal wall contractions and a negative pressure in the oral cavity show posterior crossbite.

γ-**group:** Alternate positive and negative pressure; least effect on anterior occlusion.

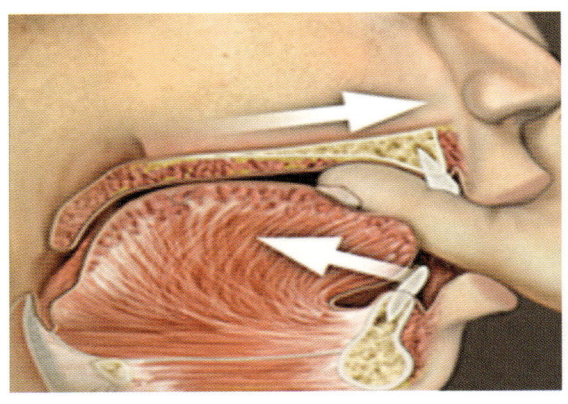 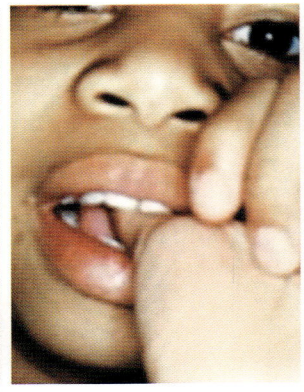 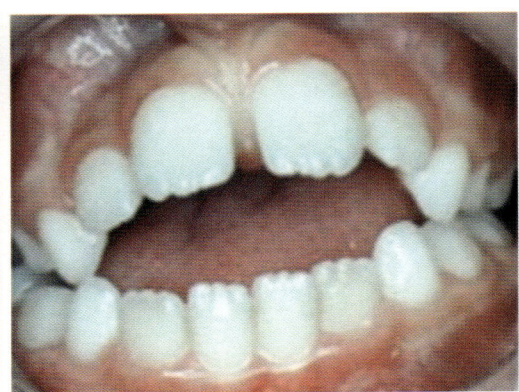

Fig. 14.7: Thumb sucking habbit

Table 14.1: Classification of NNS Habits (Johnson 1993)	
Level	Description
I (+/−)	Boys or girls of any chronological age with a habit that occurs during sleep
II (+/−)	Boys below 8 years with a habit that occurs at one setting during waking hours
III (+/−)	Boys below 8 years with a habit that occurs at multiple setting during waking hours
IV (+/−)	Girls below 8 years or boy over 8 years with a habit that occurs at one setting during waking hours
V (+/−)	Girls below 8 years or boy over 8 years with a habit that occurs at multiple setting during waking hours
VI (+/−)	Girls over 8 years with a habit during waking hours

(+/−): Designates willingness of parents to participate in treatment

2. Subtelny Classification (1973)

Type A: It is seen in almost 50% children, where in the whole digit is placed inside the mouth, with the pad of thumb pressing over the palate, while at the same time maxilla and mandible anteriors contact is present (Fig. 14.8a).

Type B: It is seen in almost 13–24% of children wherein the thumb is placed in oral cavity without touching the vault of the palate, while at same time maxillary and mandibular anteriors contact is maintained (Fig. 14.8b).

Type C: It is seen in almost 18% of children where the thumb is placed in the mouth first and contacts the hard palate and maxillary incisors but there is no contact with mandibular incisors (Fig. 14.8c).

Type D: It is seen in almost 6% of children where very little portion of thumb is placed into the mouth (Fig. 14.8d).

3. Johnson and Larson Classification

They classified non-nutritive sucking (NNS) habits and are given in Table 14.1.

4. Clinical Classification of Thumb Sucking (Table 14.2)

Based on clinical observation, thumb sucking can be classified into following two types:

1. Normal thumb sucking
2. Abnormal thumb sucking
   - Physiological
   - Habitual

Table 14.2: The clinical aspects of the problem may be divided into three distinct phases of development (Moyers)			
Phase	Clinical stage	Age of child	Inference
Phase I	Normal or subclinically significant sucking	Pre-school infant	This phase extends from child birth to about 3 years of age dpending on the child's social development. Most infants display a certain amount of thumb sucking during this period particularly at time of weaning
Phase II	Clinically significant sucking	Grade school	This phase extends from 3 to 6 years. Continued, purposeful digit sucking during this time. Deserves more serious attention because the possibility indicates a clinically significant anxiety and it is the time to solve dental problems related to digit sucking.
Phase III	Intractable sucking	Teenage child	Any thumb sucking persisting after the child's fourth year presents the dentists with a problem. A thumb sucking habit seen during this phase may require psychological therapy and an intergrated approach by the dentist

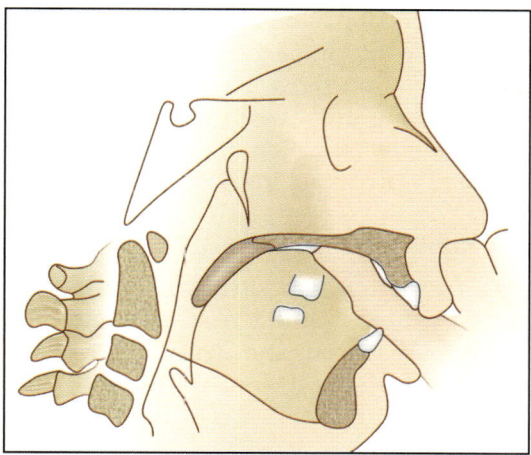

Fig. 14.8a: Type-A

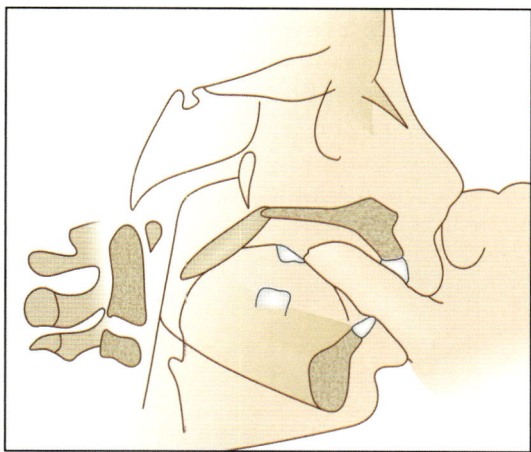

Fig. 14.8b: Type-B

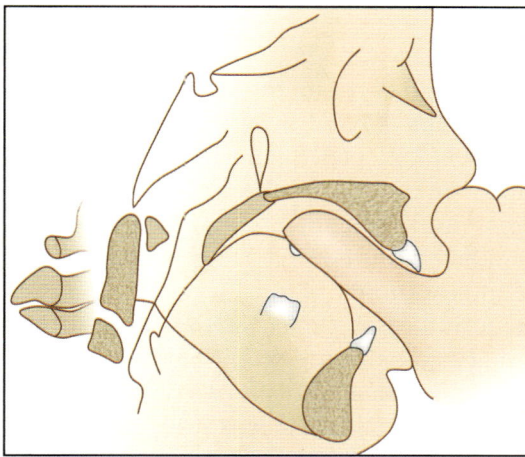

Fig. 14.8c: Type-C

Normal thumb sucking habit is usually seen to disappear after 4 years as the child matures whereas persistence of abnormal thumb sucking habit beyond the pre-school period is considered as abnormal thumb sucking habit.

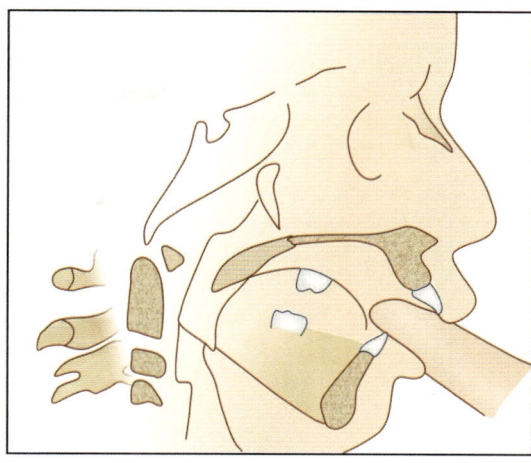

Fig. 14.8d: Type-D

5. *Thumb Sucking Habit by O' Brien*

He classified the habit into nutritive and non-nutritive sucking habit.

Nutritive sucking habit: It includes breastfeeding, and bottle feeding.

Non-nutritive sucking habit: It includes thumb sucking, finger sucking and pacifier sucking.

Digit Sucking

- *Sucking reflex:*
  – It starts at 29 weeks IU.
  – It disappears by 3–4 years.
  – It is coordinated muscular activity.
  – Psychological and nutritive need.
- *Rooting reflex (Fig. 14.9):*
  – It is well-defined sensory area around mouth.
  – Head turning and opening of mouth by stimulation

Gesell and lla of Yale's child development laboratory contend that finger sucking is perfectly normal at one

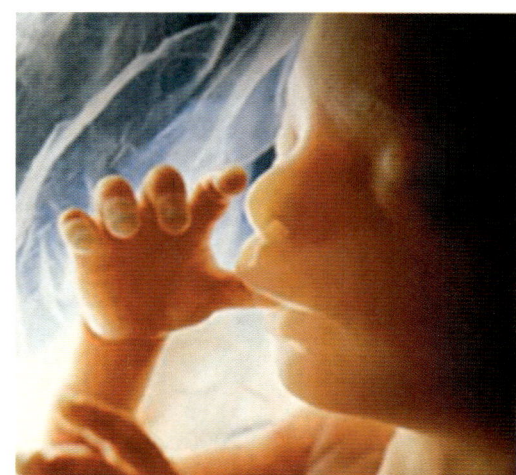

Fig. 14.9: Rooting reflex

stage of a child's development. They feel that most finger sucking and tongue sucking habits, which may be considered normal for the first year and half of life, will disappear spontaneously by the end of the second year with proper attention to nursing.

For the first three years of life, damage to the occlusion is confined largely to the anterior segment. This damage is usually temporary provided the child starts with a normal occlusion. Babies who are restricted from sucking due to disease or other factors become restless and irritable. This deprivation may motivate the child to suck thumb or finger for additional gratification.

Active Finger Sucking Habit after 4 Years

No appliance is required till the age of 4 years. But after 4 years, the active finger sucking habit cause the permanent deformation of occlusion resulting the increase of overjet with difficult swallowing procedures. The lower lip cushions to the palatal of the maxillary incisors forcing them farther forward. Swallowing creates vacuum between the dorsal surface of the tongue and the vault of the palate. But in active finger sucking habits, the swallowing requires the creation of a closing off—a partial vacuum. Since we swallow at least once a minute all day long, the lip muscle aberrations are often assisted by a compensatory tongue thrust during the swallowing act. So, the deglutitional maturation is retarded in confirmed finger suckers. The infantile suckle swallow with its plunger like function continues or the transitional period is greatly prolonged with a mixture of infantile and mature swallowing cycles. This may be the most significant deforming mechanism.

Causative Factors

- *Parents occupation:* Sucking habit commonly observed in children with working parents.
- *Socioeconomic status*
  - Child in low socioeconomic group had to suckle intensively for long time to get required nourishment thereby exhausting the sucking urge. This theory explains increased incidence of the thumb sucking in industrialized areas compared to rural areas.
  - Number of siblings
  - Order of birth of a child
  - Feeding practice
  - Cristiane, Luz (AJODO-2006): If breastfeeding is shorter than 6 months, there is a fourfold likelihood that an infant will develop a non-nutritive sucking habit that could warp its occlusal relationship into an Angle Class II dysmorphology. The association between the short duration of breastfeeding and the development of sucking habits seems to develop in response to frustration and need for contact in these children.

Trident of Habit Factors

Duration, frequency and intensity: This trident of conditioning factors must qualify conclusions of psychiatrist, pediatrician and dentist.

- Duration of the habit beyond early childhood is not only determinant. Equally important is at least two other considerations.
- The frequency of the habit during the day and night affects the end result. The child who sucks sporadically or just when going to sleep is much less likely to do any damage than who constantly has his finger in his mouth.
- The intensity of the habit is important. In some children, the sucking can be heard loudly. The perioral muscle function and facial contractions are easily visible. In others, the thumb-sucking habit is little more than a passive insertion of the finger in the mouth with no apparent buccinators activity.

Management

- Psychotherapy
- Reminder therapy
- Behavior therapy
- Appliance therapy

Psychotherapy

- Most children between the age of 4 and 8 years with a concern about habit need only reassurance.
- Once this is achieved, the positive reinforcement and friendly remainders are best possible treatments.
- Child should be made aware of the habit which is accomplished by emphasizing the positive aspects of habit cessation.
- Destructive approaches in the form of nagging, shaming and belittling ought to be strictly avoided.
- Various aids are employed to bring the habit under the notice of the child such as study models, mirrors, etc.

Behavioral Therapy

This form of therapy seeks to identify and help change potentially self-destructive or unhealthy behaviors. It functions on the idea that all behaviors are learned and unhealthy behaviors can be changed.

The therapist meets regularly with the family to monitor progress and provide support between sessions, parents practice using the skills they have learned from the therapist.

Steps in treatment are gradual and sequential
- The control of undesirable oral habits is usually begun in phase. It is wise to begin with a discussion of the problem with the child alone. No threads or shaming should be used instead; a calm friendly attempt should be made to learn about the child's attitudes towards the habit.
- The child may be shown casts or photographs of mouth of children who have had detrimental sucking habits.
- The dentist can show the treated case results to establish what can be done.
- Excellent results have been obtained by use of a card that the child is given for scoring each morning to indicate whether the thumb was sucked during the night. It should not be a printed form, but rather a card with the child's home written on especially for this purpose, two columns are drawn and labeled simply "yes" or "no" and make an appointment for the child to return in 2 weeks or less and to bring the card. Instruct the child that the thumb may be sucked. But a score must be kept for you so that you can learn about the severity of the habit.

Extraoral Approaches
- *Chemical methods:* Use of spicy, bitter flavoured preparation (Femitem Nobite) or distasteful agents preparation placed on the thumb that is sucked can make that habit distasteful. This is effective only when the habit is not firmly entrenched. Some of the available medicaments are:
  - Cayenne pepper dissolved in a volatile medium
  - Quinine
  - Asafotida
  - A commercially available product Femite composed of denatonium benzoate which is hard and bitter in taste. It should be applied on the skin and nails when the child is sleeping and allowed to dry for 10 minutes. This unpalatable compound prevents children from sucking their digits on application.
- *Mechanical methods:* This mechanical means avoid direct contact of the finger with oral cavity. They are adhesive bandage covering with cloths, gloves around wrist, nail polish and thumb guard (Fig. 14.10a). Thermoplastic thumb post was devised by Allen in 1991 where a thermoplastic material was placed on

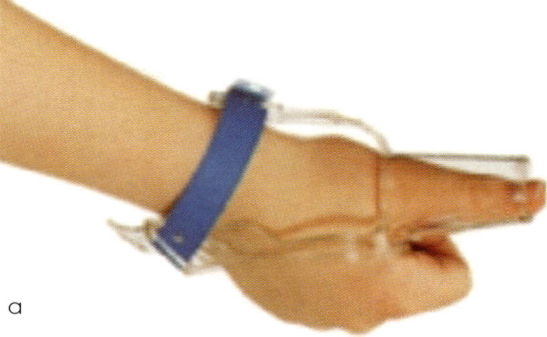

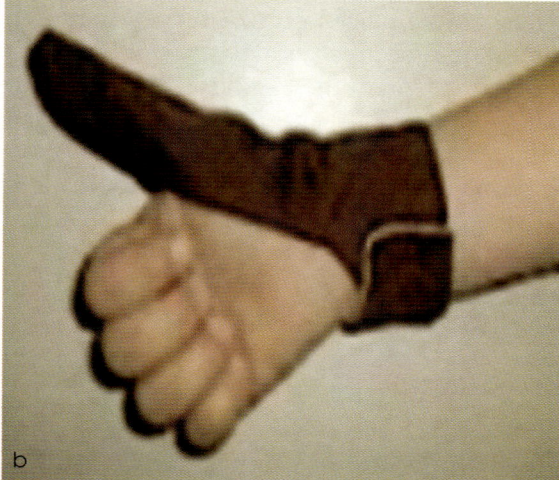

Fig. 14.10: (a) Thermoplastic thumb post; (b) Ace bandage approach

the affected digit. A total of 6 weeks of treatment time was required for elimination of habit.
- *Ace bandage approach:* It includes the use of ace bandage which is an at home program to assist children with nocturnal digit sucking habits. The program involves nightly use of an elastic bandage wrapped across the elbow. Pressure exerted by the bandage removes the digit from the mouth as the child tires and fall asleep (Fig. 14.10b).
- *Three-alarm system for mature children by Norton and Gellin:* This includes the taping of the offending digit. This is first alarm
  - Bandage is tied on the elbow of the arm with the offending digit. This is the second alarm.
  - A safety pin is placed lengthwise. Bandage is tightened, if the child persists to have the thumb sucking habit. This serves as third alarm.

Use of long sleeve night gown: This is useful in children who sincerely want to discontinue the habit and only perform during their sleep. The arms of their night suit are lengthened so that they cannot reach their thumb during night.

Thumb-home concept: This is the most recent concept. In this method, a small bag is tied around the wrist of the child during sleep. It is explained to the child that just as the child sleeps in the home, the thumb also sleeps in its house. Thus the child is restrained from thumb sucking during sleep.

Use of hand puppets: Currently, the use of hand puppets is gaining popularity. These help in eliminating thumb sucking. This helps in minimizing the damage of the finger sucking by providing a number of tools to address the habit in a phased manner.

Band aids can be placed on the thumb each night by the child to remind the thumb to put out of the mouth.

As the child enters the period of trying to control the habit alone, a talk should be with one or both parents to emphasize that no one should discuss:

- The problem with the child or it should not be a discussion in the family. Only the dentist and the child will take care of these problems.
- If the child with phase 2, the next step is the insertion of a habit correcting appliance.

Appliance Therapy

Intraoral Approaches

Various orthodontic appliances are employed to attenuate and eventually break the habit. Removable appliances used may be palatal crib, palatal arch, lingual spurs (Fig. 14.11).

Rake: The Rake is used on the patients that seem to get around all the other designs. A .040" support arch wire is soldered to bands on the first molars and a vertical rake is extended just behind the lower anteriors. The rake can be made as long or wide as the clinician desires (Fig. 14.12).

Habit with pearl: The habit with an added pearl is used on the upper arch to restrain the tongue from excessive

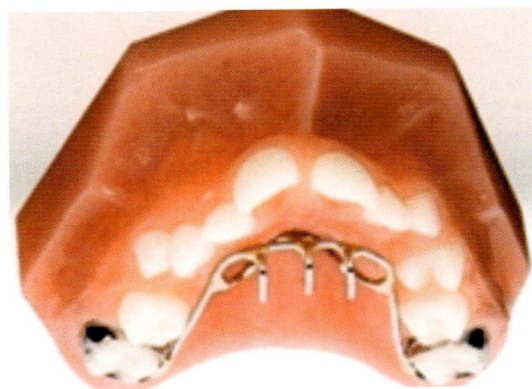

Fig. 14.12: Rakes as intraoral application

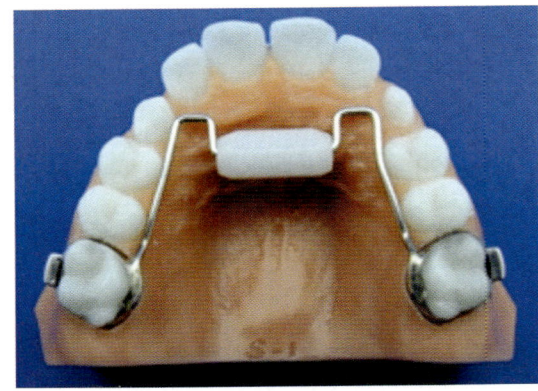

Fig. 14.13: Appliance with pearl

anterior movement. A .040" support archwire is soldered to bands on the first molars. A vertical cage is extended just behind the lower anteriors to prevent the patient from tongue thrust. A pearl is added in the vault of the palate to retrain the tongue (Fig. 14.13).

Oral screen: Oral screen is a functional appliance introduced in Newell in 1912. It produces its effect by redirecting the pressure of the muscular and soft tissue curtain of the cheeks and lips. It prevents from placing the thumb or finger into the oral cavity during sleeping hours.

Bluegrass appliance: It was developed by Bruce S Haskell in 1991. It is a fixed appliance using a teflon roller together with positive reinforcement. It is used to manage thumb-sucking habit in children between 7 and 13 years of age. The patient believes that he has acquired a new toy to play with (Fig. 14.14).

Modified Bluegrass appliance: Chris Baker in 2000 modified Bluegrass appliance. This is the modification of the original appliance with the difference being that this has two rollers of different colors and material

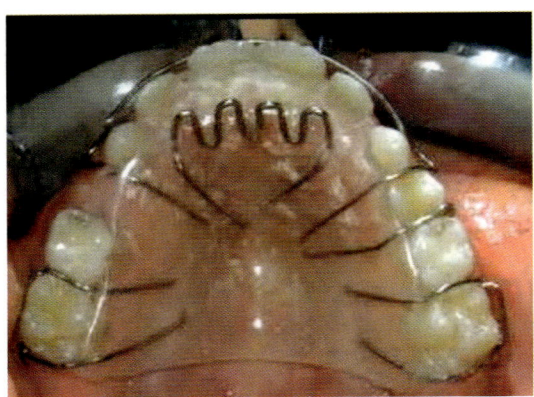

Fig. 14.11: Hawley appliance with palatal crib

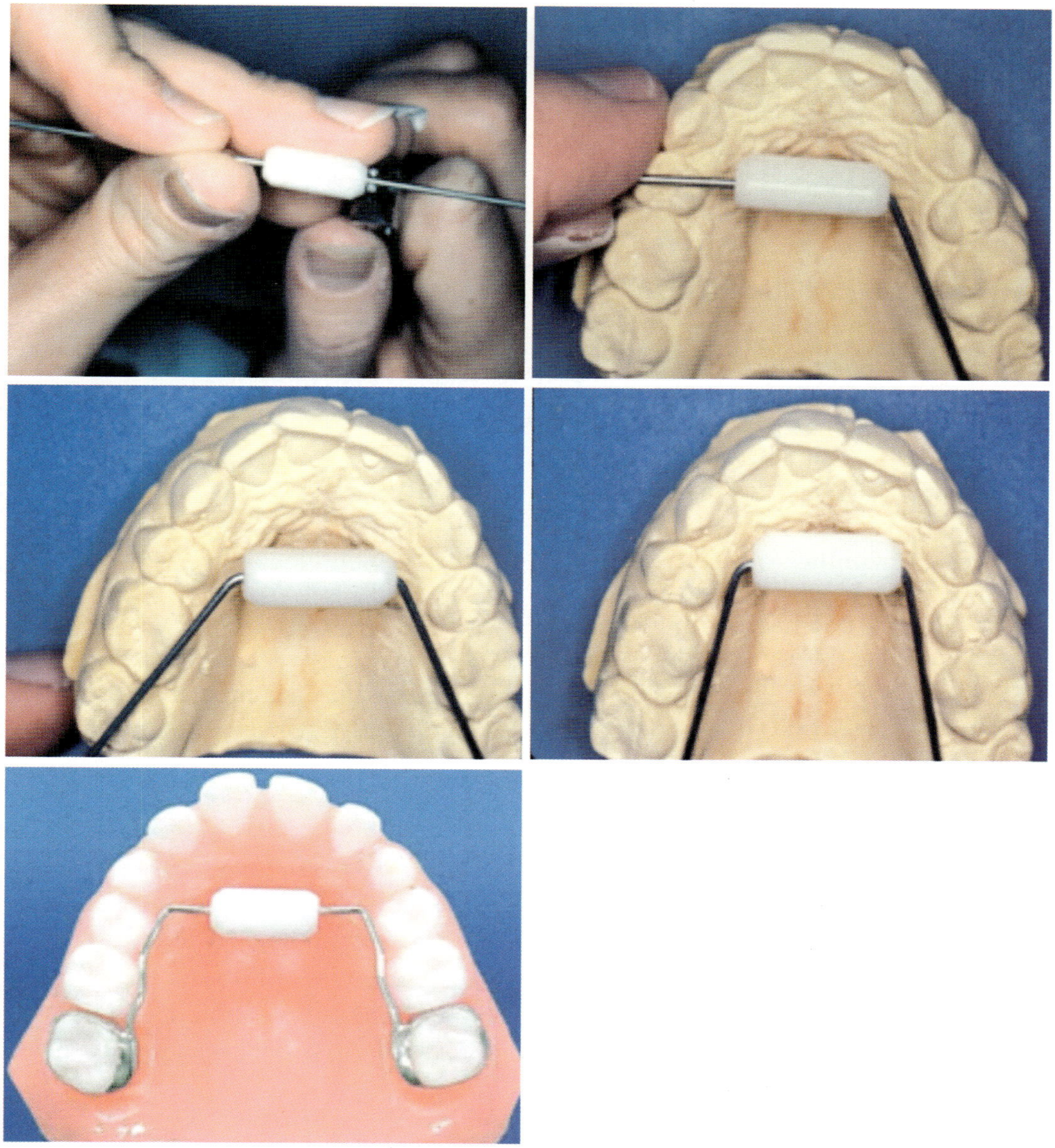

Fig. 14.14: Steps in fabricating Bluegrass appliance

instead of one. If the patient tries to suck on his thumb, the suction will not be created and the thumb will slip from the rollers thus breaking the act (Fig. 14.15).

Advantages

- It encourages the maximum neuromuscular stimulation by using two or more beads.
- It reduces bulkiness of appliance, which results in less obstruction and more stimulation of tongue function.
- Wire and beads cementd to second deciduous molar that is not seen from outside mouth. A child quickly becomes comfortable with the Bluegrass and enjoys the sensation of the tongue playing with the beads.

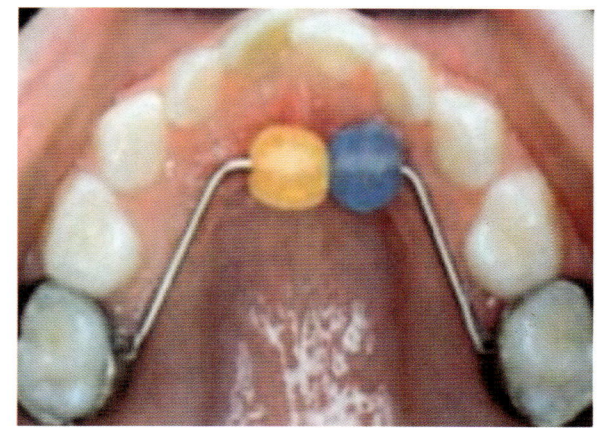

Fig. 14.15: Modified Bluegrass appliance

Graber explained the working of these appliances as given below.

- Render finger habit meaningless by breaking suction.
- Prevents finger pressure from displacing maxillary central incisors thus avoids labially from creating worse a malocclusion.
- Forces the tongue backwards changing its postural rest position, thus exerting more lateral pressures.

Triple loop connector—Viazis AJODO in 1991:

- It is simple thumb-sucking habit control appliance easily constructed by bending three consecutive loops.
- It requires minimal chairside time and can be designed to cover whole span of patient's open bite to make insertion of thumb difficult.
- This appliance works, if there is significant open bite and marked overjet (Fig. 14.16).

Dunlop's theory or beta hypothesis: It states that the best way to break a habit is by conscious, purposeful repetitions. By practicing the bad habit with the intent to stop it, one learns not to perform that undesirable act. This is especially practiced in older children between 8 years and above.

Dentofacial Changes associated with Prolonged Sucking Habit

- Increased proclination of maxillary anteriors with diastema
- Increased maxillary arch length

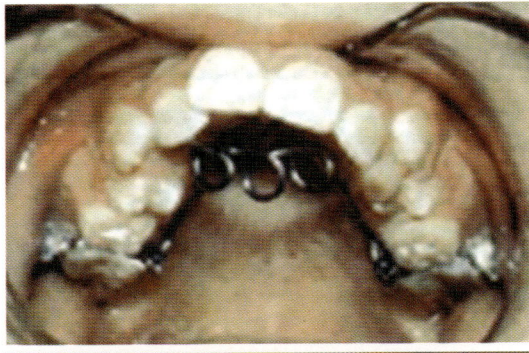

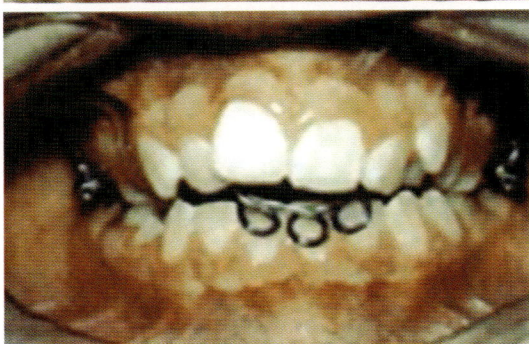

Fig. 14.16: Tripple loop connector

- Increased anterior placement of apical base of maxilla
- Increased SNA
- Increased clinical crown length of maxillary incisors
- Increased counterclockwise rotation of the occlusal plane
- Decreased SN to ANS-PNS angle
- Decreased palatal arch
- Increased atypical root resorption in primary central incisors
- Increased trauma to maxillary central incisors
- Increased proclination of mandibular incisors
- Increased mandibular intermolar distance
- Increased distal position of B point
- Increased overjet
- Decreased overbite
- Increased posterior crossbite
- Increased unilateral and bilateral Class II occlusion

Effects on Interarch Relationship

Effects on lip placement and function:

- Increased lip incompetence
- Increased lower lip function under the maxillary incisors

Effects of tongue placement and function:

- Increased tongue thrust
- Increased lip to tongue resting position
- Increased lower tongue position
- Risk to psychologic health.

Other effects

- Increased deformation of digits
- Increased risk of speech defects especially lisping

ABNORMAL SWALLOWING HABIT

Certain variations of swallowing behavior do have an orthodontic significance. This may be classified as:

- Adaptive swallowing behavior.
- Primary atypical swallowing behavior.

Adaptive Swallowing Behavior

Adaptions in swallowing behavior may occur either due to incompetent lips markedly or anomalies in the incisor relationship.

1. *Lip incompetence:* Swallowing may take place with the tongue lying over the tips of the lower incisors and with the teeth apart. If the teeth are brought into occlusion during swallowing, the tongue will be contained within the lower arch.
2. *Anomalies of incisor relationship:* When the overjet is markedly increased, it is obtained by tongue to lower

lip contact and swallowing will take place as described above. If the overjet is only moderately increased, there is forward posture of the mandible and idle swallowing will take place with the mandible in this position.

In case of anterior open bite or incomplete overbite, the malocclusion caused by thumb sucking does not always spontaneously resolve following cessation of the habit because, the adaptive position of the tongue may perpetuate the incisor malrelationship.

However, on correction of the malocclusion, swallowing anomalies of this type will readapt to the new positions.

They should be distinguished from the primary atypical pattern of swallowing behavior which is quite rare but it does a direct influence on the position of the teeth which will not adapt to correction of the incisor position.

Primary Atypical Swallowing Behavior

Rarely, the tongue is thrust quite forcibly forward against the palatal surface of the upper incisors during swallowing. This proclines the upper incisors and increases the overjet. The overbite is incomplete. During swallowing, there is usually a considerable amount of contraction.

It is important to assess the primary atypical swallowing behavior before orthodontic treatment. Because, the tongue activity will not adapt to a change in position of the upper incisors and hence relapse will follow.

MOUTH BREATHING HABIT

Definition

FM Chacker defined mouth breathing as the prolonged or continued exposure of the tissues of the anterior area of the mouth to the drying effects of inspired air.

Sassouni (1971): Mouth breathing is defined as habitual respiration through the mouth instead of the nose.

Merle (1980) suggests the term oronasal breathing instead of mouth breathing

It is common in children between 5 and 15 years of age and is estimated that 85% of mouth breathers suffer from some degree of nasal obstruction while 20% are habitual mouth breathers. Mouth breathing can occur only with failure of all the below mentioned three barriers, namely anterior oral seal formed by the lips, intermediate or middle oral seal formed by the dorsum of the tongue and the hard palate and posterior oral seal formed by soft palate and dorsum of the tongue (Fig. 14.17).

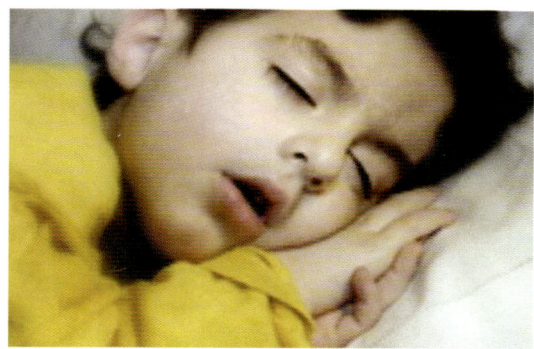

Fig. 14.17: Mouth breathing habit

Classification

Sim and Finn classified the mouth breathers into three types:
- Anatomic
- Obstructive
- Habitual

Anatomic:
- Hereditary characteristics of facial form may be a factor in size of the nasal passages and position of the septum.
- Abnormal development of nasal cavity.
- Abnormal development of nasal turbinates
- Abnormally short upper lip preventing proper lip seal
- Under development or abnormal facial musculature.
- Partial obstruction due to deviated nasal septum. It can be result of birth injuries/exogenous nasal trauma. It can cause bilateral blockage creating an 'S' shaped deformity or more typically a unilateral one creating a 'C' shaped obstruction.
- Partial obstruction due to narrow nasal passage associated with narrow maxilla.

Obstructive:
- Chronic inflammation of nasal mucosa
- Chronic atrophic rhinitis
- Sinusitis
- Nasal polyps
- Localized benign tumors

Habitual: This child breathes through his mouth by force of habit although the abnormal obstruction has since been removed.

Assessment of respiration: There are three types of breathing: Nasal, oral and oronasal.

Tests to Diagnose the Mode of Respiration (Fig. 14.18)

- *Mirror test:* A double-sided mirror is held between the nose and the mouth. Fogging on the nasal side

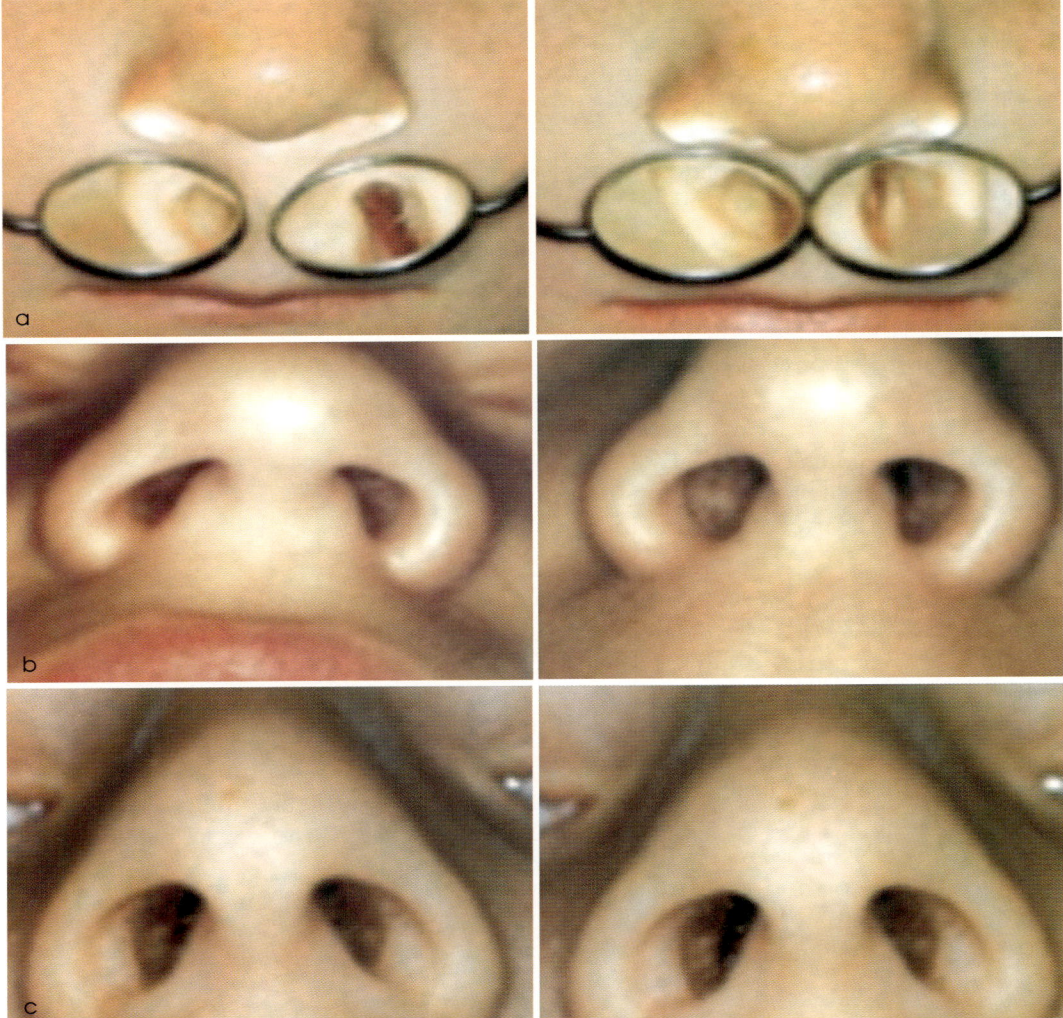

Fig. 14.18: Examination of breathing mode: (a) Mirror test; (b) Nasal respiration—observation of nostrils; (c) Oronasal respiration—inactive nares do not change their size

of the mirror indicates nasal breathing while fogging towards oral side indicates oral breathing.

- *Massler's water-holding test:* The patient is asked to hold the water in the mouth for a while. The nasal breathers accomplish this with ease whereas mouth breathers find it difficult task.
- *Butterfly test:* A butterfly-shaped cotton piece is placed over the upper lip below the nostrils. If the cotton vibrates down, it indicates nasal breathing. This test is used to determine the unilateral nasal blockage.

Mouth breathers are prone to:
- Nasal congestion
- Watery itchy eyes
- Running nose
- Enlarged tonsils
- Halitosis
- Dry cough
- Tongue thrust
- Abnormal swallowing habit
- Long face syndrome
- Speech problems
- Poor palate development

LIP HABITS

Classification

- Lip habit is classified into:
  - Wetting the lips with the tongue
  - Pulling the lips into the mouth between the teeth.
- Lip habit can be of following three types:
  - Lip sucking
  - Lip wetting
  - Lip biting

Lip-sucking habit: In lip-sucking habit, the entire lip including vermilion border is pulled into the mouth.

Lip-wetting habit: In lip-wetting habit, the tongue constantly wets the lips due to dryness/irritation which later become a habit.

Lip-biting habit: In lip-biting habit, either the upper or lower lips are bitten by the incisal edges of upper and lower incisors.

Clinical Features of Lip Habits

- Angle Class II division 1 malocclusion
- Emotional stress
- Flabby cheeks

Clinical features of lip-sucking habit

- In case of dryness of lower lip sucking:
  – Maxillary anterior proclination
  – Retroclination of mandibular anteriors
- In case of upper lip sucking
  – Retroclination of maxillary anteriors
  – Proclination of mandibular anteriors
- Vermilion border: Reddening of the vermilion border
- Cracking of lips
- Hypertrophy of lips

Clinical features of lip-wetting habit

- Dryness of lips
- Irritation of lips

Clinical features of lip-biting habit

- Abrasion of lips
- Indentation of incisors on lips
- Cuts on lips
- Proclination of maxillary anterios
- Retroclination of mandibular anteriors

Management

- Oral screen
- Lip bumper with fixed appliance helps to stop the habit by keeping lips apart each other and the teeth.

POSTURAL HABIT

Face leaning: Lateral pressure from face leaning which is an unintentional, extrinsic pressure habit, may cause lingual movement of maxillary teeth on that side. The mandible is less affected as it does not have a rigid attachment and can slide away from the pressure.

Abnormal pillowing/habitual sleeping on right or left side of face: Normally, children do not lie in one position during sleep. The movements are largely involuntary and are produced by nervous reflexes in order to prevent pressure interferences with circulation. Pillowing habits may cause flattening of the skull, and facial asymmetry in infants.

BRUXISM

Definition

Ramfjord in 1966 defined bruxism as the habitual grinding of teeth when the individual is not chewing or swallowing.

Rubina (1986): Bruxism is the term used to indicate nonfunctional contact of teeth which may include clenching, smashing, grinding and tapping of teeth.

Types

Bruxism is of two types:

1. *Diurnal bruxism/daytime bruxism:* It is conscious or subconscious grinding of teeth usually during the day.
2. *Nocturnal bruxism/night-time bruxism:* It is the subconscious grinding of teeth characterized by rhythmic pattern of masseter EMG activity.

Etiology of Bruxism

- *Psychological factors:*
  – Anxiety
  – Rage
  – Hate
  – Aggression
- Genetics
- Occlusal discrepancies
- Systemic factors
  – Mg^{++} deficiency
  – Allergies
  – Enzymatic imbalance
- *Occupational factors:* Compulsive over achievers

Clinical Features

The signs and symptoms of bruxism depends on:

- Frequency
- Intensity
- Duration
- Occlusal trauma
  – Tooth mobility
  – Bone loss
- Tooth structure
  – Attrition of upper teeth
  – Attrition of lower teeth

- Muscular tenderness
  - Tenderness of jaw muscles
  - Muscular fatigue
  - Hypertrophy of masseter
- TMJ disorder
- Headache
- Other signs and symptoms like soft tissue trauma and ulceration

Treatment

- Occlusal adjustments like correction of restoration and coronoplasty.
- Occlusal splints can be recommended to cover the occlusal surface of all teeth as treatment of bruxism.
- Restorative treatment should be carried out in case of abrasion.
- Psychotherapy: Counseling the patient can lead to decrease in tension and also create habit awareness.
- Malocclusions such as Class II and Class III when associated with functional malocclusion may create a predisposition to bruxism, such malocclusion are corrected by removable or fixed orthodontic appliance.
- Drugs like vapocoolants (ethyl chloride) to relieve pain in TMJ and diazepam to reduce sleep.
- Electrical method: Electrogalvanic stimulation for muscles relaxation is currently advocated for bruxism.
- Acupuncture technique used for muscle relaxation.

Occlusal Splint (Fig. 14.19)

Fabrication of Splints

1. Mount maxillary and mandibular models to precision articulator, i.e. SAM.
2. Prepare the model by defining the anatomical contours with a lab knife and fill voids with a quick setting stone such as Snapstone. Block out moderate undercuts using Model Bloc, Great Lakes Compound 101 or Great Lakes Block-out Gel which is light curable.
3. Open articulator about 4 mm from first tooth contact. Upper and lower cusps of the posterior dentition should not overlap.
4. Place mounted model into the center of pellet cup. If possible, place pellets around the mounted model from the rim of cup to model at:
   - Posterior segment of gingival margin.
   - Anterior segment 3 mm below incisal edges
   - Heel of model (do not cover palate/lingual areas).
5. Isofolan may be used as a model release or minor block out agent. Place a sheet of 0.10 mm Isofolan

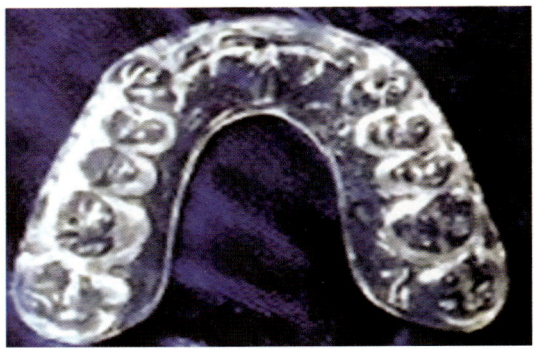

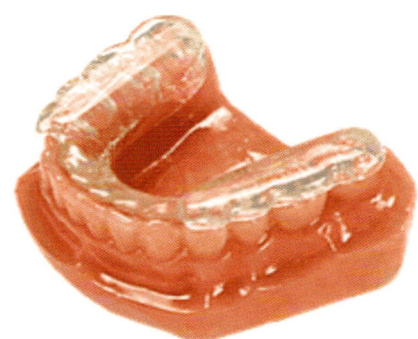

Fig. 14.19: Occlusal splint

material on the pressure chamber and securt it with the clamping frame. Enter the heating time of 25 seconds into the Ministar or Biostar and swing the heating element over the pressure chamber to initiate the heating cycle.

6. Once the heating cycle is complete, remove the heating element and swing the chamber over the model and lock the chamber in place by turning the locking handle toward the front of the machine to initiate the pressure molding/cooling cycle for 30–60 seconds.
7. At the end of the cooling phase, evacuate the air pressure from the chamber and unlock the chamber by turning the locking handle toward the back of the machine. Slide the clamping frame to the back to its open position.
8. Heat a lab knife with a torch.
9. Cut out and remove excess Isofolan material from perimeter of model.
10. The model with the Isofolan spacer in place is properly positioned in the pellets for thermal forming the splint material. Liquid separator is not needed, if Isofolan is used.
11. Use one side of 2 mm splint Biocryl disc with sandpaper in a handpiece mandrel. Place sanded side of plastic facing the inside of the chamber and clamp in place. Swing the heating element over the pressure chamber to initiate the heating cycle. Heat 2 mm material for 60 seconds.

12. Once the heating cycle is complete, remove the heating element and swing the chamber over the model and lock the chamber in place. Cool formed material under pressure for 2–3 minutes. Evacuate the pressure from the chamber. Unlock the chamber and slide the clamping frame to the left to release the formed material. Swing the chamber back to its open position.

13. Remove model with formed material from machine. Scrape excess pellets back into the pellet cup. Cut out template along pellet/model reference using a ¾ inch lightning disc with a standard mandrel in a lab handpiece.

14. Place model with template on articulator and equilibrate the template as needed to maintain the required vertical opening set on the articulator.

15. Wax-relieve opposing model with strips of 1 mm base plate wax to protect teeth during the acrylicing process. This will allow for confirmation of centric stops against splint.

16. Prime template with a thin layer of monomer to retain the acrylic which will be added.

17. Use splint Biocryl acrylic resin. Measure 20 mL powder to be mixed with 10 mL liquid. Also, place a small amount of monomer in a resimix cup to help hand-mold these materials later.

18. Mix the measured ingredients in a large resimix cup with a wax spatula.

19. Place tight-fitting gloves on hands and lubricate with Vaseline. When mixed resin reaches a dough like consistency, hand form to a horseshoe shape.

20. Apply horseshoe-shaped resin to the occlusal surface of the template.

21. Close the articulator to incisal pin setting. Finger form acrylic resin to the facial and lingual areas. Use monomer to help finger-form resin.

22. Cure acrylic in humid pressure pot for 5 minutes. Pressure pot temperature should be approximately 120°F and pressure regulated at 20 psi. Remove from the pot and open articulator.

23. Identify lower buccal cusp tip and incisal speed lathe.

24. Rough trim acrylic with grinding stone on a high speed lathe.

25. Reduce occlusal acrylic with a grinding stone, then with a carbide taper bur in a lab handpiece. If constructing a flat plane splint, trim occlusal acrylic around entire arch to centric contacts. For a splint with a ramp, flatten only centric stops of occluding posteriors. Moderate indexing is removed.

26. Trim the anterior acrylic creating an incisal guide ramp for excursive movements.

27. Reduce incisor and cuspid indexing to minimal contact and identify protrusive and lateral movements against the acrylic ramp using articulating paper.

28. Remove high acrylic areas to achieve even contact of occluding anteriors along ramp during excursive movements. Continue this process until the desired contacts are achieved. Close the lower model into the upper splint on the articulator to check shallow references of the mandibular buccal cusp tips.

29. Lightly trim lower anterior contacts for minimal indexing. This will prevent anterior interferences during eccentric movements. Horseshoe lingual area 3–5 mm below the gingival margin. Trim the posterior section (facially) 1.5 mm gingival to the height of contour of the clinical crowns. Reduce acrylic along the anteriors (facially) to maintain a 2–3 mm overlap.

30. With a mandrel and 150 gnt sandpaper, smooth trimmed acrylic areas. Make sure the anterior guide ramp and posterior centric stops are lightly sanded so the guidance is not altered.

31. Smooth acrylic using medium grade pumice with a wet rag wheel on a low speed lathe. Again, caution must be taken not to over pumice which could alter the splint's guidance. Rinse pumice from the appliance and dry with a towel.

32. After polishing, place the splint back onto articulated models and recheck centric stop contacts and eccentric movements.

33. Finished full contact splint with anterior ramp. Mount mamodels to precision articulator, i.e. SAM.

BIBLIOGRAPHY

1. Ayer WJ. Psychology and thumbsucking. J Am Dent Assoc 1970;80:1335–7.
2. Bakwin H. Persistent finger sucking in twins. Dev Med Child Neurol 1971;13:308–9.
3. Good.S. Mouth habits-mouth breathing, J India Dent Assoc 1966;38:132–5.
4. Popovich FF. Prevalance of sucking habits and relation to malocclusion. Oral Health 1967;57:498–9.
5. Tewari A. Abnormal habits and malocclusion. J Indiana Dent Assoc 1970; 42:1–4.

PREVIOUS YEAR'S UNIVERSITY QUESTIONS

Essay

1. Classify mouth breathers. What are the investigations to identify mouth breathers and their orthodontic management?

2. What are the intraoral and extraoral approaches to correct thumb-sucking habit?

3. List and discuss the various classification of abnormal oral habits.

Short Questions

1. Speech sounds
2. Abnormal pressure habit
3. Bruxism
4. Tongue thrusting habit
5. Abnormal swallowing habit
6. Differences between infantile and mature swallow

MCQ

1. *Management of bruxism includes:*
   a. Occlusal adjustments
   b. Occlusal splint
   c. Psychotherapy and acupuncture technique
   d. All of the above   **(Ans: d)**

Appliances

15.1 REMOVABLE ORTHODONTIC APPLIANCES

Chapter Outline

- Definitions
- Classification of appliance
- Development of removable appliances
- Components of removable appliance
- Bite planes

DEFINITIONS

Lischer defined an orthodontic appliance as, "an orthodontic appliance is a mechanism for the application of force to the teeth and their supporting tissues, to produce changes in their relations and to control the growth and development of these structure.

Graber defined as a device through which an optimal orthodontic force is delivered to a tooth or a group of teeth in a predetermined direction.

Attributes

Appliance should possess the following qualities:
- Simple to fabricate
- Less expensive
- Ease of repair and comfortable for the patient to use as well as to clean.
- Able to deliver an optimal or orthodontic force so that periodontal ligament is not compressed much.
- Able to perform almost all the possible types of tooth movement.
- Should be free of inherent qualities harmful to the oral tissues and should not be easily injured by oral secretions.
- Should be as light and inconspicuous as possible and strong enough to withstand stress of mastication and ordinary wear.

- Appliance is able to carry an additional auxiliary springs or coils for effective tooth movement.
  The design should be such that the tooth movement can be controlled by dentist or orthodontist.

CLASSIFICATION OF APPLIANCES

It is classified into:
1. Mechanical appliances
2. Removable appliances
3. Fixed appliances
4. Combination of removable and fixed appliance

Mechanical appliances: It may be defined as device through which an optimal orthodontic force is delivered to the alveolar bone via teeth in a predetermined direction by means of screws, elastics and springs.

Removable appliances: Removable orthodontic appliances have many advantages like:
- Majority of cases will require only simple tipping of teeth.
- It can incorporate bite platforms to eliminate occlusal interferences and displacement.
- Simple to fabricate and easy to maintain
- Adjustments are possible by an educated patient.
- Inexpensive and any dentist can deal with appliance.
- Less visible and easy repair.

These advantages for both the patient and the dentist have ensured a continuing interest in removable appliances. There are also obvious disadvantages:

- The response to treatment is heavily depended on patient compliance.
- Bodily movement and multiple rotations are not possible to correct.
- In extraction cases, uprighting of roots of canine and 2nd premolar is not possible.
- Not indicated in certain skeletal cases.
- The amount of activation is minimal which in turn affect tooth movement.

Because of their limitations, removable appliances are most useful for the first of two phases of treatment and contemporary comprehensive treatment is dominated by fixed, not removable appliances.

DEVELOPMENT OF REMOVABLE APPLIANCES

In the limited states, Victor Hugo Jackson was the chief proponent of removable appliances among the pioneer orthodontics of the early 20th century. At that time, neither the modern plastics for base plate materials nor stainless steel wires for claps and springs were available nor were the appliances rather clumsy combinations of vulcanite bases and precious metal or nickel-silver wires.

In early 1900s, George Crozet developed a removable appliance fabricated entirely of precious metal that is still used occasionally. The Crozet appliance attracted a small but devoted following primarily in the area around New Orleans. It is still used by some practitioners, but had little impact on the mainstream of American orthodontic thought and practice, from the beginning the emphasis in American orthodontic has been on fixed appliances and the steady progression of fixed appliance techniques in the US is described.

For a variety of reasons, development of removable appliances continued in Europe despite then neglect in the US. A major part of European removable appliance orthodontics of this period was functional appliances for guidance of growth.

Within the past 20 years, the dichotomy between European and American orthodontics has largely disappeared. European style removable appliances, particularly for grown modification during first stage mixed dentition treatment, have become widely used in the United States. The fixed appliances have largely replaced removable for comprehensive treatment in Europe and elsewhere throughout the world.

At present, removable appliances are indicated primarily for three major uses:

1. Growth modification during mixed dentition
2. Limited tooth movements, especially for arch expansion or correction of individual tooth position.
3. Retention after comprehensive.

COMPONENTS OF REMOVABLE APPLIANCE
(Flowchart 15.1)

It consists of:

- Active components—bows/springs/elastics/screws
- Retentive components—clasps
- Base plates—provide framework to hold clasps and springs in position and also anchorage.

Flowchart 15.1: Components of removable orthodontic appliance

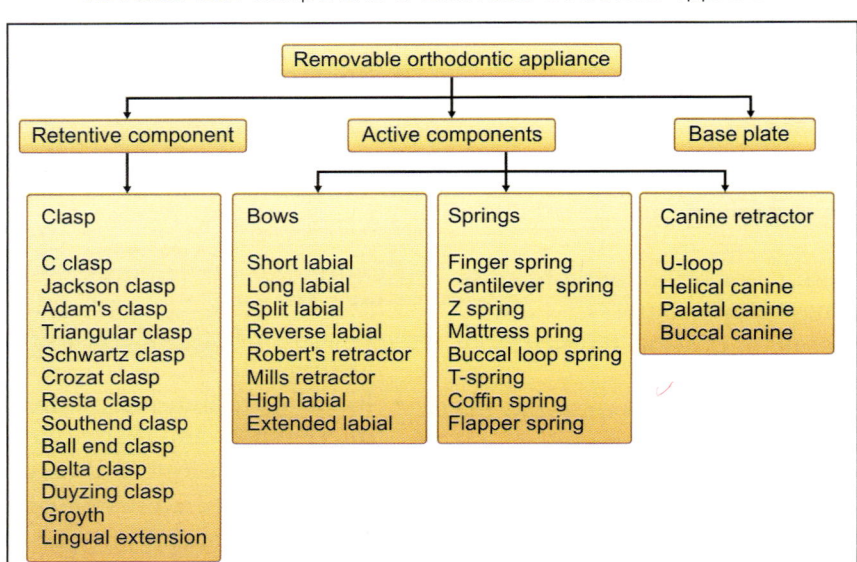

Bows

Labial bows are used for following purposes:

- To limit the labial movement of incisors
- To reinforce the anchorage
- Media through which pressure exerted a lingual direction
- To carry an auxiliary springs and soldered attachments for headgear
- To modify the labial bow for engaging the elastics
- It is used as retainer

Types

Short labial bow: It is made from 0.7 mm wire. It carries a vertical loop which passes over the interdental contact points distal to canine. Both loops should be indentical. The height of vertical loop is determined by the clinical crown height. The upper part of loop is located just 3 mm above the cervical line. The distance between the two arms of loop is again determined by mesiodistal dimensions of canine (Fig. 15.1).

For small size of canine: A bend is started for loop near distal half of lateral incisors.

For bigger size: It is started at mesial angle of canine.

It is placed at the junction of incisal and middle third of crown. It is activated by compressing the each loop by 0.5 mm. It is indicated where there is minor tooth movement, for the purpose of retention and for attachment of whip spring to correct single tooth rotation.

Long labial bow: It is similar to short labial bow except that it covers 1st premolar also. It is mainly used to close the space between canine and premolar and to control the canine position (Fig. 15.2).

Split labial bow: A short labial bow is split into halves. Each loop embraces the incisor of opposite side to close the mild midline diastema and minor rotation (Fig. 15.3).

Mills retractor: It is made up to 0.7 mm. It is used to correct severe protrusion of upper teeth. It is activated

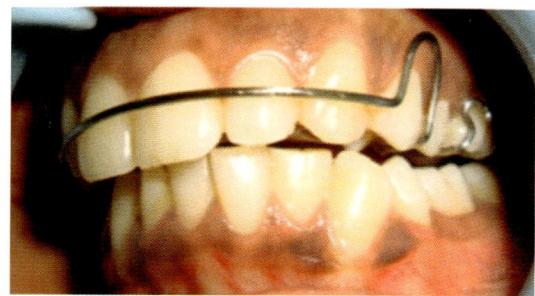

Fig. 15.2: Long labial bow

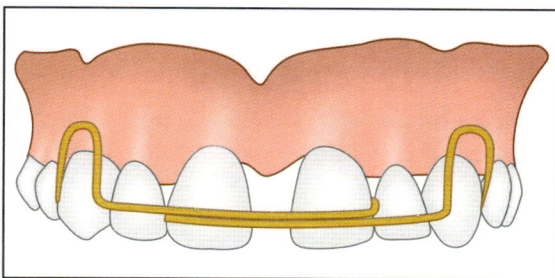

Fig. 15.3: Split labial bow

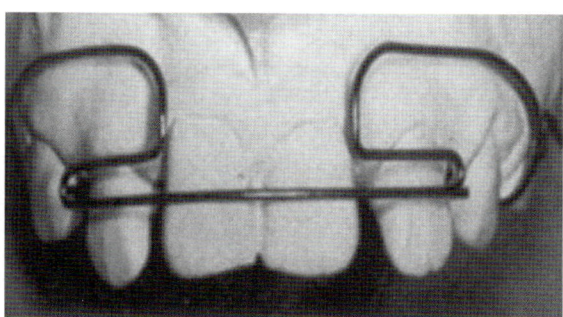

Fig. 15.4: Mills retractor

by compressing the horizontal loops. Minor alignment of tooth irregularities can be corrected (Fig. 15.4).

Robert's retractor: It is made up of 0.5 mm. It is used for correction of severe proclination of upper teeth. It is activated by closing the coil. It is modified by adding tubing in the distal part of the coil in order to strengthen the wire while activating this retractor is not like short and long labial bows but the loops carry coil and it is shaped like '^' (Fig. 15.5).

Extended labial bow: It is made up of 0.7 mm. It is used for controlling the high canine and slight rotation of canine and correction of proclined anteriors too. The labial bow is extended on the canine carrying the horizontal loop and after finishing the horizontal loop, the loop is continued as vertical loop. The both horizontal and vertical loops are activated simultaneously or

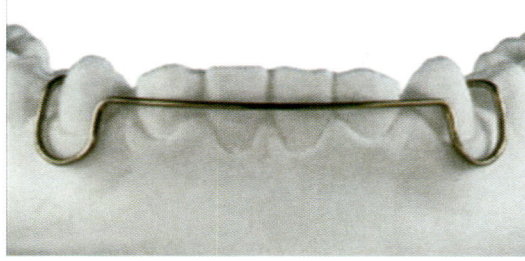

Fig. 15.1: Short labial bow

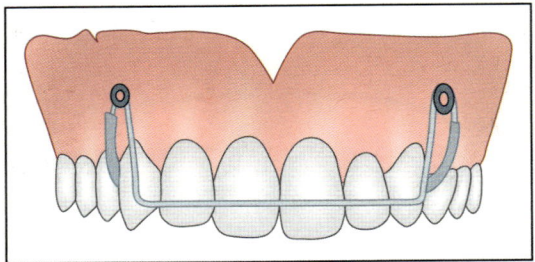

Fig. 15.5: Robert's retractor

individually. There are two types of extended labial bow:

- Extended labial bow without coil (Fig. 15.6a and b)
- Extended labial bow with coil (Fig. 15.7a and b)

Reverse loop labial bow: It is made up of 0.7 mm. The loop is reversed passing in between first premolar and canine. The loop is activated by opening the loop (Fig. 15.8).

High labial bow with apron spring: High labial bow acts as a base onto which apron springs (made from 0.4 mm wire) are attached/wound. It is made up of thick wire of 0.9 mm or 1 mm. The high labial bow is

constructed by extending till the vestibular sulcus and giving relief for frenum. The wire is passed between canine and premolar. In cases where there is abnormal frenal attachment, the high labial bow can be split in the midline and the free ends can be circled. Apron springs help in retraction of one or more upper anterior. This type of bow is made highly flexible because of the springs and is, therefore, used for retraction in cases with large overjet (Fig. 15.9a to c).

The apron spring is made by winding one end 0.4 mm wire onto the base wire tightly and free end is soldered. It is formed as apron for one or two group of teeth. The other end of apron is wound in the opposite direction and the free end is soldered.

Labial bow with hook: A hook is attached to the short labial bow. Distal arm by the loop an either side to carry the elastics. This is indicated where the activation by labial bow is not sufficient to close the spaces (Fig. 15.10).

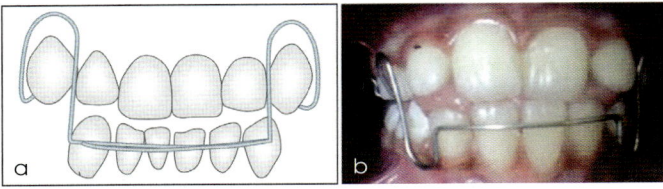

Fig. 15.6: Extended labial bow without coil

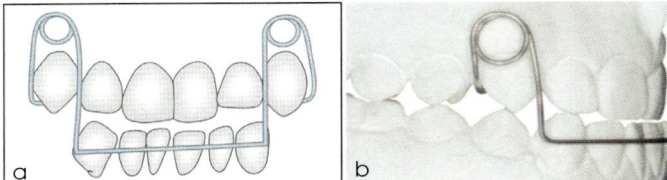

Fig. 15.7: Extended labial bow with helices in the loop

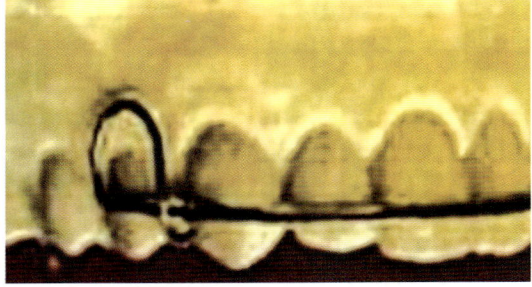

Fig. 15.8: Reverse loop labial bow

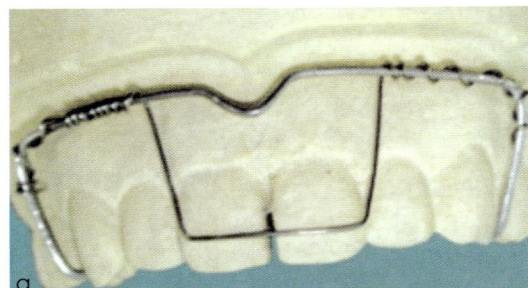

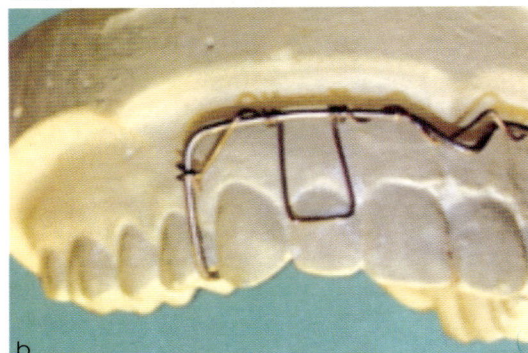

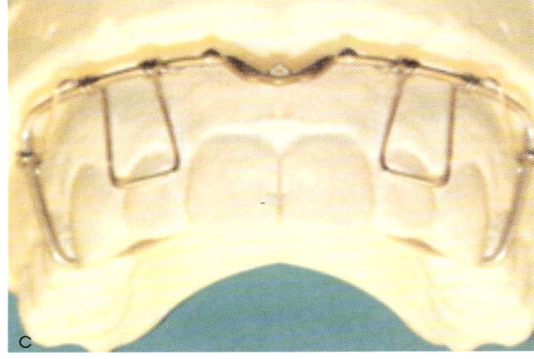

Fig. 15.9a to c: High labial bow with apron spring

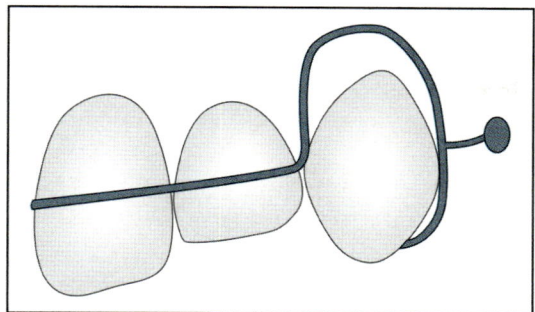

Fig. 15.10: Labial bow with distal hook for elastic bands

Fitted labial bow: It is made up of 0.7 mm wire and is similar to short labial bow except that horizontal bow part is closely adapted onto the labial surface of the teeth. It is mainly used to control the corrected teeth as retentive device (Fig. 15.11).

Soldered labial bow: The distal arm of the loop is not passed in between canine and premolar but it is extended posteriorly and the free end is soldered onto bridge of the Adam's clasp. It is indicated for retention of teeth after the active treatment is completed. The loop can be either passive or active. The loops can be activated, if the extracted space gets opened up (Fig. 15.12).

Wraparound retainer: The labial bow which is used as retentive device here is not like short or other labial

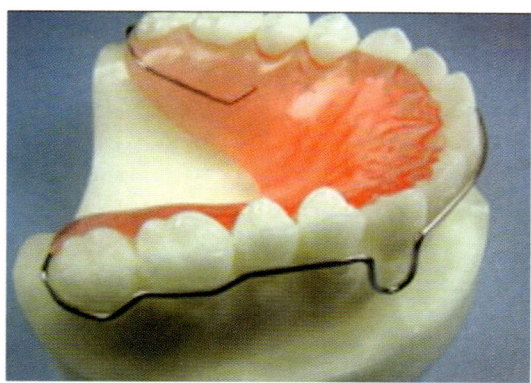

Fig. 15.13: Wraparound retainer

bow. A single piece by wire is constructed with the loop at the extraction site and is extended on to the molar as clasp (Fig. 15.13).

Labial bow for 'J' hook attachment: Eyelets or hooks can be soldered onto the labial bow near the spot by distal part of the lateral incisors, for engaging the 'J' hooks of extraoral traction (Fig. 15.14).

Hooks may be soldered in the horizontal section.

Asymmetrical labial bow: One side loop on the canine and other side on the 1st premolar. It is indicated where one side canine is either rotated or any space present distal to canine.

A—Labial wire with vertical M-loops (Fig. 15.15a).

B—Hooks for elastic bands can be either on mesial or distal leg (Fig. 15.15b and e).

C—Vertical loop combined with horizontal loop for canine control (Fig. 15.15c).

D—Modified loop at the canine. The horizontal segment is stabilized by the crossover (Fig. 15.15d).

E—Labial wire with distal leg on the loop for anterior elastics (Fig. 15.15e).

F—Labial wire sheathed in acrylic.

G—Maxillary and mandibular labial wires in activator.

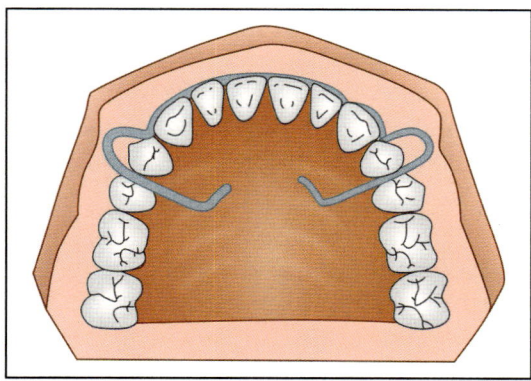

Fig. 15.11: Fitted labial bow

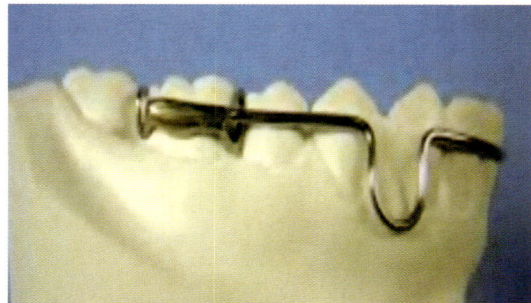

Fig. 15.12: Soldered labial bow

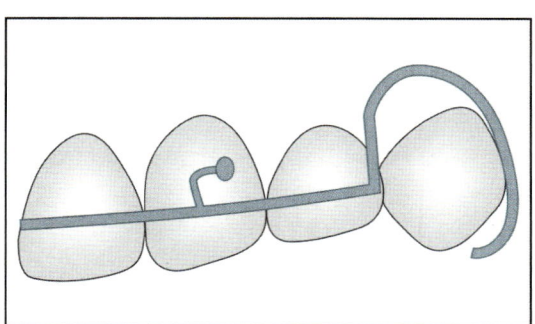

Fig. 15.14: Labial bow for 'J' hook attachment

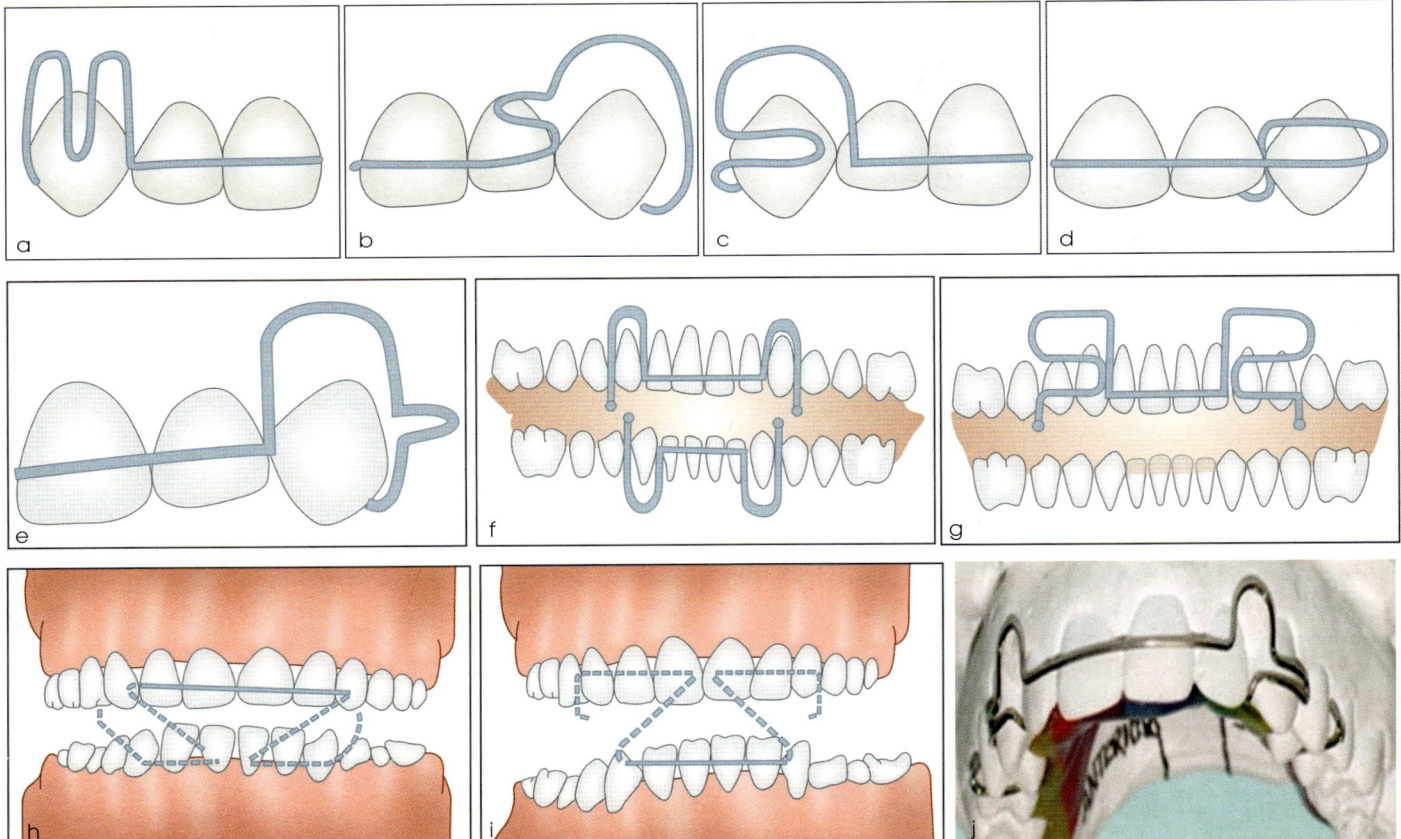

Fig. 15.15 a to j: Other types of labial bow

Note the distal arm of loop passes in the center of wax bite block to avoid damage of the wire during trimming of activator (Fig. 15.15f).

H—A canine loop design (Eschler 1971) can also be altered to move the lateral incisor (Fig. 15.15g).

I—The positive segment contacts the maxillary incisors. The negative segment resides in the mandibular labial vestibule (Fig. 15.15h).

J—The positive segment contacts the mandibular incisors. The negative segment is in the maxillary vestibule (Fig. 15.15i).

Rickett's labial bow (Fig. 15.15j)
- 0.028 inch wire crosses occlusion mesial to cuspids.
- Alternative design to Hawley bow when minimal or no occlusal freeway space is present distal to cuspids.
- It may be used when greater anterior retention is required.

Clasp

- Clasp literally means to fasten or grasp. It is an attachment or a device used for fixation, stabilization or retention of an appliance.
- Lawson and Blazuki defined it as a part of an appliance that partially encircles the abutment teeth and aids in retention and stabilization.
- Originally, the term crib was used to loosely denote a clasp. Crib is metal framework enclosure.

Significance of Using a Clasp

- It maintains mechanical efficiency of the appliance by ensuring that springs are continuously held in accurate position.
- It helps in patient adaptation to the appliance by providing a firm fit. Discourages habits, movements and initial difficulty with speech and eating are minimized.
- Extraoral traction may be added without any risk of displacement.
- Contribution by base plate is maximized by preventing forward sliding of acrylic plate down the curvature of the palate.

Requisites of a Clasp

- It should provide adequate retention for the appliance.

- It should not cause irritation to the buccal and gingival mucosa.
- It should be devoid of occlusal interferences. Occlusal interferences can be eliminated by proper occlusal crossover, straight across the occlusal embrasure. Or it can be directed to fit into the occlusal embrasure.
- Wedging or separation of teeth by clasps is undesirable.
- It should engage either undercut or embrasure area.
- Retentive arm should be 1 to 1.5 mm away from the represented tissue surface on the cast.
- Claps should be biocompatible.

Wire should be gently contoured into the desired form. Sharp bends and overworking render it prone to breakage. They should not be overworked or stressed. Since clasps are used in removable appliances, they should spring over the maximum contour of the teeth.

Solder joints should be avoided since they are potential sources of weakness. Such joints lead to corrosion and breakages. If solders have to be advocated, they have to be polished well. Clasps should be passive unless otherwise indicated. If activated, they cause tooth movement and distortion and breakage. They should be strong enough to withstand masticatory forces.

Selection and Design of Clasp

The selection and design of clasp depends on the case being treated. Since each is different, it is essential to visualize the condition. Design of a clasp is directed by:

- Amount of retention to be provided or factors tending to displace the appliance
- Condition of abutment teeth
- Partially erupted
- Fully erupted
- Presence of gingival recession

In case of partially erupted teeth, the gingival tissue represented on the cast is carved to follow the contour of the future tooth.

In case of gingival recession, cementoenamel junction is not engaged where maximum undercut is present. If it is engaged, clasp does not spring out.

- Contact area
- Occlusal and gingival embrasures
- Undercut area
- Morphology of the tooth—cervical ridge or curvatures which are invariably present on most teeth.

Classification of Clasps

Based on number of retentive arms

Single armed clasps:
- Ball end clasp
- Lingual extension clasp
- Triangular clasp
- Eyelet clasp
- Groth clasp

Double armed clasps:
- Jackson's clasp
- Crozat's clasp
- Southend clasp
- Adam's clasp
- Arrowhead clasp

Based on the presence or absence of arrowheads

Arrowhead clasps:
- Adam's clasp
- Schwartz arrowhead clasp
- Single arrowhead clasps

Non-arrowhead clasps:
- Lingual extension clasp
- Ball end clasp

Description of Individual Clasps with their Modifications and Applications

Circumferential clasp (C clasp or ¾ clasps): It is known as ¾ clasp because it engages three surfaces—the mesial, the buccal undercut and the distal surfaces of the teeth. Mainly used for 2nd molars and occasionally for canines. It is easier to keep out of occlusal contact than Adam's clasp. It is a supportive element rather than retentive. It has a single arm embedded into acrylic (Figs 15.16a and 15.16b).

Modification of C-clasp (Fig. 15.18) and (Fig. 15.16c).

Soldered 'C' clasp—for securing either upper or lower appliances (when posterior clasp is not practical): A

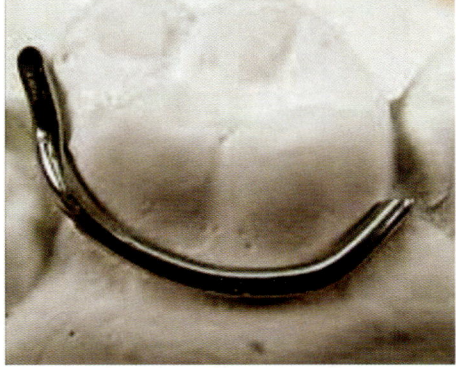

Fig. 15.16a: 'C' clasp

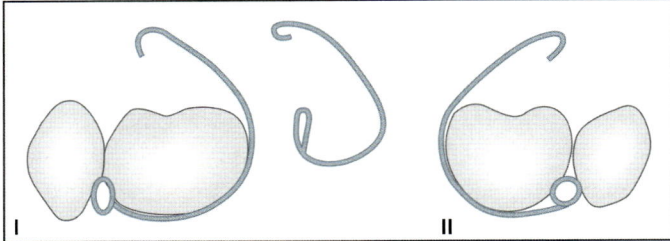

Fig. 15.16b: C clasp modification. **I.** 'C' Clasp with vertical end loop. **II.** 'C' clasp with horizontal end loop

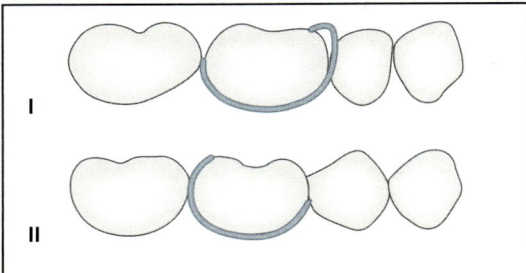

Fig. 15.16c: I. Mesial 'C' clasp in case of crowding (anterior; II. Distal 'C' claspin case of spacing (anterior)

piece of wire can be soldered at the tip of 'C' clasp acting as ball end clasp for extra retention. Eyelet in the center of 'C' clasp is used for mild intrusion of molar by engaging the elastic band to the spur in the high arch labial bow (1 mm) (Fig. 15.17).

Jackson's clasp: This clasp was introduced by Jackson in 1906. It is also called 'U' clasp or full mouth clasp. It is squared mesially and distally so that it makes contact with the mesial and distal undercuts (Fig. 15.19).

Crozat's clasp: Crozat's clasp also makes use of mesial and distal undercuts. To an ordinary orthodontic loop, an additional piece of wire is welded or soldered which runs into the mesial and distal undercuts (Fig. 15.20).

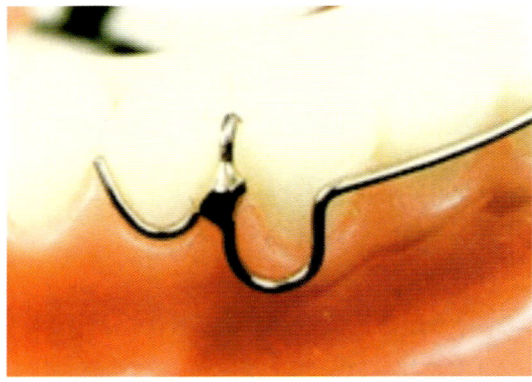

Fig. 15.17: Soldered 'C' clasp—for securing either upper or lower appliances (when posterior clasp is not practical)

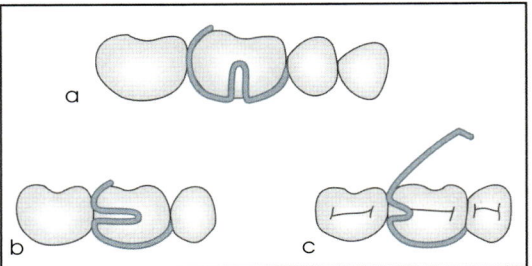

Fig. 15.18: Modifications. a. 'C' clasp with vertical spur for molar control or spur may be activated to move palatally to certain extends. b. 'C' clasp with horizontal spur for molar rotation control to certain extends. c. 'C' clasp carries an occlusal rest to prevent supraeruption of molar

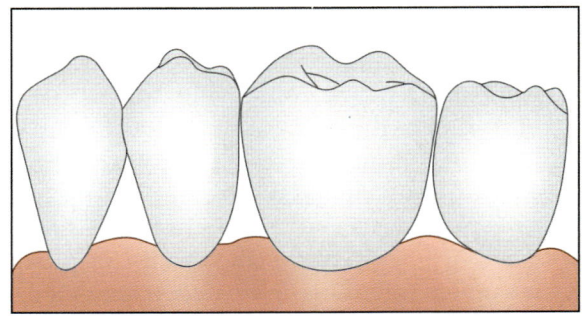

Fig. 15.19: Jackson's clasp

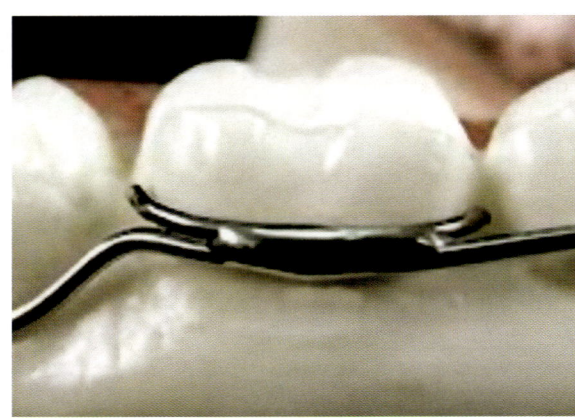

Fig. 15.20: Crozat's clasp

Arrowhead clasp (Schwarz, 1935): It is a retentive element which finds wide application in primary, mixed and permanent dentition. It is fabricated with specially designed pliers a combination of two pliers (Fig. 15.21).

For superior results in individual cases as embrasure area is different between any set of given two adjacent teeth, manual fabrication with flat beaked plier is preferred. To make an arrowhead clasp, a 23 guage wire is used.

Arrowhead must be bent in a horizontal plane perpendicular to the long axis of the tooth. For optimal

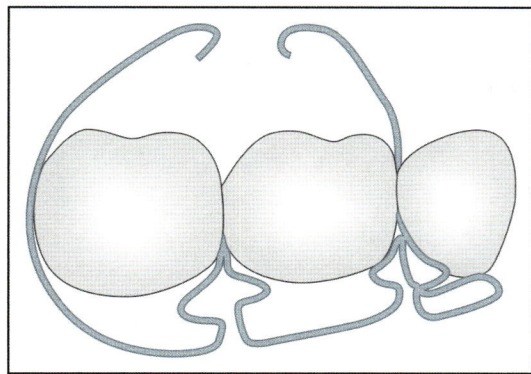

Fig. 15.21: Arrowhead clasp

retention, arrowhead is adapted to the anatomic contour. Small tapered arrowheads are not preferred since they lie too deep into the interdental space where papillae are traumatized.

Clasp arm should make a sweeping curve from the base of the arrowhead to its insertion as pointed out by Sthal (1958). In doing so, the length of the wire is increased for adjustments by the operator.

If short, it becomes stiff and exerts more force on interdental papillae and dislodges the plate. Arrowheads are continuous, 2 between 3 teeth or 3 between 4 teeth.

Uses: It is incorporated into a removable appliance which is to be used for extraoral anchorage, to provide high quality retention.

Disadvantages: It causes separation of teeth.

Ball end clasp: It uses the mesial and the distal undercuts of the teeth and can be fabricated using commercially available ball end wires or by adding a drop of solder at the end of the wire (Fig. 15.22).

The wire is sprung into the angular undercuts as shown. Ball clasps formed with a short arm have less potential for adjustments. The wire is before bent at 45° toward the interdental space. Ball end also finds application as C-clasps. 21-gauge wire is used.

Advantages: It is easy to fabricate.

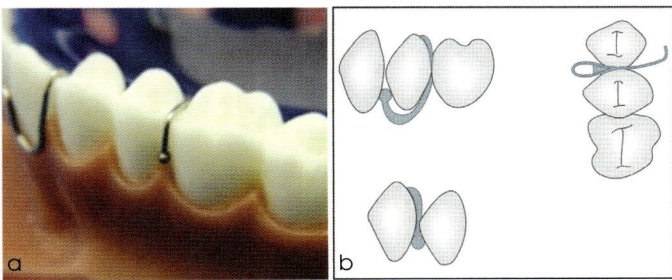

Fig. 15.22: (a) Ball clasp; (b) Ball clasp bent as a 'C' form

Disadvantages:
- It has a short span and so it is stiff.
- Undercuts are not deeply engaged. Only limited demands can be placed on them.

Duyzing's clasp: Two stainless steel wires are bent over the maximum contour of the tooth from the mesial and distal aspect and then curved back below the maximum contour and ends are sprung. 21-guage wire is used (Fig. 15.23).

Lingual extention clasp: It is designed to prevent occlusal interferences (idealistic). Theoretically, it is feasible by extending a spring element (of 25 or 26 guage wire) into the gingival embrasure area from the palatal aspect between the upper 2nd premolar and 1st molar. Practically, it is inefficient. It provides enough retention for maxillary retainer.

Advantages: No occlusal interferences.

Disadvantages
- Impossible to adjust
- Prone to breakages
- Tissue irritation
- Tooth separation

Triangular clasp (Zimmer, 1949): It uses interdental space gingiva to the contact point or embrasure area. It is larger than ball end. It occlusally project 1.5–2 mm before being bent back into the gingival embrasure and this extension is used for adjustments (Fig. 15.24).

It is used between premolar areas because morphology presents adequate embrasure space for retention. 21-guage wire is used. Elastics can be engaged.

Eyelet clasp (Fig. 15.25): It can be single or continuous and uses the interdental space gingiva to contact. Its length is increased because occlusal part of the clasp

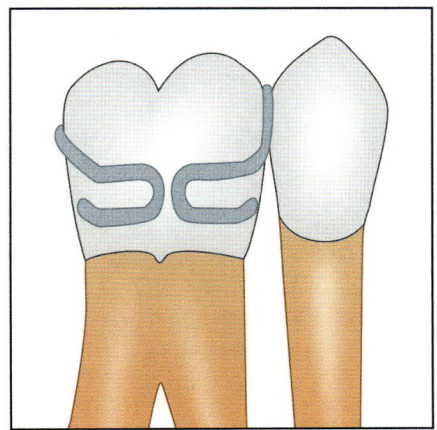

Fig. 15.23: Duyzing clasp

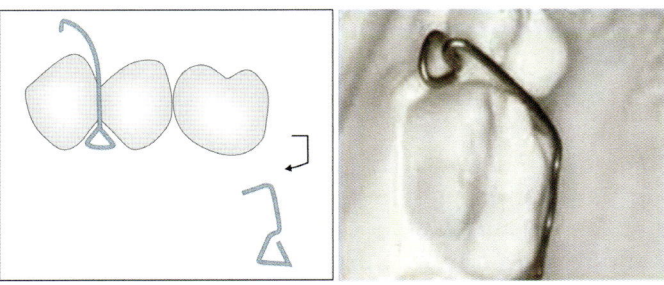

Fig. 15.24: Zimmer's—triangular clasp

arm projects 1.5–2 mm bucally before being bent back toward the gingival aspect. Eyelet fits perpendicular to the long axis of the tooth into the interdental space.

21-gauge wire is used. When extraoral traction is applied retention is increased by multiple eyelets, between the posterior teeth.

Groth clasp: It has a small inverted 'V' reaching deep into the interdental space for anchorage. A long bow-shaped arm is present on the buccal aspect for adjustments. It is an ideal for securing plates in primary dentition. 21-guage wire is used (Fig. 15.26).

Southend clasp: It is designed by Di Biase and Leavis and described by Stephans in 1979. It is fabricated on central incisors for retention with 19/21-guage wire.

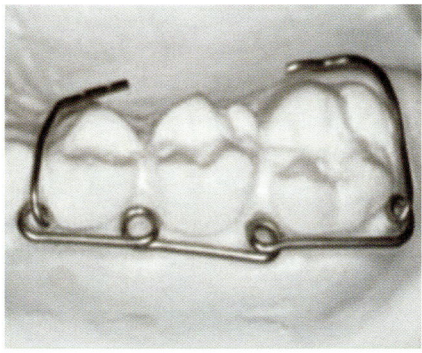

Fig. 15.25: Eyelet clasp

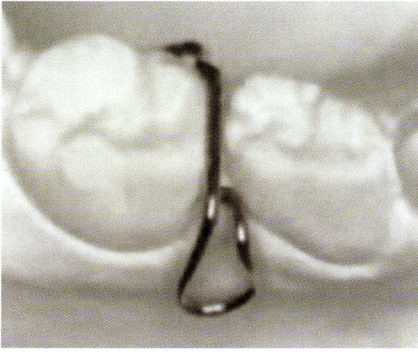

Fig. 15.26: Groth clasp

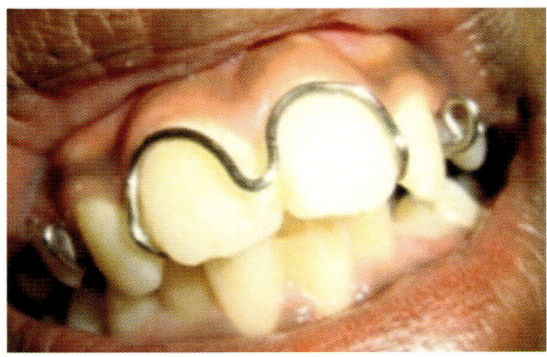

Fig. 15.27: Southend clasp

It follows the contour of gingiva but interdentally bent towards the gingival embrasure area, forming a kind of arrowhead. It engages the undercut in gingival 3rd. It has two arms which go into acrylic plate. It is prepared for stability of removable appliances in the absence of lateral incisors. It is tightened by pushing it at interdental crest (Fig. 15.27).

Uses:
- Habit-breaking appliance
- Space maintainer
- Retainer

In young patients, there is a short clinical crown, so the C-clasp is engaged close to the gingival margin for adequate retention. In mixed dentition over the 1st molar, C-clasp is combined with ball or eyelet for increasing retention.

Adam's clasp (introduced by CP Adam, 1949): It is a modification of Schwarz arrowhead clasp. Most popular retentive device without removable appliance therapy would be less successful. It is also known as *the Liverpool clasp (universal clasp) or modified arrowhead clasp.* It contains bridge, arrowhead and retentive arms. It engages mesiobuccal and distobuccal undercuts of the tooth rather than the embrasure area. Thus, it does not separate the teeth (Fig. 15.28).

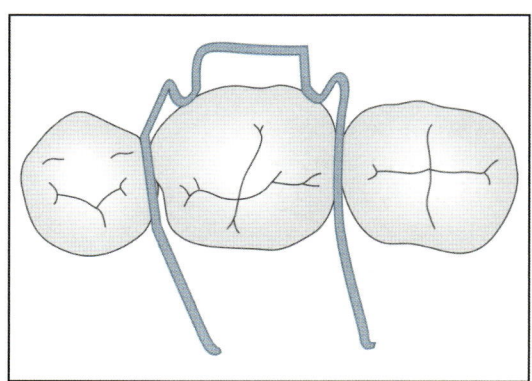

Fig. 15.28: Adam's clasp

Prior to fabrication of clasp, the cast for the tooth position, eruption and undercut is studied. The Adam's universal plier and 21-guage wire is used. A piece of wire approximately 12 cm is straightened. The width of the bridge is said to be two-thirds the maximum mesiodistal width of the tooth.

Ideally maximum width of the tooth is in its middle third where it contacts the adjacent teeth but if two-thirds this width is used one can visualize that the arrowheads will lie in the embrasure area rather than the undercut areas, which is not the requirement of an Adam's clasp.

The posterior teeth are somewhat spheroidal in their buccal and lingual views. They taper from the point of contact, both occlusally and (more) gingivally so that two-thirds of the mesiodistal width of the occlusal surface, corresponds to the undercut area we need to engage and is adequate (and not the cementoenamel junction).

After estimating the width of the bridge, two right-angled bends are given and then made acute so as to overlap.

Arrowhead bend is made such that bridge will lie in the middle third of the tooth. To make an arrowhead first, a sharp bend is made parallel to the bridge.

The bridge of the clasp is laid against the back of the plier and the tip of the plier engages the first arm of the arrowhead to bend the arrowhead outside the beak of the plier. Similarly, the second arrowhead is made.

The arrowheads are squeezed and adjusted but while doing so outward pressure is exerted so that the arms of the arrowhead remain parallel and then checked on the tooth. Arrowheads are bent 45° toothward, to align them with the contour at the undercut. Also a downward and toothward thrust is laid for the same reason. The clasp is tried on the tooth for fit.

A bend is given on the retentive arm such that the length of the second arm of the arrowhead is half the first arm. After laying, the bridge across the beak and grasping the arrowhead at the suitable level. A bend is given in a direction parallel to the bridge.

Essential features of Adam's clasp
- Bridge should be straight.
- Bridge is halfway between the occlusal surface of the tooth and the gum margin.
- Bridge stands away from the tooth surface—2 mm.
- Bridge should be parallel to the buccal segment and not the buccal surface of the tooth.
- Arrowheads are parallel.
- Arrowheads should contact the tooth only at the extreme ends.

- Uniform space is left between the tags and the represented tissue surface of the cast.
- Excessive sharp bends weaken the wire and so are avoided.
- Arrowhead should be sufficiently long:
  - 0.6 mm for canine (22-guage)
  - 0.7 mm for molar (21-guage)

Precautions: Erupting teeth, recession of gingiva.

Clinical adjustments: The clinical adjustments can be carried out at the following:
- At first occlusal bend (CP Adams)
- At the second occlusal bend or point of attachment
- By directing arrowhead points towards tooth
- Bridge is bent towards or away from the tooth surface.

Advantages of Adam's clasp
- Makes use of undercuts mesiobuccal and distabuccal and not embrasure area and so can be used in isolated teeth.
- Small, neat, unobtrusive. Occupies minimum space in bucal sulcus and base plates.
- Universally applicable any tooth deciduous, permanent and semi-erupted teeth.
- Strong firm, resists distorting and masticatory forces
- No special pliers are required
- Can be easily repaired
- Can be modified to suit the needs

Modifications of Adam's clasp
1. Modified Adam's clasp (Fig. 15.29)
2. Clasp with single arrowhead—Resta clasp (Fig. 15.30)
3. Adam's clasp with eyelet on the bridge (Fig. 15.31)
4. Adam's clasp with inverted question mark soldered onto the bridge (Fig. 15.32)
5. Adam's clasp with horizontal loop (Fig. 15.33)
6. Labial wire is soldered to the bridge of Adam's clasp (Fig. 15.34)

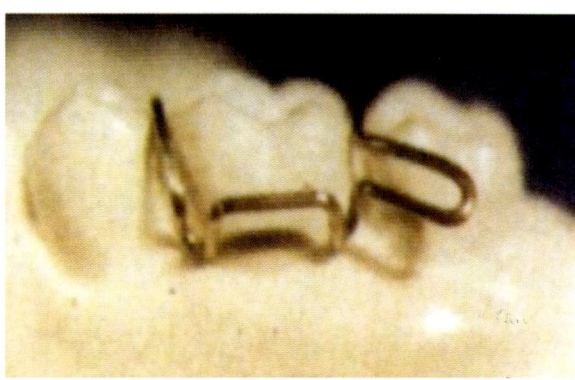

Fig. 15.29: Modified Adam's clasp

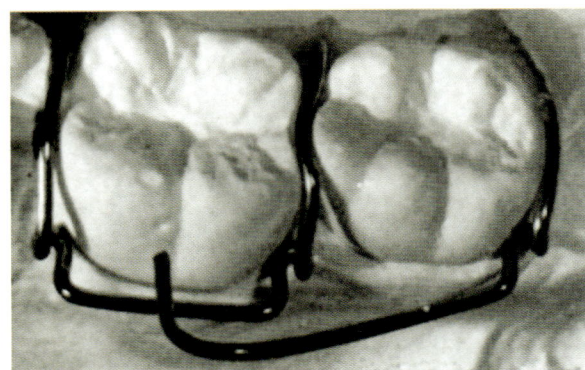

Fig. 15.30: Resta clasp

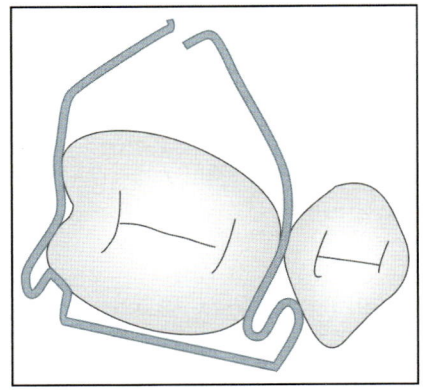

Fig. 15.33: Adam's clasp with horizontal loop

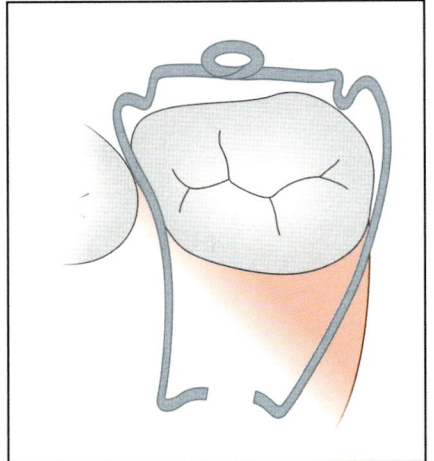

Fig. 15.31: Adam's clasp with eyelet on the bridge

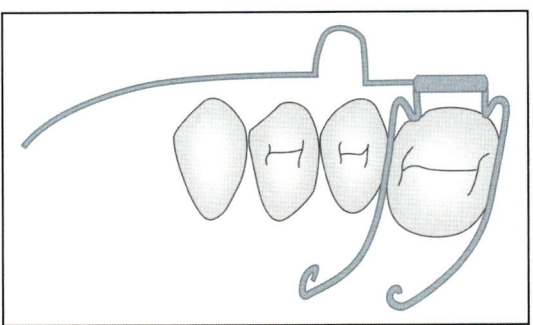

Fig. 15.34: Labial wire soldered to Adam's clasp

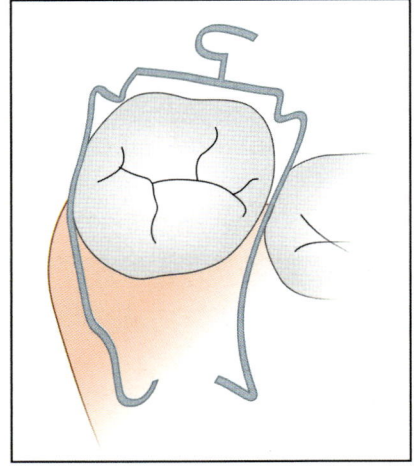

Fig. 15.32: Adam's clasp with inverted question mark soldere

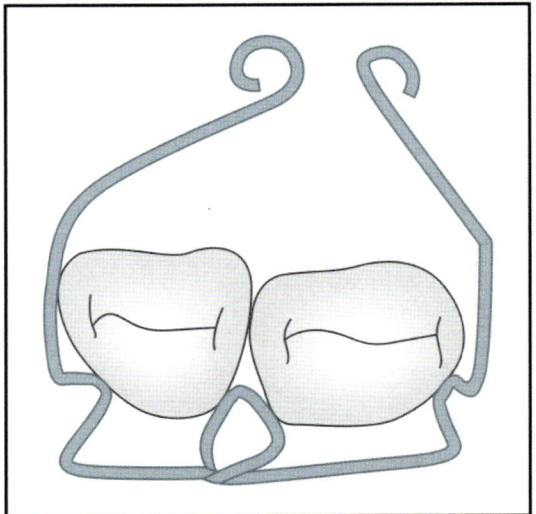

Fig. 15.35: Adam's clasp with a triangular clasp

7. Adam's clasp with a triangular clasp (Fig. 15.35)
8. Adam's clasp with arrow head clasp (Fig. 15.36)
9. Double Adam's clasp on two central incisors (Fig. 15.37)
10. Adam's clasp covering two buccal teeth (Fig. 15.38)
11. Double Adam's clasp carrying coils fabricated on the bridge for insertion by inner facebow (Fig. 15.39)
12. Adam's clasp with eyelet facing embrasure (Fig. 15.40)

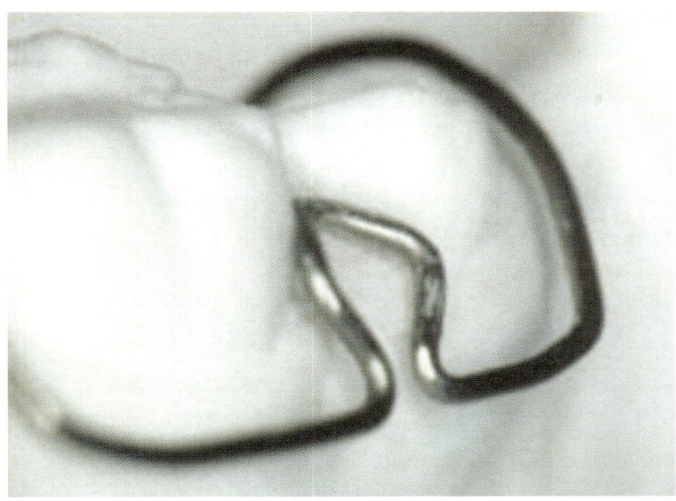

Fig. 15.36: Adam's clasp with arrowhead clasp

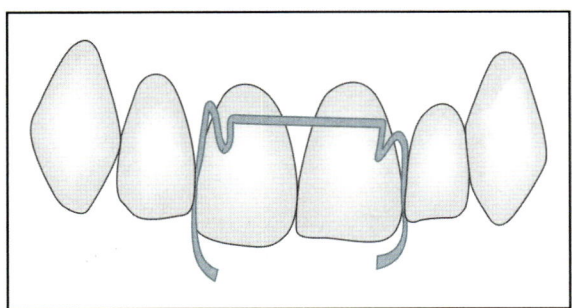

Fig. 15.37: Double Adam's clasp on two central incisors

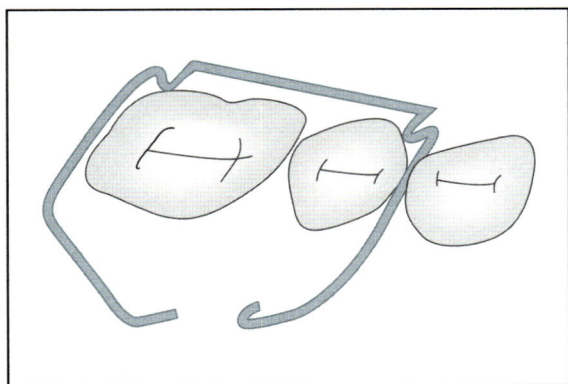

Fig. 15.38: Adam's clasp covering two buccal teeth

Limitations of Adam's clasp: According to CP Adams, the temptation to use Adam's clasp on anterior teeth should be resisted and because its clasping efficiency is the best when used on single tooth. Adam's clasp is unsatisfactory step for proclined incisors. When retentive arrowhead is required in two teeth need to be clasped, an accessory clasp is used but solder joint is a potential source of weakness.

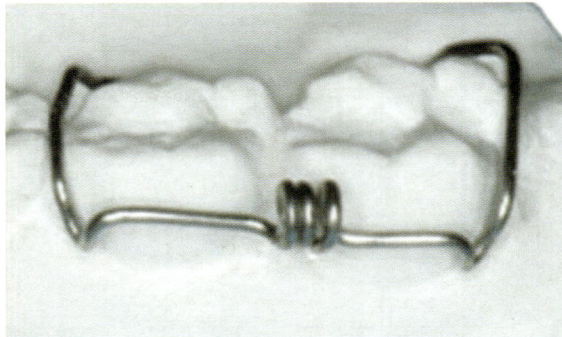

Fig. 15.39: Double Adam's clasp carrying coils fabricated on the bridge for insertion by inner facebow

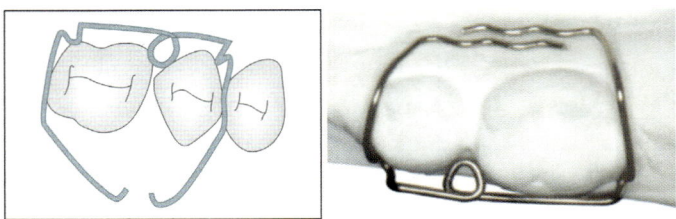

Fig. 15.40: Adam's clasp with eyelet facing embrasure

Resta clasp: It is a modified version of the Adam's clasp. It uses the arrowhead retentive point from the Adam's clasp and the ball from a ball clasp to engage two undercut areas on the buccal surface of the anchor tooth. This clasp is useful when interocclusal clearance or space available on only the mesial or distal side of the tooth to be clasped (Fig. 15.30).

Single arrowhead clasp: It is indicated in a situation as above. A single arrowhead clasp is made up of 0.8 mm straight wire. It is placed in mesiobuccal corner of the upper 2nd premolar. The thicker gauge gives so stronger. Avoidance of solder has less chances of breakage.

Incisor clasp: Adam's clasp is not suitable for anterior teeth and thus alternative clasps, incisor clasp can be used.

Universal clasp: It is similar to Adam's clasp. Instead of arrowhead, helix incorporated in the undercut. Here it is in combination with buccal adjustment loop (Fig. 15.41).

Delta clasp (Fig. 15.42)
- It is designed by WJ Clark of Scotland.
- It is made up of 0.8 mm wire, i.e. 20-guage wire.
- It provides excellent retention for lower premolar. Requires minimal adjustments.
- It is used in twin block functional orthopedic appliance.

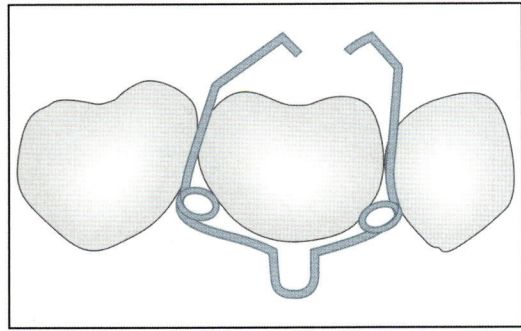

Fig. 15.41: Universal clasp

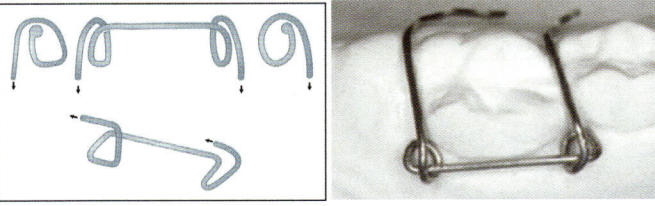

Fig. 15.42: Delta clasp

Axillary Methods of Increasing Retention

- By cutting grooves in the enamel of a tooth, undercut was created to accept a clasp arm.
- A bend with artificial undercut such as a buccal tube provides undercut.
- Bonded plastic (composite resins) to create horizontal ledge.
- Direct bonded buttons and brackets from fixed armamentarium.

Springs

In designing springs to move a too the facially, lingually or mesiodistally within the arch, a few important principles must be kept in mind. Ideal qualities of orthodontic wires to form a spring are (1) flexibility, (2) spring back action and (3) formability. The wire should be bent at any configuration.

Physical properties of wire:
- Rigidity
- Resistance to distortion

Susceptibility to fracture: The flexibility of wire depends on the length by wire and its diameters. The effective length is increased by incorporating a coil at least 3 mm in diameter. If a thin wire is used, deflection will be doubled.

Classification of Springs

Based on the direction of tooth movement brought about by the springs, they can be classified as:
- Springs used for mesiodistal tooth movement

- Springs used for labial movement
- Springs used for lingual movement and expansion of arches
- Springs used for expansion of arches

Based on the nature of support required for their action, orthodontic springs can be broadly classified as:
- Self-supporting spring
- Guided spring
- Auxiliary spring

Self-supporting spring:
- Buccal canine retractor
- Helical canine retractor
- Palatal canine retractor
- Reverse loop canine retraction
- 'U' loop canine retractor

Guided spring:
- Finger spring
- Cantilever spring

Auxiliary spring: High labial bow with apron spring for any retractor, there are active arm and passive arm.

Self-supported Spring

Buccal canine retractor: It is indicated where a buccally placed canine is to be moved distally as well as palatally. It is not popular because liable to cause discomfort for the patient. It is difficult to adjust and unstable in the vertical direction. However, it can be adjusted with the precautions. The free end should be adapted in such a way that it encircles the canine at the cervical third. After every activation, the free end is cut and readapted. The activation is by closing the coil by 1 mm. Since the 0.7 mm wire is used, deflection is small and hence frequent adjustments are necessary. The retractor carries a helix which lies at the extraction site and the free end passes through mesial aspect 2nd premolar. Tubing should be done to support the passive arm of retractor (Fig. 15.43).

Helical canine retractor: It is made up of 0.5 mm wire. the active arm lies below and it carries a 11/2 coil helix and the passive arm lies over the active arm and passes through the mesial aspect of second premolars. The both arms of the helix should be parallel. The activation is by opening the coil and the arms of the loop unparallel after activation. The free end is cut by 1 mm after every activation. The free end should engage the canine at the embrasure and should be readapted every time. It is indicated where the canine lies in the occlusal plane. The helix is placed 3–4 mm below the gingival margin (Fig. 15.44).

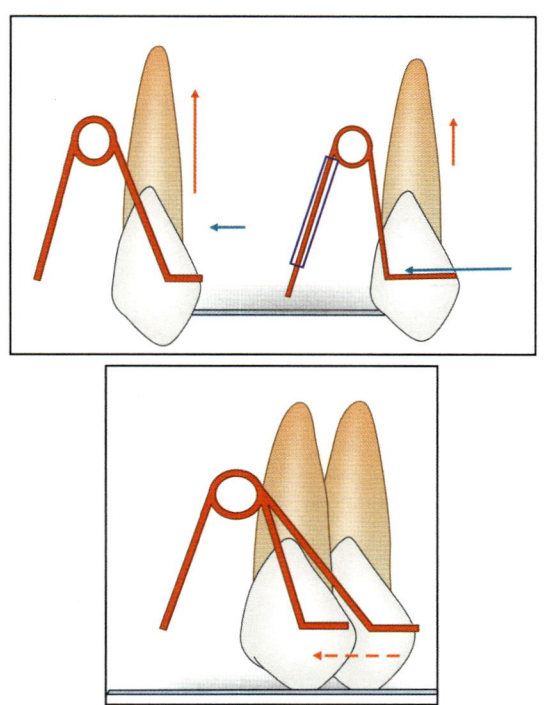

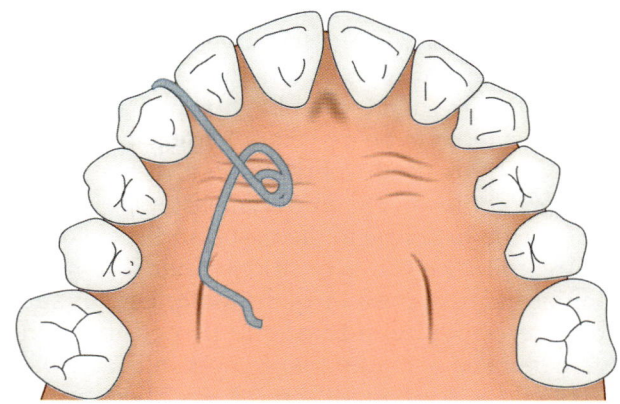

Fig. 15.45: Platal canine retractor

Palatal canine retractor: Helical canine retractor is given on the side but palatal canine retractor is given for retraction of palatally placed positioned canines (Fig. 15.45).

'U' loop canine retractor: It is made up 0.7 mm wire and activation is by compressing the loop or by cutting the free end of the active arm by 2 mm and readapting it. The other feature of the retractor remains the same as other retractor. It is given on the buccal side (Fig. 15.46).

Guided Spring

The use by thinner wire gets distorted by the tongue forces. Hence the spring has to be guided.

Finger spring: Parts of finger spring
- One helix—diameter 3 mm
- Active arm—it is about 12 to 15 mm long
- Retentive arm—it is about 4 to 5 mm long
- Retentive tag

Fig. 15.43: (a) Supported buccal canine retractor; (b) Activation

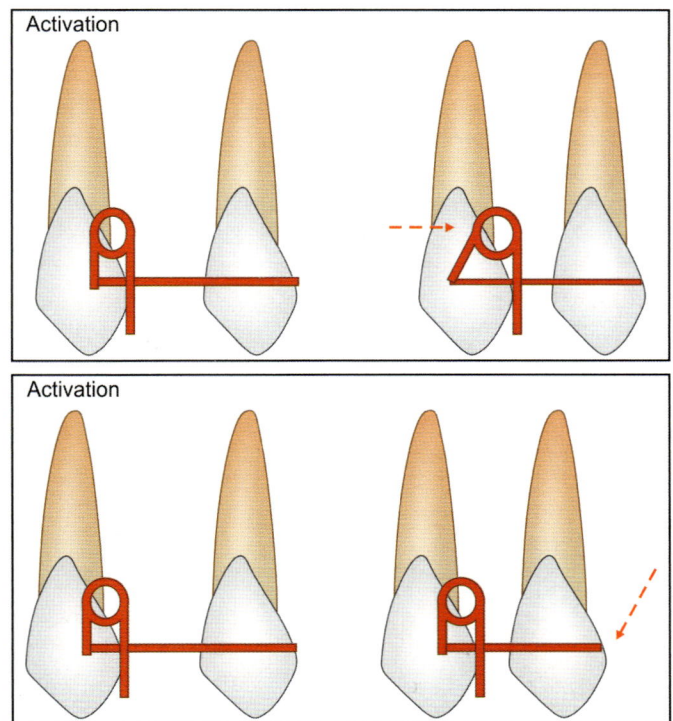

Fig. 15.44: Helical canine retractor

Reverse loop canine retractor: It is same as helical canine retractor but it is given for lower teeth.

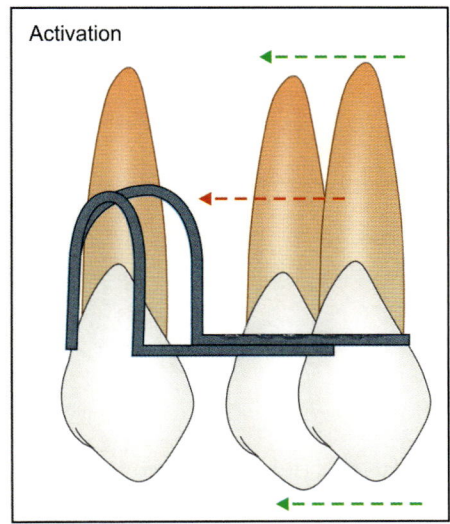

Fig. 15.46: 'U' loop canine retractor

It should be constructed such that the helix lies along the long axis of the tooth to be moved. Helix and active arm of finger spring are boxed in the wax to support the thin wire. It is activated either by moving the active arm towards the tooth to be moved or by opening the helix.

This spring is used to bring about mesial or distal movements of teeth, e.g. midline diastema. The active arm of spring lies close to the tissue and carry one and half turn coil. The coil is positioned midway between the initial and final position of the tooth. The coil should be on the opposite side of the direction of tooth movement. The activation is by opening the coil and the free end is readapted (Fig. 15.47). There are other methods also as shown in Figs 15.48 and Fig. 15.49.

Helical coil springs are used for mesial or distal movement after the teeth have drifted into an edentulous area (Fig. 15.47).

Cantilever spring

- Single cantilever spring
- Double cantilever spring
- Cranked spring
- 'Z' spring without coil.

Single cantilever spring: It is made out by 0.5 mm wire and active arm should be parallel to the occlusal plane or at right angle to the long axis of the tooth. The active arm lies below and carry one and half coil. It is indicated for correction of labial movement by single tooth, e.g. anterior crossbite or lingually placed anterior tooth. It is activated by opening the coil. While activating, it is ensured that the active arm lies always at right angle to the tooth which is to be corrected (Figs 15.50 and 15.51).

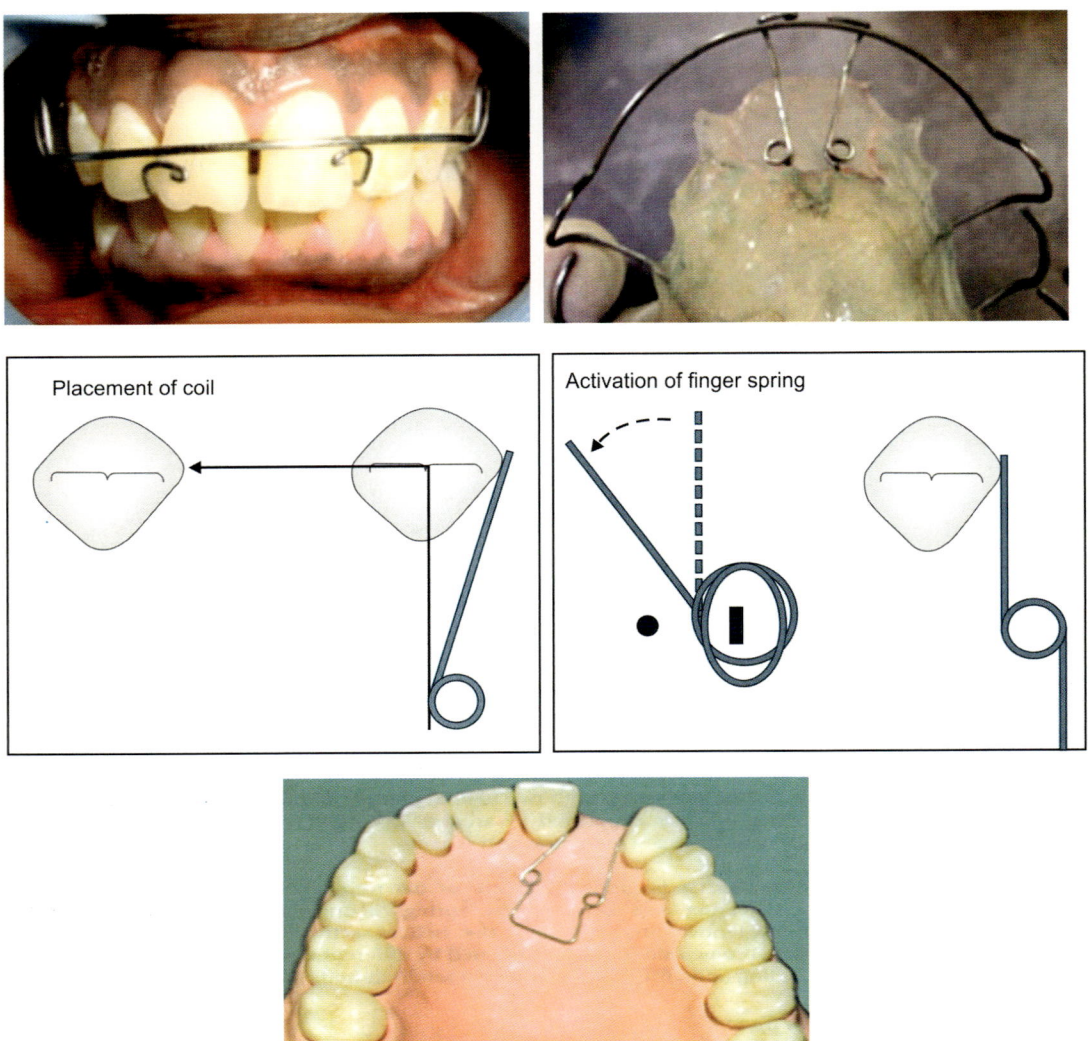

Fig. 15.47: Midline diastema correction—first method and placement of coil and activation

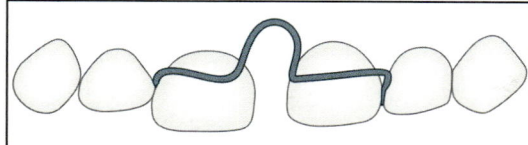

Fig. 15.48: Second method—closed proximal

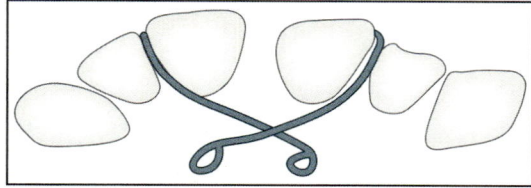

Fig. 15.49: Third method—crossed retention arms

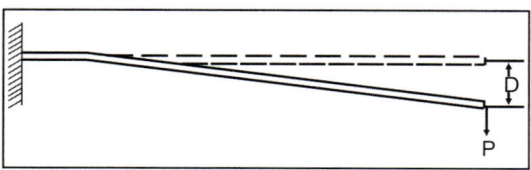

Fig. 15.50: Single cantilever spring: It is fixed at one end and free at the other end

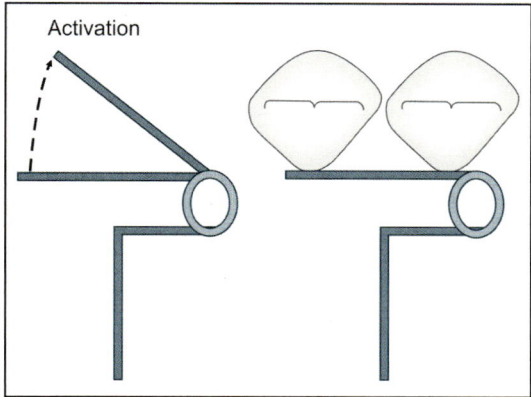

Fig. 15.51: Cantilever spring with coil at the point of attachment to the base plate

- A cantilever spring is fixed at one end and free to move at the other which deflects under pressure and delivers a gradually diminishing pressure in returning to its original form.
- If the thickness of the spring is reduced to one-half, the amount of deflection becomes 16 times as great for the same amount of pressure.
- The degree of pressure is proportional to the amount of deflection.
- If the length of the spring is doubled, the degree of deflection becomes eight times as great of the same amount of pressure.

Double cantilever spring: It is similar to single cantilever spring except it carries double helices. The passive arm of the first coil becomes active arm of the second coil. The activation is done by opening both coils. It is indicated in anterior crossbite, e.g. two teeth involvement (Figs 15.52–15.55). This spring can be boxed with a layer of wax and acrylized over the boxing. This raised flatform of acrylic acts as anterior bite plane.

Cranked spring: A longer active arm is made and an offset is placed so that the active arm of the spring can be precisely adapted to the tooth (Fig. 15.54).

Z spring without coil can also be designed. The activation is at the loop by openly the loop (Fig. 15.55).

Mattress spring: It is made up of 0.6 mm diameter wire. It is shaped like a mattress with 'U' loops extending till the retentive arm. It engages the tooth close to the gingival margin (Fig. 15.55).

Auxiliary spring: It is discussed already in the labial bow chapter (high labial bow with apron spring).

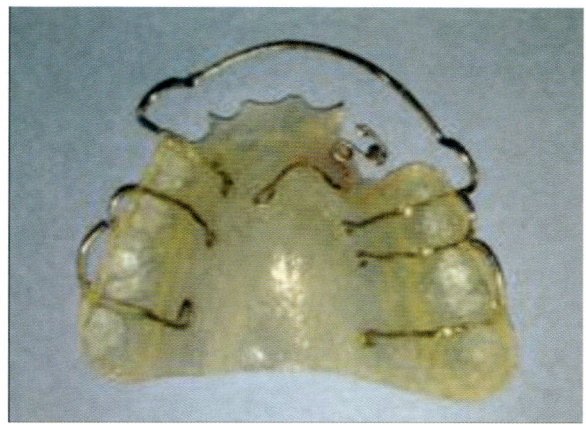

Fig. 15.52: Double cantilever spring

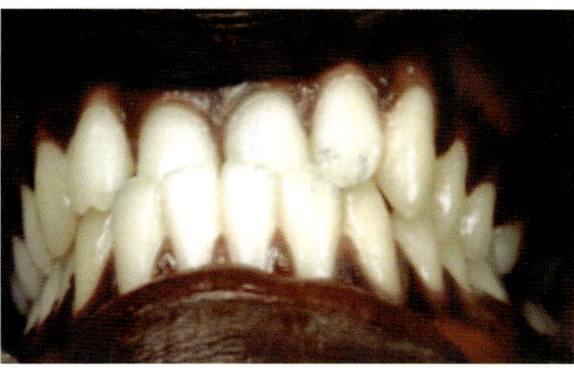

Fig. 15.53a: Developed crossbite appliance with double cantilever spring and bilateral posterior bite plane

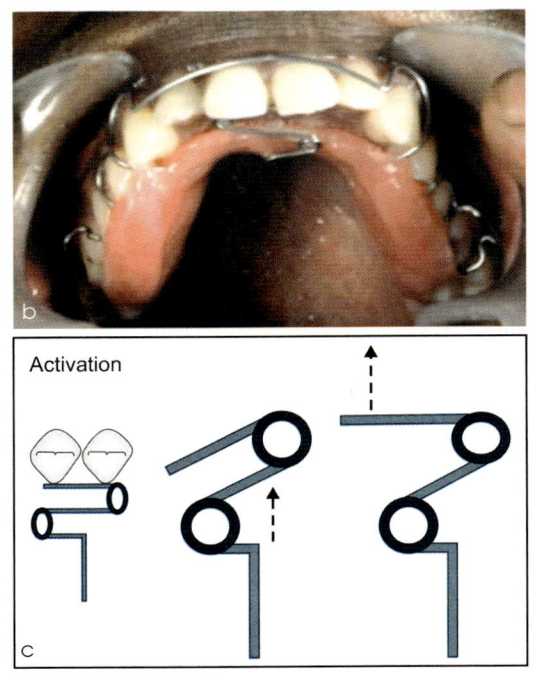

Fig. 15.53b and c: Activation of double cantilever spring

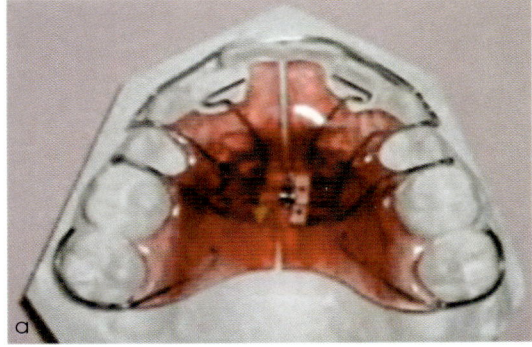

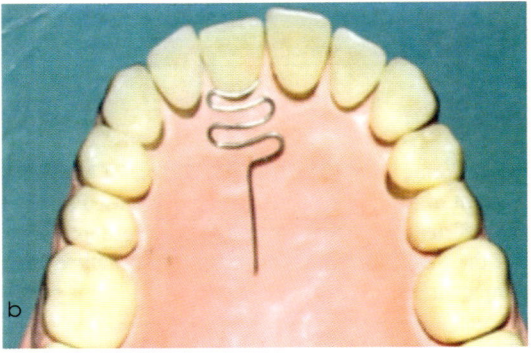

Fig. 15.55: (a) Cantilever without coils; (b) Mattress spring

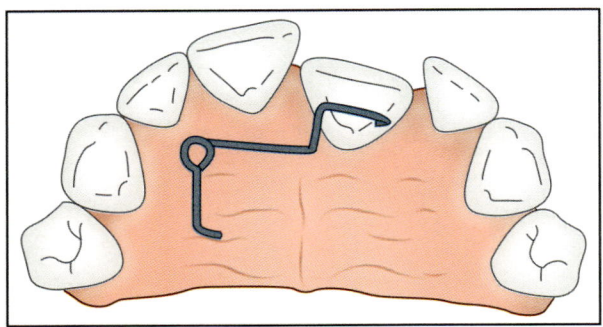

Fig. 15.54: Cranked spring

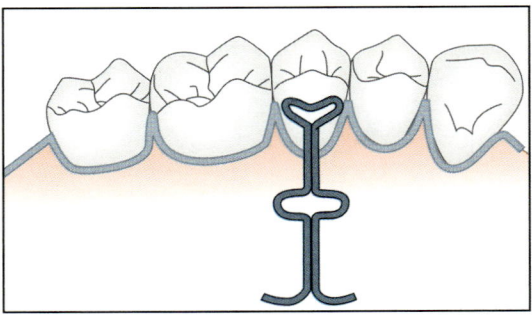

Fig. 15.56: T-spring

T-spring

It is indicated in premolar or molar crossbite. It is made out of 0.5 mm wire and kept on the palatal side to move palatobuccal direction. It is adjusted with additional loops incorporated, so that spring can be elongated as the tooth moves. It is adjusted by straightening the loop. It is activated by pulling the free end of the 'T' towards the intended direction of tooth movement (Fig. 15.56).

Coffin Spring

Coffin in 1881 introduced the spring and hence it is named after his name. It is fabricated with the wire of 1.25 mm or 1 mm. It is indicated in bilateral and unilateral crossbite for lateral expansion.

Boxing

The two ways of fixing the flexible springs like cantilever and finger spring to avoid distortion of the wire are (1) to give guide and (2) to box the springs.

Fabrication of boxing

- First the spring is fixed and a layer of wax is placed on the spring to act as spacer.
- The acrylic can be fruit up over the spacer as flat form which act as bite plane in case of deep bite.
- The main disadvantage of boxing is the accumulating of food particles and difficulty in cleaning. The second disadvantage in the difficulty in activating the coil.

- If the boxing method is adopted, there is no need to have a guide.

BITE PLANES

Bite planes may be divided into planes which lie parallel to the occlusal plane and planes inclined at an angle to the occlusal plane.

Anterior bite planes lying parallel to the occlusal plane (some times called horizontal bite planes) are designed to produce mainly axial stresses on the teeth. Such planes are intended either to proof the bite temporarily to facilitate certain teeth movements or to cause certain adjustments of the vertical relationships of the teeth.

Clinical Management

Appliance with anterior bite plane is indicated in the case of deep bite. When the appliance is worn in the mouth the posteriors are disengaged so that it will supraerupt. Once the supraeruption is complete, the anteriorly deep bite is opened. This is called opening the bite. Initially, the labial bow should not be activated and once the bite is opened, then only labial bow should be activated. Otherwise the anterior should be loose within the socket due to the pressure from the labial

bow anteriorly and on the palatal side the anterior part of anterior bite plane, restricts the tooth movement palatally. As the labial bow is activated, the anterior part of the anterior bite plane is trimmed 2 mm every time. While trimming the care should be taken to maintain the semicircle shape of acrylic anteriorly. The thickness of the acrylic should be sufficient to disengage the posteriors about 2 to 3 mm (Fig. 15.57).

Bite plane with groove for mandibular incisors (for mandibular orientation): To treat the pairs associated with the TMJ, the anterior bite plane is designed to free the existing occlusal contacts which often are abnormal due to the loss of the teeth and tilting of the remaining teeth and the presence of high spots on the occlusal plane due to faulty orthodontic treatment.

Problems with Anterior Bite Planes

If the lower incisors are severely proclined or retroclined, unwanted changes in their position may occur. If it arises, the inclined bite plane is given so that the surface is perpendicular to the long axis of lower anterior (sved bite plate).

Anterior bite plane with capped maxillary incisor gives an additional anchorage to the maxillary plane. If it is worn for longer period, a sinking of the appliance

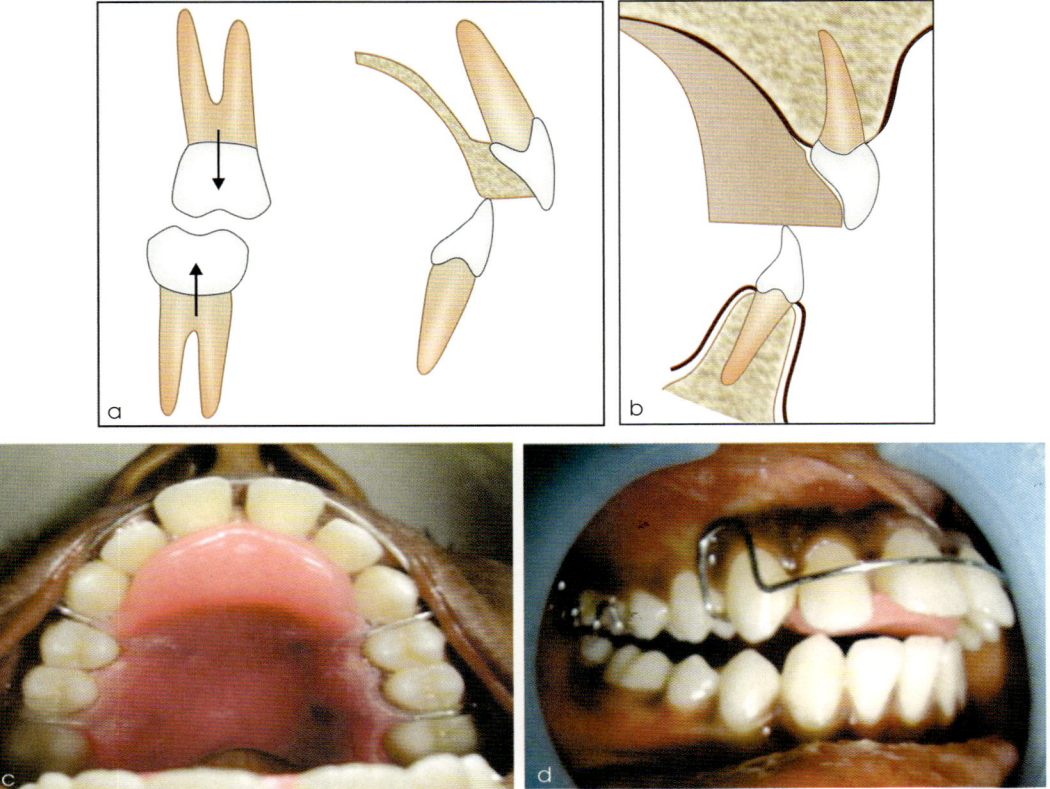

Fig. 15.57: Anterior bite plane

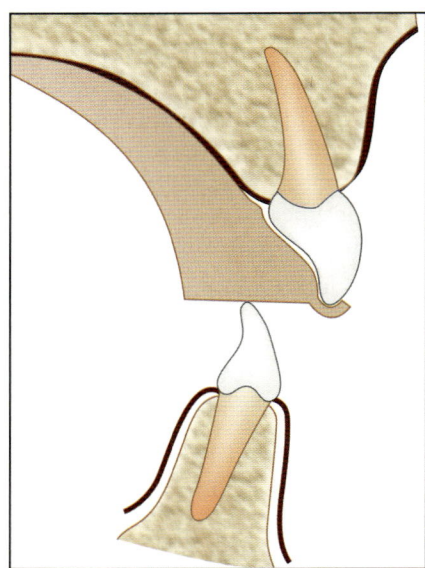

Fig. 15.58: Sved bite plane

takes place anteriorly causing upper anteriors proclined. If the bite plane sinks, the labial bow moves forward with it and cannot restrain the upper incisors.

A sved bited plane transmits the pressure axially to the upper incisors. Any forward component is restricted because the sved bite plate prevents tipping labially of the upper incisors (Fig. 15.58).

Fixed Anterior Bite Planes

It can be built with glass ionomer cement. A palatal arch is soldered on the lingual aspect of upper molar band on the anterior part of the palatal arch a mesh wire is soldered over which it carries glass ionomer anterior bite plane.

The second method is like the first method except glass ionomer bite plane. Instead of glass ionomer bite plane acrylic bite plane is added with short labial bow attached on the acrylic (Fig. 15.59).

Anterior Inclined Bite Plane

Instead of being flat, the bite plane is inclined it faces downward and forward at an angle of 60° to the occlusal plane and engages the lower incisors and canines when the jaws are approximated guiding the mandible forward.

The inclined bite plane reinforces the anchorage and proclines the lower anterior teeth in addition to the correction of anterior deep bite (Fig. 15.60).

When the mandible is brought into centric occlusion, the lower incisor is slided over the guide plane to bring the mandible forward. This may be act as mandibular repositioning splint.

Posterior Bites Plane

The posterior bite planes can be given either bilaterally or unilaterally. The unilateral posterior bite plane is indicated for correction of unilateral crossbite of simple or two or group of posterior teeth. The expansion appliance is given with unilateral posterior bite plane.

Bilateral posterior bite plane is given where there is mature anterior crossbite. The base is carried onto the occlusal surface of posterior till the buccal cusps of all the posteriors. The thickness of the bite plane should be sufficient to disengage the anterior which is cross bite. The posterior bite plane should not be too bulky. Otherwise the patient cannot close the mouth, causing inconvenient to the patient. While constructing the posterior bite plane, the care should be taken not to increase the same thickness of acrylic at the posterior end. Otherwise excess acrylic trimming may be necessary to maintain the sufficient disengagement (Fig. 15.61).

The fixed posterior bite plane can be used on the lower molar occlusal surfaces with glass ionomer filling materials. This is indicated along with fixed appliances.

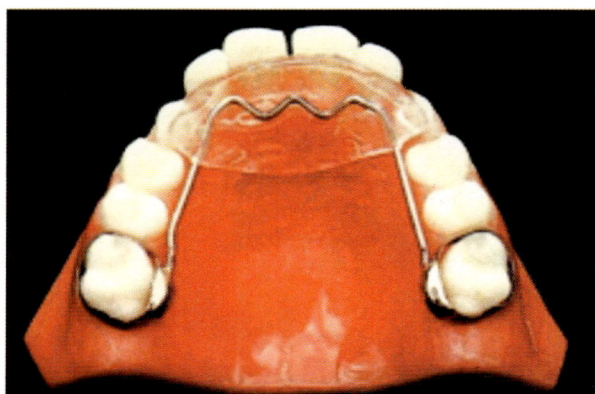

Fig. 15.59: Fixed anterior bite plane

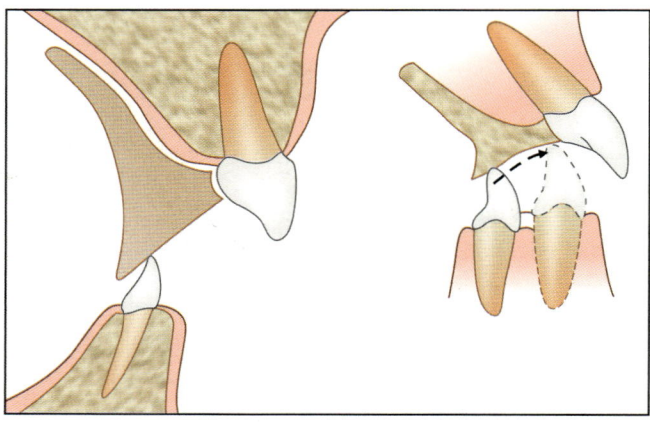

Fig. 15.60: Upper anterior inclined plane

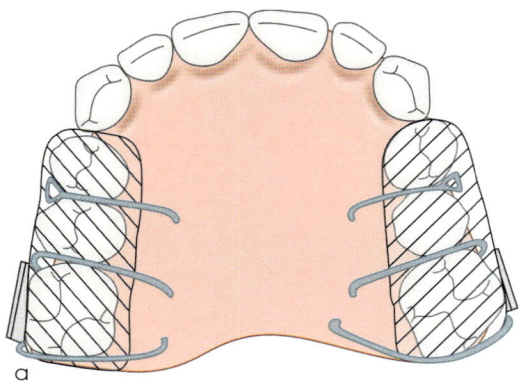

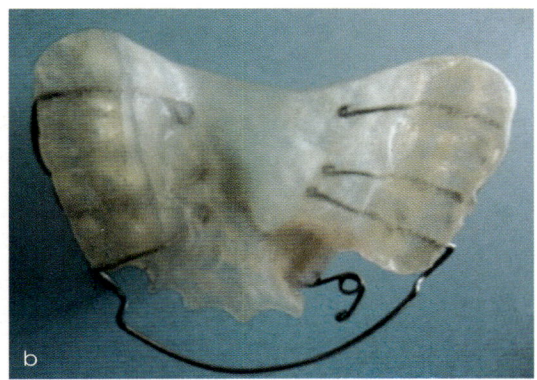

Fig. 15.61a and b: Bilateral bite plane

Once the crossbite correction is over, the posterior bite plane should be trimmed completely and keep the base plate alone.

Fixed bilateral or unilateral bite plane can be processed with glass ionomer cement on the occlusal surface.

Base Plates

The functions of the base plates are:
- They carry all the wire components.
- They anchor the appliance.
- They carry anterior bite plane, posterior bite plane and other acrylic extensions.
- They extend the acrylic over the finger spring and cantilever spring as boxing.
- They carry the expansion screw.
- They act as Nance button to hold the arch (Nance holding arch—combination of fixed and acrylic)
- In case of molar distalization acrylic button on the slope of palate is processed (combination of fixed and acrylic plate).

Elastics in Removable Appliance

- Elastics in conjunction with removable appliance are used for the movement of single and groups of teeth and for intermaxillary traction

- They can be used to move impacted canine to proper place along with the Hawley appliance.
- Use of elastics in moving the canine distally along with screw appliances.

BIBLIOGRAPHY

1. Adams CP. The modified arrowhead clasp-some further considerations. Dent Record 1953;73:333–2.
2. Graber TM, Neumann B. Removable Orthodontic Appliances. Philadelphia: WB Saunders, 1984.
3. Profitt WR. Contemporary Orthodontics St Louis: CV Mosby, 1986.
4. Schwartz AM, Gratzinger M. Removable Orthodontic Appliances. Philadelphia: WB Saunders, 1966.

PREVIOUS YEAR'S UNIVERSITY QUESTIONS

Essay

1. How do you classify orthodontic appliance? Add a note on ideal requirements of an orthodontic appliance.
2. Define appliance. What are the components of a removable appliance? Add a note on labial bows.
3. How do you classify springs? Write about canine retractors in detail.

Short Questions

1. Anterior and posterior bite planes
2. Single and double cantilever springs
3. Self-supported spring
4. Adam's clasp and its modifications
5. Labial bow and its modification
6. Boxing
7. Bite plane

MCQs

1. *Anchorage in a removable appliance is provided by:*
   a. Labial bow
   b. Finger springs
   c. Clasps
   d. Acrylic plate   **(Ans: d)**

2. *Inclined plane is constructed:*
   a. 90° to occlusal plane
   b. 45° to the occlusal plane
   c. 30° to occlusal plane
   d. 70° to occlusal plane   **(Ans: b)**

3. *Which clasp is used in anterior segment?*
   a. Adam's clasp
   b. South end clasp

c. Both a and b
d. None of the above   (Ans: c)

4. *Which clasp is used as accessary clasp?*
   a. Ball end clasp
   b. Triangular clasp
   c. C-clasp
   d. Both a and b   (Ans: d)

5. *How do you activate short labial bow?*
   a. Compression of U loop
   b. Opening the U loop
   c. Twisting the U loop
   d. All of the above (Ans: a)

6. *Mill's retractor is also called:*
   a. It is in the shape of a Mill
   b. Extensive labial bow
   c. Both a and b
   d. None of the bow   (Ans: b)

7. *Saved bite plane is modification of the following:*
   a. Lower anterior inclined plane
   b. Upper anterior inclined bite plane
   c. Both a and b
   d. None of the above   (Ans: b)

8. *Anterior bite plane is used to correct the following:*
   a. Scissors bite
   b. Deep bite
   c. Open bite
   d. Crossbite   (Ans: b)

9. *What are the other names for Jackson clasp?*
   a. Full clasp
   b. U-clasp
   c. Both of the above
   d. None of the above   (Ans: c)

15.2 EXPANSION APPLIANCE

Chapter Outline

- Introduction
- Classification
- Slow expansion appliance
- Types of expansion screw

- Transverse expansion
- Anterior and posterior expansion
- Rapid maxillary expansion appliances

INTRODUCTION

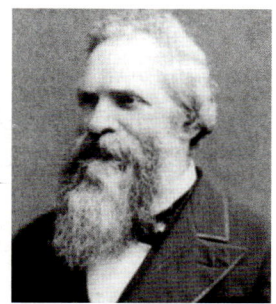

Emesson C Angel is regarded as the 'father of expansion appliances'. He developed Bandelette expansion appliance and he was the first to advocate the opening of mid-palatal suture to expand the dental arch. William Lintott introduced the expansion screws. Walter Coffin introduced the

Emesson C Angel

Coffin spring in 1875. In 1947, Rickett introduced the quad helix. And in 1993, Wendell V Arndt introduced nickel–titanium palatal expander.

It is a mechanical appliance through which the orthodontic forces are transmitted by a screw called an expansion appliance. It is divided into slow and rapid expansion appliance.

CLASSIFICATION

It is classified:

According to the jaws involved
- Maxillary expansion—slows and rapid expander
- Mandibular expansion—Schwarz plate, lip bumper

According to the rate of activation: Rapid and slow

According to type of expansion:
- Orthodontic
- Orthopedic
- Passive—lip bumper, vestibular shield

According to direction:
- Anterior
- Posterior
- Unilateral
- Bilateral
- Three-dimensional
- Individual tooth

According to type of appliance:
- Removable
- Fixed—banded or bonded
- Tooth-borne—Hyrax, Issacson
- Tooth and tissue borne—Hass appliance

According to active element:
- Screws
- Dental expansion—Schwarz appliance
- Skeletal—Hyrax
- Springs/coils—Coffin spring, W-arch or Porter appliance, Quad helix

Indications

- Cleft palate
- Syndromes associated with cleft palate
- Class III malocclusion where there is a defeat in the maxilla—bilateral and unilateral crossbite (Fig. 15.62).
- To help activator therapy, Norwegian screws are attached in the center of activator where there is severe constriction of upper arch.
- Real and relative maxillary deficiencies
- Cases of inadequate nasal capacity exhibiting chronic nasal respiratory problems
- In a clinical condition where there is bilateral buccal crossbite and single tooth and double teeth anterior crossbite (Fig. 15.63)

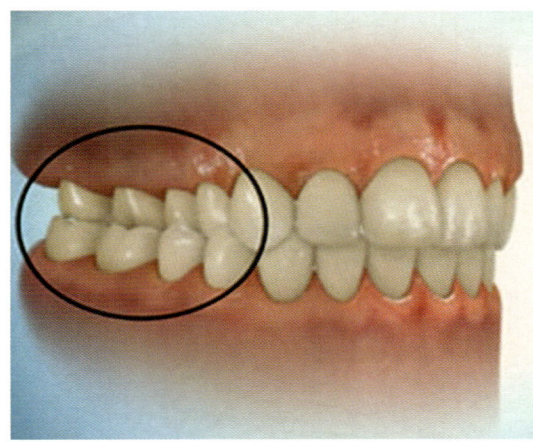

Fig. 15.62: Unilateral posterior crossbite

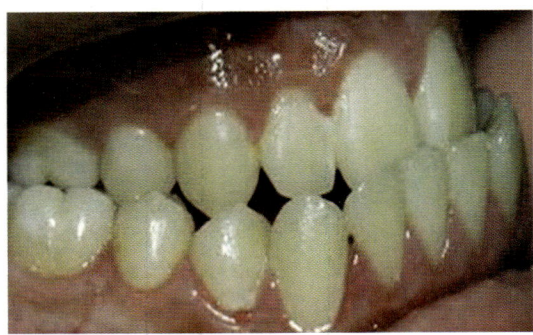

Fig. 15.63: Total crossbite

- In a clinical condition where there are anterior crossbite involving six teeth.

SLOW EXPANSION APPLIANCE

Different Ways of Expansion

- By using screws of different type
- By using Coffin's spring
- By using Portar appliance—modified form of Coffin's spring.
- By using W-arch appliance
- Quad helix appliance
- Memory screw appliance
- NiTi palatal expander
- Transpalatal arch
- RME (rapid maxillary expansion)

TYPES OF EXPANSION SCREW (Table 15.1)

Slow Type

1. Skeleton type—maximum:
   - 7 mm expansion
   - 3–4 mm expansion
   - 5 mm expansion
2. Three-dimensional screws—to correct total crossbite

3. Fan type expansion screw for anterior movement of maxilla
4. Mandibular bow screw (lateral and sagittal anterior expansion of the mandible)
5. Telescopic screws are to move a tooth or group of teeth and lateral expansion of upper and lower jaws
6. Spring loaded screws
7. Norwegian plate screw in Class III malocclusion
8. Standard expansion screws for lateral expansion of the maxilla
9. Sectional screws for distal movements in upper and lower jaws
10. Expansion by magnet
11. Traction screw

Advantages of Screw over Spring (Fig. 15.64)

- Appliances with screw are easier to manage than those with springs. Therefore, they are useful in the less skillful patient.
- Screws are activated by the patient at regular intervals using a key, and therefore, they are more valuable in patients who cannot visit the dentist frequently.
- Appliance with a screw has fewer tendencies to get dislodged than those with springs. Therefore, they offer more stability for moving several adjacent teeth in same direction.
- Forces generated can be controlled, based on the amount of activation done.

The patient or the parent using a key activates the screw. Activations may be done once or twice a week or more frequently depending upon the type and amount of tooth movement required. Ideal tooth movement is achieved by turning the screw a quarter turn every 3 to 7 days. Most screws produce 0.2–0.25 mm movement per quarter turn. The movement produced is a direct function of the thread height. More the thread height, more the opening and higher the forces generated. The amount of force applied to each

	Table 15.1 Difference between slow and rapid expander	
	Slow	*Rapid*
1	Slow in action	Rapid in action
2	Expansion is achieved in a few weeks	Expansion is achieved in 21 days
3	A weekly single quarter turn produces 0.25 mm of tooth movement	One turn in the morning and another turn in the evening on the first day followed by one activation every day
4	Expansion is 1 mm per month	7–11 mm expansion in 21 days
5	No pain and it is physiological	It is painful and pathological
6	Orthodontic force	Orthopedic force
7	Dentoalveolar expansion	Skeletal expansion
8	No midline diastema seen	Clinically midline diastema noticed
9	Less chances of relapse	Results are not stable, more chances of relapse

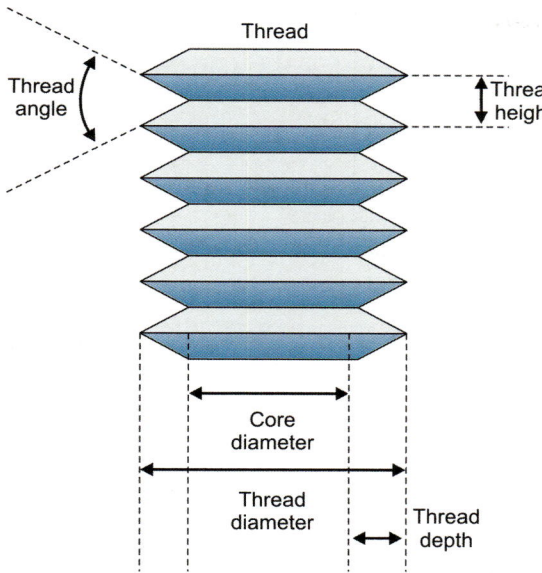

Fig. 15.64: Cut section of expansion screw showing thread

tooth by a screw appliance also depends on the number of teeth being moved, each tooth receiving a part of the total force. Screw should not be budged too much out of the acrylic. Based on the location of the screw and the acrylic splint, three types of tooth movement can be brought about by screw appliances (Fig. 15.65).

• Arch expansion-screw planed in the center of the arch. It is used to correct upper anterior crossbite by delivering upper Hawley's appliance with

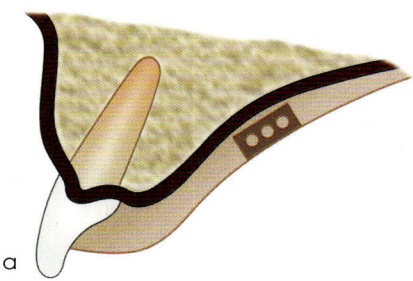

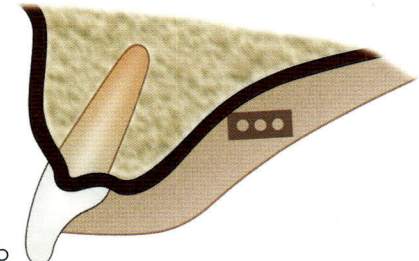

Fig. 15.65: (a) Correct placement of expansion screw; (b) Incorrect placement of expansion screw

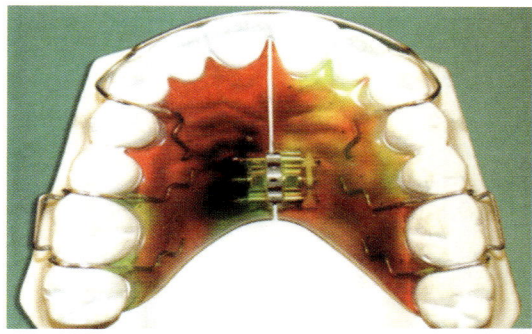

Fig. 15.66: Upper Hawley's appliance incorporating universal screw for bilateral expansion

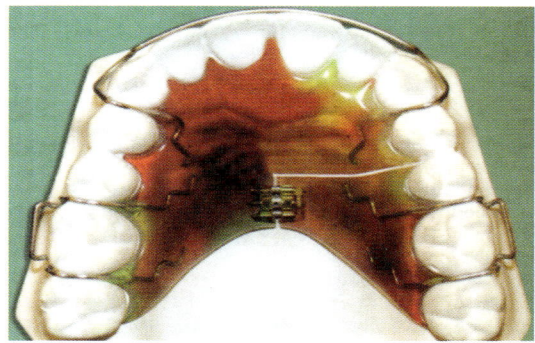

Fig. 15.67: Removable appliance for buccal movement of a group of teeth

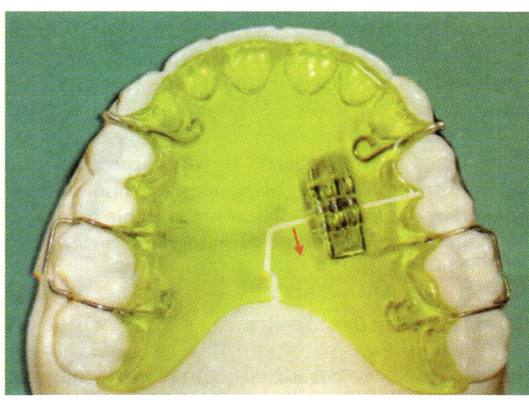

Fig. 15.68: Removable appliance for distal movement of teeth

expansion screw and bilateral posterior bite plane (Fig. 15.66).

• Labial/buccal movement of one or group of teeth (Fig. 15.67).

• Mesial/distal movement of one or more teeth (Fig. 15.68).

TRANSVERSE EXPANSION

The most common circumstance in which arch expansion needed is a constricted maxillary arch with a tendency towards buccal crossbite.

An active plate split in the midline will expand the arch almost totally by tipping the posterior teeth buccally, not by opening the mid-palatal suture and widening the maxilla itself for this reason, removable plates are not indicated for skeletal crossbite or for dental expansion of more than 4 to 5 mm. Excellent clasping is required to prevent displacement of the plate.

Lateral expansion of the mandibular arch with a removable appliance is much more difficult than maxillary expansion, because the screw must be placed more anteriorly. Expanding the mandibular intercanine distance with an anteriorly positioned screw in a removable appliance is not recommended, because the force is concentrated against the incisor and canine so that excessive forces easily can be produced and because mandibular intercanine expansion is notoriously unstable.

ANTERIOR AND POSTERIOR EXPANSION

The Sagittal Appliance

An early forerunner of the sagittal appliance was referred to as the y-plate because of the shape of the cuts on the base plate separating the plate into its component parts. Most of the early model y-plates or lateral expansion active plates of that era had a labial bow and one which is constructed that way today still bear the name of 'Schwarz plate' after the man Schwarz in 1938 who brought their use to such high level of proficiency.

The word sagittal is derived from the original Latin root *Sagitta* which means 'arrow'. It must be remembered that like an arrow, the appliance is designed primarily for front to back expansion of the dental arch in a linear direction. This implies that if it is used to correct a narrow, short arch of crowded teeth, the end result will be narrow, longer arch of uncrowded teeth.

If the second molar is intact, the primary direction of the development of the arch will be in an anterior direction. This is especially useful in the development and expansion of a crowded or retruded premaxilla as in a Class II division 2 cases. However, if 2nd molars are removed, the primary direction of the movement of the teeth will be of the posterior segments in a distal direction. This is exceptionally useful in cases of severe anterior crowding. Of course, the appliance itself expands in both directions about 80% anteriorly and with the second molars out, the expansion is about 80% posteriorly.

Sagittal I

The sagittal I appliance is designed to distalize one or both posterior segments to varying degrees as necessary to relieve anterior crowding, which usually expresses itself in the form of blocked out cuspids in Cl crowded cases and it also may be used for the same purpose in Class II division 1 cases.

Sagittal II

All but identical in appearance to the sagittal I, sagittal II appliance is used for expansion of the arch in the completely opposite direction. Instead of distalizing teeth posteriorly, it develops them anteriorly using second molars as anchorage and by means of the appropriate adjustments, the sagittal II can be used to apply labial crown torque to the anterior teeth (Fig. 15.69).

Sagittal III

The anterior plane should extend slightly forward of the upper incisors, so as to contact the lower incisors in bite occlusion. This is an excellent for pseudo Class III cases with a reversed overbite (Fig. 15.70).

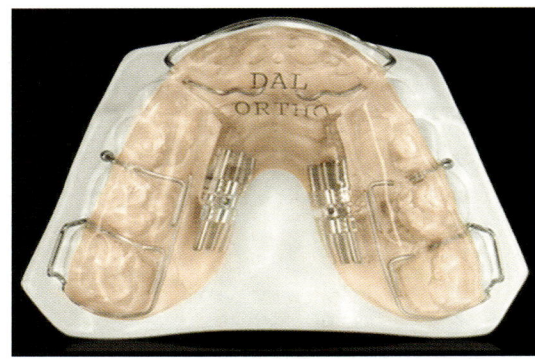

Fig. 15.69: Sagittal II appliance

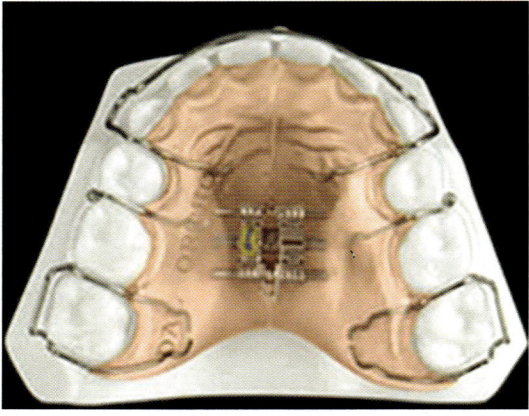

Fig. 15.70: Sagittal III appliance

W-Arch Appliance

The bilateral posterior crossbites are corrected in preadolescent children by using W-arch appliance and quad-helix appliance. The active spring is in the shape of W and is activated by simply opening the apices of W. It is made up of 0.09 mm wire or 20 gauge wire which is soldered to molar bands. It brings both dental and skeletal changes. It moves both primary and permanent teeth. Expansion should continue at the rate of 2 mm per month. Usually 2–3 months of active treatment followed by retention for 2 months is required (Fig. 15.71).

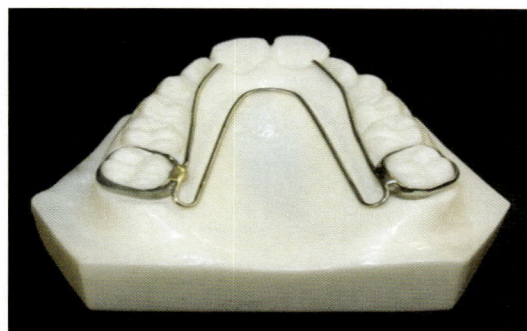

Fig. 15.71: W-arch appliance

Coffin Spring

The appliance consists of an omega-shaped wire made out of 1.25 mm thickness. The base of omega is placed posteriorly with the free ends of the omega wire embedded in acrylic plate covering slopes of the palate. The spring is activated by pulling the two sides apart manually. This should be done first in the premolar region and in the molar region (Fig. 15.72).

Quad Helix Appliance

The quad helix incorporates 4 helices that increase the wire length. Therefore, the flexibility and range of action of this appliance is more. It is made up of 1 mm or 19 gauges and it consists of anterior helices and a pair of posterior helices.

The quad helix consists of a pair of anterior helices and a pair of posterior helices. The portion of wire between the two anterior helices is called the anterior bridge. The free wire ends adjacent to the posterior helices are called outer arms.

They rest against the lingual surface of the buccal teeth and are soldered onto the lingual aspect of the molar bands.

The quad helix can be used to expand a narrow arch as well as to bring about rotation of molars. It can be prefabricated by stretching the two molar bands apart prior to cementation or by using 3 prong pliers. When

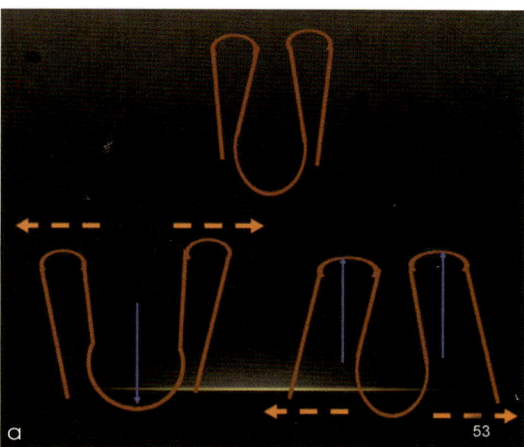
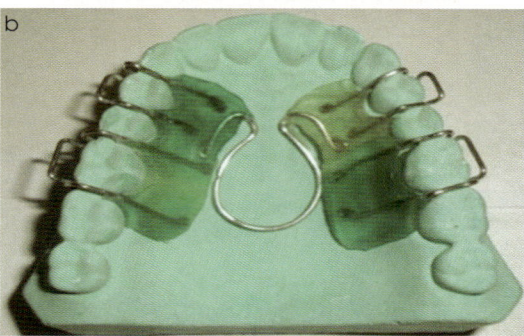

Fig. 15.72: (a) Coffin spring activation; (b) Coffin spring fabricated on model

used in mixed dentition a skeletal mid-palatal splitting can be achieved (Fig. 15.73).

Two Ways of Activation

- Intraoral activation
- Extraoral activation (Fig. 15.73)

The first activation is done out of the mouth before the appliance is cemented. The appliance is expanded about 8 mm maintaining the lateral arms palallel in order to have the same magnitude expansion on both sides.

The first activation will generate 400 g of force approximately. It is scheduled for 6 more weeks.

A second activation is done inside the mouth on the anterior bridge with a 3-prong plier, where the single prong of the plier must be in front. This way the posterior sector is expanded and the molars rotate mesially.

The third and last activation is done in the posterior bridges, to produce rotation of the molars and expansion of the lateral arms.

Advantages

- Patient cooperation is not required because it is a fixed appliance.

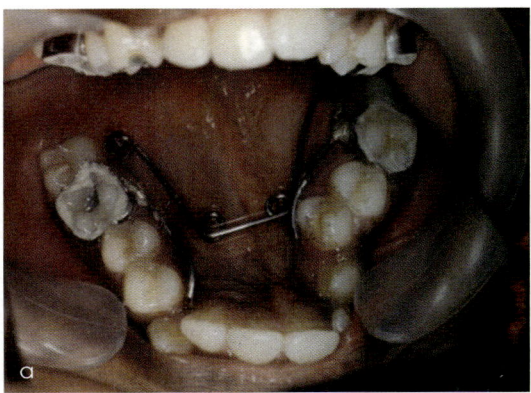

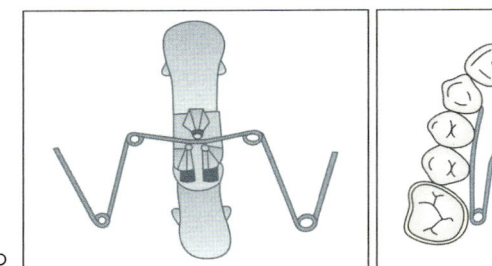 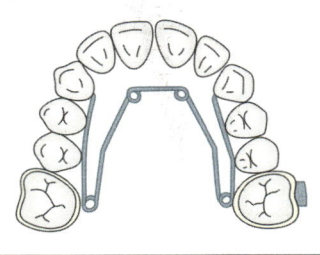 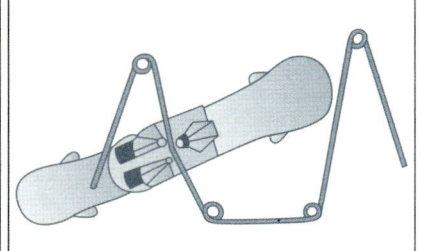

Fig. 15.73: (a) Quad helix appliance; (b) Activation of quad helix appliance

- It produces continuous and light physiologic forces.
- It produces up to 6 mm of intermolar and inter-canine width increase.
- In young patients, 3 to 4 mm mid-palatal suture separation can be obtained.
- Generally, the expansion and the rotations are obtained within 60 to 90 days.
- After the expansion has taken place, the appliance must remain passive for 6 months and the same appliance can be used as retention appliance.

Modifications

The QH appliance may be modified a number of ways. Modifications usually fall into one or more of the following categories.

- *Increased no. of helices:* For anteroposterior expansion, extra helices may be added to procline the upper incisor teeth.
- *Decreased number of helices:* The anterior helices may be omitted and a palatal button substituted, if space maintenance and molar rotation rather than upper arch expansion are the objectives of treatment. By convention, the term bihelix refers to an appliance with posterior helices only which is placed in the lower arch.
- *Addition of light wire springs:* Sandham (1979) has described the addition of light wire spring to a QH, to effect minor teeth movements.

- *Addition of habit breaking auxillaries:* Bench et al 1978 described the addition of tongue spurs grids to discourage digits or tongue sucking habits.

Nickel Titanium Expander

Nickel titanium can be processed into a set shape to which it constantly tends to return when deformed. This is called shape memory. Nickel titanium can be alloyed to produce a metal with a specific transition temperature. (Ortho organizers transition temperature is 94°F). At temperature above the transition temperature, the interatomic forces bind the atoms tighter, producing a stiffer metal. At temperature below transition temperature, the interatomic forces weaken producing a metal much more flexible. Clinically, expander should be chilled to make it flexible.

As the mouth begins to warm the appliances (and subsequently reaches 98°F), device becomes stiffer. The shape memory is restored and the expander exerts continuous low forces as the teeth and mid-palatal suture to produce expansion as the expansion begins to take place. The stiffness in the appliance can cause discomfort which may be relieved by sipping a cold fluid.

Selection of NiTi Expander

A kit is available which contains one expander each of the following 8 sizes ranging from 26 to 47 mm in every 3 mm increments. It also contains the ice spray and one blue cold pack.

Research has indicated that approximately 90% of the cases needing palatal expansion require a 4 mm expansion of the upper 1st molars (2 mm per side).

Measure with a Boley gauge, lingual the upper first molars at the location where the lingual sheaths will be placed, e.g. if the intermolar width is 31 mm and then add 4 mm to the above measurement to equal 35 mm. It is ideal to select 35 mm expander. If 1 to 2 mm additional expansion is required, it can be achieved by placing ortho organizers plier 200–450 in the loop of the distal wire. 1–2 mm reduction can also be achieved by squeezing the loop of the distal wire. If total 6 mm of more expansion is needed, two separate expanders in 3 mm increments should be used sequentially when desired expansion has been achieved, cut and remove the mesial looped wire to create to retainer.

The **Nitanium palatal expander** can be used in:
- Primary dentition
- Mixed dentition
- Adult dentition
- Cleft palate patient
- Surgery cases
- Class III cases
- TMJ cases

It is excellent for:
- Maxillary deficiency
- Total crossbite correction (Fig. 15.74)
- Distal rotation and expansion of molars
- Molar stabilization
- Auxiliary placement for habit correction
- Intrusion of molars
- Three-way sagittal with utility arch
- Alignment before functional appliance
- Aiding Class II correction
- Retainer, etc.

Advatages of NiTi Palatal Expander

- Histologic findings show greater respiratory reaction and greater stability than the RPE.
- Requires no adjustment by the patient.
- Can program appliance to exact expansion required and will stop at that point.
- No effect on speech or eating.
- Does not require frequent adjustments.
- Rotates molars buccally and distally.
- Can be placed directly, does not require costly lab procedures.
- No real apparent suture splitting
- Light, gentle, continuous force
- No patient discomfort
- Total operator control
- Can widen the suture slightly for favorable fibroblastic, and osteoblastic response
- Influence the direction of maxillary and mandibular growth.
- Less retention time required usually 6–8 weeks.
- Less tipping of abutment teeth—less relapse.
- Takes only 2 well-fitted bands and is easy to insert
- Very hygienic.
- Can be used with headgear, utility arches or continuous archwires.
- Will cause orthodontic and orthopedic changes.
- Greater stability.

Preparation for Placing the Nitanium Palatal Expansion Appliance

- Separate molars with elastic modules or brass wire.
- Fit and festoon bands (mesial-gingival and distal-occlusal) that have both buccal tubes and lingual sheaths attached.
- Assemble the expander with the bands as one unit and secure with ligature wire. It is very important to secure appliance and bands as one unit prior to cementing appliance.
- Mix cement on a chilled slab to incorporate maximum amount of powder for a strong mix. Dry teeth and place cotton rolls. Apply cement to bands.
- You are now ready to use the ice spray, which makes the appliance 'dead soft' for placement. Connect the red spray straw to nozzle of ice spray, and then spray the center bends of the nitanium wires.

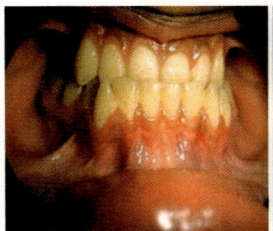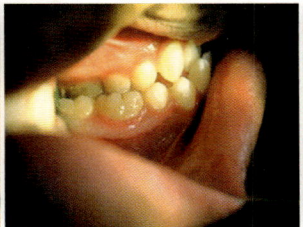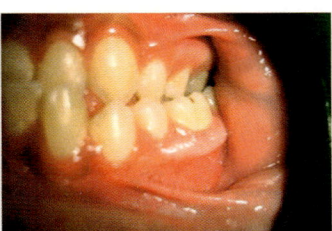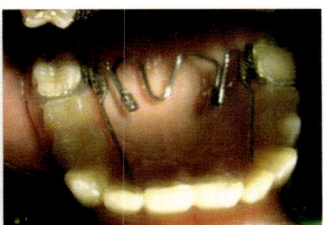

Fig. 15.74: NiTi expander in total crossbite case

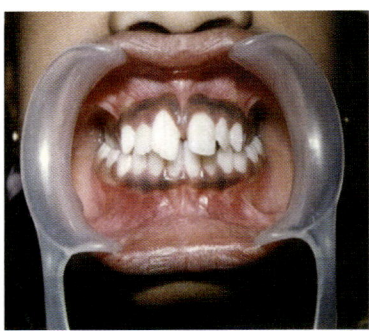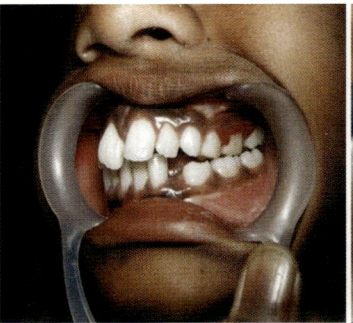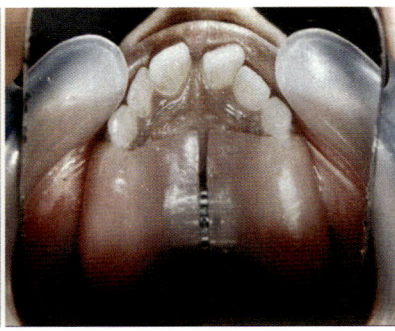

Fig. 15.75: Bilateral posterior crossbite case—memory screw appliance

- While the wires are pasive, seat one band and let it cure. Then seat the other band. Make certain bands are completely seated. Wipe-off excess cement with cotton rolls. Patient can also bite down on cotton rolls as cement is setting. This will allow for easier clean up.

Optional methods, if ice spray is not available:

Option 1. Keep blue ice pack (supplied) in freezer until needed then remove from freezer. Place NPE on frozen blue ice pack and let it chill for 3 to 5 minutes before insertion.

Option 2. Place the NPE in freezer prior to application for 3 to 5 minutes.

Although the chilling effects will not last as long as the ice spray, the above techniques will give you some working time while the appliance has less spring tension.

Memory Screw

The new memory transversal expansion screw offers more patient comfort with a fewer adjustments and less patient cooperation. This has an invisible incorporated superflexible spring.

A constant force of approximately 500 g is applied to the tooth by a spring range of 0.8 mm via 1.5 turn of the spindle. Readjustment is necessary, only if the spring is fully extended. It gives 5 mm expansion. An elastic biomechanical force is exerted constantly over the teeth via a memory spring and this makes for substantially shorter treatment times approximately 6 weeks.

Visits are spaced at weak intervals. A weekly activation of 1 spindle turn is particularly effective. It is processed into the cold cure acrylic appliance in the same way as any other transverse expansion screw. The use of heat-cure acrylic is not recommended. With MTES, both orthodontic and orthopedic changes can be achieved particularly in late deciduous and early mixed dentition period with span of six weeks. After correction, the appliance can be inactivated as retainer (Fig. 15.75).

RAPID MAXILLARY EXPANSION (RME) APPLIANCES

Applied Anatomy

The morphology of the mid-palatal suture has been studied by Melsen (1975).

Stages of Development used by Bjork and Helm

First stage: Covering the infantile period. The suture is very broad and Y-shaped with the vomerine bone placed in a V-shaped groove between the two halves of the maxilla (Fig. 15.76).

Second stage: Juvenile period, the suture is found to be wavier (Fig. 15.77).

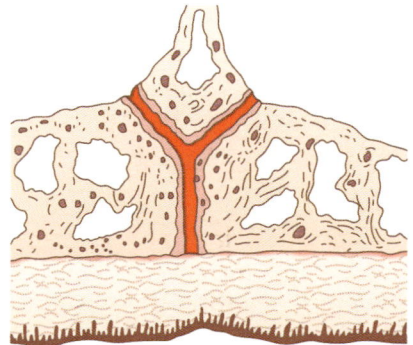

Fig. 15.76: First stage—'Y' shaped pattern

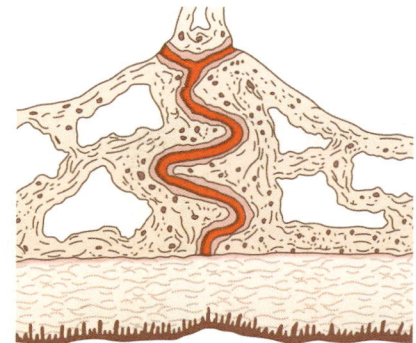

Fig. 15.77: Second stage—juvenile period

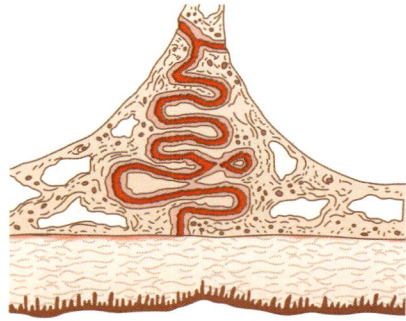

Fig. 15.78: Third stage—tortuous course

Third stage: Adolescent period, the suture is characterized by a more tortuous course with increasing interdigitations (Fig. 15.78).

The fixed rapid expanders can be classified into banded and bonded appliances. Banded appliances are again divided into (Table 15.2).

- Tooth-borne
- Both tooth- and tissue-borne

Most commonly used fixed expander of tooth- and tissue-borne appliances are:

- Derichsweiler type
- Haas type

Tooth-borne appliances are:

- Hyrax
- Isaacson type

Banded Tooth- and Tissue-Borne Appliances

Derichsweiler Appliance

This is both tissue- and tooth-borne appliance. Molar and premolar bands are fabricated and fitted, wire tags are soldered onto the palatal aspect of the bands. The tags do not directly contact the screw. These wire tags and the screw at the center is inserted into split palatal acrylic plates.

This appliance is a rigid appliance which not only transmits forces onto the teeth but also onto the palatal shelves directly. Thus it is both a tissue- and tooth-borne appliance. It has a ridged wire framework of stainless steel of 1.2 mm diameter. The wire soldered on the buccal and lingual aspects connecting the premolar and molar bands.

Table 15.2: Fixed rapid expander	
Banded—tooth-borne appliances	*Banded—tooth-and tissue-borne appliances*
• Isaacson	• Derichsweiler type
• Biedermann type or Hyrax type	• Haas type

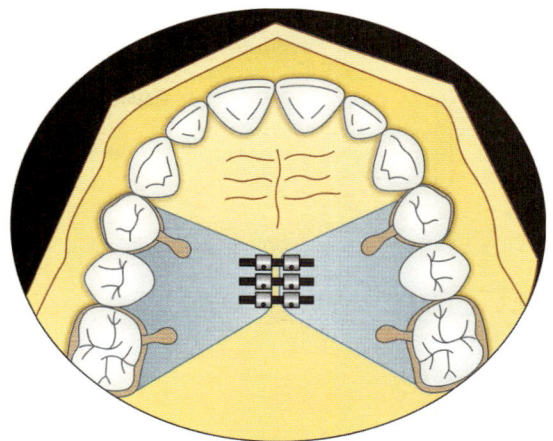

Fig. 15.79: Derichsweiler appliance

These palatal extensions of the 1.2 mm diameter wire are incorporated in the acrylic plate which contains an expansion screw in the midline. The palatal wire is kept longer so as to extend past the bands both anteriorly and posteriorly. The plate does not extend over the rugae area. One of the main disadvantages is the inflammation of the palatal tissue (Fig. 15.79).

Haas Type Expander

Haas expander was designed and popularized by Andrew Haas in the year 1961. It consists of molar bands on the right and left permanent molars and premolars. A jack screw is incorporated in the midline into the two acrylic pads that closely contact the palatal mucosa. Support wires also extend anteriorly from the molars along the buccal and lingual surfaces of the posterior teeth to add rigidity to the appliance permitting the forces to be generalized not only against the teeth but also against the underlying soft and hard palatal tissues.

Haas states that more bodily movement and less dental tipping is produced when acrylic palatal coverage is added to support the appliance thus permitting the forces to be generalized not only against the teeth but also against the underlying soft and hard palatal tissues (Fig.15.80).

Tooth-Borne Appliances

Isaacson RME Appliances

The Isaacson type of appliance consists of a metal framework soldered both labially as well as palatally on the first premolar and molar bands. This is a tooth-borne appliance without any acrylic palatal covering. A spring-loaded screw often called the Minne expander (developed at the University of Minnesota, Dental School) is soldered on the palatal extension of the metal

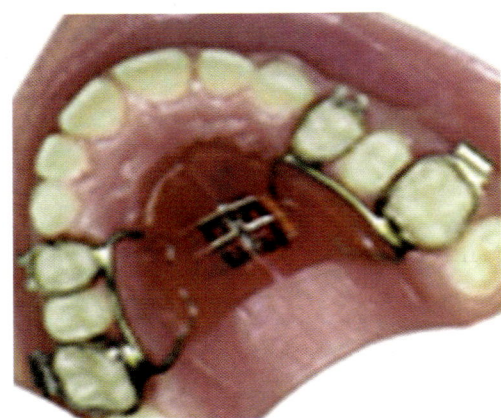

Fig. 15.80: Haas RME

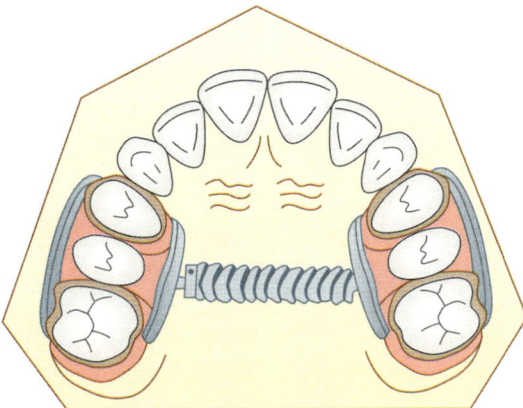

Fig. 15.81: Isaacson RME appliance

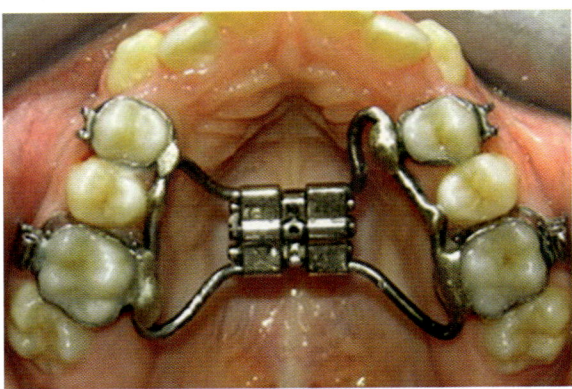

Fig. 15.82: Hyrax

In case the premolars have not erupted yet, the extension arms are contoured up to the first primary molar.

Advantages

* It is hygienic because it does not have acrylic.
* Depending on the transversal requirements of the patient, we can choose among 8 mm, 11 mm and 13 mm screws.
* It is very effective appliance.
* The addition of acrylic on the occlusal aspects of the molars and premolars will prevent the over inclination of the teeth that serve as anchorage.
* Expansion up to 10 to 12 mm is possible. It improves the respiratory capacity of the patients due to the descent of the nasal cavity.

Clinical management:

* Daily activation of 0.5 mm (¾ of a turn per day), one activation in the morning and another in the night which is tolerable measure for the patient (¼ of a turn = 0.25 mm).
* It should be activated 30 minutes after the appliance has been cemented to allow the complete setting of the cement.
* Once the expansion has ended, use the appliance as a fixed retainer for 3 to 6 months. It takes 3 months for the mid-palatal suture to reossifie and the same appliance should be retained as retainer.
* Once the appliance is removed, a transpalatal arch on the upper molars is fixed.

framework. The expander consists of a coil spring and a nut that compresses this spring on closing. This coil spring with the nut extends between the soldered lingual metal flanges. The expander is activated by closing the nut so that the spring gets compressed and exerts pressure in opposite direction (Fig. 15.81).

Biedermann Type or Hyrax (Fig. 15.82)

It is the most commonly used rapid maxillary expansion screw in patients that are in the mixed or early permanent dentition. It was designed by Briedermann and it is totally made of stainless steel and does not have any acrylic, so it is hygienic.

Fabrication of appliance

* Four bands, two on the first premolars and two on the first permanent molars.
* An expansion screw placed on the midline of the palate separated 3 mm from the palatal mucosa. When th maxilla is separated, the palatal vault descends.
* It also has two palatal support arches soldered to the band providing more rigidity to the appliance.

Bonded RME (Fig. 15.83)

They have the splint covering over occlusal and buccal surfaces of posterior teeth on either side to which jack screws is attached. These bonded appliances expand and interfere with freeway space by its vertical thickness acting as a functional appliance. Elevator musculature is stretched gives stretch and reflex, thus

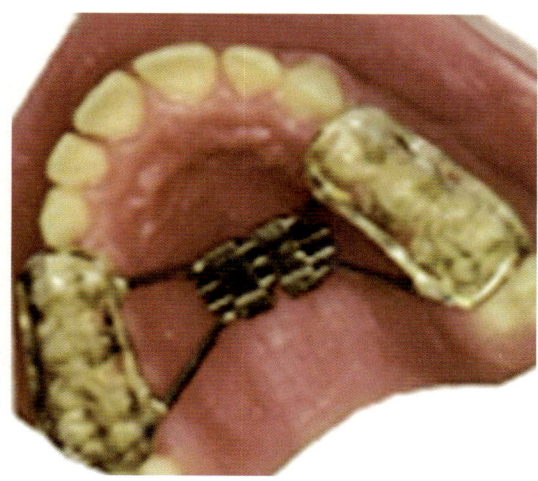

Fig. 15.83: Bonded RME

giving apically directed force on maxillary and mandibular teeth.

The bonded expander produces changes in transverse as well as vertical and anteroposterior direction. The acrylic occlusal coverage opens the bite posteriorly, facilitating correction of anterior crossbite. A slight superior movement of the posterior aspect of the palatal plane occurs with these appliances. Usually this type of appliance is given in facemask therapy.

Effects of Rapid Maxillary Expansion

Effect of rapid on maxillary skeletal base: Triangular or fan-shaped opening of the mid-palatal suture with maximum opening in the maxillary incisor region and gradually diminishing towards the posterior part of the palate.

According to Korbs:
- In sagittal plane, the maxilla rotates in a downward and forward direction.
- In coronal plane, the two halves of the maxilla rotate away from each other.

Effect of RME on Maxillary Anterior

It causes the separation of incisors in the midline resulting in midline diastema which indicates that expansion has been taken place. This midline diastema later will be closed as a result of the transseptal fiber traction in about 3–5 months.
- *Effect of RME on maxillary posterior teeth:* There will be buccal tilting of the maxillary posterior teeth and extrusion of maxillary posterior teeth to some extent.
- *Effect of RME on mandible:* Activation results in a downward and backward rotation of the mandible due to extrusion of maxillary posterior teeth.

- Alveolar bone bends buccally due to the compression of periodontal ligament fibers on activation of RME.
- Adjacent cranial bones such as parietal and occipital bones are found to be displaced.
- Activation results in increased intranasal space due to separation of outer walls of the nasal cavity
- Expansion is achieved up to 10 mm with the rate of 0.2–0.5 mm/day.

Hazards, Indications and Contraindications

- Oral hygiene; not so serious threat
- Length of fixation.
- If the oral hygiene is satisfactory, the usual period of up to 4 months where the palate has been covered by the appliance it may become spongy and hemorrhagic but this will return to normal after a few days. In general, a recovery period of 2–3 days only is needed between removal of fixed splints and removable retention appliance.
- Dislodgement and breakage.
- *Tissue damage:* To avoid damage to the deeper tissues, it is advised that the rate of expansion to 0.5 mm per day.
- *Infection:* An invasion of pathogenic organisms in the mouth represents a true hazard in RME, especially if the appliance used consists of cap splints and covers large portions of the palate. Beneath such an appliance, organisms can flourish in perfect incubator conditions and in this event, the appliance must be removed immediately to permit cleaning.
- *Failure of suture to open:* Pain is a symptom of force build-up, which may stem from unyielding maxillae because of midpalatal sutural resistance and general skeletal rigidity. Damage is done, if expansion is carried into the alveolus. For this reason, it is advised that the maxillary centrals not be capped. By leaving them free, they can indicate sutural opening by forming a median diastema. On no account should expansion be that has not been opened. Finally, it should never be forgotten that mid-palatal synostosis has been reported as early as 14 years of age.

BIBLIOGRAPHY

1. Hass. Rapid expansion of the maxillary dental arch and the nasal cavity by opening the mid palatal suture. Angle Orthod 1961;31:73–90.
2. Hass. Treatment of maxillary deficiency by opening the midpalatal suture. Angle Orthod 1968;200–217.
3. James P Moss. Rapid expansion of the maxillary arch. J Clin Orthod 1968;215–223.
4. Spolyar J. A full coverage rapid maxillary expansion appliance, Am J Orthod 1997;219–5.

PREVIOUS YEAR'S UNIVERSITY QUESTIONS

Essay

1. Classify expansion. List out the different ways of expansion and write in detail about quad helix appliance.
2. Write the difference between slow and rapid expansion appliance. Discuss in detail about hyrax appliance
3. Write in detail about hazards, indications and contraindications. Write notes on effect of RME on maxilla and mandible.

Short Questions

1. NiTi expander
2. Indications, advantages and selection of NiTi expander
3. Bonded RME

MCQs

1. *Who is regarded as the Father of expansion appliances?*
   a. Emesson C Angel
   b. Walter Coffin
   c. Andrew Haas
   d. Isaacson   **(Ans: a)**

2. *Who developed the appliance called Coffin spring?*
   a. Emesson C Angel
   b. Walter Coffin
   c. Andrew Haas
   d. Isaacson   **(Ans: b)**

3. *According to Korbs, what are the effects of RME on the maxillary skeletal base?*
   a. In sagittal plane, maxilla rotates in a downward and forward direction
   b. In coronal plane, the two halves of the maxilla rotate away from each other.
   c. Both a and b
   d. None of the above   **(Ans: c)**

4. *How much expansion can be achieved with RME?*
   a. Up to 10 mm
   b. Up to 15 mm
   c. Up to 20 mm
   d. Up to 25 mm   **(Ans: c)**

5. *What is the rate of expansion with RME?*
   a. 0.2–0.5 mm/day
   b. 0.5 mm/day
   c. 1–2 mm/day
   d. 3–4 mm/day   **(Ans: c)**

6. *What is Timm's schedule of activation of expansion screw for the patients aged up to 15 years?*
   a. 90° 2 times in a day
   b. 45° 2 times in a day
   c. 90° 4 times in a day
   d. 45° 4 times in a day   **(Ans: a)**

7. *What is Timm's schedule of activation of expansion screw for the patients aged above 15 years?*
   a. 90° 2 times in a day
   b. 45° 2 times in a day
   c. 90° 4 times in a day
   d. 45° 4 times in a day   **(Ans: d)**

8. *Quad helix is activated by using:*
   a. Three-prong plier
   b. Universal plier
   c. Light wire plier
   d. Adam's plier   **(Ans: a)**

9. *Retention followed by RME should be:*
   a. Not less than 3–6 months
   b. 2–5 months
   c. 5–6 months
   d. Only one month   **(Ans: a)**

15.3 REMOVABLE FUNCTIONAL APPLIANCES

Chapter Outline

- Classification of functional appliances
- Incline plane
- Vestibular screen
- Removable functional appliance—functional regulator

- Activator
- Bionator
- Twin block appliance

DEFINITIONS

By Moyer: Functional appliances are loose removable appliances designed to alter the neuromuscular environment of the orofacial region to improve occlusal development and/or craniofacial skeletal growth.

By Proffit: Functional appliances are appliances which alter the posture of mandible, holding it open or closed and forward or backward.

Functional appliances are appliances which either harnessing the muscular forces or by preventing aberrant muscular forces. Andresen was the first to develop functional orthodontic appliance.

CLASSIFICATION OF FUNCTIONAL APPLIANCES

Functional appliances can be divided into removable functional appliance or fixed functional appliance. Removable functional appliances are further classified into removable tooth-borne functional and removable tissue-borne functional appliances. The fixed functional appliances are tooth borne.

First Classification

All the functional appliances were grouped together, where considered to be a subclass of removable appliance.

Second Classification

Put forth by Tom Graber, when functional appliances were still removable.

Group A: Teeth-supported appliances, e.g. Catalan's, inclined planes, etc.

Group B: Teeth-/tissues-supported appliances, e.g. activator, bionator, etc.

Group C: Vestibular-positioned appliance, e.g. oral screen Frankel, lip bumpers.

Third Classification

With the advent of fixed functional appliances, a third classification evolved.

a. Removable functionals, e.g. activator, Frankel, etc.
b. Semifixed functionals, e.g. Den Holtz, Bass appliance
c. Fixed functionals, e.g. Herbst, Jasper Jumper

Fourth Classification

With the awareness and acceptance of the concept of hybridism by Peter Vig, functional appliances could be further classified as:

a. Classic functional appliances like activator, Catalan's, Frankel, etc.
b. Hybrid appliances like propulsor, double oral screen, hybrid bionators, activators.

A further dimension of active and passive appliances was incorporated and a new system of classification advocated.

1. Tooth-borne passive appliance—also known as myotonic appliances:
   i. Andreson/Harpal activator
   ii. Herren activator
   iii. Woodside activator
   iv. Balters bionator
2. Tooth-borne active appliances—also known as myodynamic appliances:
   i. EOA (elastic open activator) or Klammpt activator
   ii. Bimler appliances
   iii. Modified bionator
   iv. Stockfish appliances
   v. Kinetor
3. Tissue-borne passive appliances, e.g. oral screen, lip plummers.
4. Tissue-borne active appliances—Frankel's appliances

Advantages

- Can be used in mixed dentition
- Very effective in vertical control of increased overbite
- Require minimal chairside adjustment

Disadvantages

- Depends on patient cooperation.
- Precise tooth movement is not possible with functional appliances.
- Treatment duration is prolonged.
- Functional appliances often need two phases to complete the treatment.

Visual Treatment Objective (VTO)

One of the important criteria in case selection for the functional appliance therapy is eliciting a positive visual treatment objective (VTO). VTO is said to be positive, if the profile of the patient improves noticeably when the patient advances the mandible voluntarily to correct the overjet. A negative VTO, i.e. patient whose profile does not improve/worsens on voluntary forward posturing of the mandible, are not good candidates for the functional appliance therapy. In case the profile worsens, then other treatment modalities have to be considered (Fig. 15.84).

INCLINE PLANE

Lower inclined plane was first introduced by Catalan more than 150 years ago. Simplest functional appliance used for the correction of a developing anterior crossbite (Fig. 15.85).

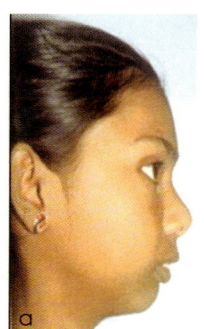
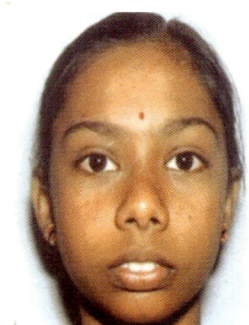
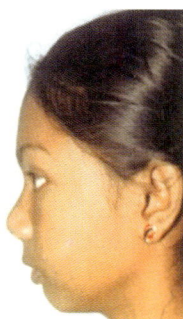
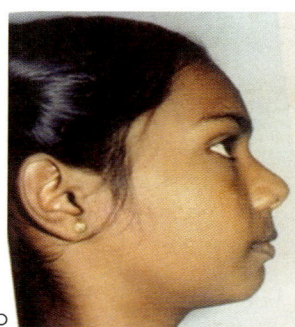

Fig. 15.84: Positive VTO: (a) Before; (b) After

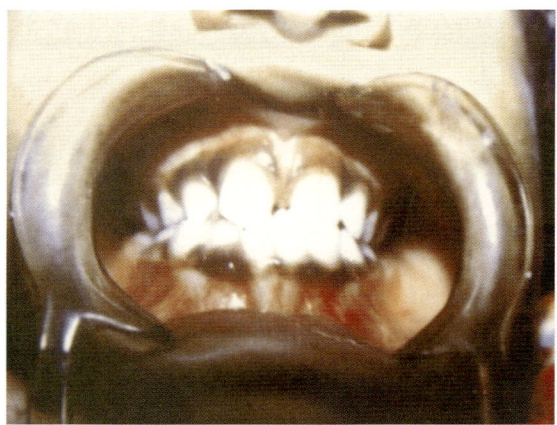

Fig. 15.85: Developing anterior crossbite

It is used on lower anterior teeth. Incisal capping may be processed in acrylic resin or cast in silver alloy and is cemented to lower incisors (Fig. 15.86).

Indications

- Good degree of overbite.
- Sufficient space in the arch (non-extraction case).
- In young patients whose permanent molars have not yet erupted but who have had the deciduous molars extracted and have lost all the molar occlusal contact. In such cases, it is often impossible to obtain fixation or anchorage for a removable orthodontic appliance carrying springs or screws.
- It is to be used only in cases where crossbite is due to a palatally displaced maxillary incisor.

Contraindications

- Crossbite which is due to true mandibular prognathism.
- Where the degree of overbite is less.
- In cases with periodontally weakened teeth.
- When there is lack of sufficient space in the arch.

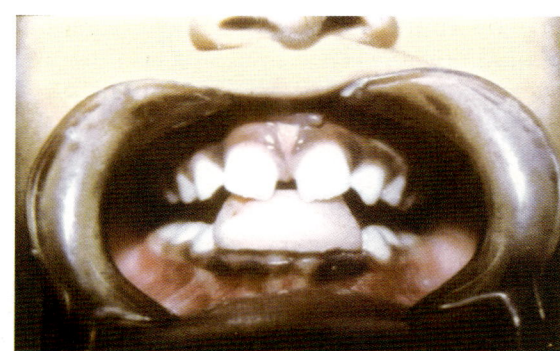

Fig. 15.86: Inclined plane in the mouth

- In cases where crossbite has completely developed and after growth period is complete.
- In cases where there is an end-to-end overbite relationship or an open bite tendency.

Types

- Incisal capping with clasps on lower first permanent molars.
- Incisal capping with clasps on lower first permanent molars and a labial bow.
- Incisal capping with lingual acrylic extension up to the lingual aspect of lower first permanent molar.
- Oppenheim splint: The original Oppenheim splint is fabricated out of vulcanite, with a polished metal incline incorporated on the inclined surface which is in contact with the tooth/teeth in crossbite.

Placement of the incline on the lingually malposed tooth itself:

- Cast incline
- Inclined crown (sved appliance)
- Banded incline

Cemented Type of Inclined Plane (Fig. 15.87)

- Make a working cast from a well extended impression.
- Block out the undercuts present in the anterior region with modelling wax.
- Draw the outline of the inclined plane extending it to take support form at least one tooth on either side of the tooth in crossbite.
- Acrylize the inclined plane using self-curing or autopolymerising acrylic resin.
- After polymerization, complete the finishing and polishing before cementing it onto the teeth.

Angulation of Inclined Plane (Fig. 15.88)

- The steeper the plane, greater the forward pressure on maxillary incisors.

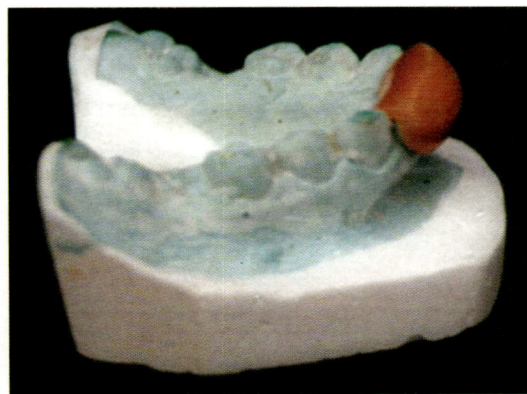

Fig. 15.87: Inclined plane fabricated on model

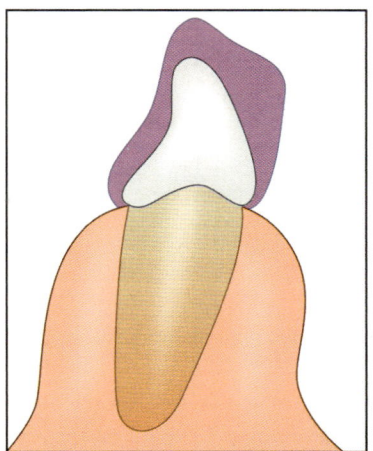

Fig. 15.88: Angulation of inclined plane

- Normally, it should be between 45 and 60°.
- Angulation of less than 45° causes intrusion of the maxillary incisors.
- Angulation more than 45° causes extrusion of the maxillary incisors.

Duration of Treatment

- It takes about 15 days for the correction of crossbite.
- The appliance should be used for a maximum period of 2 to 3 weeks.
- If used for a longer period, the posterior teeth may become supraerupted, and gagging of these teeth may produce an anterior open bite with lack of incisal overbite essential for the retention of the upper incisor in their new position.

Mechanism of Action

- Appliance has contact only in the anterior region where there is crossbite.
- During functional movements like swallowing, due to the lack of contact of the posterior teeth, all the muscle forces are transmitted to the region of contact which guides the teeth to erupt into normal position.

Instructions to Prevent Relapse

- Patient is instructed in the intense use of tongue blade to maintain the crossbite correction and to bring about the normal alignment of the malposed tooth.
- An hour or two a day for 10–14 days following removal of guide plane.
- Use of Barton bandage or vertical pull chins cap assists in keeping teeth in occlusion.
- Orthobite plastic retainer will permit further correction of malposed teeth.

Advantages

- Ease of fabrication
- Rapidity of correction using functional and muscle forces.
- Lack of soreness or looseness of teeth during movement.
- Rarity of relapse.

Disadvantages

- Patient encounters problems in speech during the therapy.
- Patient has to put up with dietary restrictions.
- If the appliance is used for more than 6 weeks, it can result in anterior open bite due to the supraeruption of the posteriors.
- Appliance may need frequent recementation.
- Imperfect alignment of the malposed tooth when the appliance is removed.

VESTIBULAR SCREEN

The vestibular screen or oral screen is a functional appliance introduced by Newell in 1912. It acts as a screen between the teeth and the surrounding musculature. It comes into contact with the most protruding anterior teeth. When the teeth are not proclined, the oral screen does not contact any teeth and it is called a vestibular screen (Fig. 15.89a and b).

Indications

- If the oral screen is indicated in mouth breathing habit, holes should be made in the oral screen so that the child can breathe through the holes.
- In thumb sucking, tongue thrusting.
- It can be used to perform muscle exercises. It helps to strengthen and re-train the hypotonic labial and buccal muscles.
- Developing Class II malocclusion with mild proclination of anterior.

Mechanism of Action

- Oral screen shields off the buccal musculature away from exerting its force during functional movements on the buccal aspect of posteriors. The lingual tongue force acting from within on the posterior teeth is no longer counteracted by the forces of perioral musculature resulting in the expansion of the arches.
- If it is designed to contact the labial surface of proclined incisors only, then the forces of perioral musculature are transferred onto it and help in bringing about the retraction of anterior teeth.

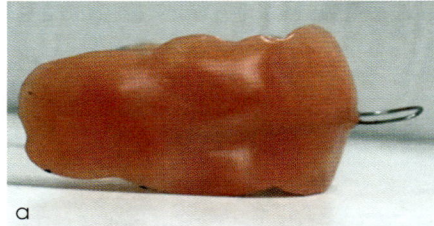

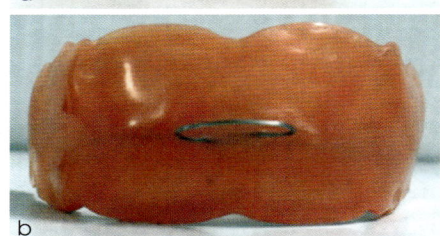

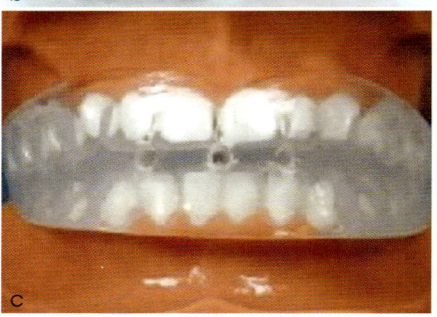

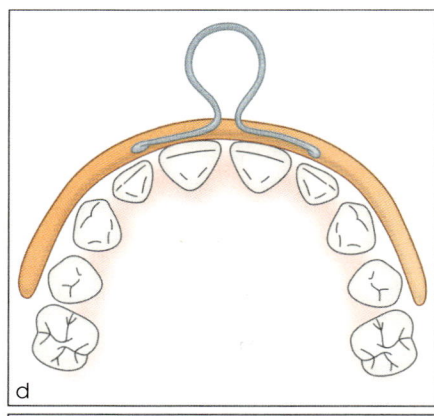

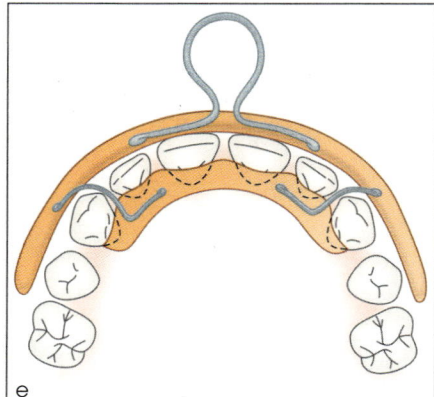

Fig. 15.89: (a and b) Vestibular screen; (c) Oral screen for mouth breather where holes are given in the oral screen; (d) Oral screen; (e) Double oral screen

Steps in Fabrication of Oral Screen

- Upper and lower impressions are made and casts are poured.
- If there is mild proclination of anterior, the construction bite is built by advancing the mandible to the desired level so that Class II molar relationship is also corrected.
- The upper and lower casts are seated with thin wax sheet on the occlusal surface in normal intercuspation.
- A single sheet of modeling wax to be used as a spacer is adapted onto the labial and buccal surfaces of teeth extending well into the functional depth of the sulcus. Frenum relief should be given. Posteriorly the spacer should extend up to the mesial half of the buccal surface of the last erupted tooth.
- A window is cut and wax relief is remved to expose the incisal one-third of the teeth. This makes the acrylic screen come into direct contact with the most proclined incisors.
- The appliance is fabricated and finishing should be done to check for the fit of the appliance.

Clinical Management

The patient is instructed to wear the appliance fulltime at nights and minimum of 3–4 hours during the daytime. The patient is asked to close the lips tightly to maintain the proper lip seal.

Modifications of Oral Screen

- *Hotz modification:* It is fabricated with ring projecting between the upper and lower lips on the labial side to aid in carrying out muscle exercises.
- Another modification of Hotz of oral screen includes incorporating an acrylic projection or wire extending onto the lingual aspect to keep the tongue away in cases of open bite.

Double oral screen is recommended by Kraus in case of tongue-thrusting habit, an additional screen is placed on the lingual aspect of teeth. This additional screen is attached to the vestibular screen by means of a 0.9 mm stainless wire that runs through the bite in the lateral incisor region (Fig. 15.89e).

In case of mouth breathing, the number of holes should be made in the oral screen initially. The holes are gradually closed once the mouth-breathing habit is corrected (Fig. 15.89c).

REMOVABLE FUNCTIONAL APPLIANCE— FUNCTIONAL REGULATOR (FR)

Function regulator appliances were developed by Rolf Frankel (Germany). According to him, the buccinator mechanism and orbicularis oris have a major role in the development of skeletal and dentofacial deformities. Hence, he developed FR as orthopedic exercise device to aid in the maturation, training and reprogramming of the orofacial neuromuscular system.

Frankel Philosophy

1. *Vestibular area of operation:* Shields of the appliance extend to the vestibule and this prevents the abnormal muscle function.
2. *Sagittal correction via tooth-borne maxillary anchorage:* Appliance is fixed on the upper arch by grooves mesial to the first permanent molar and distal to the canine in the mixed dentition period. Presence of the lingual pad acts as proprioceptive stimulus and helps in the forward posturing of the mandible.
3. *Differential eruption guidance:* FR is placed on the upper teeth. Lower posterior teeth are free to erupt and their unrestricted upward and forward movement contributes to both vertical as well as horizontal correction of the malocclusion.
4. Periosteal pull by buccal shields and lip pad exerts the periosteal pull which helps in bone formation and lateral expansion of the maxillary apical base.
5. *Minimal maxillary basal effect:* Downward and forward growth of maxilla seems to be restricted even though lateral maxillary expansion is seen.

Frankel hypothesizes that:
Vertical extension of the shields
↓
Stretch on the alveolar mucosa
↓
Subsequent tension produced on the periosteum
↓
New bone deposition occurring on
the lateral borders of alveolus

The appliance can utilize the ability of an erupting tooth to act as a 'matrix' for alveolar growth. Arch expansion is best achieved with this appliance when used before and during the eruption of the canines and premolars.

Mode of Action

1. Increase in transverse and sagittal directions by use of buccal shields and lip pads.
2. Increase in vertical direction by supraeruption of lower teeth.
3. Muscles adaptation by form and extension of the buccal shields and lip pads along with the prescribed exercises corrects the abnormal perioral muscle activity.

Classification of FR

It has been listed in Table 15.3.

Table 15.3: Classification of FR	
Types	Indications
FR I	• Used for Class I and Class II division 1
	• FR Ia—used for Class I moderate crowding and deep bite (Fig. 15.96a)
	• FR Ib- used for Class II division 1 overjet less than 7 mm (Fig. 15.96b)
	• FR Ic-used for Class II division 1overjet more than 7 mm (Fig. 15.96c)
FR II	Used for Class II division 2 and division 1
FR III	Used for Class III
FR IV	Used for cases with open bite and bimaxillary protrusion
FR V	FR with headgear

Steps in Fabrication

- Impression
- Construction of wax bite
- Trimmimg the casts
- Placement of seating grooves/notching the teeth (Figs 15.91 and 15.92)
- Mounting the casts
- Wax relief (Fig. 15.93)
- Fabrication of the appliance

Construction Bite (Fig. 15.90)

For minor sagittal problems, the construction bite is taken in an edge-to-edge incisal relationship.

In case of severe retrognathism, the mandible should be brought into edge-to-edge bite about 4 to 6 mm with vertical clearance of 2.5 to 3 mm while registering the bite for FR I and FR II.

While construction the bite for FR III, the mandible should be in the most retruded position with 1 to 2 mm vertical clearance.

Trimming of cast is done in the following regions (Figs 15.91 and 15.92)

1. Maxillary tuberosity region

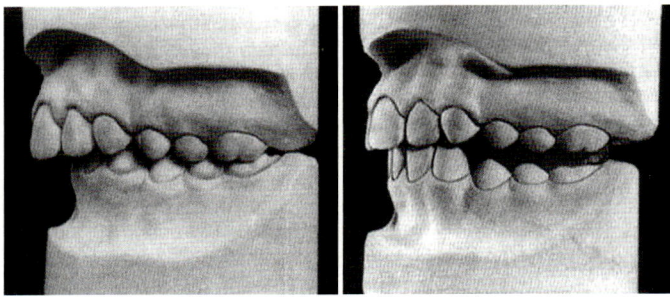

Fig. 15.90: Construction bite

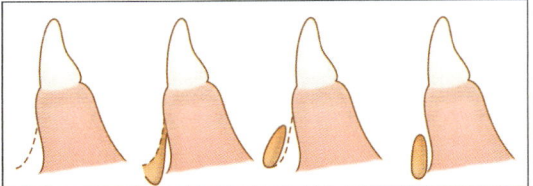

Fig. 15.91: Sulcus trimming and position of lower lip pad

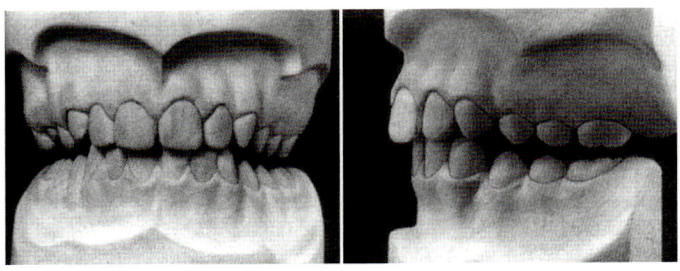

Fig. 15.92: Properly carved working models

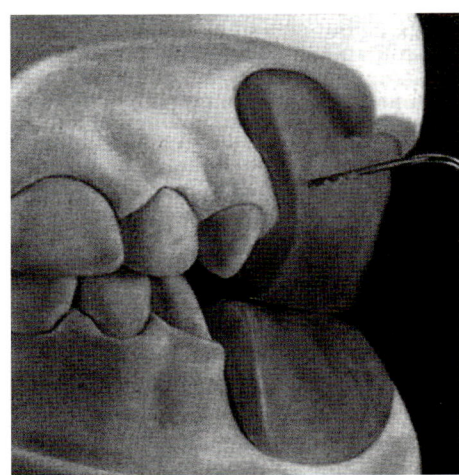

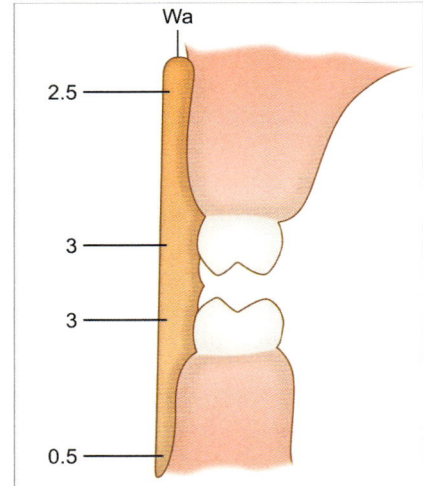

Fig. 15.93: Wax padding under the buccal shield to allow for dentoalveolar expansion

2. Maxillary first premolar or first deciduous molar area anterior to buccal frenum
3. Mandibular pad region
4. Maxillary lip pad region

Separation and Seating Grooves

Space has to be provided for the passage of the wires of lingual bow, canine clasp and the palatal bow in order to allow proper seating of the appliance and to provide intermaxillary anchorage. This can be done by using heavy elastic separators or by cutting seating grooves/notching the teeth.

Before making the impressions, elastic separators are placed in the maxillary canine—first deciduous molar embrasure and in the deciduous 2nd molar—first permanent molar embrasure. There should be sufficient separation for the seating of the crossover wires. If necessary, slicing of the deciduous teeth at the contact points can be done to create the required space (Fig. 15.94).

Components of FR

- Acrylic
- Wire components
- Buccal shield
- Lip pads
- Lingual shield

Acrylic Components

Vestibular or Buccal Shield

Buccal shields are located in the vestibular area buccal to the posterior teeth. The shields should well extend deep into the sulcus up to the tolerance limit of the patient. The buccal shields should be in contact with the buccal surfaces of posterior teeth if expansion is not desired. If expansion is desired, the buccal shields

should be shielded off from the dentoalveolar structures by providing wax relief during fabrication.

Purpose of vestibular shield: The vestibular shield eliminates restrictive force of the perioral musculature on the dentition and brings about the expansion of dental arches due to outward thrust of tongue pressure. It trains the cheek musculature to a more relaxed level of tonicity.

The shields which are extended in the region of first premolar and maxillary tuberosity area stretch the periosteum and cause tension and result in the deposition of bone along the lateral aspects of maxilla.

Lower Lip Pad (Fig.15.95)

The lower lip pad assembly has two acrylic pads, rhomboidal in shape.

- It is located 5 mm from greatest curvature of alveolar base to ensure optimum extension.
- Lower relief should be 12 mm below gingival margin.

FR-I Appliance

1. ***FR-Ia:*** It is indicated in treating Angle's Class I malocclusion with deep bite.
2. ***FR-Ib:*** It is indicated for Angle's Class II division 1 where the overjet does not exceed 5 mm.
3. ***FR-Ic:*** Indicated for treating cases of Angle's Class II division 1 and Class II division 2 (Fig. 15.96)

FR-II Appliance

Wire Components (Figs 15.97 and 15.98)

1. ***Labial bow:*** The labial bow used for FR II is a passive type and it runs in the middle third of the labial surface of the maxillary incisors. The labial bow turns gingivally at the right angle from the distal margin of the lateral incisor. The labial bow should be bent

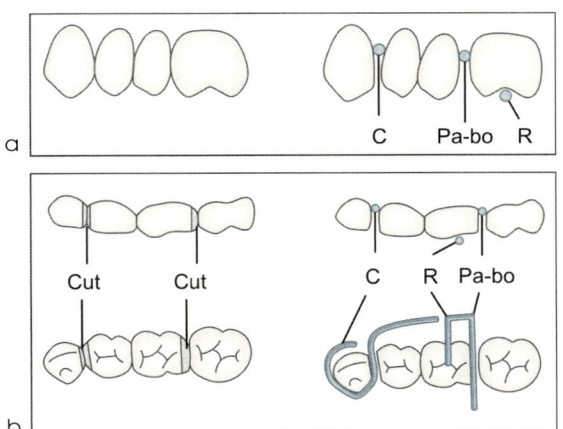

Fig. 15.94a and b: Seating grooves are cut in the maxillary model in FR I and FR II in the permanent dentition

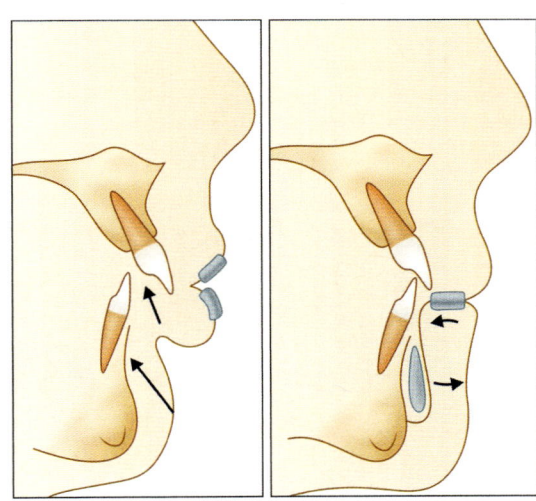

Fig. 15.95: Lip pads

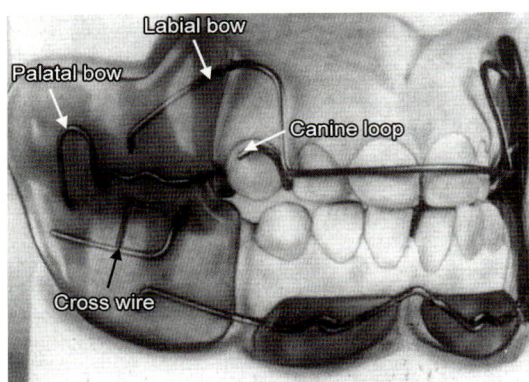

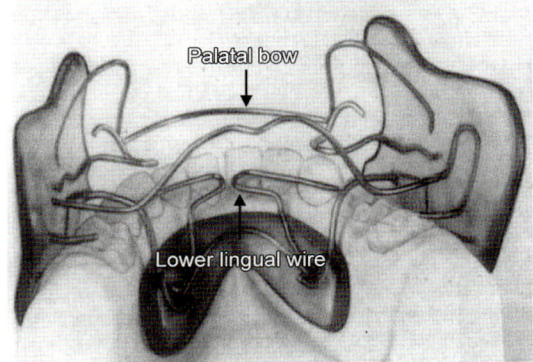

Fig. 15.96a: FR-Ia

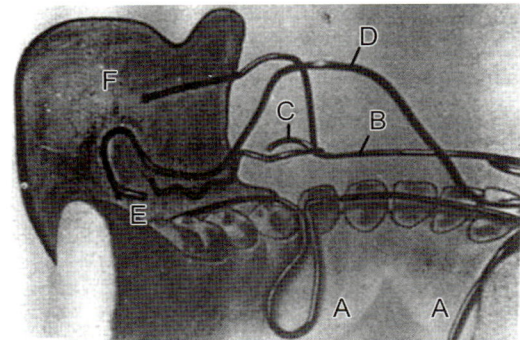

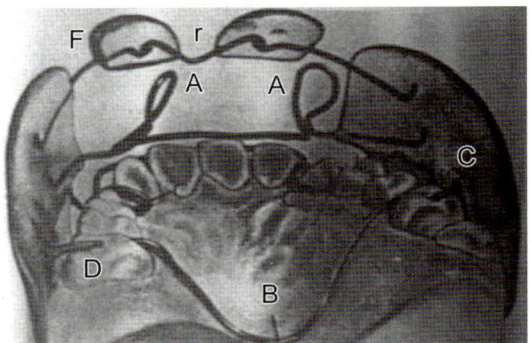

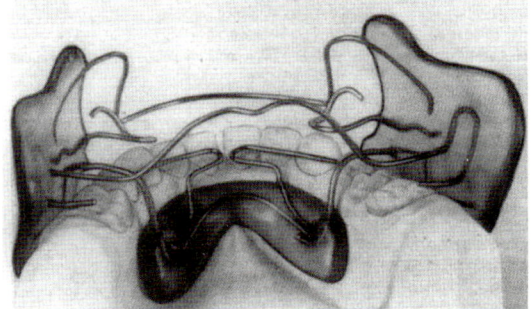

Fig-15.96b: FR-Ib

in an ideal contour and not in the contour of malaligned teeth, and then it ends in the vestibular shield on either side.

2. *Canine extensions:*
   a. Canine extensions are also called canine guards.
   b. Loop of the canine extensions hooks to the distal surface of the canine and extends distally about 2–3 mm away from the buccal surface of canine and ends in the vestibular shield.
   c. They are two in number one on right permanent canine and another on left permanent canine.

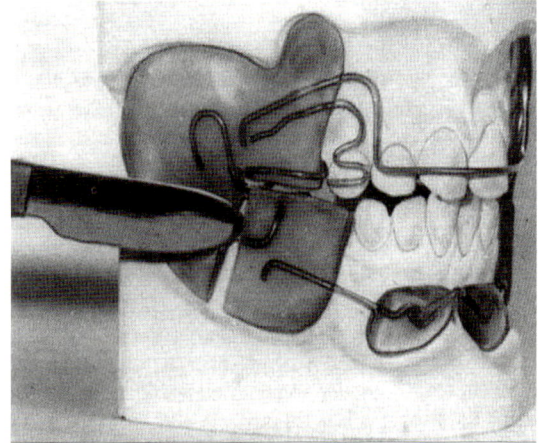

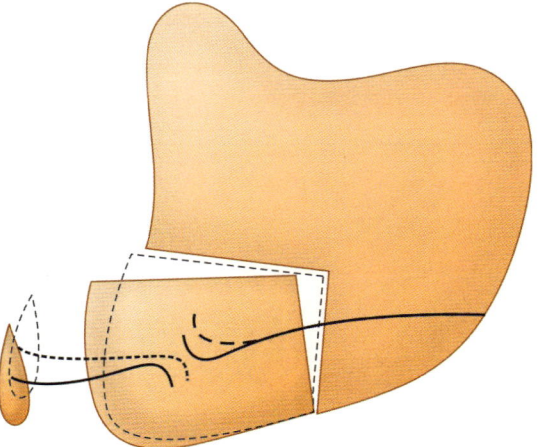

Fig. 15.96c: FR-Ic

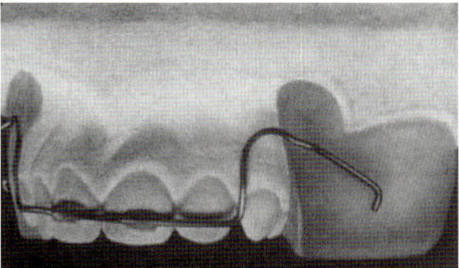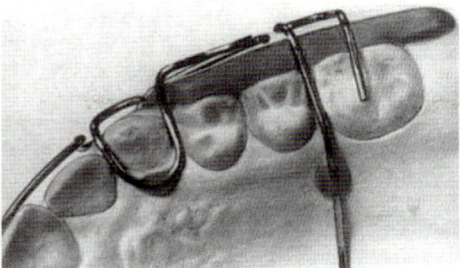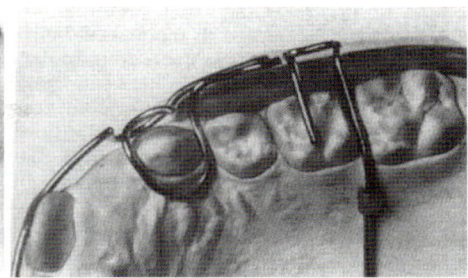

Fig. 15.97: Correct position of wires on the maxillary work model

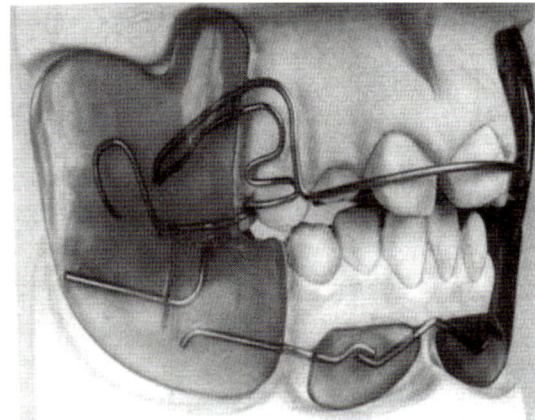

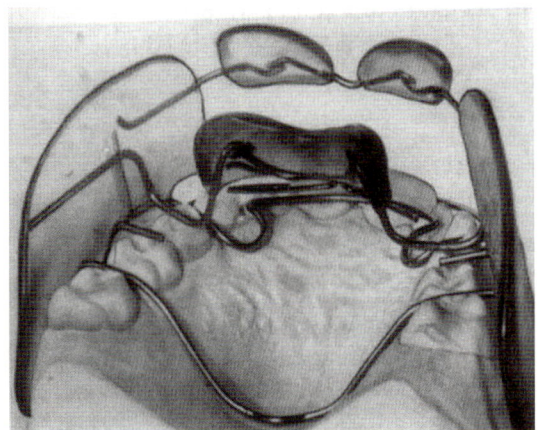

Fig. 15.98: FR-II

d. They help in the elimination of restrictive muscle function and helping in transverse development in the canine region.

3. *Palatal bow:* It should follow the curvature of the palate and should have a clearance of 2–3 mm between the bow and the palatal tissue. Lateral extensions of the bow cross interdentally between mesial to first permanent molar and distal to the second permanent premolar and enter the acrylic buccal shield. The recurved ends of the bow terminate as occlusal rest on the buccal surface between the mesiobuccal and distobuccal cusps of first permanent molar. Similarly palatal bow transverses on another side of the same arch.

4. *Upper lingual wire:* It is also called lingual stabilizing wire or protrusion bow. The wire prevents tilting of maxillary incisors. It is a sort of labial bow fabricated on palatal surface of maxillary anterior teeth. It orginates from vestibular shield and reaches palatal surface by passing distal to canine. The loop is fabricated on canine, then passes on the palatal surface of anterior teeh at the level of the cingulum till it reaches distal marginal ridge of other side lateral incisor and then another loop is fabricated. The distal arm of the loop enters the vestibular shield by passing through the distal surface of another canine.

5. *Lingual crossover wire:* Lingual crossover wire follows the contour of the lingual mucosa 3–4 mm below the lingual margin of the mandibular incisors.

6. *Lower lingual springs:* They are also called so because they are made to rest on the lingual surface of the mandibular anterior teeth and they are used to prevent the supraeruption of lower incisor and also to procline the lower anteriors, when the lower anteriors are retroclined.

7. *Support wire of lip pads.*

Treatment Effects Produced by FR II

1. *Effects on dentoalveolar development:*
   a. The cheek is held away from the dentition by the vestibular shield.
   b. The tongue becomes relatively more of a force because the counterbalancing force of cheek musculature is shielded.
   c. This effect is a result of the vertical extension of the vestibular shields.

2. *Effects on skeletal growth:*
   a. Correction of malocclusion
   b. Increases in the mandibular length
   c. Increased posterior facial height (ramus length)
   d. Facial axis angle is closed

e. A more horizontal vector of facial growth
f. Increases in lower anterior facial height
g. Dental arch expansion

FR III Appliance

FR III has two upper lip pads. The lip pads are teardrop shaped, larger and more extended than the lower pads of FR II. The purpose of lip pads is to eliminate the restrictive pressure of lip on the underdeveloped maxilla. They also exert tension on the tissues and periosteal attachments in the depth of the sulcus to stimulate bone growth. The buccal shields stand away from the maxillary posterior dentoalveolar structure by about 3 mm but are made to contact with the mandibular apical bone. They serve to eliminate the buccinators muscle force and also cause a periosteal pull leading to bone growth. Protrusion bow is seen behind the upper incisors to stimulate forward movement of these teeth (Fig. 15.99a to c).

FR-IV Appliance

The FR IV is used for correction of open bites and bimaxillary protrusion. Its use is almost exclusively restricted to mixed dentition. The FR IV has the same vestibular configuration as FR I and II. It lacks canine

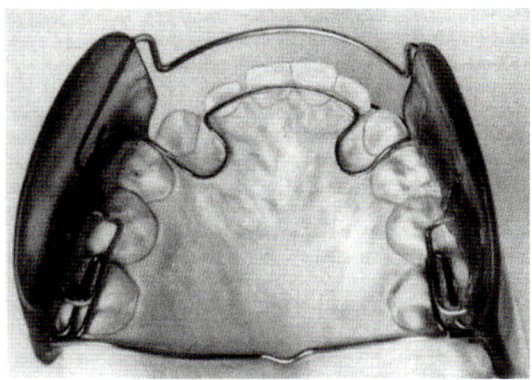

Fig. 15.99c: Palatal bow and occlusal rest in FR-III

loops and protrusion bows. It consists of IV occlusal rests on the maxillary first molars and first deciduous molars to prevent tipping of the appliance. The palatal bow is like in FR III placed distal to last molar.

It consists of lower labial pad and buccal shields, upper labial bow, four occlusal rests and palatal bow (Fig. 15.100).

FR V Appliance

This FR V incorporates headgear. The appliance consists of posterior acrylic bite blocks to prevent molar eruption due to the action of elevator muscles of mandible. They are indicated in patients with long face

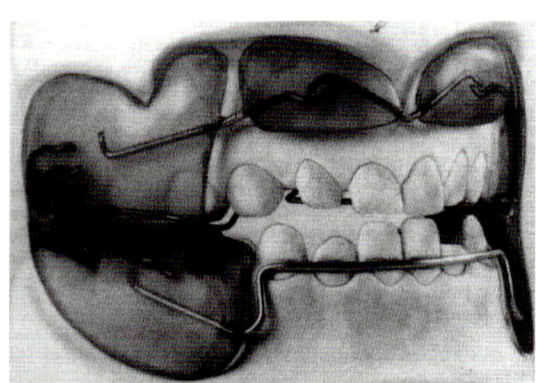

Fig. 15.99a: FR-III

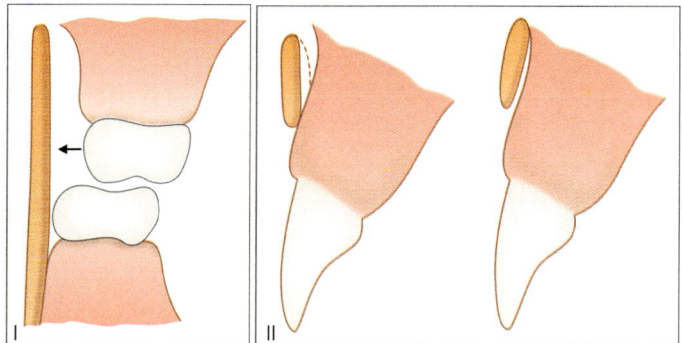

Fig. 15.99b: I. Buccal shield in FR-III; II. Lip pads in FR-III

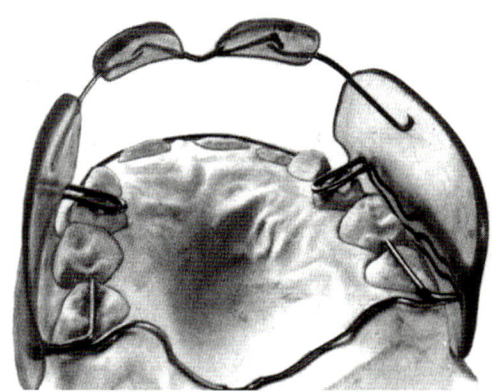

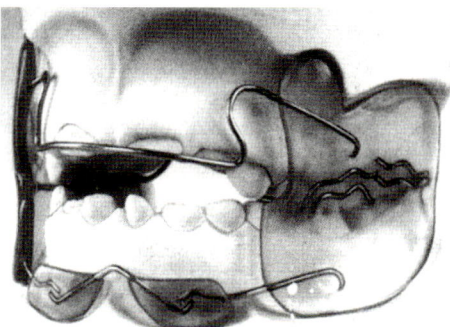

Fig. 15.100: FR-IV

syndrome having high mandibular plane angle and vertical maxillary excess.

ACTIVATOR

Norman Kingsley used vulcanite plate with the anterior inclined plane and introduced the term and the concept of 'Jumping the bite' in 1879 which influenced the development of functional jaw orthopedics.

Hotz used modified Kingsley plate or 'Vorbiss plate' in cases of deep bite retrognathism.

Pierre Robin devised an appliance called *monobloc* consisting of a single block of upper and lower appliance. The present activator was originally developed by **Viggo Andresen of Denmark** in 1908. He developed a loose-fitting appliance. It was termed as activator due to its ability to activate muscle forces. It is also known as Andersen appliance or Norwegian appliance (Fig. 15.101). Since Norwegian screw is incorporated in the activator for expansion of arches, it is called Norwegian appliance. It is also called noctournal appliance.

- Impressed by Kingsley ideas, Viggo Andresen developed a mobile loose fitting appliance that transferred functioning muscle stimuli to the jaws, tooth and supporting structures. He made a modified Hawley type of retainer on the maxillary arch to which he added a lower lingual horseshoe-shaped flange which helped in positioning the mandible forward.
- Used as retainer for his daughter to wear while at summer camp. On her return three months later, he found and was surprised to see improvement in sagittal jaw relationship.

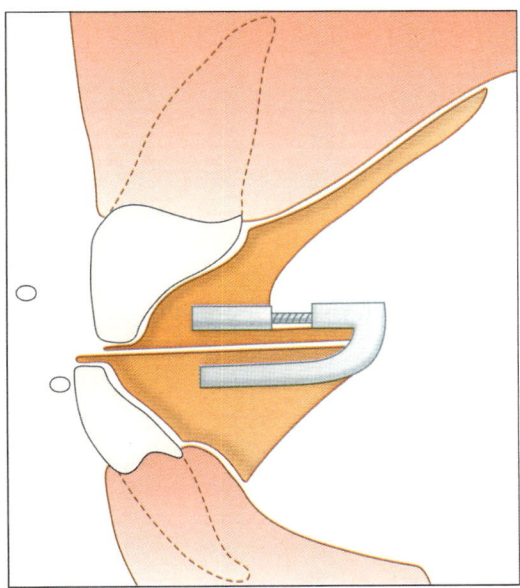

Fig. 15.101: Norwegian screw

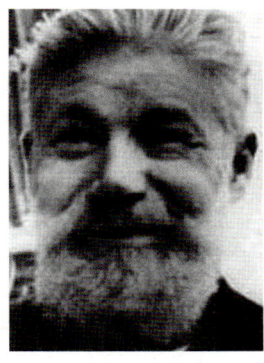

Viggo Andresen

- When Andersen moved from Denmark to Norway, he got associated with Haupl, at Oslo University
- Haupl became convinced that the appliance-induced growth changes in physiologic manner and stimulated or transformed the natural forces with an intermittent functional action transmitted to jaw, teeth and investing tissues.
- They called it as activator because of its ability to activate the muscle forces.
- According to Haupl, goal of activator is to help patient achieve optimal size of mandible consistent with morphogenetic pattern.
- Activator cannot create a large mandible from small one.

Synonyms

- Biomechanic working retainer
- Andersen appliance
- Nocturnal airway patency appliance
- Norwegian appliance
- Monobloc
- Kingsley or bite jumping appliance

Andresen and Haupl Concept

- According to Andresen and Haupl, the bite is not opened beyond the postural rest position (i.e. no more than 4 mm).
- Forward positioning of mandible induces myotactic reflex actively and isometric muscle contraction

| These muscle contraction forces are transmitted by the appliance to move the teeth. | Stimulate the LPM and retrodiscal pad thus bring about bone remodeling and condylar adaptation. |

Thus, activator relies mainly on the muscle activity during biting and swallowing and thus works by using kinetic energy.

Concept of Viscoelastic Property

- The concept was to overcome the drawback of previous theory.
- If the mandible opens beyond the 4 mm limit, the appliance does not work in the manner Anderson and Haupl had suggested.

- Clasp-knife reflex is initiated that builds up potential energy.
  - Herren overextends in the sagittal plane moving mandible into anterior crossbite position.
  - Woodside opens as much as 10–15 mm beyond the postural rest position.

Viscoelastic Activity

Viscoelastic Reaction

- Emptying the vessels
- Pressing out of interstitial fluid
- Stretching of fibers
- Elastic deformation of bone
- Bioplastic adaptation

Types of Activator

- *Class II activator:* In Class II division 1 and Class II division 2 malocclusion after aligning incisors
- *Class III activator:* Class III malocclusion and open bite cases

Over the years, various modifications have been made to the original design of Andresen's appliance such as:

- The bow activator of AM Schwarz
- Wanderer's modification
- The propulsor
- Cut out or palate free activator
- The reduced activator or cybernator of Schmuth
- Kawetzky modification
- Herren's modification of the activator

Disadvantages

- It requires good patient cooperation.
- Perfect finishing is not possible with activator and it should be followed by fixed appliance therapy.
- Pretreatment fixed appliance is needed in case of lower anterior crowding.
- Activator acts in backward and downward rotation of the mandible. Thus, activators are contraindicated in patients with already excessive lower facial height.
- It is bulkier.
- Patients cannot wear it fulltime. It is indicated in night only.

Effects produced by activator are categorized into following two categories: Dental and skeletal changes.

Dental Changes

a. *Incisor changes:* The overjet and overbite are reduced by retroclination of upper incisors and proclination of lower incisors.

b. *Vertical molar changes:* The design of the activator permits removal of occlusal acrylic above the lower molar and premolars. This facilitates upward and forward eruption of the lower molars and makes the activator a logical choice for low Angle Class II division 1 where there is a need for the molars to be free to erupt into the freeway space.

c. *Upper molars expansion:* The activator with an incorporated expansion screw produces expansion in the upper molar region.

d. *Changes in lower facial height:* There is an increase in lower facial height by reduction of deep bite.

Skeletal Changes

a. It produces a downward and forward growth of the mandible.

b. Changes on the growth of the maxilla: Upper anteriors retrocline during Andresen wear and point "A" can move distally with the incisor roots. This indicates an apparent maxillary skeletal change where point "A" is used to assess the position of maxilla.

Construction Bite

- In case of large overjet, the forward advancement should be done step-wise in 2 phases instead of full advancement at a stretch.
- Optimally, the vertical opening of the construction bite should be approximately 2 mm in excess of the resting position of the mandible.
- In case of more horizontal advancement, it is called H-activaor. This type of activator is given in severely retruded mandible. The optimal forward movement for recording the bite is half of the maximum distance to which the mandible can move forward during protrusion. It is approximately about 5 mm.
- In case of more vertical opening, it is called V-activator which is given in deep bite cases.
- If the horizontal advancement of mandible is 6 mm, vertical opening should be 2 mm and vice versa.
- In case of Class III, vertical opening of 5 mm and a posterior positioning of about 2 mm is recommended.

Wire Component

The labial bow is fabricated in 0.9 mm stainless steel wire. The labial bow is designed in such a way so that the distal arm of the loop should be adopted close the model. When it is fixed into the constructed wax bite, it should be in the mid-point of thickness of the wax block. The lower capping should be done in order to preserve the advanced position of incisors. If the lower

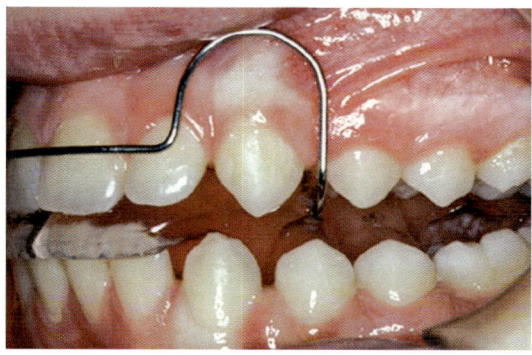

Fig. 15.102: Activator

capping is not done, then the lower labial bow is constructed (Fig. 15.102).

Trimming the Activator for Vertical Control

Intrusion of teeth (Fig. 15.103)

Incisors: Can be achieved by loading the incisal edges of teeth, the labial bow should be below the area of greatest convexity or on incisal third.

Molars: Performed by loading only the cusps. The pits and fossae are cleared to eliminate any possible incline plane effect.

Extrusion of teeth (Fig. 15.104)

Incisors: It requires loading the acrylic above the area of greatest concavity in the maxilla and below this area in the mandible. Although it is not effective, it can be enhanced by placing the labial bow above the area of greatest convexity.

Indicated in open bite problems

Molars: It is done by loading the lingual surface of these teeth above the area of greatest convexity in maxilla and below this area for mandible.

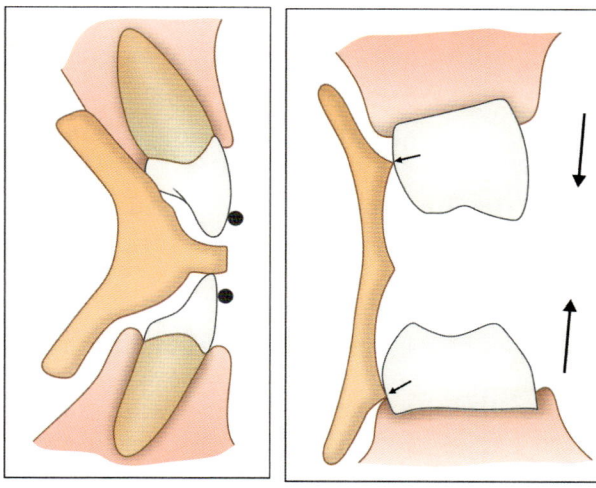

Fig. 15.104: Indicated in deep bite cases

Protrusion of incisors (Fig. 15.105)

Incisors can be protruded by loading their lingual surface and screening lip strain by passive labial bow.
1. Entire lingual surface loaded
2. Incisal third of lingual surface is loaded.

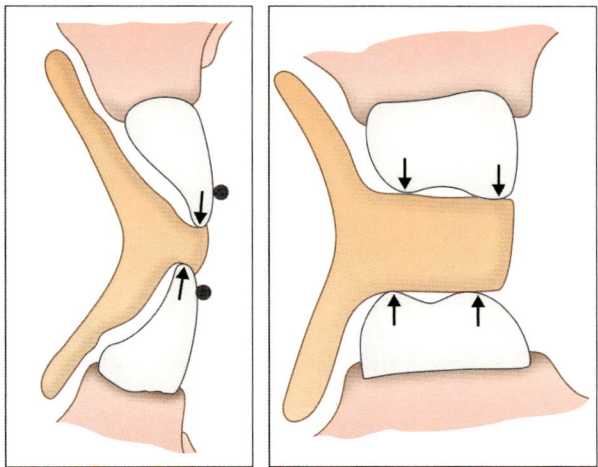

Fig. 15.103: Trimming for intrusion of teeth

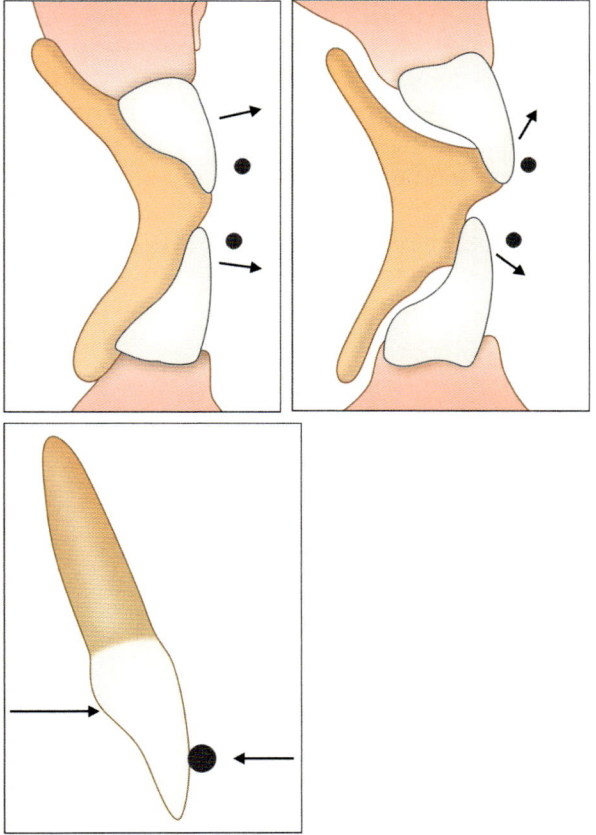

Fig. 15.105: Correction of protrusion of incisors

Retrusion of incisors (Fig. 15.106)
- Acrylic is trimmed from the back of incisor
- Active labial bow is incorporated

Upper (Fig. 15.107): Trimming for upper should be: Distobucco-occlusal direction—DBO.

Lower: Trimming for lower: Mesiobucco-occlusal direction—MBO

BIONATOR

The bulkiness of the activator and its limitation to night-time wear was a major drawback. The appliance is too bulky for daytime wear. Morever, during sleep, the function is minimized. This led to the development of the bionator a less bulky appliance and the palate is free for proprioceptive contact with the tongue and the buccinators wire loops hold away the potentially deforming muscles.

The bionator was developed in Germany by Wilhelm Balter in the early 1950s to increase patient's comfort and facilitate daytime wear to increase the functional use of the appliance. Balter accomplished this by drastically reducing acrylic bulk of the appliance.

Philosophy of Bionator

According to Balters, the equilibrium between the tongue and the circumoral muscles is responsible for the shape of the dental arches and that the functional space for the tongue is essential for the normal development of the orofacial system. He designed the appliance with omega loop to take advantage of tongue posture. Through the bite registration, the forward positioning of the mandible brings the dorsum of the tongue in contact with the soft palate. Thus, the principle of bionator is not to activate the muscles but

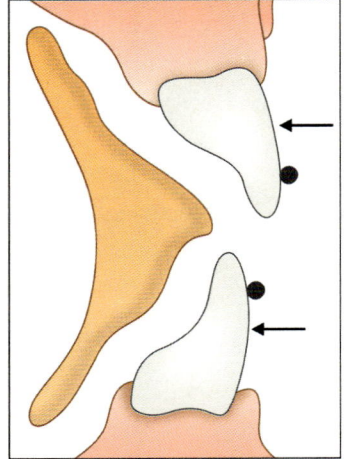

Fig. 15.106: Correction for retrusion of incisor

to modulate the muscle activity, thereby enhancing the normal development of the inherent growth pattern and eliminate abnormal and potentially deforming environmental factors.

Bionator—Types
- Standard appliance
- Bionator for open bite
- Reverse or Class III bionator

Standard Appliance

It consists of a lower horseshoe-shaped acrylic lingual plate extending from the distal of the last erupted molar to the corresponding point on the other side. The appliance has only posterior lingual extensions that cover upper molar and premolar regions. The anterior portion is open from canine-to-canine. The upper and lower parts which are joined interocclusally extend

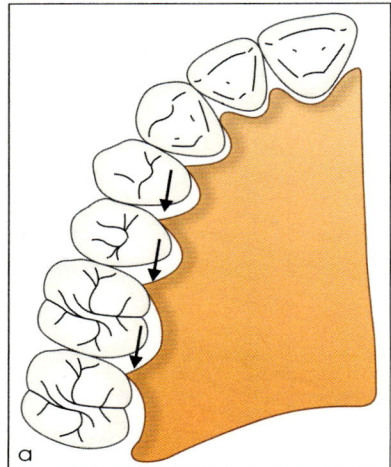
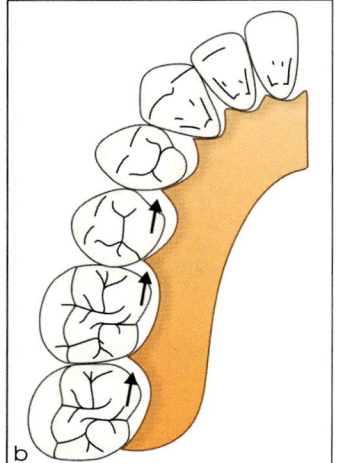
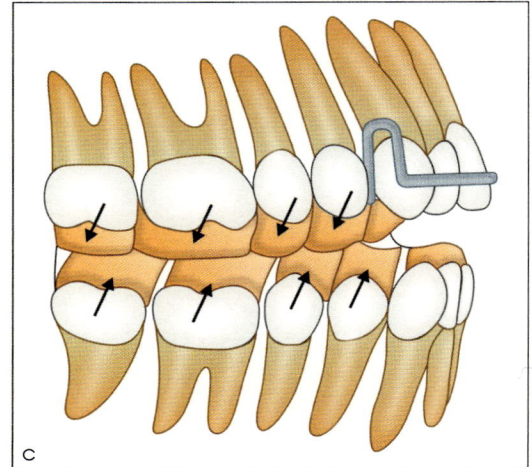

Fig. 15.107: Trimming: (a) Upper—DBO; (b) Lower—MBO; (c) Occlusal

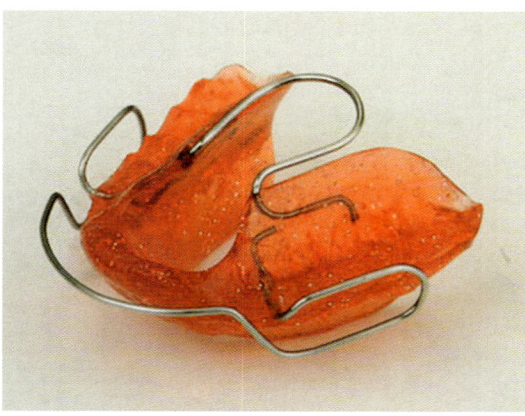

Fig. 15.108: Bionator

2 mm above the upper gingival margin and 2 mm below the lower gingival margin.

The palatal bar is formed of 1.2 mm hard stainless steel wire extending from the top edges of the lingual acrylic flanges in the middle area of the deciduous first molars. The palatal bar forms an oval posteriorly directed loop that orients the tongue and the mandible anteriorly to achieve a Class I relationship.

The labial bow is made from 0.9 mm hard stainless steel. It starts above the contact point between the canine and deciduous upper first molar/premolar. It extends vertically making a rounded 90° bend to the distal along the middle of the crowns of the posterior teeth and extends as far as the embrasure between deciduous second molar and permanent first molar. It then makes a gentle downward and forward curve running anteriorly till the lower canine. From there, it forms a sharp curve extending obliquely till the upper canine, bends to level at approximately the incisal third of the incisors and extends to the canine on the opposite side (Fig. 15.108).

Open Bite Appliance

The construction bite is kept as low as possible with acrylic bite blocks between the posterior teeth to prevent their extrusion. The acrylic portion of the lower lingual part extends up to the upper incisor region as lingual shield to prevent tongue movements. The palatal bar has the same configuration. The labial bow is quite similar with the exception that the wire runs approximately between the incisal edges.

Class III Bionator

The bite is taken in most possible retruded position to allow labial movement of the maxillary incisors and reciprocally a slight restrictive effect on the lower arch. The bite is opened about 2 mm only in the interincisal region.

The palatal bar configuration runs forward instead of posterior direction with the loop extending as far as the deciduous first molar or premolar. The labial bow runs infront of the lower incisors rather than in front of the upper incisor.

Trimming

Terminologies used:
A. *Articular plane:* Extends from the tips of the cusps of upper first molars, premolars and canines to the mesial margin of upper central incisors.
   - Runs parallel to ala-tragal line.
B. *Loading area:* Palatal/lingual cusps of deciduous molars and permanent first molars are relieved in acrylic part of appliance (Figs 15.109 and 15.110).
C. *Tooth bed:* Some parts of loading areas are trimmed away to articular plane. Acrylic surfaces prepared in this manner are termed tooth bed.
D. *Nose:* Interdental acrylic finger-like projections. Act as guiding surface and source of anchorage (Fig. 15.111).
E. *Ledge:* Reduced plastic extension placed only on occlusal third of interdental area is called a ledge (Fig. 15.112).

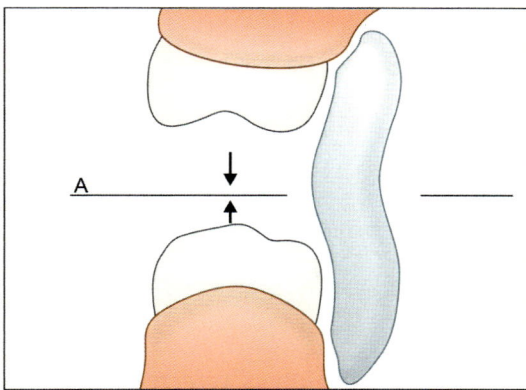

Fig. 15.109: Unloading of upper and lower molars for extrusion

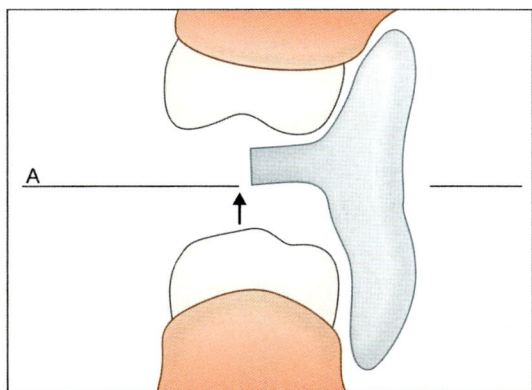

Fig. 15.110: Loading of the upper and unloading of the lower molars

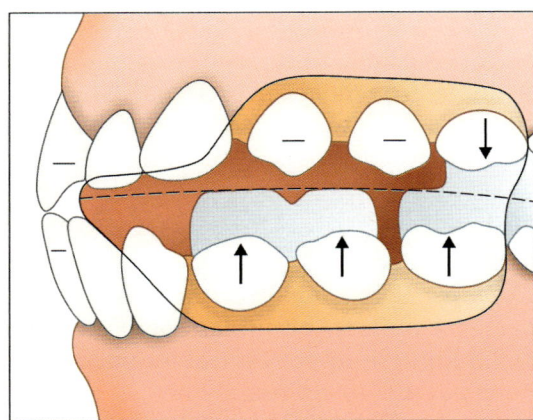

Fig. 15.111: Nose in the molar region

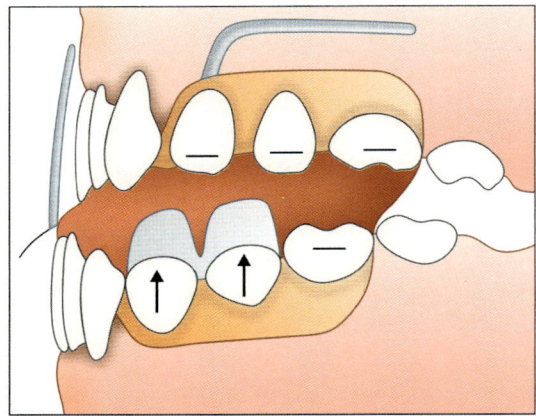

Fig. 15.112: Ledge between premolars

Nose is mostly on mesial margin of first permanent molars, whereas ledge is between premolars, or deciduous molars.

According to Balter

- Simulation of eruption is referred as unloading/promotion of growth.
- Prevention of eruption-loading/inhibition of growth.
- Because of need to anchor the appliance, trimming cannot be performed in all areas at same time. Thus periodic loading and unloading of same area are necessary.

TWIN BLOCK APPLIANCE

The twin block appliance was developed by Clark in 1977 as a two-piece appliance resembling a Schwarz double plate and a split activator. In comparision with other functional appliances, a number of advantages result from using separate upper and lower appliances with occlusal bite blocks. Occlusal inclined plane gives greater freedom of movement in anterior and lateral excursion and causeless interference with normal function.

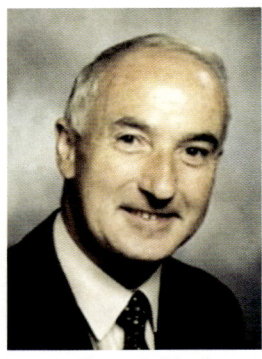

William J Clark

Twin blocks are constructed in protrusive bite that effectively modifies the occlusal inclined plane by means of acrylic inclined planes on occlusal bite blocks. The occlusal inclined plane acts as a guiding mechanism, displacing the mandible down and forward.

Twin blocks are designed for full time wear to take advantage of all functional forces applied to dentition, including the forces of mastication. The bite blocks interlock at 70° angle, usually covering the upper and lower teeth in buccal segments (Fig. 15.113).

The twin block design may be varied to treat individual patient differences in skeletal pattern and dental relationships. A major advantage of twin block is that it may be integrated with fixed, removable and functional jaw orthopedic mechanics for variable, specific, controlled, predictable clinical management and outcome.

- Occlusal forces transmitted through the dentition provide a constant proprioceptive stimulus to influence the rate of growth and trabecular structure of supporting bone.
- The functional appliance therapy aims to improve the functional relationship of the dentofacial structures by eliminating unfavorable developmental factors and improving the muscle environment that envelops the developing occlusion.

Design and Construction

- Tooth- and tissue-borne type of appliance
- Designed to link teeth together as anchor units to maximize orthopedic response.
- Limits tipping and displacement of individual teeth.

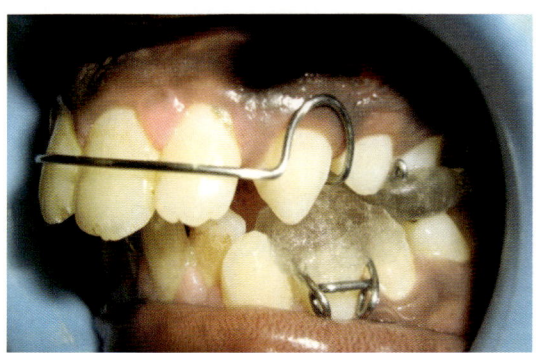

Fig. 15.113: Twin block

Original Design (Fig. 15.114)

- Adam's clasp—upper molars and premolars
- Midline screw
- Upper labial bow (optional)
- Occlusal bite blocks
- Ball clasp on lower incisors
- Springs to move individual teeth (if necessary)
- Provision for extraoral traction (if necessary)
- Method of fixation is most important.
- Adam's clasp—requires routine adjustment.
- Delta clasp (Clark 1985) (Fig. 15.115):
  - Improved retention
  - Minimum adjustments
  - Reduces metal fatigue

Clasps are given according to area of retention:
1. Mesial and distal undercuts
2. Interdental undercut.
- Used on:
  - Upper first permanent molar
  - Lower first premolar
- Ball end clasps
  - Mesial to lower canines
  - Upper premolar
  - Deciduous molar

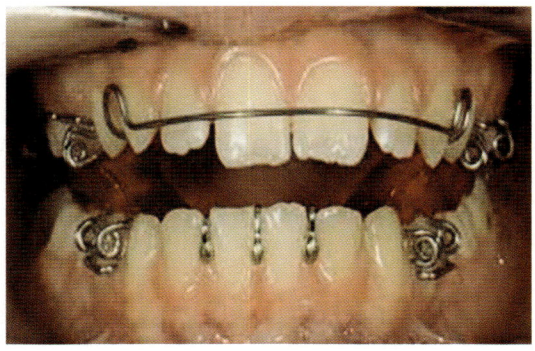

Fig. 15.114: Standard twin block

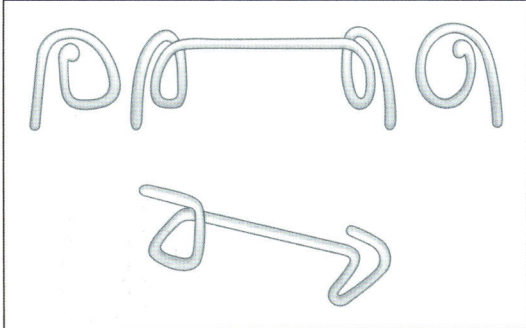

Fig. 15.115: Delta clasp

- C clasp
  - Deciduous molar
  - Canines
- Labial bow—over correction of incisor angulation, acts as a barrier and limits functional correction by mandibular advancement.
- Base plate—two types: Heat-cure and cold-cure material
- Occlusal inclined planes—70°
- Inclined plane on the lower bite block is angled from the mesial surface of the second premolar or deciduous molars.
- Reduce in canine region.
- Upper inclined plane is angled from mesial surface of the upper second premolar.

Bite Registration

- Most important step in the fabrication of the appliance.
- Equal importance for both sagittal and vertical activations.
- Overjet greater than 10 mm—initial activation of 7–8 mm followed by further activation.
- Vertical dimension—blocks should be thick enough to open the bite slightly beyond the freeway space.

Stages of Twin Block

Three stages;
1. Active phase—sagittal and vertical dimensions are established.
2. Support phase—support the corrected position as teeth settle in occlusion.
3. Retention

Active phase: Aim is to correct:
- Distal occlusion
- Overjet
- Overbite
Duration: 6–9 months

Support phase
Aim: To maintain corrected incisor relation until buccal segment occlusion is fully interdigitated.

Duration: 3–6 months

Retention phase
Duration: 9 months.

Management of Deep Bite

- This is achieved by trimming the occlusal block, so as to encourage eruption of the lower molars (Fig. 15.116):
  - Trimming: 1–2 mm/visit

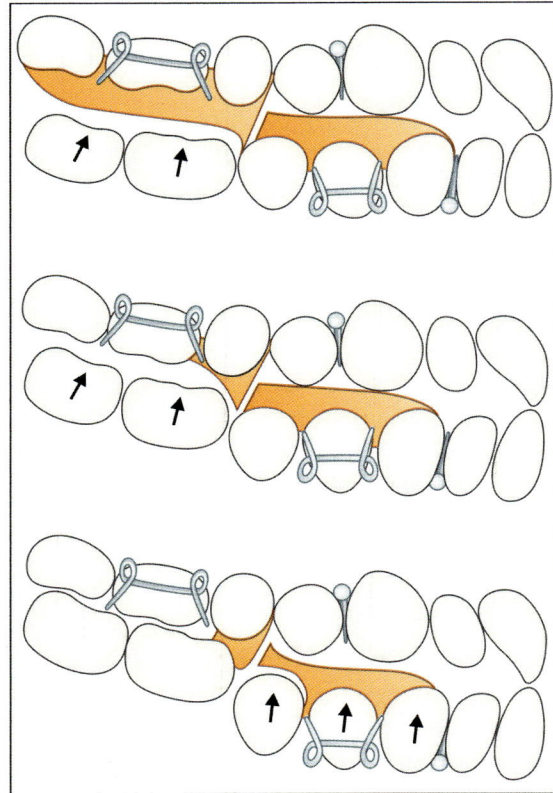

Fig. 15.116: Triming of twin block

– Molars supra erupt 6–9 months
– Triangular wedge shaped area
– Eruption of the premolar
- Intergingival height—used to establish correct vertical dimension.
- Comfort zone: 17–19 mm.
- This is used as a guide to establish the correct vertical dimension during treatment.
- Patients whose intergingival width varies significantly from comfort zone are at greater risk of developing TMJ dysfunction.

Reactivation of Twin Block (Fig. 15.117)

- In case of larger overjet
- Full correction not achieved with initial activation.
- Growth is less favorable (vertical)
- In adult treatment
- In TMJ therapy

Transition Twin Block

Passive eruption of teeth can be time consuming process which taxes both the patient and clinician. It is usually helpful to accelerate treatment and to achieve objectives in the least time. To complete twin block stage I step 3

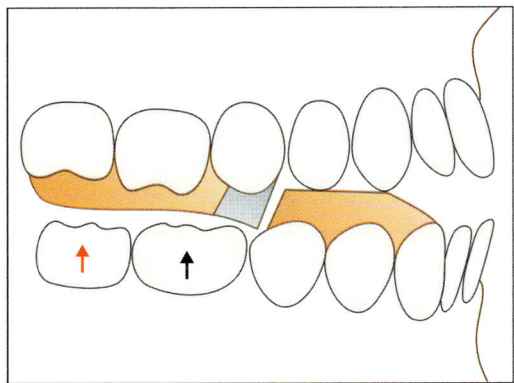

Fig. 15.117: Reactivation of twin block

and stage II objectives more quickly, the author developed the transitional twin block management. It is as follows:

Twin Block Stage I

- *Comfort design:* Patient cooperation is excellent because the tongue has freedom of speech.
- *Segmental mechanics:* Posterior fixed braces. Fixed braces may be placed before of following twin block construction.
- Vertical interarch elastics complete stage I-step 3
- Air rotor slenderizing per need
- Achieve bite stabilization with class I buccal segments with teeth in occlusion

Twin Block Stage II

- Convert stage I upper twin block into stage II support appliance.
- Complete lower fixed braces and archwires to align teeth, level curve of Spee, and close lateral open bite in premolar–cuspid region.

Fixed Braces

- Place fixed on upper anterior teeth
- Archwire to align teeth and close any residual spaces
- Case finishing. In most cases, the final detailing of upper anterior teeth is accomplished with six months of fixed appliances.
- Achieve orthodontic goals.

BIBLIOGRAPHY

1. Dentofacial orthopedics with functional appliance- Graber, Rakosi & Petrovic.
2. Twin Block Functional Therapy- Applications in Dentofacial Orthopedics. William Clark
3. WJ Clark. The twin blocks technique. A functional orthopedic appliance system. AJODO 1988; 93(1):1–18.

4. Turkkahraman H, Sayin MO ; Effects of activator and activator headgear treatment: comparison with untreated Class II subjects. Eur J Orthod. 2006 Feb; 28(1):27–34.
5. Haralabakis NB, Halazonetis DJ, Sifakakis IB; Activator versus cervical headgear: superimpositional cephalometric comparison. AJO 2003; 123(3):296–305.

PREVIOUS YEAR'S UNIVERSITY QUESTIONS

Essay

1. Write about the indications and contraindications of function appliances.
2. Classify functional appliances and write in detail about any one tissue-borne functional appliance.
3. What is growth modulation? Describe the principles on which the functional appliances work.
4. Classify functional appliances and write in detail about activator.

Short Questions

1. VTO
2. Twin block appliance
3. Oral screen
4. Philosophy of bionator
5. Vestibular screen
6. Modifications of activator
7. FR III appliance

MCQs

1. *An example of fixed tooth-borne appliance is:*
   a. Activator
   b. Frankel appliance
   c. Jasper jumper
   d. All of the above   **(Ans: c)**

2. *Who designed the activator?*
   a. Viggo Anderson
   b. EH Angle
   c. Farrar
   d. Hunter   **(Ans: a)**

3. *Activator is also known as:*
   a. Monoblock appliance
   b. Andreson appliance
   c. Both a and b
   d. None of the above   **(Ans: c)**

4. *Where bionator appliance was developed?*
   a. Germany
   b. France
   c. Switzerland
   d. England   **(Ans: a)**

5. *Who developed bionator?*
   a. Wilhelm Balter
   b. Coffin
   c. Pierre Robin
   d. Hapul   **(Ans: a)**

6. *FR-IV appliance of Frankel is indicated in:*
   a. For treating bimaxillary protrusion
   b. For treating open bite
   c. Both a and b
   d. None of the above   **(Ans: c)**

7. *Who developed oral screen?*
   a. Newell
   b. Pierre Robin
   c. Haupl
   d. Andersen   **(Ans: a)**

8. *An example of removable tissue-borne functional appliance is:*
   a. Activator
   b. Frankel appliance
   c. Herbst appliance
   d. All of the above   **(Ans: b)**

15.4 FIXED APPLIANCES

Chapter Outline

- Components of fixed appliance
- Wires
- Brackets
- Springs
- Techniques

William E. Magill was first to band the teeth for active tooth movement. Fixed mechanical appliances are the most common and versatile appliances used in orthodontics. Appliances that are fixed or fitted onto the teeth by the operator and cannot be removed by the patient at will are called fixed appliances. Fixed appliance can bring about varied tooth movements such as bodily movement, rotation, tipping, intrusion, extrusion, etc. all at the same time, if required.

Indications

- Fixed appliances are indicated when precise tooth movements are required.
- Correction of mild to moderate skeletal discrepancies
- Intrusion/extrusion of teeth
- Correction of rotation
- Overbite reduction by intrusion of incisors
- Multiple tooth movements required in one arch
- *Active closure of spaces:* Extraction spaces/hypodontia
- In surgical orthodontics.

Advantages

- Duration of activation is more compared to removable appliances thus the number of visits by the patients is reduced.
- Multiple tooth movements are possible within the given time frame.

- Precise tooth control is possible to move the individual teeth in three planes of space to achieve functional occlusion.
- Need not depend on patient's co-operation.

COMPONENTS OF FIXED APPLIANCE (Flowchart 15.2)

- Active component
- Passive component

Separators

Separators are of two types—**slow** and **rapid.**
- Brass wire separators
- Kesling's spring separator
- Ring separators
- Dumb-bell separators.

Brass Wire Separators (Fig. 15.118)

Soft brass wire of thickness 0.5 mm is passed around the contact and ends are twisted tightly together. The end is cut short and tucked interdentally between the teeth.

Kesling's Spring Separator

This is a spring type separator that effectivley separates the contact area. These are made of 0.016 or 0.018 special plus Australian wire with helices the closed end. The spring consists of coil and two arms. The longer is

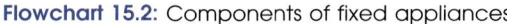

Flowchart 15.2: Components of fixed appliances

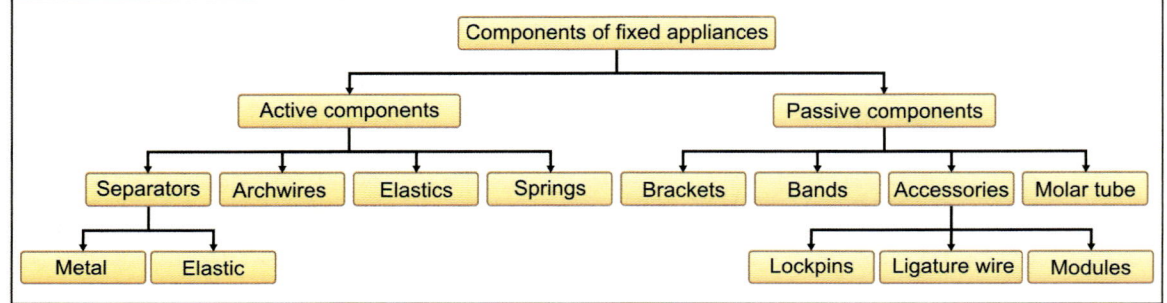

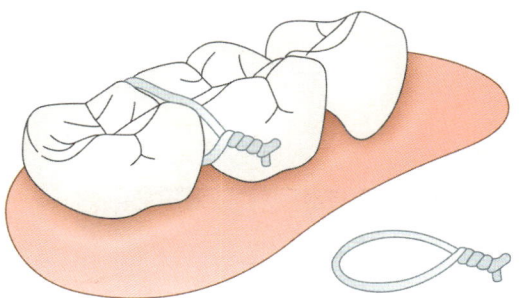

Fig. 15.118: Brass wire separator

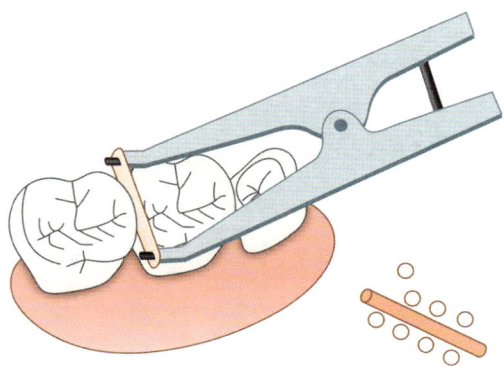

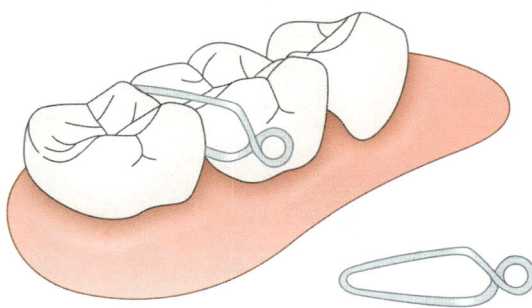

Fig. 15.119: Kesling spring separator

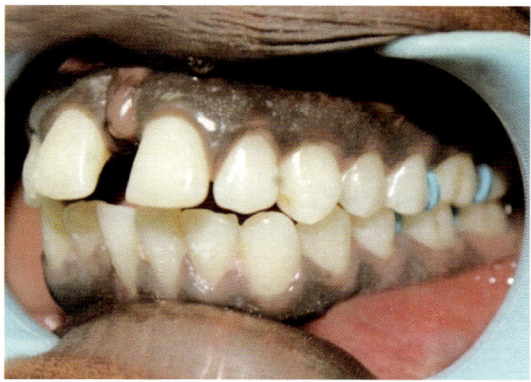

Fig. 15.120: Ring separators

hooked and rests above the contact while the shorter is passed below the contact (Fig. 15.119).

Ring Separators

They are small thick elastic rings that are passed forcibly through the contact using special pliers. The stretched ring encircles the interdental area and teeth are separated (Fig. 15.120).

Dumb-bell Separator

This is elastic type of separator with dumb-bell shape. The elastic is stretched and passed through the interdental contact. The separation is achieved when it tries to regain its shape (Fig. 15.121).

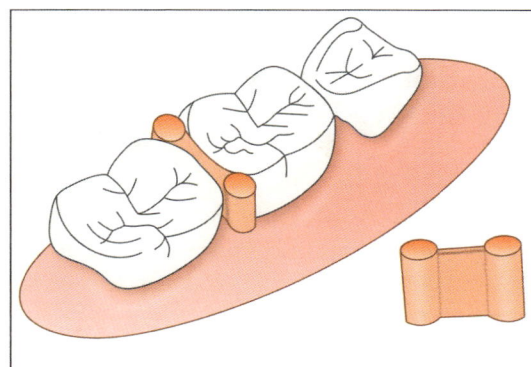

Fig. 15.121: Dumb-bell separator

Elastics and Elastomerics

Celvin case discussed the use of intermaxillary elastics at the Columbia Dental Congress. However, in 1893, Henry A Baker was credited with originating the use of intermaxillary elastics with rubber bands and named it as Baker anchorage.

Elastics are commonly used as active components of fixed orthodontic appliance. They are used in the form of simple elastic rings, elastic chains, elastic threads and elastic modules.

Elastics generate light continuous force for:
- Correction of rotations
- Closure of spaces
- Retracting canines
- Correction of open bite
- Correction of posterior crossbites.

The following are some of the applications of elastics: Elastics can be latex or non-latex. Non-latex deteriorates less than latex in oral environment.

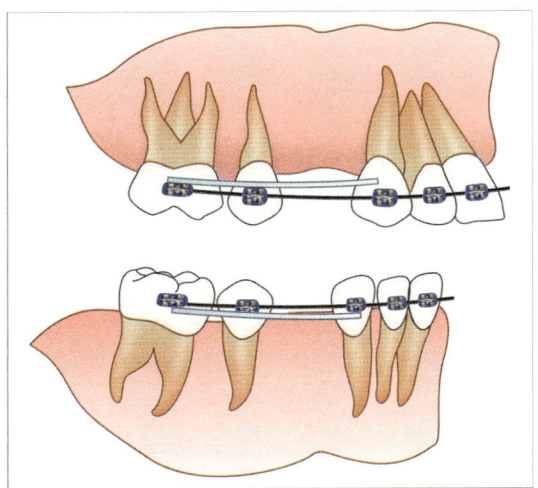

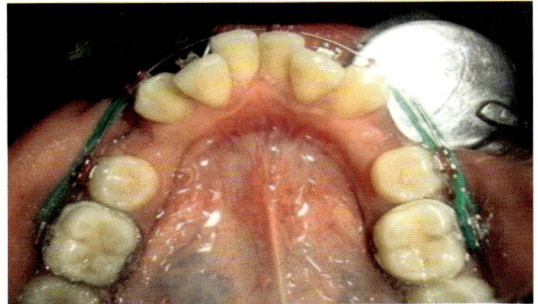

Fig. 15.122: Class I elastics

Different Size Elastics

- 3/16"—X-small—4.76 mm—red color
- 1/4"—small—6.35 mm—blue color
- 5/16"—medium—7.94 mm—yellow color
- 3/8"—large—9.35 mm—pink color

Elastics are made of synthetic latex and of uniform sizes and applying uniform forces when stretched to required length. These elastics come in different sizes of internal diameter and different thickness of their wall. Thinner-walled elastics are called light elastics and thick-walled elastics are called heavy elastics. These elastics exert a force equal to between 60 and 70 gm when they are new and first placed.

Class I Elastics (Fig.15.122)

They are intra-arch elastics stretched between the molars at posterior end and anterior teeth at the other end. They close the interdental spaces, extraction space and retraction of teeth.

Class II Elastics

They are intermaxillary elastics (1 to 2 Oz) stretched between the lower molars and upper anteriors to be worn full time. It is used to retract the upper anteriors. Overbite reduction is more effective with a more distal application of elastic to the molar which better resists distal crown tip and encourage fuller expression of the anchor bends to the anterior segment (Fig. 15.123).

Class III Elastics

They are intermaxillary elastics to bring about mesial movement of upper buccal teeth and retraction of lower anteriors.

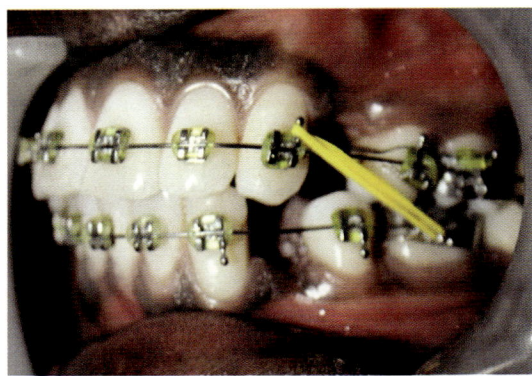

Fig. 15.123: Class II elastics

- It prevents advancement of mandibular incisors
- It advances the maxillary dentition or retract mandibular dentition
- It corrects anterior dental crossbite

Crossbite Elastics

They extend between the palatal surface of upper molars and premolars to buccal surface of lower molars and premolars.

They are worn bilaterally in the case of double posterior crossbite and worn on the abnormal side in the unilateral crossbite. The correction of posterior crossbite is largely due to elastic force (Fig. 15.124).

Box Elastics

They are worn in the form of box between the upper and lower anterior teeth. They are used for correction of open bite. Dental open bite is corrected with fixed appliance either with vertical elastic or triangular elastic or box elastic (Fig. 15.125).

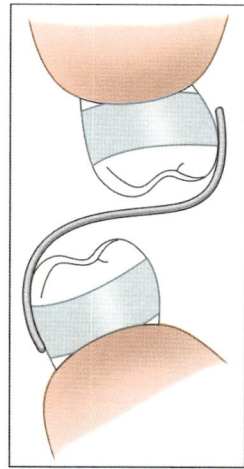

Fig. 15.124: Crossbite elastics

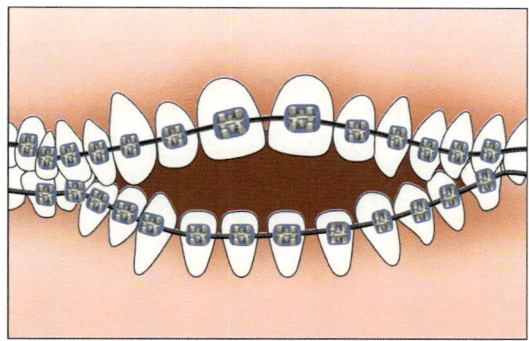

Fig. 15.125: Box elastics

- It is used to improve the overbite relationship of incisor teeth.
- Open bite up to 2 mm may be corrected with these elastics.
- They may extend from the lower lateral incisor to the upper laterals or central incisor teeth or from the lower cuspid to the upper laterals.
- It is used in conjunction with a plain archwire for closing spaces between anteriors. It produces a reciprocal free tipping of anterior crown which closes the space.

Diagonal Elastics

They are used to correct midline deviations.

Settling Elastics

They are used in the final stage of settling the occlusion (Fig. 15.126).

Triangular Elastics

- They aid in the improvement of Class I cuspid intercuspation.

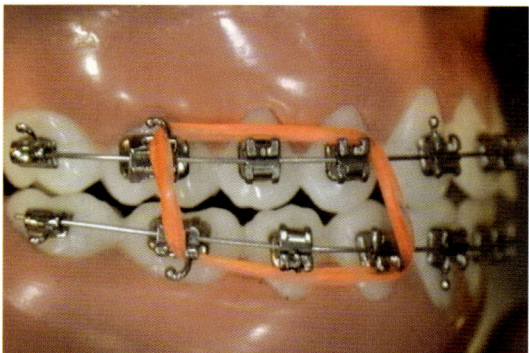

Fig. 15.126: Settling elastics

- They increase the overbite relationship anteriorly by closing open bite in the range of 0.5 to 1.5 mm.
- They extended from upper cuspid to the lower cuspid and first bicuspid teeth.
- They are used for similar reasons of box elastics, but including only 3 teeth.

Up and Down Elastics (Fig. 15.127)

- 'W' with a tail in Class II cases
- 'M' with a tail in Class III cases

Cross-Palate Elastics

This is to correct the undesired expansion of the upper molars during third stage of Begg appliance. This is placed between the lingual aspects of the upper molars. Upper molar expansion during the third stage of Begg appliance is usually bilateral, the cross-palate elastics is appropriate because the force it exerts in pulling one molar lingually is equal and opposite to the force it exerts in pulling the other lingually.

Elastic Chain

They are synthetic polyurethane elastics with inter-connected rings. They are continuous or closed, short and long. They are used to close interdental spaces (Fig. 15.128).

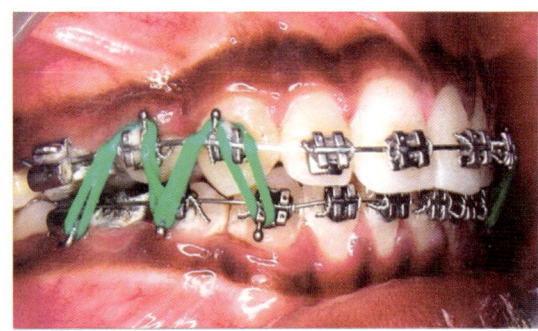

Fig. 15.127: Up and down elastics

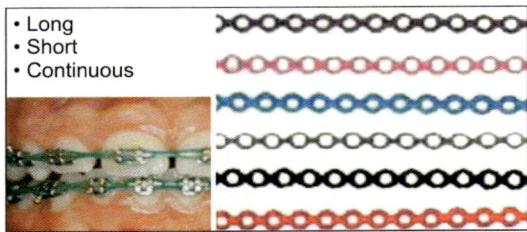

Fig. 15.128: Elastic chain

Elastic Thread

It is used to correct rotations, close spaces. It is inserted under the archwire in a figure of 8 configurations from the canine to premolar and firmly knotted. It is available in long lengths or spools. Elastic thread is obtainable in two different forms:

- Cotton covered
- *Plain uncovered elastic:* The sizes available are 0.625 mm (0.025") and 0.75 mm (0.030").

The cotton covered elastic is easier to knot firmly but become dirty in use. The uncovered elastic remains clean in mouth but with passage of time can loosen.

Elastic Modules

They are used to close the spaces and de rotation of teeth (Fig. 15.129).

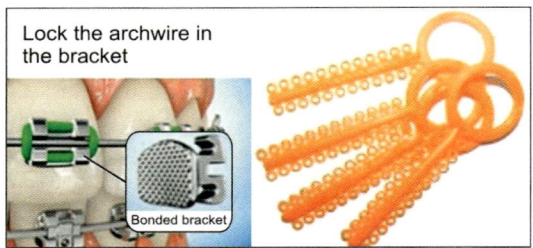

Fig. 15.129: Elastic modules

Open and Closed Coil Springs

They are made up of stainless steel wire or NiTi wire. Coil springs were introduced in orthodontics in 1931.

- *Open coil spring:* It is used for opening the space (Fig. 15.130).
- *Closed coil spring:* It is used for closing space.

Different Ways of Using Coil Springs

- Coil spring is an excellent method of closing upper incisor spaces/central diastema using the force exerted by the reciprocal action of the coil spring.
- Coil spring is compressed between central incisor and canine bracket.

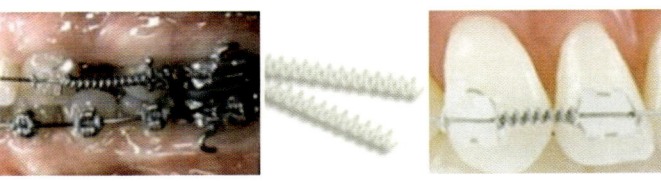

Fig. 15.130: Open coil spring—used to open space

- Coil springs compressed by a tie back ligature:
  a. 3–4 mm length of closed coil spring opened to twice their length then compressed are threaded to the archwire to lie mesial to the cnines (Fig. 15.131)
  b. Using soft SS ligature is placed mesial to springs twisted and tied to premolars
  c. Archwire should be rigid and should fill the slot.

Lingual Attachments

- *Lingual cleat:* It is used for attachments of elastics or elastomerics. It is welded in the middle with ends being open and is available with a mesh base for bonding (Fig. 15.132).
- *Lingual button:* Buttons with variable shaped bases for attachment of elastics or elastomerics. Flat base for centering on molars, curved for mesial or distal placement on molars or extra-curved for use on premolars (Fig. 15.133).

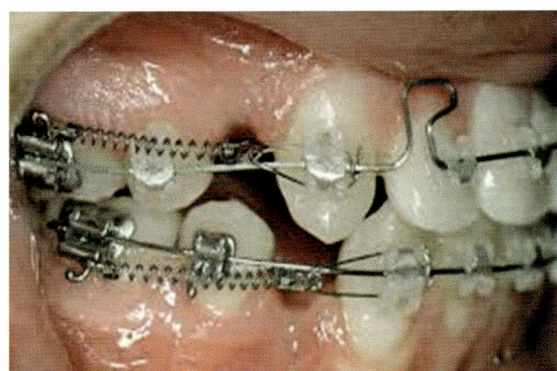

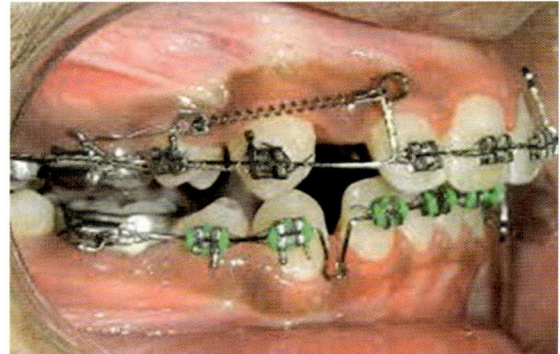

Fig. 15.131: Closed coil spring

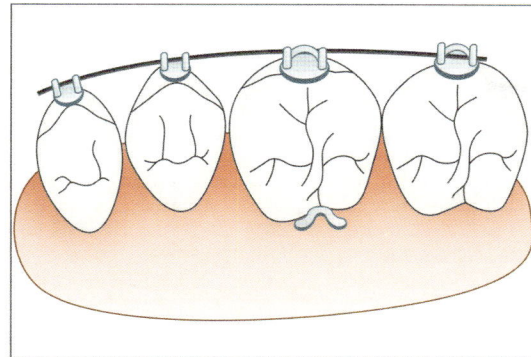

Fig. 15.132: Lingual cleat

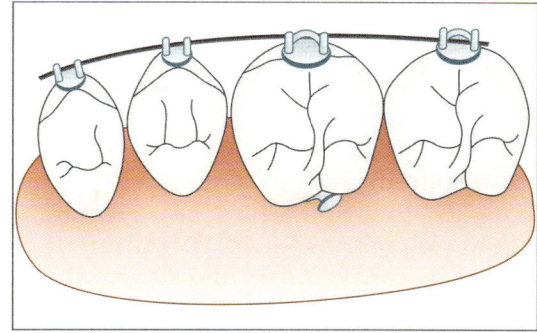

Fig. 15.135: Eyelet

- *Lingual ball hooks:* These are small balls attached to a weldable flat arm. The offset can be mesial or distal. They are used to attach elastics or elastomeric chains/rings from the lingual aspect (Fig. 15.134).
- *Lingual eyelets:* They are used to tie elastic threads or ligature wires. Hollow in the middle and welded on the two sides (Fig. 15.135).
- *Lingual sheaths:* They are used for attaching accessories such as transpalatal arches, NiTi molar rotators and expanders.

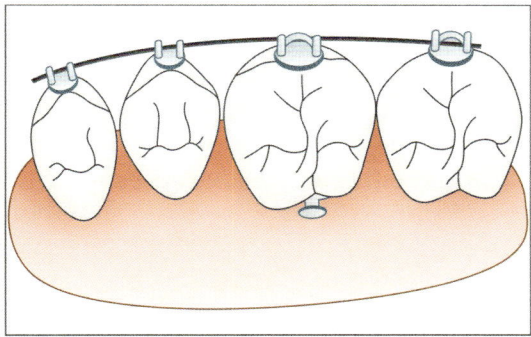

Fig. 15.133: Lingual button

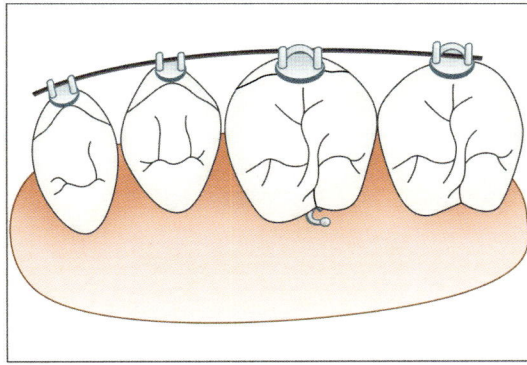

Fig. 15.134: Ball and hook

Buccal Tubes

Classification

1. Buccal tubes can be classified into following two types based on the mode of attachment:
   a. *Weldable buccal tubes:* Weldable buccal tubes have a flat contoured metal flange base and are welded to the bands that are cemented on the molars.
   b. *Bondable buccal tubes:* The bondable buccal tube has a mesh base and is bonded directly to the tooth surface.

   Buccal tubes can be welded to the bands or directly bonded to the tooth surface.
2. Based on number of tubes, they can be classified as:
   a. Single buccal tube
   b. Double buccal tube
   c. Trible buccal tube
3. Buccal tubes are of two types based on their shape in the cross-section:
   a. Round
   b. Flat-oval.

Bands (Fig. 15.136)

The band is cemented to individual tooth and provides a place for attachment of other auxiliaries like buccal tubes, lingual buttons, etc. These auxiliaries can be either welded or soldered to the bands.

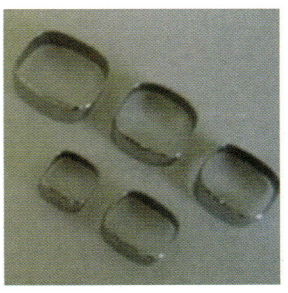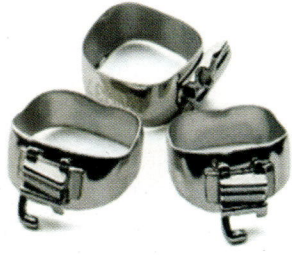

Fig. 15.136: Bands

Bands can be either custom fabricated for individual teeth or selected from the various sizes available commercially for different teeth.
- Molar band thickness: 0.005 × 0.180"
- Premolar band thickness: 0.004 × 0.150"
- Anterior band thickness: 0.003 × 0.125"

Bands are thin strips of stainless steel which are adapted to the contours of the tooth to which attachments are welded or soldered.

Types
1. Performed
2. Custom made
   a. Molar bands
   b. Premolars
   c. Incisors

Ligature Wires

Ligature wires are soft stainless steel wires of 0.008 to 0.010 inch in diameter. These may be used to secure the archwire in the slot of bracket or to tie the segment of teeth together (Fig. 15.137).

Ligature wire can also be placed in the fashion of figure of eight around the bracket to prevent opening of space between.

Lock Pins (Fig. 15.138)

Lock pins are mainly used in Begg's technique for securing archwire in the ribbon arch/bracket. Lock pins are made up of brass or soft stainless steel. Lock pins are of five types based on their use in the stages of Begg's technique.

1. Stage I
2. Stage II

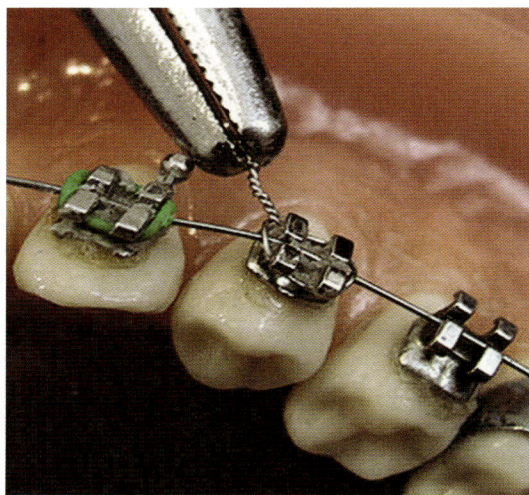

Fig. 15.137: Ligature wire

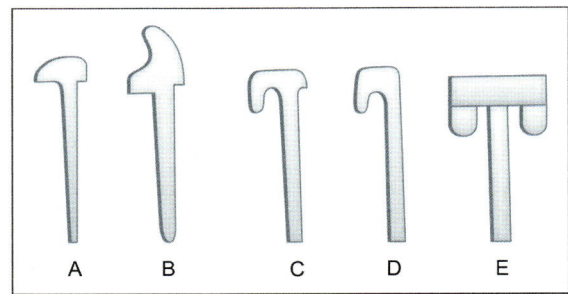

Fig. 15.138: Lock pins: (a) One point safety pin; (b) High hat safely pin; (c) Double safety pin; (d) Hook pin; (e) Universal T-pin

3. Stage III
4. High hat pin
5. T-pin

Brackets (Fig. 15.139)

Brackets are of various types depending upon the technique used:
- Banded
- Bonded attachment

Bonded attachment: Mechanical locking of an adhesive to irregularities in the enamel surface of the tooth and to mechanical locks formed in base of the orthodontic attachment.

Components of the system:
1. Tooth surface and its preparation
2. The design of the attachement base
3. Bonding material itself

Brackets can either be welded to bands which are then cemented to individual tooth or can be bonded.

AUSTRALIAN WIRES (AJ WILCOCK WIRES)

Arthur J. Wilcock of Victoria, Australia, introduced these wires. These are round austentic stainless steel wires which are heat-treated and cold drawn to proper diameter from round wires of larger diameter to give

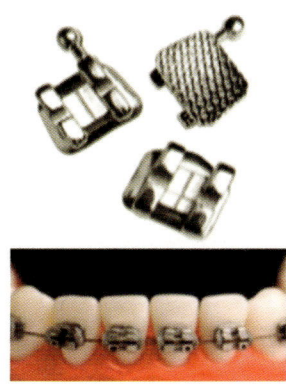

Fig. 15.139: Brackets

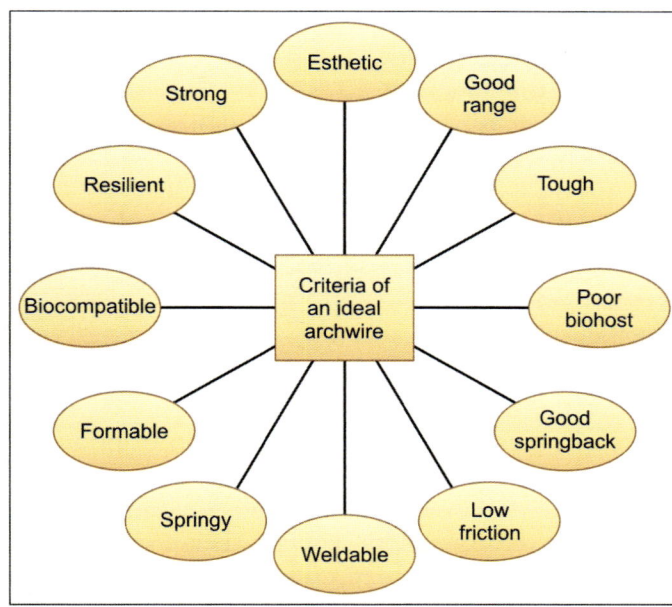

Fig. 15.140: In search of the ideal archwire

required resilience, toughness and strength. The fundamental difference for superior properties of these wires is due to manufacturing process of pulse straightening and spinner straightening.

Ideal requirements of archwire are listed in Fig. 15.140.

Grades of AJ Wilcock Wires

Spinner Straightened Wire

Regular grade (white level)
- Lowest grade wires
- Used for wire bending practise
- Can be used in patients when distortion of wire and bite opening is not a problem.
- Available in 0.012", 0.014", 0.016", 0.018", 0.020" diameter.

Regular plus grade (green level)
- Stiffness is more compared to regular grade.
- Available in 0.014", 0.016", 0.018", 0.020" diameter.

Special grade (black level)
- Have high tensile strength but complicated bends can be given with little danger of breakage
- Available in 0.014", 0.016", 0.018", 0.020" diameter.

Special plus grade (orange level)
- Better hardness
- Better resiliency
- Good for supporting anchorage and reducing deep bites
- Available in 0.014", 0.016", 0.018", 0.020" diameter.

Pulse Straightened Wires

Premium grade (blue level)
- Also called extra special plus wires
- Better tensile strength
- Better stiffness
- Available in 0.014", 0.016", 0.018", 0.020" diameter.

Premium plus grade (blue level)
- Called supreme wires
- Used in early treatment of rotation, alignment and levelling.
- Available in 0.012", 0.014", 0.016", 0.018" diameter.

Supreme grade (lavender level)
- Most effective during early phase of treatment for initial alignment in conjuction with anterior intrusion.
- Correction of anterior crowding, mini-uprighting springs.
- Good strength and stiffness
- More resilient
- Can be welded and biocompatible.
- Available in 0.09", 0.010", 0.011" diameter.
  Cobalt chromium wire as shown in Table 15.4.

Table 15.4: Cobalt chromium wires		
Gradation		
Types	Level	Property
Type 1	Blue	Soft
Type 2	Yellow	Ductile
Type 3	Green	Semi-resilient
Type 4	Red	Resilient or hard

Esthetic Wires

Optiflex
- This is made up of top coating optical glass fiber (pure silicon dioxide) with a hot melt adhesive and nylon skin. The silicon dioxide core provides force for moving teeth. Silicon resin middle layer protects the core from moisture and adds strength. Provides lighter force, no deformation. Effective in alignment of crowding teeth.
- Sharp bends must be avoided, since they could fracture the core.

Made of clear optical fibre; comprises of three layers:
1. A silicon dioxide core
2. A silicon resin middle layer
3. A stain resistant nylon outer layer

Precautions to be taken with optiflex

- Use elastomeric ligatures
- No sharp bends
- Avoid using instruments with sharp edges, like the scalers etc., to force the wire into the bracket slot.
- Use the (501) minidistal end cutter (AEZ)
- No rough diet
- Do not 'cinch back'

Polynorborgen

A shape memory plastic developed in japan.The glass transition temperature is 35°C. Once the temperature exceeds the glass transition temperature, it begins to display an elastic property and returns to its original shape. At 50°C, it can be stretched 2 times its original length and deliver 29–150 gm force on the teeth.

Fiber-Reinforced Polymeric Wires

It is composed of ceramic fibres that are embedded in a linear or cross-linked polymeric matrix. The matrix is either epoxy resin or dental resin.

These wires are as strong as piano wire. When compared to nickel titanium wires, resilience and springback are comparable. When elastic failure of these wires occur, it loses its stiffness and remains intact. Different characteristics of wire can be varied during manufacturing without any change in the dimension by process known as pultrusion.

Teflon-Coated Wires

These are metal wires with white-coated teflon or epoxy resin on their surface. They provide excellent esthetics.

BRACKETS

Brackets can be classified in a number of ways as listed below:

I. *Based on materials:*

A. Metal brackets
- Stainless steel brackets
- Gold-coated brackets
- Platinum-coated brackets
- Titanium brackets

B. Plastic brackets
- Polycarbonate bracket
- Polyurethane composite brackets
- Thermoplastic polyurethane bracket

C. Ceramic brackets
- Monocrystalline alumina
- Polycrystalline alumina
- Polycrystalline zirconia

II. *Depending on mode of attachment:*
- Weldable brackets
- Bondable brackets

III. *Depending on technique for which they are used*
- Ribbon arch brackets
- Begg's modified ribbon arch brackets
- Tip-edge brackets
- Preadjusted edgewise brackets
- Lingual brackets
- Self-ligating brackets (Fig. 15.141)

Metal Brackets

- Metal brackets are routinely used in orthodontic practice.
  Of which steel brackets are the most frequently used. Although biocompatible, gold brackets are expensive.
- Titanium brackets are recently introduced and have high biocompatibility and low friction.

Advantages of metal brackets: These include:
a. They can be sterilized.
b. They can be recycled.
c. They resist deformation and low fracture.
d. Exhibit less friction with the archwire.
e. They are comparatively less expensive (cost-effective).

Disadvantages: These include:
a. Easily noticeable, metallic brackets are esthetically not pleasant.
b. They may corrode and cause stainig of the teeth.

Plastic Brackets

Plastic brackets made of polycarbonate and other related materials were introduced to improve esthetics. However, they are not preferred.

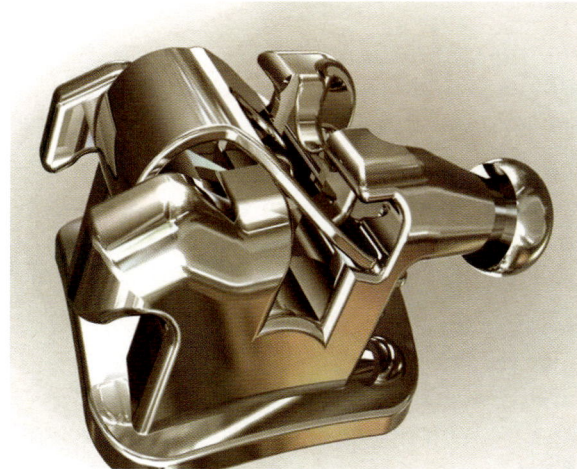

Fig. 15.141: Self-ligating bracket

As they have a number of disadvantages, such as:

1. They tend to get discolored easily, especially in patients who smoke or drink coffee, tea, etc.
2. They have poor dimensional stability.
3. Their slots tend to distort.
4. There is a high amount of friction between plastic brackets and metal archwire.

Ceramic Brackets

Ceramic brackets were introduced in 1987 and offer a good alternative when esthetics is a major concern while undergoing orthodontic treatment. Transparent and available and opaque tooth-colored ceramic brackets are available and are generally made of alumina or zirconium-based products (Fig. 15.142).

Advantages of ceramic brackets:

1. They are highly esthetics and not easily noticeable.
2. Resist discoloration unlike plastic brackets.
3. Dimensionally stable, do not distort in oral cavity.

Disadvandages: These include:

1. They are very brittle and thus tend to fracture easily during active treatment and also while debondig.
2. Exhibit greater friction at wire/brackets interface then metallic brackets.
3. High cost of material, they are highly expensive.

Weldable Brackets

- They are either welded or soldered to the band, which is then cemented over the teeth.
- Weldable brackets have metal flanges on the base to facilitable welding.

Bondable Brackets

- They are directly bonded onto the teeth using bonding adhesives.

- Base of these brackets generally exhibit meshwork or indentations to facilitate bonding with the adhesive material.

Ribbon Arch Brackets

- Ribbon arch brackers had a simple design with occlusally facing vertical slot in it.
- They were used in ribbon arch technique.

Modified Ribbon Arch Brackets in Begg Technique (Fig. 15.143)

- Begg technique uses modified ribbon arch brackets in which the vertical slot is facing gingivally rather than occlusally.
- This modification allowed easy tipping of the teeth.

Tip-edge Brackets

They are used in the tip-edge technique. Bracket design is a modification of the conventional edgewise brackets where two diagonally opposite corners of the conventional edgewise bracket slot are removed and a vertical rectsngular slot is also added.

Edgewise Brackets

Edgewise brackets and their modifications become the mainstay in orthodontic practice today. They are employed in edgewise technique. Most edgewise brackets have rectangular horizontal slot with four wings—two gingival and two occlusal.

The rings help in securing archwire in the slot and brackets may also have hooks for attaching auxiliaries, such as elastics. They are available as a set of different brackets for different teeth.

Preadjusted Edgewise Brackets

They are modified edgewise brackets with inbuilt tip, torque angulations incorporated in their design.

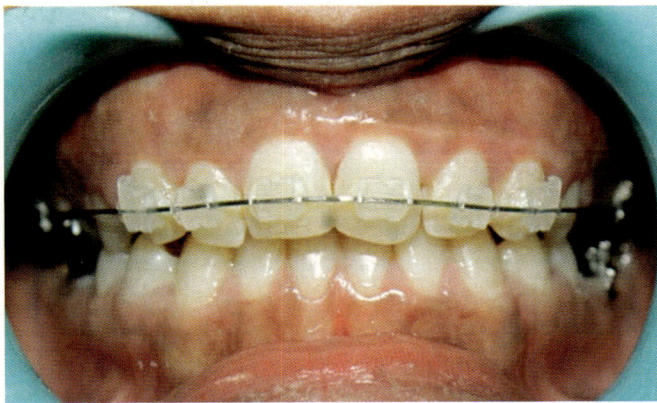

Fig. 15.142: Ceramic bracket

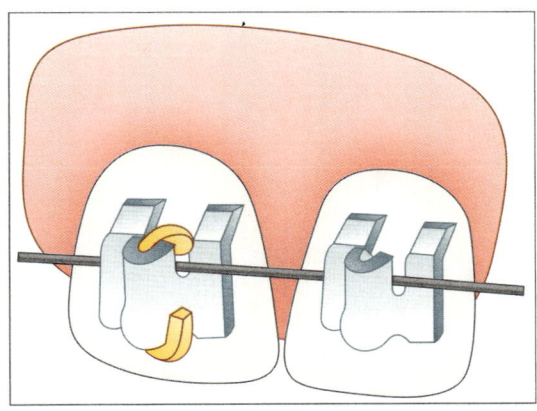

Fig. 15.143: Modified ribbon arch bracket

Lingual Brackets

They are used in lingual orthodontic technique where the breackets are attached to the lingual aspects of the teeth. Indirect bonding procedure is preferred for attaching these onto the teeth, due to inadequate visibility of lingual aspects.

SPRINGS

Uprighting springs: They are the springs which move the root in mesial or distal directions (Fig. 15.144).

Rotating springs: They are used in first stage of Begg's technique. Used in labiolingual rotation of teeth (Fig. 15.145).

Torquing springs: They move the root in lingual or palatal direction. It is used in begg's therapy (Fig. 15.146).

TECHNIQUES

Begg Appliance or Light Force Technique or Differential Force Technique

Raymond Begg of Australia introduced this technique. He received his training in Angle's School of Orthodontics in the early 1900s. Later he returned to

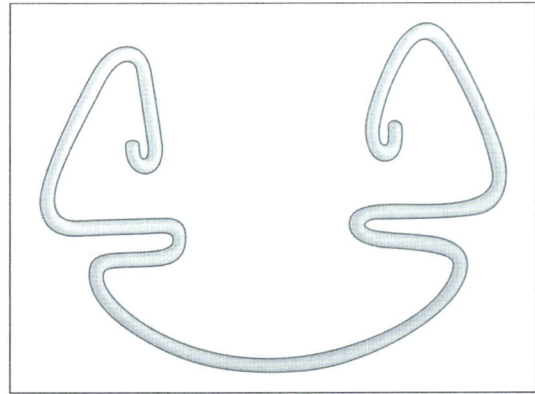

Fig. 15.146: Torquing spring—occlusal view

Australia in 1925 and practiced the edgewise technique. Begg modified the Angle's ribbon arch technique and introduced the Begg light wire differential force technique. This appliance used the concept of differential force and tipping of teeth rather than bodily movement. The Begg appliance used high strength heat-treated stainless steel wires manufactured by Wilcock Company. These basal archwires are used with a number of auxiliaries and springs to achieve the desired tooth movement. This technique utilizes round wires with vertical slot brackets. The buccal tube is round or oval in cross-section (Fig. 15.147).

It is carried in three stages. The first two stages involve crown tipping and the third stage is restricted to root tipping or torquing.

Stage 1: It is concerned with alignment, correction of crowding, rotation correction, closure of anterior spaces and achieving an edge-to-edge anterior bite. The bite is opened in order to reduce the overjet. Usually, 0.016" stainless round archwire plain or with loops, NiTi wire or coaxial wire is used. Intermaxillary elastics are used usually and intramaxillary or class I elastics are not used at this stage.

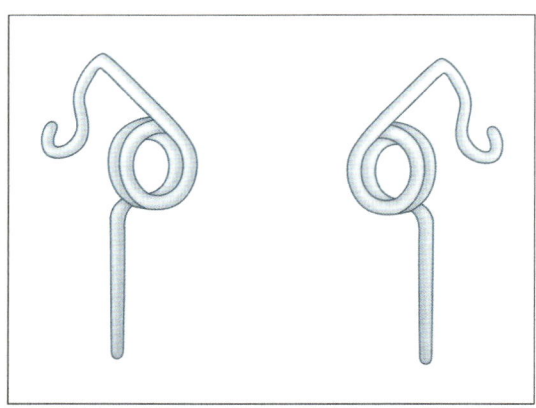

Fig. 15.144: Uprighting springs

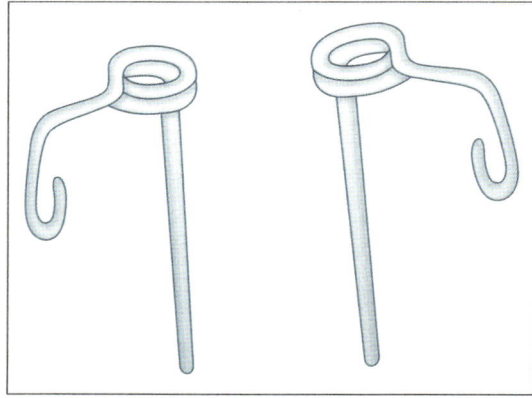

Fig. 15.145: Rotation spring

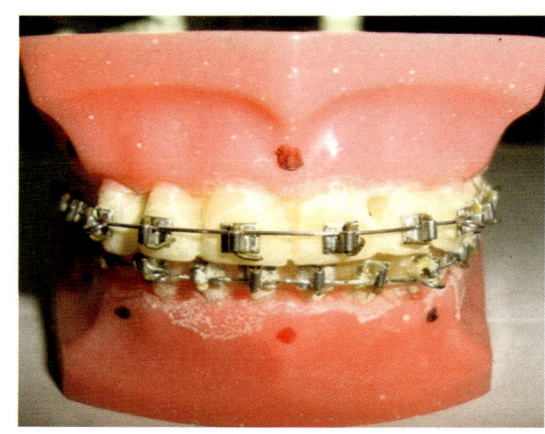

Fig. 15.147: Begg technique

In *stage two*, the remaining extraction spaces are closed while maintaining the previous corrections that have been achieved. Usually 0.018" stainless steel round plain archwire is used. Both intra- and intermaxillary elastics are used.

In the *final stage*, uprighting and torquing is carried out to achieve normal axial inclination of the teeth. A basal round wire of 0.020" stainless steel wire with 0.012 or 0.014" torquing auxiliary is utilized. Uprighting springs are also used in this stage (Table 15.5).

Table 15.5: Begg's technique	
Advantages	*Disadvantages*
• Continuous light forces which are within the physiologic limits	• Difficult to control the tooth movement in all three planes effectively
• Rapid alignment and overbite correction	• Difficult to achieve molar control
• Minimal friction between the wire and the brackets	• Precise root positioning is difficult to achieve
• The appliance does not strain the anchorage	• Excessive tipping of anterior occurs during stage II giving dishing in appearance to the face
• Extraoral forces are not required to conserve anchorage	

Lingual Technique

The lingual edgewise technique was introduced by Craven Kurz in 1976. Both edgewise and Begg's principles are employed in lingual orthodontic technique. Kurz developed edgewise lingual appliance technique and Fujita of Japan developed light wire lingual appliance known as Mushroom appliance. Brackets are placed on palatal and lingual aspects of teeth. Lingual technique is highly esthetic, poor access in speech and oral hygeine (Fig. 15.148).

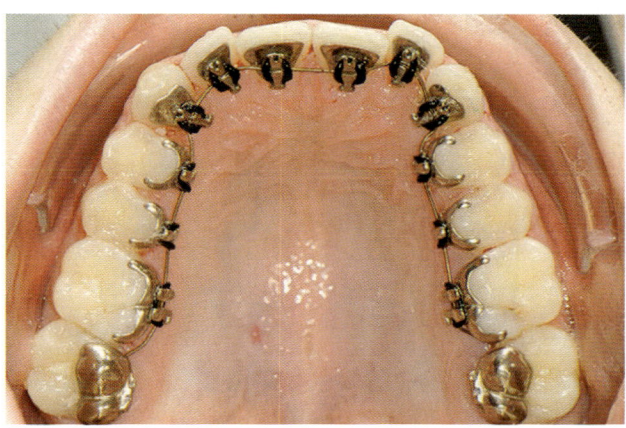

Fig. 15.148: Lingual technique

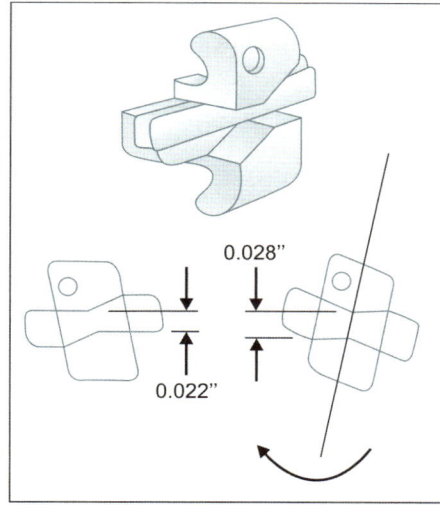

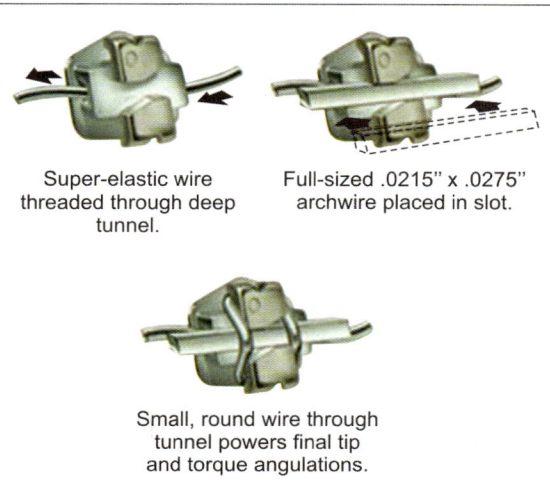

Super-elastic wire threaded through deep tunnel.

Full-sized .0215" x .0275" archwire placed in slot.

Small, round wire through tunnel powers final tip and torque angulations.

Fig. 15.149: Tip edge bracket

Tip Edge Technique

This is a combination technique which utilizes the advantages of both the edgewise and Begg appliance hence the tip edge or differential straight arch technique. It was introduced by Peter C Kesling. The bracket design has both the features of vertical as well as horizontal slot.

The advantages include rapid opening of the bite as well as reduced treatment time and at the same time there is good control over tooth movement.

Peter C Kesling developed the tip edge bracket by removing opposite corners of the edgewise bracket to allow mesial and distal crown tipping during initial stages and engagement of rectangular wires for torque control during finishing stages (Fig. 15.149).

Features of Tip Edge Appliance

• Labially facing archwire slots—improved manipulation with elastomeric ties

- Light force—2 oz
- Reduced strain on anchorage
- With rectangular slot, a 3D control is afforded.
- Facilitate intrusion of teeth.

Advanatages of Tip Edge over Edgewise Technique

1. Archwire slots open and close.
2. Ease of archwire changes.
3. Prevents undesirable couples on anterior.
4. Diminished anchorage bends
5. Light forces are used—anterior teeth retracted by crown tipping.

Straight Wire Technique

The straight wire technique is a modification of the edgewise appliance. This was introduced by Lawrence F Andrews in 1970s based on his six keys to normal occlusion. Andrews developed straight wire appliances by series of 14 research works which led development of six keys of optimal occlusion, concept of straight wire.

Basically, the brackets have rectangular slots similar to standard edgewise brackets. The basic concept was to preprogram the bracket such that the first, second and third order components are inbuilt in the brackets itself. This incorporation of the bends in the design of the bracket eliminates the need of a wire to have any complex bending as required in standard edgewise appliance. Hence it is called preadjusted edgewise appliance (PEA). It requires a plain straight wire in the arch form to be inserted in his brackets. Hence, it is called as straight wire appliance. However, minor wire bending or fabrication is required for ideal finishing.

Andrews developed straight wire appliances by series of 14 research works which led development of six keys of optimal occlusion, concept of straight wire (Fig. 15.150).

Advantages

- Precise control—premolar and molar torque
- Bilateral symmetry—buccolabial inclination readily obtained
- Reduced nends in the archwire
- Finishing is good

Direct Bonding Technique

Bonding of brackets to acid-etched enamel has become a universally accepted technique in clinical orthodontics ever since the introduction of the technique by **Bounocore in 1955.**

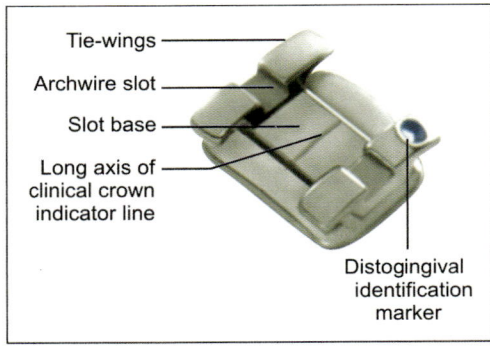

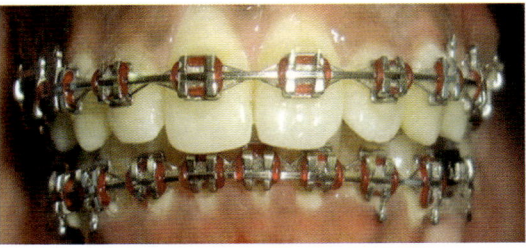

Fig. 15.150: Straight wire technique

Etching of enamel with phosphoric acid results in surface roughness and subsurface porous zones into which the flow of resins results in the bonding of resin to enamel surface. The depths of the etch or the amount of surface enamel lost is dependent on the type of acid used, the concentration, the duration of etching, the chemical composition of the enamel and also the area of the facial surface of tooth (Figs 15.151 and 15.152).

To control the permanent loss of enamel and at the same time to achieve adequate bond strength, it has been suggested that there should be changes in acid concentration and etching times.

Enamel Pretreatment

Conventional adhesive systems use three different agents—enamel conditioner, primer solution and adhesive resin—in the process of bonding orthodontic brackets to enamel. Untouched enamel surface is hydro-

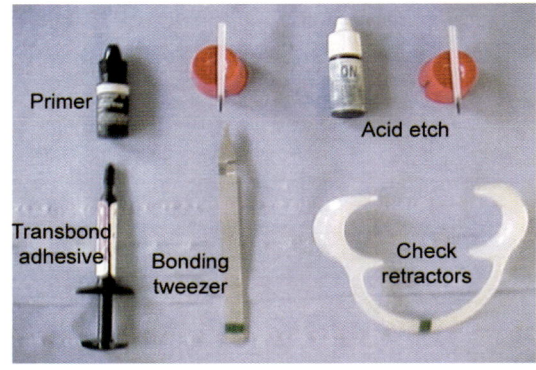

Fig. 15.151: Armamentarium

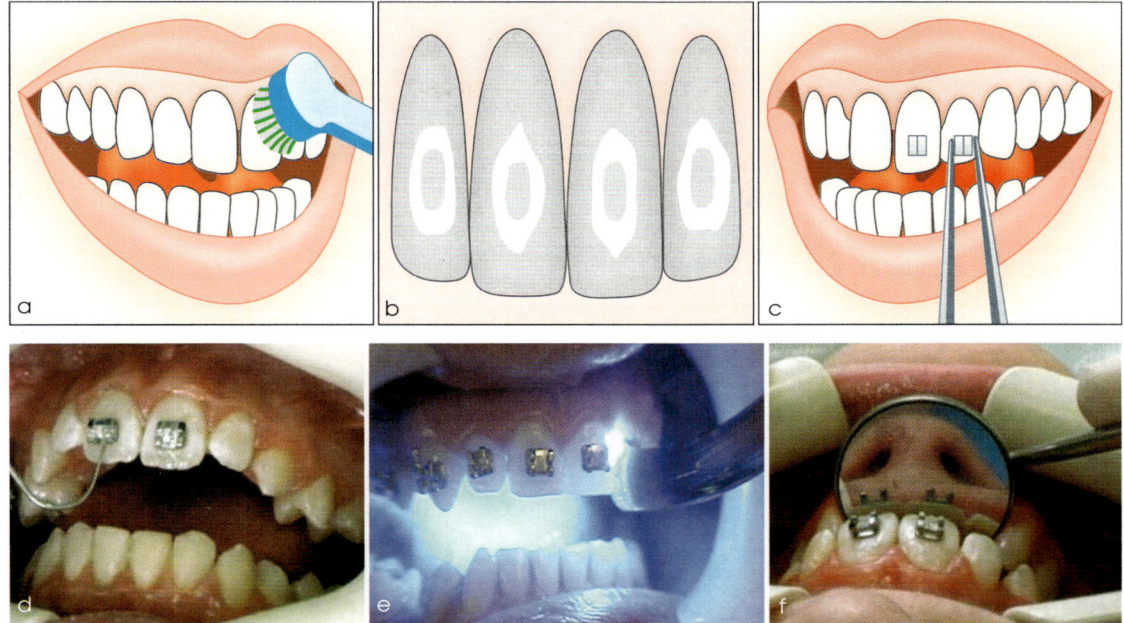

Fig. 15.152: Direct bonding technique: (a) Cleaning; (b) Acid etching; (c) Bracket fixing; (d) Removal of excess bond material from around the bracket; (e) A cordless light used to activate adhesive bonding process; (f) The bracket is bonded in place

phobic and wetting is limited. This makes bonding to intimate enamel surface a challenging procedure. Enamel pretreatment or surface conditioning is necessary to make successful bond usually accomplished by etching the surface by various acids.

Different Acid-Etching Methods

37% orthophosphoric acid: Bonding to enamel with acid etching creates microporosities of enamel surface that result in a micromechanical bond. It is applied over the enamel surface for 30 seconds after careful isolation of the operating field. The etching time can range from 15 to 60 seconds. But 15 seconds is adequate for etching young permanent teeth.

At the end of etching period, the bulk of the etchant is rinsed with abundant water spray. A powerful evacuator is crucial for increased efficiency in collecting the etchant–water rinse. The teeth are then thoroughly dried with a moisture-free and oil-free air source to obtain the well known frosty appearance.

Teeth that do not appear frosty should be re-etched. Saliva contamination does not require rerinsing, but blood contamination decreses shear bond strength.

The teeth contaminated with blood should be rerinsed and dried. Etchant is available in the form of gel or acid. The clinical advantage of gel over the liquid is the possibility of better control in placing the gel on the required area of the enamel surface. While the acid gels require longer wash time after etching procedure is completed; acid liquids can be washed off in shorter time.

Use of milder acid: 10% maleic acid decreases mineral loss alone and may produce similar bond strength to 37% orthophosphoric acid. However, the use of maleic acid has been popularized.

Laser etching: Laser treatment of dental enamel causes thermally induced changes within the enamel to a depth of 10 to 20 µm. Depending on the type of laser and the energy applied to the enamel surface, laser etching involves a process of continuous vaporization and microexplosions caused by vaporizing the water trapped within the hydroxyapatite matrix. The degree of surface roughening depends on the system used and the wavelength of laser.

Sandblasting: Even the enamel loss resulting from sandblasting at low pressure and short exposure time was found to be smaller than in acid etching. The bond strength achieved with sandblasting alone is not clinically acceptable.

Crystal growth: This system consists of polyacrylic acid treatment liquid contining a sulfate component that reacts with the calcium in the enamel surface to form a dense growth of small needle-shaped crystals. The crystal build up on the enamel serves as an additional retentive mechanism for the resin that bonds the orthodontic attachment to the teeth.

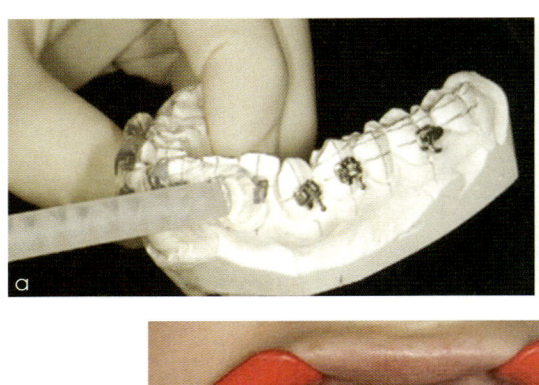
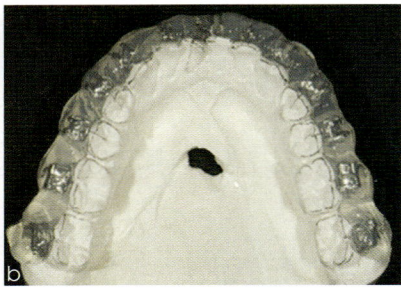
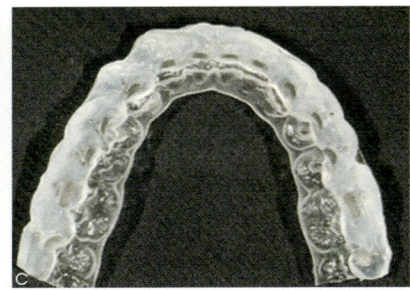
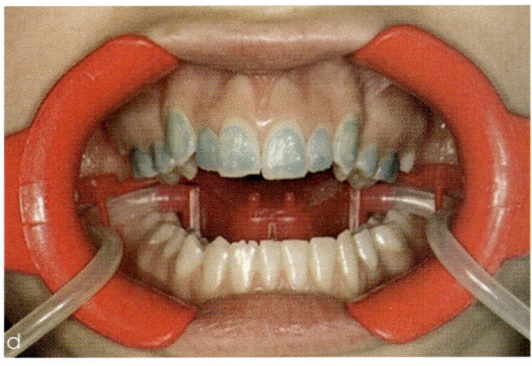
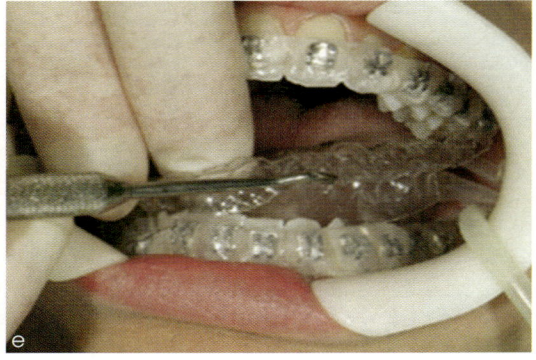

Fig. 15.153: Indirect bonding: (a) Brackets are placed precisely on a cast of the teeth and held in place with a fitted resin; (b) After the brackets are cured in the ideal position, a transfer tray is formed and placed on the working cast; (c) The trays are removed from the working cast after soaking in warm water and trimmed; (d) The teeth are isolated, etched, and a chemically cured two-paste resin is painted on the etched enamel and brackets. (e) After the resin has completely set, the trays are carefully removed, leaving the brackets bonded to the teeth

Self-etching primers: Combining conditioning and priming into a single treatment step results in improved chairside efficiency and cost-effectiveness for the children and save time for patients. In a self-etching primer, the active ingredient is a methacrylated phosphoric acid ester. The phosphoric acid and methacrylated group are combined into a molecule that etches and primes at the same time. The phosphate group dissolves the calcium and removes it from the hydroxyapatite. The removed calcium forms a complex with the phosphate group and is incorporated into the network when the primer polymerizes.

Etching and monomer penetration to the exposed enamel rods are simultaneous. In this manner, the depth of etch and depth of the primer penetrates and identical.

Application of Acid Etching in Orthodontics

- Bonding of brackets and other orthodontic attachements to enamel surface in labial and lingual orthodontics.
- Prior to fixing of lingual bonded retainers after the orthodontic treatment.
- In the cases of bonded space maintainers.
- Acid-etching and bonding offers a range of esthetic techniques for the solution of problems with anterior teeth.

- Splinting of traumatized teeth for stabilization and to prevent damages to the periodontal structures.
- In case of missing tooth, etching and bonding is required to fix semipermanent bonded replacement.

Indirect Bonding (Fig. 15.153)

1. Brackets are placed precisely on a cast of the teeth and held in place with a fitted resin.
2. After the brackets are cured in the ideal position, a transfer tray is formed and placed on the working cast.
3. The trays are removed from the working cast after soaking in warm water and trimmed.
4. The teeth are isolated, etched, and a chemically cured two-paste resin is painted on the etched enamel and brackets.
5. After the resin has completely set, the trays are carefully removed, leaving the brackets bonded to the teeth.

BIBLIOGRAPHY

1. Graber TM. Orthodontic: Principles and Practice. WB Saunders, 1998.
2. Harradine NW. Self-ligating brackets and treatment efficiency. Clin Orthod 2003; 30:262–73.
3. Roth RH. Treatment mechanics for the straight wire appliance: In: Graber TM, Swain BF (Eds). Orthodontics: Current Principles and Techniques. The CV Mosby Company, St Louis, 1966.

PREVIOUS YEAR'S UNIVERSITY QUESTIONS

Essay

1. Classify orthodontic appliance. What are the advantages and disadvantages of fixed appliance? And add a note on elastics.
2. Enumerate the different components of fixed appliance and a note on passive components.

Short Questions

1. Separators
2. Coil springs.
3. Direct bonding technique
4. Elastics
5. Lingual orthodontics
6. Tip-edge technique

MCQs

1. *An example for tooth-colored brackets is:*
   a. Ceramic bracket
   b. Polyacrylic bracket
   c. Ceram flex bracket
   d. All of the above   **(Ans: d)**

2. *Rotation of teeth is best corrected by:*
   a. Hawley's appliance
   b. Buccal retractor
   c. Fixed appliance
   d. All of the above   **(Ans: c)**

3. *Disadvantages of bonding over banding:*
   a. Bonded attachments are weaker than banded attachments
   b. Enamel loss
   c. Increased risk of demineralization
   d. All of the above   **(Ans: d)**

4. *Acid etch technique was introduced by:*
   a. Buonocore

b. Jon Golberg
c. CJ Burstone
d. MF Tolass   **(Ans: a)**

5. *Banding is indicated:*
   a. In case of posterior teeth where moisture control is a problem for bonding.
   b. In tooth that requires buccal as well as lingual attachment
   c. When bands are likely to resist heavy force as in case of extraoral device.
   d. In porcelain or gold restoration of crown
   e. All of the above   **(Ans: e)**

6. *What is the significance of leveling and alignment?*
   a. Bracket alignment in buccal and lingual space
   b. Bracket alignment in vertical and lingual space
   c. Bracket alignment in occlusal and vertical space
   d. Bracket alignment in vertical and horizontal space   **(Ans: d)**

7. *Nickel titanium alloys were introduced to orthodontic world by:*
   a. Williams Buchler
   b. Anderson
   c. Goldberg
   d. Burstone   **(Ans: b)**

8. *Which type of bracket does not permit tipping of teeth?*
   a. Ribbon arch bracket
   b. Metallic bracket
   c. Edgewise type of bracket
   d. Weldable and bondable brackets   **(Ans: c)**

9. *Which one of the following is a passive component of fixed appliances?*
   a. Buccal tube
   b. Springs
   c. Separators
   d. Archwires   **(Ans: a)**

15.5 FIXED FUNCTIONAL APPLIANCES

Chapter Outline

- Herbst appliance
- Jasper Jumper appliance
- Forsus fatigue resistant device

- Fixed lingual mandibular growth modificator
- Power scope

INTRODUCTION

A prerequisite for attainment of excellent results in orthodontics is patient co-operation. Deficiencies in this area are the ubiquitous concern of orthodontics. Specifically, are those patients who fall to commit themselves to faithful wearing of functional appliances, possibly because of bulk, discomfort or inconvenience and those who do not wear consistently intermaxillary elastics.

The uniqueness of functional appliances lies in their mode of force application. A force can produce the desired orthodontic effect, only if it has a certain duration, direction and magnitude.

- *Duration of force:* In most removable functional appliances, treatment is interrupted because the appliance is usually not worn constantly but only for 12–16 hours per day.
- *Direction of force:* The movement of teeth should be consistent. Functional forces may stimulate tooth movement in one direction. But the forces of intercuspation and occlusion may drive the teeth in the opposite direction. When the appliance is not being worn, such jiggling effects should be eliminated.
- *Magnitude of force:* The magnitude of force is small further more; the treatment time with these appliances is prolonged over several years making it difficult to differentiate between the treatment effects and normal growth changes.

Failure to adhere to prescribed schedule, removable appliance wear will result in the slow treatment response or no response at all. On the other hand, it is possible with fixed functional appliance (FFA) to get short time.

CLASSIFICATION

Fixed functional appliance can be classified as given in Table 15.6.

In this text, a few appliances are described.

HERBST APPLIANCE

Emil Herbst developed the Herbst bite jumping mechanism in the early 1900s. The appliance can be compared to an artificial joint working between the maxilla and mandible. A bilateral telescope mechanism attached to orthodontic bands keeps the mandible mechanically in a continuous anterior jumped position.

Each telescope device consists of (Fig. 15.154):
- A tube
- A plunger
- Two pivots—one on each side
- Two screws

Anchorage for the Herbst Aappliance

The anchorage system of the Herbst consists basically of the following:
- In the maxillary arch, the first premolars and the permanent first molars are banded and are interconnected on each side with a half round (1.5 × 0.75 mm) lingual or buccal sectional archwire.
- In the mandibular dental arch, the first premolars are banded and soldered with a half round (1.5 × 0.75 mm) lingual sectional archwire touching the lingual surfaces of the front teeth. This form of anchorage is called partial anchorage.

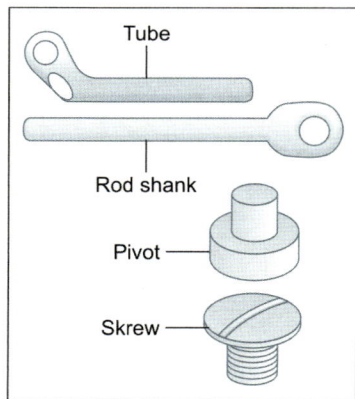

Fig. 15.154: Parts of herbst appliance

Table 15.6: Classification of functional appliances

Appliance	Author	Year
Regid fixed functional appliances		
1. Herbst Appliance	Pancherz	1979
2. Mandibular Advancing Repositioning Splint (MARS)	Clements & Jacobson	1982
3. Mandibular Corrector Appliance (MCA)	Jones	1985
4. The Cantilevered Bite Jumper	Mayes	1996
5. MALU Herbst Appliance	Schiavoni et al	1996
6. Flip Lock Herbst Appliance	Miller	1996
7. The Ventral Telescope		
8. The Magnetic Telescopic Device	Ritto	1997
9. The Mandibular Protraction Appliance (MPA)		
Type I	Coelho Filho	1995
Type II	Coelho Filho	1997
Type III	Coelho Filho	1998
Type IV	Coelho Filho	2001
10. The Universal Bite Jumper (UBJ)	Calvez	1998
11. Mandibular Anterior Repositioning Appliance (MARA)	Eckhart	1998
12. Molar Moving Bite Jumper	Mayes	1998
13. The Biopedic Appliance		
14. Integrated Snoring Therapy (IST)		
15. Ritto Appliance	Ritto Orthod Cyber-J Archives	
16. Functional Mandibular Advancer (FMA)	Kinzinger et al	2002
Flexible fixed functional appliances		
1. Jasper Jumper	Jasper	1987
2. Scandee Tubular Jumper		
3. Amoric Torsion Coils	Amoric	1994
4. Adjustable Bite Corrector	West	1995
5. Churro Jumper	Castanon et al	1998
6. Bite Fixer	Awbrey	1999
7. Klapper Super Spring	Klapper	1999
8. Forsus Nitinol Flat Spring	Heinig & Goz	2001
9. Flex Developer	Winsauer	2002
Hybrid appliances		
1. Eureka Spring	DeVincenzo	1997
2. Sabbagh Universal Spring		
3. Forsus Fatique Resistant Device		
4. Twin-force Bite Corrector	Corbett & Molina	2001
Appliances acting as substitute for elastics		
1. Saif Spring	Starnes	1998
2. The Calibrated force Module Alpren Class II closers		

- In several instances, this type of anchorage is insufficient and is, therefore, increased by the incorporation of additional dental units. In the maxillary dental arch, a labial archwire is ligated to brackets on the first premolars, canines and incisors. In the mandibular arch, the lingual sectional wire is extended to the permanent first molars which are also banded. This form of anchorage is called total anchorage.

- The pivot for the tube is usually soldered to the maxillary permanent first molar band and the pivot for the plunger to the mandibular first premolar band. The screws prevent the telescoping parts from slipping off the pivots. The length of the tube determines the amount of bite jumping. Usually, the mandible is retained in an incisal end-to-end relationship. The length of plunger is kept at a maximum in order to prevent it from slipping out of the tube when the mouth is opened wide. If the plunger is too long, it may protrude for behind the tube and injure the buccal mucosa distal to the maxillary permanent first molar. The mechanisms permit vertical opening movements and when properly constructed also lateral movements of the mandible (Fig. 15.155).

Advantages

Neglected patients: The patients who have passed maximal pubertal growth may be too old for removable functional appliances, because treatment with these appliances is extended over a long time period (2–3 years). Treatment with the Herbst appliance, on the other hand, can be finished within 6–8 months, thus making is possible to use the residual growth left in older patients.

Permanent dentition: It is ideal appliance for adult aged patients. Even though there was a restriction in the lateral jaw movement, the patient was comfortable with this appliance.

Mouth breathers: Nasal airway obstructions will not interfere with the correct functioning of the Herbst appliance.

Uncooperative patients: Since it is fixed, it works 24 hours a day without patient assistance.

Multiple design possibilities: Acrylic Herbst splint, cantelever bite jumper, etc.

Disadvantages

- It is expensive and rigid.

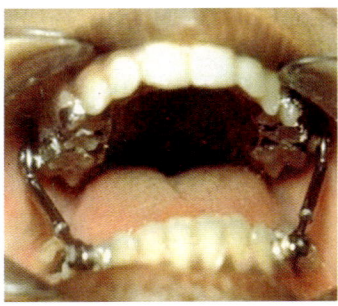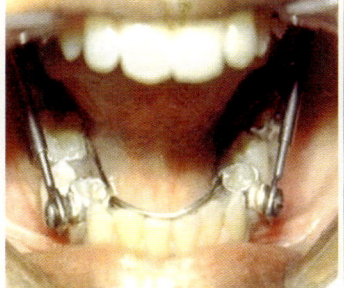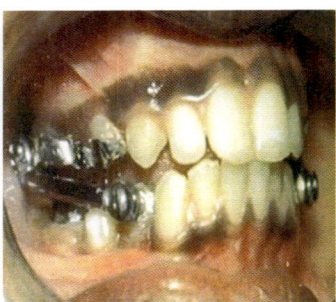

Fig. 15.155: Herbst appliance

- Permanent changes in condylar position cannot be expected when treating adults.
- Herbst affects the maxilla minimally; therefore, it cannot be used when Class II malocclusion is due to protracted maxilla.
- In such case, fixed appliance therapy should be started.

JASPER JUMPER APPLIANCE

JJ Jasper in 1980 introduced this new flexible fixed tooth-borne appliance.

This appliance produces both sagittal and intrusive forces like Herbst appliance, but affords the patients much more freedom of mandibular movement. The Jasper Jumper is new auxiliary capable of producing rapid change in occlusal relationships. It is flexible which delivers light continuous force. Its modular system can be attached to most commonly use fixed appliances (Fig. 15.156).

This system is composed of two parts—the force modules and the anchor units.

This is a coated intermaxillary torsion spring sold in a kit which includes the spring, the covering, the connectors, the ballpins and the glue. There is no distinction between left and right. The orthodontist constructs the appliance, cutting the spring to the length seen fit. When a fracture occurs, it is only necessary to

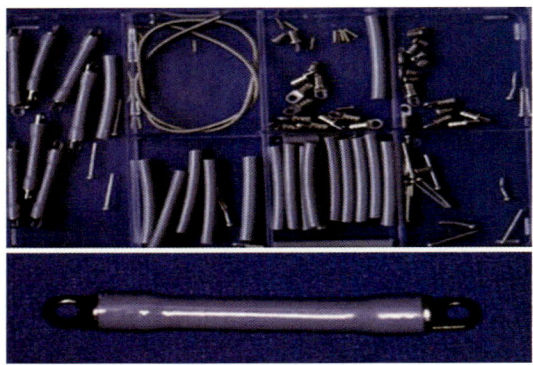

Fig. 15.157: The scandee tubular jumper

replace individual components. It has the drawback of being thick after the covering is applied (Fig. 15.157).

Force Module

Stainless steel coil or spring that is attached at both ends to stainless steel end caps, is surrounded by an opaque polyurethane covering. Seven lengths ranging from 26 to 38 mm in 2 mm increment (Fig. 15.158).

Anchor Units (Fig. 15.159a–d)

Clinical Management

It is divided into three phases as advocated by Dr. Jasper:
- Leveling and anchorage preparation

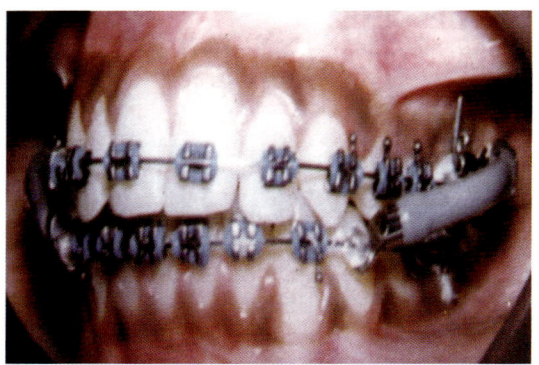

Fig. 15.156: Jasper appliance

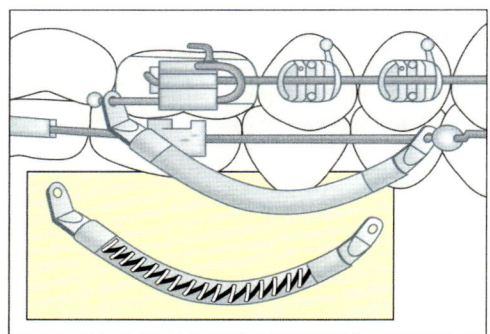

Fig. 15.158: Force module

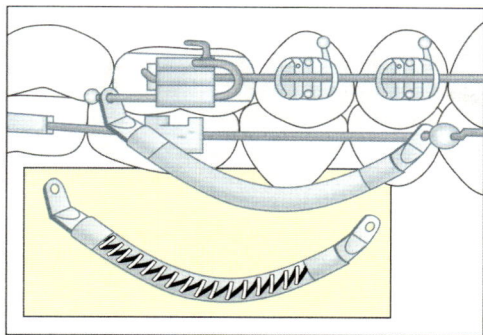

Fig. 15.159a: Attachment to the main archwire

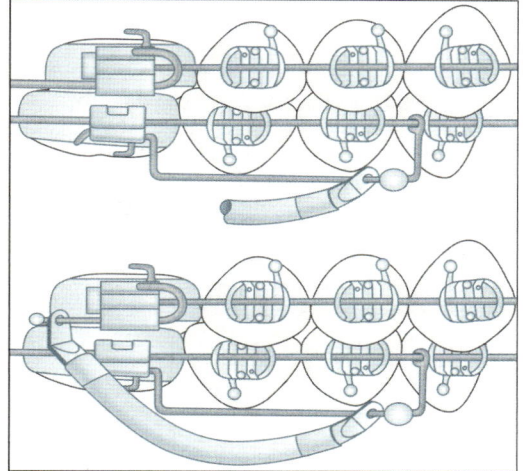

Fig. 15.159b: Attachment to auxiliary archwires

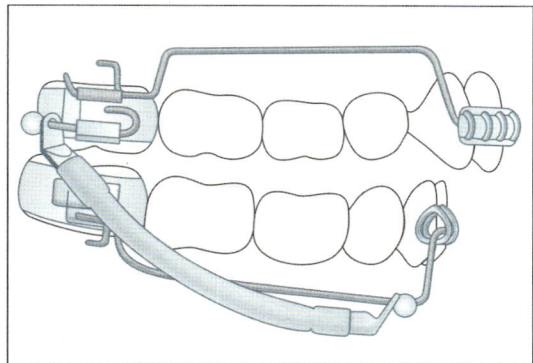

Fig. 15.159c: Attachment in the mixed dentition

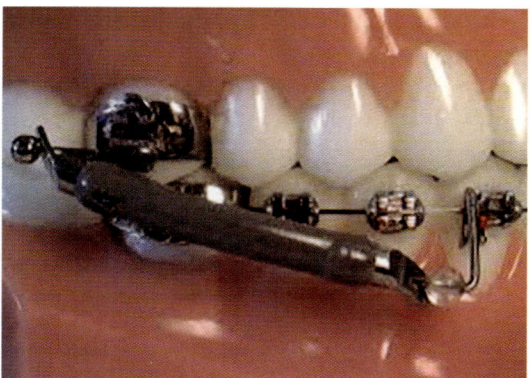

Fig. 15.159d: Jasper jumper

Note: The activation of the module is done by placing the jumper in such a way that only 2–4 ounces of force is produced by the module. In growing patients, in whom orthopedic repositioning of the mandible is desired, higher forces (6–8 ounces) are used continuously (Fig. 15.160).

Indications

- Dental Class II malocclusion.
- Skeletal Class II with maxillary excess as opposed to mandibular deficiency.
- Deep bite with retroclined mandibular incisors.

Contraindications

- Cases predisposed to root resorption.
- Dental and skeletal open bites.
- Vertical growth with high mandibular plane angle and excess lower facial height.
- Minimum buccal vestibular space.

Types of Forces Produced

- *Sagittal forces*—distalize the posterior anchor unit (max 1st and 2nd molars). Apply anterior force to mandible and mandibular dentition.

- Period of Jasper Jumper use (6–9 months)
- Period of finishing (12 months)

In patients with high mandibular plane angles, the pin is cinched to achieve approximately 2 mm of module deflection (150 gm per side). In patients, with normal or low mandibular plane angles, the ball pin is cinched forward to achieve 4 mm of module deflection (300 gm of force per side).

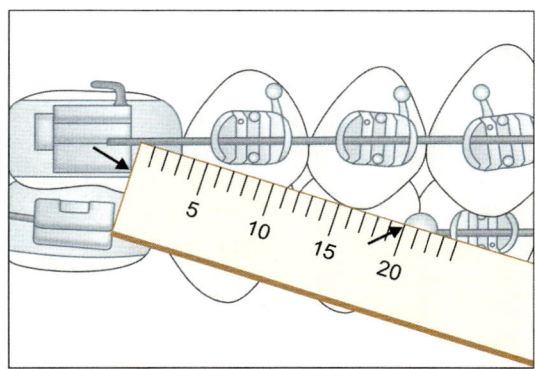

Fig. 15.160: Selection and installation of the modules

- *Intrusive forces*—in the max posterior and mandibular anterior regions.
- *Buccal forces*—due to intrusive force acting along the buccal surfaces of the maxillary teeth (produce maxillary arch expansion).
- *Modules curving outward*—vestibular shielding effect.

Jasper's 'theory of two' suggested that Class II correction with jasper jumper can be equally partitioned between five components:

1. 20% due to maxillary basal restraint.
2. 20% due to backward maxillary dentoalveolar movement.
3. 20% due to forward mandibular dentoalveolar movement.
4. 20% due to condylar growth stimulation.
5. 20% due to forward/downward glenoid fossa remodeling.

FORSUS FATIGUE RESISTANT DEVICE

The Forsus fatigue resistant device (FRD) is an interarch push spring that produces about 200 g of force when fully compressed. Unlike other push-spring appliances, such as the Herbst, the FRD can intrude the maxillary first molars and thus correct a Class II malocclusion without opening the bite (Fig. 15.161).

Componenets of FRD (Fig. 15.162)

Telescoping cylinder with outer and inner sliding tubes:
1. Open coil spring

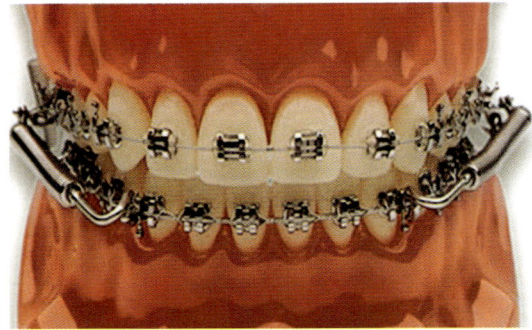

Fig. 15.161: Forsus fatigue resistant device

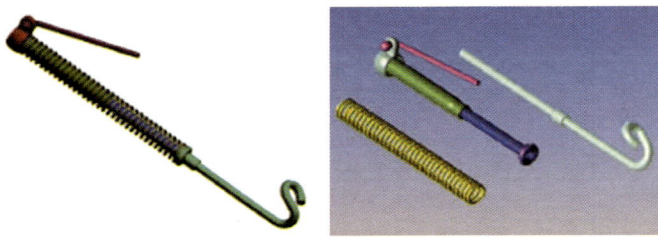

Fig. 15.162: Components of FRD

2. Push rod
3. L-pin

Installation of FRD (Fig. 15.163)

Attachment of L-pin from telescoping cylinder to maxillary molar tube.

Because the open-coil spring can be compressed about 10 mm, the FRD is capable of moving the maxillary molars with a force level of 200 g. They should be continued until the incisors are edge-to-edge and not be overcorrected into crossbite, because there may not be enough subsequent relapse. On average, the FRD corrects a full Class II malocclusion in 6 months (Fig. 15.164).

RECENT ADVANCES OF FFD

Fixed Lingual Mandibular Growth Modificator— A New Appliance for Class II Correction

Double plate system that was introduced for first time by Schwarz in early 1940s is a reliable means for treating Angle Class II, division 1 malocclusion.

Advantages

- Permanent effect, independent of patient compliance, as it is fixed.
- Esthetics, as it is small and lingually located.
- Eliminates the need for two separate treatment phases, as it is suitable for use in parallel with complete multibracket appliance in both arches.
- Flexibility in treatment timing, as it can be used anytime during the mixed and permanent dentition.
- No interference with occlusal development.
- Wide and comfortable range of mastication movements, as the appliance consists of two separate parts with no permanent and physical intermaxillary connection.
- Construction bite is unnecessary because of the easy and quick chairside reactivation and progressive advancement of the mandible in small increments.
- Easy to handle because its insertion, clipping, and removal are very simple.
- Economic and cost-effective, because it does not involve readymade components, and only one appliance is necessary for entire orthopedic phase.

Appliance Design

The fixed lingual mandibular growth modificator (FLMGM) consists of two separate and fixed parts. The upper one is palatally positioned but bucally clipped to traditional upper molar bands, while the lower is lingually welded to traditional lower molar bands (Fig. 15.165).

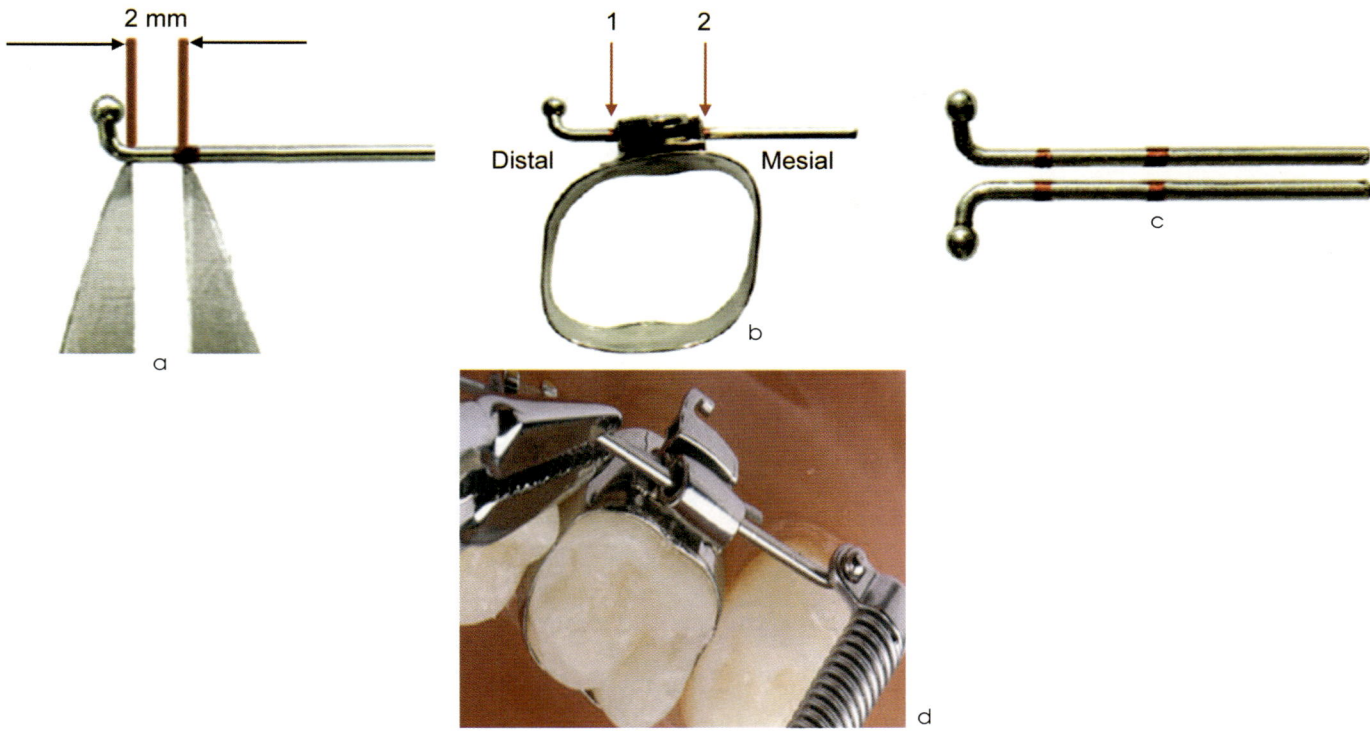

Fig. 15.163a to d: Attachment of crimpable hook from push rod to mandibular archwire

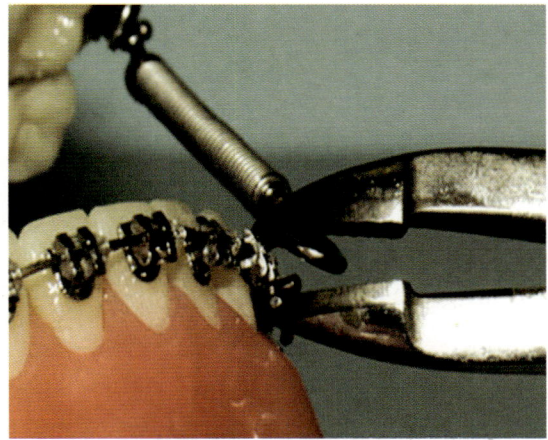

Fig. 15.164: Compression of open coil spring

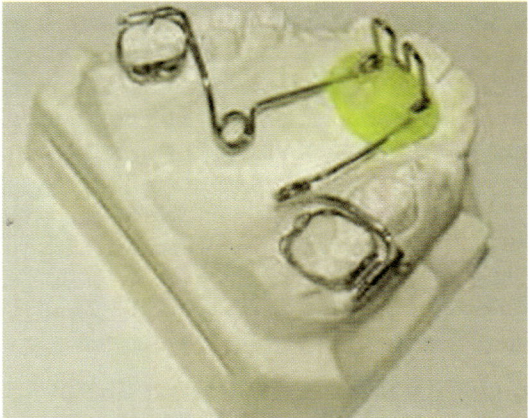

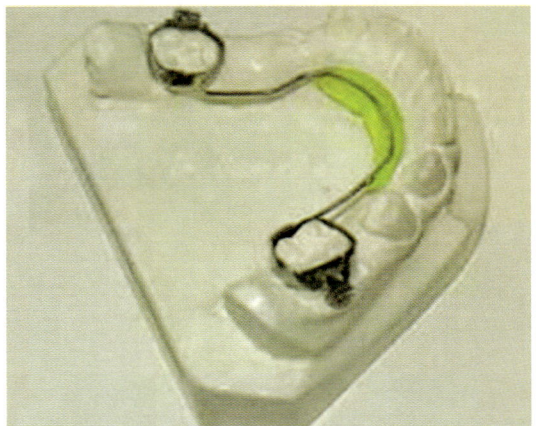

Fig. 15.165: FLMGM

Maxillary part (Fig. 15.166): It has following components:

- *Acrylic button:* It is similar to Nance button, and designed to connect wire elements of the maxillary part, preventing them from embedding into the mucosa.

- *Two retention wires:* One in each side, specifically it is designed by the author to give excellent retention to facilitate dealing with the appliance, and to enhance oral hygiene condition. They are fabricated with round 1 mm thick stainless steel orthodontic wire. The wires are anteriorly embedded into the acrylic button, run posteriorly without any contact with

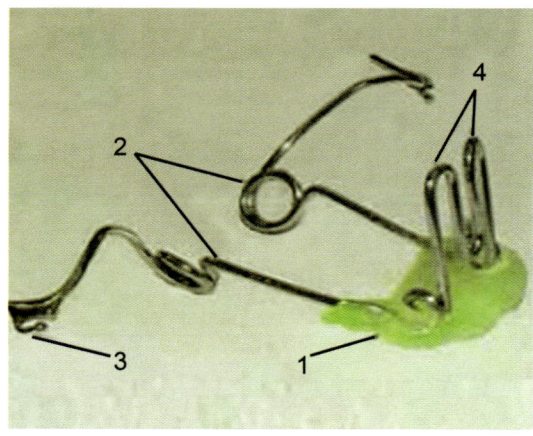

Fig. 15.166: FLMGM—maxillary part

palatal mucosa, and each one contains a "U" loop with coil (giving some flexibility to help in easy insertion and removal) at the level of second upper premolar. After the coils, the wires should run perpendicular to the midline towards the vestibule at the level of the mesial surface of upper first molar through the interdental space. Then, in the vestibule, the wires should run posteriorly to enter into the headgear tube.

- *Two retention hooks:* One in each side, have a ball end to avoid irritation, and are directed anteriorly and welded to the retention wire before entering the headgear tube.
- *Advancement loops:* Wire projection embedded in the acrylic button and extended towards the mandible. They consist of two consecutive long "U" loops, contain small protection coils where the wire exits the acrylic button, and are fabricated with round 1 mm thick hard stainless steel wire. The inclination of these advancing loops to the occlusal plane is about 70°, measured posteriorly.

Mandibular part (Fig. 15.167): It is made in a similar manner to a standard lingual arch with 1 mm stainless

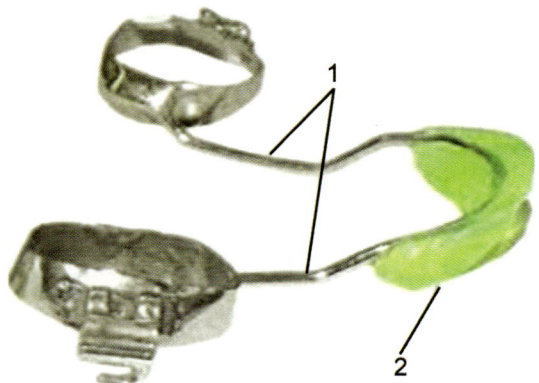

Fig. 15.167: FLMGM—mandibular part

steel hard wire welded to the lingual aspect of first molars band, and has the following features:

Its level in the anterior region must be 3–4 mm below the gingival margins of the incisors. It includes an inclined guiding plane, made of acrylic resin, fixed on the anterior part of lingual arch, seated on the lingual alveolar mucosa below the level of incisors necks till the level of mouth floor, and it is smooth to allow sliding against the advancement loops during mandibular closing movement to reach its anterior position.

Reactivation: Reactivation is generally required about every 2–3 months, and is carried out at the chairside, intra- or extraorally, by bending the advancement loops using orthodontic pliers.

Power Scope

Power scope is the latest innovation in Class II correction. This appliance addresses critical needs of the orthodontist, including patient comfort and acceptance, extensive range of motion, simple installation and much more. Power scope goes from package to mouth in just seconds and unlike other Class II correctors, there is no need for assembly, measuring or appliance manipulation. This wire-to-wire device delivers unmatched patient comfort, eliminates the need for headgear tubes or special band assemblies and can be used with either banded or bonded molar tubes. Power scope is simple, efficient and patient friendly Class II correction. Internal NiTi spring mechanism delivers 260 gm of force for continuous activation during treatment (Fig. 15.168).

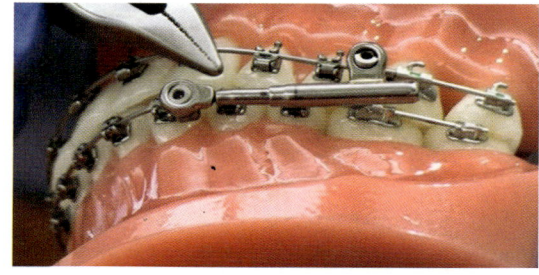

Fig. 15.168: Power scope

BIBLIOGRAPHY

1. Korrodi Ritto. Fixed Functional Appliances—A Classification Updated. 2015:1–30.
2. Hans Pancherz, Sabine Ruf. The Herbst Appliance Research-based Clinical Management. Pg 1–65.
3. Class II malocclusion treatment using Jasper Jumper appliance associated to intermaxillary elastics: a case report. Dental Press J 2013; 18(2).
4. Nazan Kucukkeles, Isil llhan, Ata orgun. Treatment efficiency in skeletal class II patients treated with the Jasper Jumper. Angle Orthodontist 2007; 77 (3): 449–456.

15.6 ORTHOPEDIC APPLIANCES

Chapter Outline

- Cervical headgear
- Reverse pull headgear
- High pull headgear

- Chin cup appliance
- Straight pull headgear

INTRODUCTION

There are two types of forces used in orthodontics.

Orthodontic forces: When applied bring about dental changes. They are light forces about 50–100 gm bringing about tooth movement.

Orthopedic forces: When applied bring about the skeletal changes. They are heavy forces (300–500 gm) that bring about changes in the magnitude and direction of bone growth. The treatment result depends on the following:

1. *Amount of force:* The force magnitude should be high i.e. at least greater than 400 gm per side to a maximum total of 2–3 lb to make sure that only skeletal and no dental movement takes place. Such high forces produce hyalinization leading to undermining resorption, which prevents tooth movement and this force is thus transmitted to skeletal element via dental units and hence only an orthopedic movement is seen.

2. *Duration of force:* The intermittent forces produce skeletal change whereas continuous forces produce dental movement. Extraoral appliances should be worn for about 12–14 hours/day to bring about the desired effect. Increasing the duration beyond the optimum range increases the dental effects. Also an intermittent heavy force is less harmful to the teeth and periodontium than a continuous force.

3. *Direction of force:* The direction of force application should be such as to maximize the skeletal effect. Depending on the requirement, the force vector may pass through center of resistance or above or below the center of resistance of skeletal unit involved like maxilla or mandible. A favorable skeletal effect is seen when a force is directed posteriorly and superiorly through the center of resistance of the maxilla. The extraoral anchor unit can be cervical or occipital to produce a low or high force vector. The length of the outer bow can also be altered to change the force vector. A cervical headgear produces extrusion of the molars along with distalization;

intermediate pull produces bodily movement of molars whereas an occipital attachment produces intrusion, which is favorable in Class II correction.

4. *Age of the patient:* Orthopedic appliances are most effective during the mixed dentition period as it takes advantage of the prepubertal growth spurt. However, treatment/retention should be maintained till growth is complete as these appliances change only the expression of growth and not the underlying growth.

5. *Timing of force application:* There is evidence that there is an increase in the release of growth hormones more during the evening and night and is associated with the sleep onset. Therefore, it is advisable for the child to wear the headgear in the evening and throughout the night. Generally, the child is more likely to wear the appliance at night.

Functional jaw orthopedics is the use of appliances which works by forward positioning of the mandible. This results in altering the activity of postural muscles of the craniofacial complex causing changes in skeletal and dental relationships. The goal is to enhance mandibular growth by allowing the full expression of the genetic potential and encouraging remodeling at the glenoid fossa.

The mandible is translated downward and forward by the appliance with resulting growth at the condyle and posterior surface of the ramus. Since the lateral pterygoid activity decreases after 6 to 8 weeks, repeated advancement of the appliance is required. Typical results from functional jaw orthopedics therapy show the following:

- *Condylar growth during treatment:* 1–3 mm.
- *Fossa displacement, growth and adaptation:* 3–5 mm with a dominant vertical vector.
- *More favorable growth direction:* 0.5–1.5 mm.
- *Withholding of downward and forward maxillary growth:* 1–1.5 mm.
- *Differential upward and forward eruption of lower buccal segments:* 1.5–2.5 mm.
- *Headgear effect:* 0.5 mm.

Dentofacial orthopedic appliances have been designed for:
- To affect neuromuscular and functional changes
- To impede or enhance growth or growth direction
- To achieve tooth movement

Orthopedic appliances generally use the teeth as via mediator to transmit forces to the underlying skeletal structures.

Headgear is used for delivering a posteriorly directed extraoral force to the maxilla. It is used to modify the growth of maxilla, to distalize and to protract the maxillary teeth, or to reinforce anchorage.

When headgear is used for skeletal growth modification, heavier forces are recommended. Such heavier forces bring about compression on the sutures of the maxilla, changing the magnitude and direction of their growth and modifying the pattern of bone apposition at these sites, while the mandible grow normally.

Following are the types of headgear:
- Cervical headgear
- Occipital headgear
- High pull headgear
- Reverse pull headgear
- Combination of occipital, cervical and straight pull headgear

HEADGEAR

Headgears are the most common among all the orthopedic appliances. They are ideally indicated in patients with excessive horizontal growth of the maxilla with or without vertical changes along with some proclination of the maxillary teeth, reasonably good mandibular dental and skeletal morphology. They are most effective in the prepubertal period. Headgears can also be used to distalize the maxillary dentition along with the maxilla. They are an important adjunct to gain or maintain anchorage.

Components
- Force delivering unit—face bow, J-hook
- Force generating unit
- Anchor unit—head cap, neck strap

J-Hook

Two separate curved wires are formed on their to small hooks, both of which attach directly to the anterior part of the maxillary archwire having soldered hooks. This type of headgear is more commonly used for retraction of canines or en masse retraction of anterior or for augmenting anchorage rather than orthopedic purposes.

Face Bow

One of the most important components helps in delivering extraoral force to the posterior teeth. The face bow consists of the following:

Outer bow/whisker bow: It is made up of round stainless steel wire 0.051" or 0.062" in dimension and is contoured around the face. It is the component which can be modified according to desired force vector by contoring it or by using either of the three sizes.
The outer bow may be:
1. Short—outer bow is shorter than inner bow.
2. Medium—outer bow is the same length as the inner bow.
3. Long—outer bow is longer than inner bow.

Inner bow: It is made up of 0.045" or 0.052" round stainless steel wire and inserts into the round buccal tube on the maxillary first molars. The inner bow is adapted according to the shape of the arch 'stops' in the form of 'U' loop, beyond bends and friction soldered stops are placed in the low mesial to the buccal tube to prevent it from sliding too far distally through the tube.

Junction: It is the point of attachment of the inner and outer bows which may be soldered or welded (Fig. 15.170). It is usually positioned at the midline of the two bows, however, it may be shifted to one side in case of asymmetric face bows.

Force Generating Unit

This connects the face bow to the anchor unit and delivers the force to the teeth and the underlying skeletal structures. The force element may be springs or elastics. Springs are preferred as they provide a constant force whereas elastics undergo force decay.

Anchor Unit

This is in the form of a head cap or a neck strap, which makes use of anchorage from the skull or back of the neck respectively. A combination of the two may also be used.

Headgears can be divided as follows:
1. According to the direction of force:
   a. Distal force
   b. Mesial force
2. According to the location of anchor unit:
   a. Cervical pull
   b. Occipital pull
   c. High pull
   d. Combination pull
3. According to asymmetric length of outer bow:
   a. Asymmetric headgear

CERVICAL HEADGEAR

Dr. Silas J Kloehn first described it in 1947. It is also known as the the Kloehn headgear. He reported the use of headgear attached by means of hooks to an upper 0.045' archwire stopped against the upper permanent first molars giving a reasonably well-controlled force action with a cervical neck strap to general force.

The decision to treat with cervical headgear needs to be based on a complete understanding of the desired tooth movement and the force system that is produced with this headgear.

Line of force moment (LFO) is a line from the strap force application point through the maxillary center of resistance

The different moments and forces produced by the cervical headgear depend on the situation of the outer bow in relation to the LFO.

The cervical (low-pull or Kloehn) headgear is used most frequently in patients of Class II malocclusions with decreased lower anterior facial height. The inner bow anchored to tubes that are placed on the buccal surfaces of molar bands (Fig. 15.169a and b).

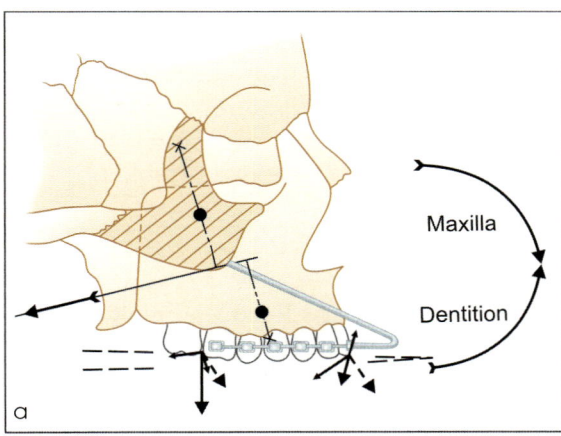

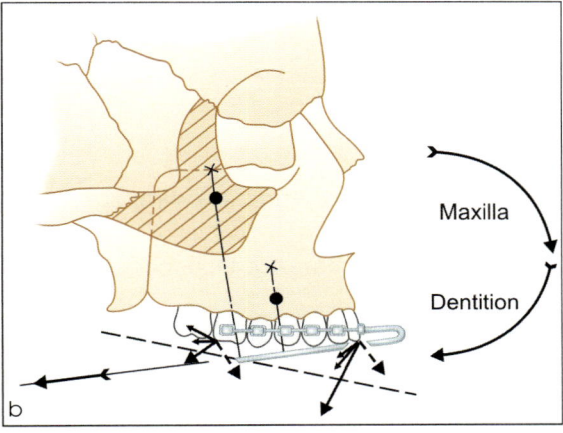

Fig. 15.169a and b: Cervical pull—effect of cervical pull headgear on dentition and maxilla

It inhibits forward displacement of the maxilla or maxillary teeth, while the rest of the dentofacial structures continue their normal growth. This can cause a change in the intermaxillary relationship from Class II to Class I. It tips the molar crown distally. It causes extrusion of upper molars, but desirable in patients with short lower facial height.

The downward and backward force of the cervical headgear intermittently extrudes the upper molars and carries them distally. The upper incisors tip lingually from the apex. This occurs when the overjet has been reduced enough for the lower lip to close over the upper incisors causing a functional retraction of these teeth.

Effect of different positions of the outer bow when the outer bow is bent upwards:
- A distalizing force to the upper teeth is done which is good for correction of Class II relation. When the outer bow is bent upwards bringing it down to the occlusal plane tends to produce a negative moment that flattens the occlusal plane. Hence the steepening effect of the cervical headgear is nullified.
- Eruption of the entire upper arch tends to increase the mandibular plane angle and tends to worsen the Class II skeletal relationship, this type is good for patients with forward growth rotation.

When the outer bow is bent downward:
- Positive moment on the occlusal plane is seen that tends to steepen the occlusal plane since the pull is below.
- Extrusive force and a distalizing force.

When the outer bow and inner bow are in the same level: No moment is produced and there is a net distalizing and extrusive force.

When the outer bow is shorter than inner bow: The head gear strap hook is placed too far anteriorly. This results in a greater tendency to steepen the occlusal plane when the straps are engaged. The pull of the bow is further forward from the Cres and this tends to steepen the occlusal plane.

When the outer bow is long, there is a tendency to flatten the occlusal plane.

Ricketts also observed the following findings:
- There was retraction of maxillary complex as measured at point A.
- Palate rotated in a clockwise direction.
- There was minimal extrusion of upper 1st molars and incisor teeth.
- Occlusal plane rotated in anticlockwise direction.
- Minimal or no adverse rotation

Advantage: Direction of pull is advantageous in treatment of short face Class II maxillary protrusive cases with low MPA and deep bites.

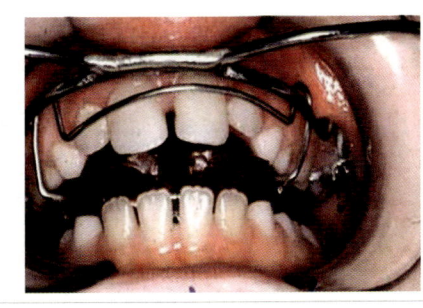

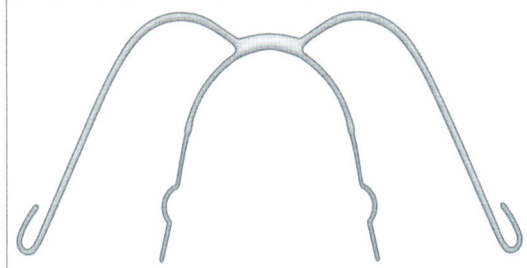

Fig. 15.170: Inner and outer face bow

Disadvantage: It normally causes extrusion of the upper molars. This movement is seldom desirable except in patients with reduced lower anterior facial height. It is contraindicated in patients with steep mandibular planes and in open bite cases.

Orthopedic Changes in Class III Malocclusion (Fig. 15.171)

- Stimulation of maxillary growth
- Inhibition of mandibular projection

Effects of Chin Cup

- Redirection of mandibular growth in a downward and backward direction.

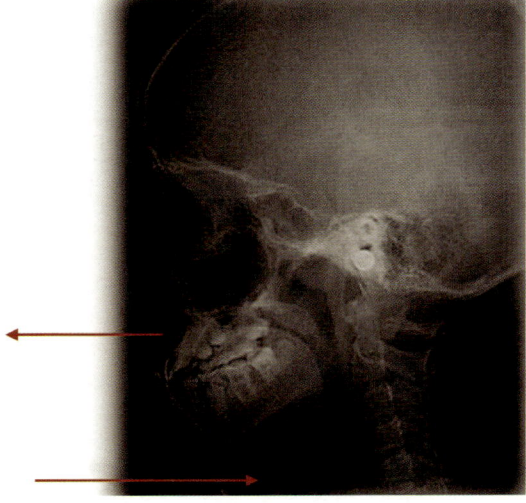

Fig. 15.171: Effect of chin cup on maxilla and mandible

- Remodeling of the mandible and a decrease in mandibular plane angle and gonial angle
- Lingual tipping of lower incisors
- Improvement in skeletal and soft tissue profile.

Therefore, chin cup works well in patients with ewduced or normal lower anterior face height but is contraindicated in long patients (Fig. 15.171).

REVERSE PULL HEADGEAR

It was developed by Hickham in 1991 using the top of the head and chin as support. The headband and chin cap are connected with the arms parallel to the mandibular bases on both sides.

Maxillary protraction is recommended for skeletal Class III patients with maxillary deficiency. Delaire and others used face mask for maxillary protraction. Petit later modified Delaire's concept by increasing the amount of force generated and thus reducing the overall treatment time. In 1987, McNamara introduced the use of bonded acrylic expansion appliance with the occlusal coverage for maxillary protraction. Turley improved patient's cooperation by fabricating customized face masks.

It is used to apply an anteriorly directed force via elastics on the maxillary teeth and maxilla. It is also useful in Class III associated with a CLP anomaly and hypodontia where forward movement of the buccal segment teeth to close space is desirable (Figs 15.172a to e).

Indications

- Mild to moderate Class II skeletal malocclusion due to maxillary retrusion, reverse pull headgear works best in young, growing children (around 8 years).
- Ideal patients for face mask should have:
    a. Normal or retrusive but not protrusive maxillary teeth as face mask causes forward movement of the maxillary teeth relative to the maxilla
    b. Short

Side Effects

- It includes downward and backward rotation of the mandible.
- Lingual tipping of mandibular incisors.

Parts of Face Mask

It is made up of following components:
- Metal framework
- Chin cup/pad
- Froehead cap

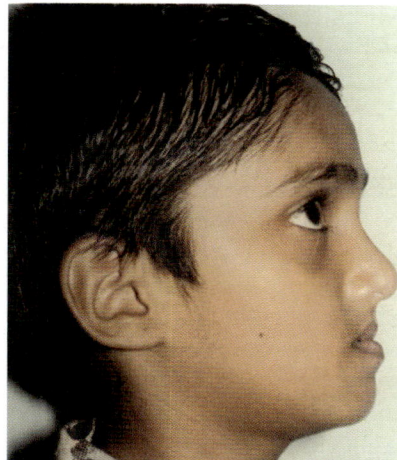

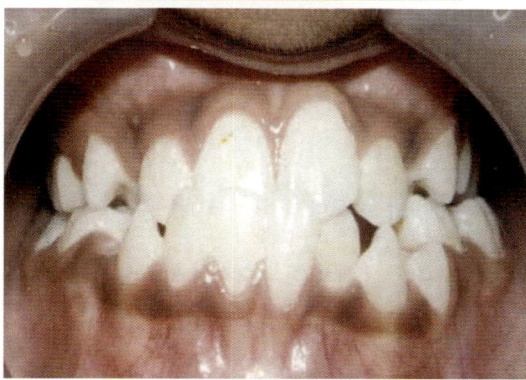

Fig. 15.172a: Extraoral and intraoral photographs for reverse pull headgear

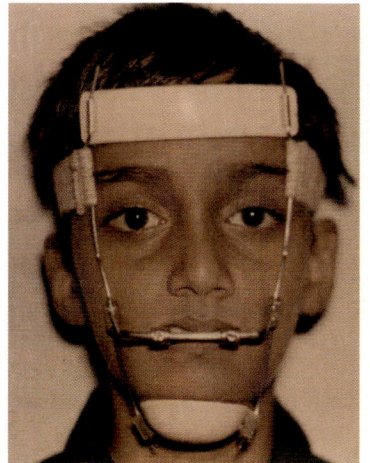 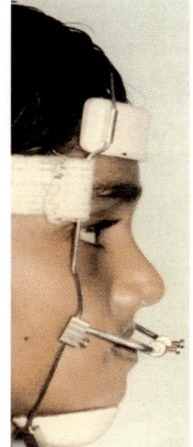

Fig. 15.172b: Face mask appliance in position

- Intraoral appliance
- Heavy elastics

The reverse pull headgear is made up of a rigid extraoral framework connecting two pads that contact the soft tissues in the forehead and chin regions. The pads are usually adjustable through the screws. The

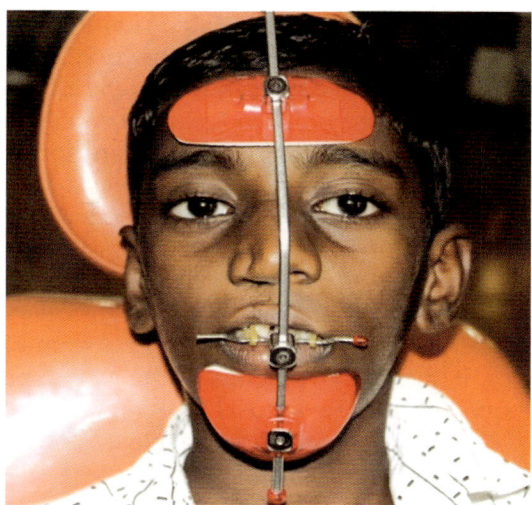

Fig. 15.172c: Reverse pull headgear

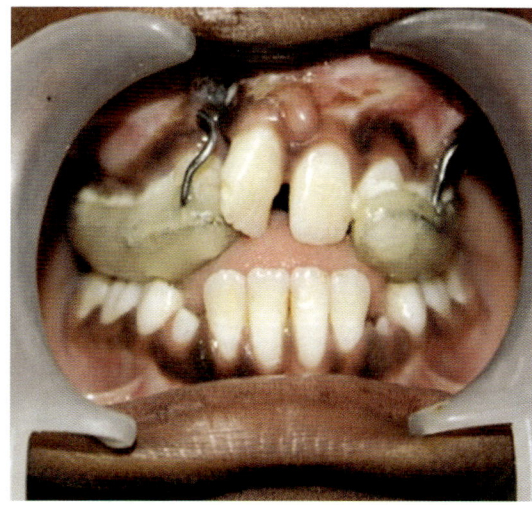

Fig. 15.172d: Bonded RME using Hyrax—front view

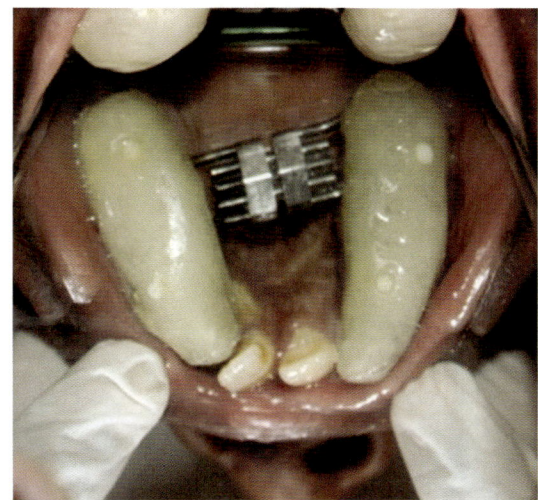

Fig. 15.172e: Bonded RME using Hyrax—occlusal view

elastics are attached to an adjustable anterior wire with hooks which is connected to the framework. Anchorage is usually derived from both chin and forehead, however, some forms of reverse pull headgears deliver anchorage from only chin or forehead. Two sites of anchorage have advantages that anchorage is spread over a large area thus reducing the amount of force exerted. Along with the face mask, banded or bonded palatal expansion appliance may also be used to correct crossbite. To resist tooth movement, it is better to splint the maxillary teeth together as a single unit. Whatever the maxillary appliance, it should have hooks in the canine primary molar region above the occlusal level for attachment of elastics. This places the force vector closer to the center of resistance of the maxilla and helps in pure translation.

The heavy elastics apply a forward traction on the upper arch. Elastics attached from the vertical posts of the chin cup to the molar tubes or soldered hook can bring about tooth movement

Biomechanical Considerations

The maxilla can be advanced 2–4 mm forward over a period of 8–12 months. The amount of maxillary movement is influenced by a number of factors like:

a. *Amount of force:* Successful maxillary protraction can be brought by 300–500 gm of force per side in the primary or mixed dentition.

b. *Direction of force:* According to most authors, a 15–20° downward pull to the occlusal plane is required to produce forward maxillary movement. In most cases of maxillary deficiency, maxilla is deficient in the vertical plane as well, therefore, a slight downward direction of force is usually desirable. The line of force passes below the center of resistance of the maxilla and dentition producing a counterclockwise moment on the maxilla and dentition. This results in a possible extrusion of maxillary teeth leading to a downward and backward rotation of the mandible. However, in patients with increased anterior facial height, downward pull is contraindicated.

c. *Duration of force:* On an average, at least 8–12 months of wear is required to produce the desired effect.

d. Frequency of use is 12–14 hours/day.

e. *Age of patient:* Optimal results are seen when face mask is used in the primary or early mixed dentition period. An optimal time to intervene an early Class III malocclusion is at the time of eruption of permanent maxillary central incisors. The anchor molars are also erupted by this time.

f. *Anchorage systems:* Palatal arches or palatal expansion appliances may be used as anchorage for maxillary protraction. Various authors recommend palatal expansion before protraction as expansion is supposed to disarticulate the maxilla making it favorable to respond to protraction forces.

Different Types

• *Protraction headgear:* In the early 1960s, Hickham developed the protraction headgear for forward maxillary traction. It is made up of 2 long and 2 short arms all of which originate from the chin cup. The long arms run parallel to the lower border of the mandible and then bend up vertically at the angle of the mandible to end behind the ears. These ends give attachment to an elastic strap which encircles the head. The short arms are used to engage the elastics. The advantage of this appliance is its ability to apply unilateral force, better esthetics and comfort.

• *Delaire face mask:* It is made up of a rigid, square-shaped metal framework which connects a chin cap to the forehead pad and has a wire for elastic attachment.

• *Petit type of face mask:* Petit modified Delaire's face mask by increasing the amount of force generated by the appliance, thus decreasing the overall treatment time. The appliance is made up of a single midline rod connecting the forehead and chin. In this appliance, the forehead cap, chin cup and crossbar can be adjusted according to the patient's needs.

• *Tubinger model of face mask:* It is a modified version of face mask in which the forehead caps and chin cup are connected with the help of two midline metal rods. An adjustable crossbar is attached in front of the mouth to engage elastics.

CHIN CUP APPLIANCE

It covers the chin and is connected to headgear. It is used to restrict the forward and downward growth of the mandible.

It is possible to use a chin to deliberately rotate the mandible downward and backward redirecting rather than restraining the mandibular growth this reduces the chin prominence at the expense of increasing the anterior face height. But controlling excessive mandibular growth is still a problem in orthodontics.

There are two types of chin cup appliances:

• Occipital pull chin cup
• Vertical pull chin cup

Occipital pull chin cup (Fig. 15.173): The anchorage is derived from the occipital region. It is used in Class III malocclusions associated with mild to moderate mandibular prognathism. It is used in patients with short anterior lower facial height, pull of chin is below the condyle. It is also indicated in patients with slightly

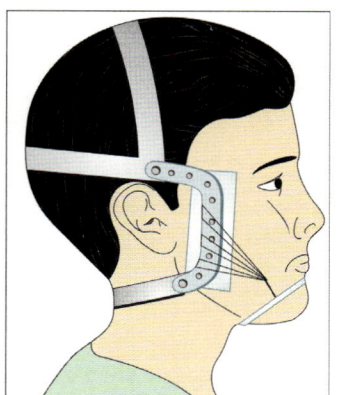 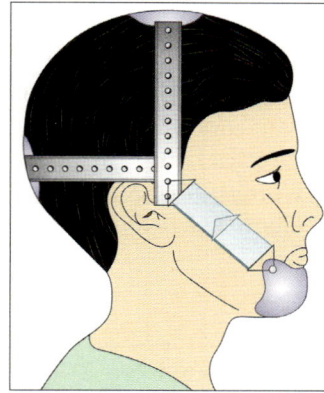

Fig. 15.173: Occipital pull chin cap

protrusive lower incisors as they invariably produce lingual tipping of the lower incisors.

Vertical pull chin cup (Fig. 15.174): It is indicated in patients with steep mandibular plane angle and excessive lower facial height. It derives anchorage from the parietal regions.

Philosophy of Chin Cup Therapy

Mandible grows by apposition of bone at the condyle and along its free posterior border. Condyle is not growth center and condylar growth is largely a response to translation of surrounding tissues. This contemporary view offers a more optimistic view of the possibilities for growth restraint of the mandible, as with chin cup therapy.

Basic Chin Cup Appliance Design

It utilizes a head cap which is fitted/seated on the posterosuperior aspects of the cranium as anchorage and has attachments for the placement and activation of the chin cup. It consists of the following:
1. *Force module:* Elastic/metal spring that provides the desired tension levels on the chin cup.

2. *Chin cup:* Custom made or performed, hard or soft. A hard chin cup can be custom made from plastic using a chin impression. A soft cup can be made from a football helmet chinstrap. A commercial metal or plastic cup can be used, if it fits well enough. Soft cups produce more tooth movement than hard ones.

Line of Direction of Force

There are two ways to use chin cup:
1. Line of force acting directly through the condyle with the indent of impeding mandibular growth in the same way that extraoral force against the maxilla impedes its growth. This method causes no opening of the mandibular plane angle.
2. Line of force acting below the condyle:
   a. Chin is rotated downward and backward
   b. Less force is required.
   c. Increase in facial height is achieved for a decrease in the prominence of the chin.

Vertical force on the chin
a. Decrease in the mandibular plane angle
b. Decrease in gonial angle
c. Increase in posterior facial height.

Biomechanics of Vertical Pull Headgear (Fig. 15.175)

- If the bow is hooked to the head cap so that the line of force is perpendicular to the occlusal plane and through the CR, there will be pure intrusion taking place.
- If the outer bow is placed anywhere in the anterior compartment, there will be counterclockwise moment; intrusive and posterior force.
- If the outer bow is placed anywhere in the posterior section, there will be clockwise moment, vertical intrusive and horizontal forward forces.

STRAIGHT PULL HEADGEAR (Fig. 15.176)

It is indicated in Class II malocclusion with no vertical problems. It prevents anterior migration of maxillary teeth and translates them posteriorly. The buccal force

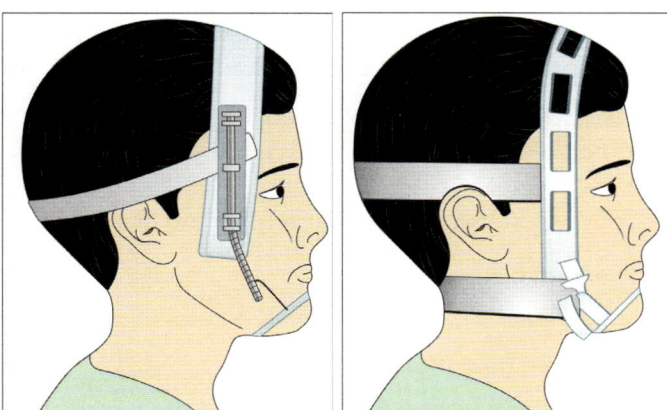

Fig. 15.174: Vertical pull chin cup

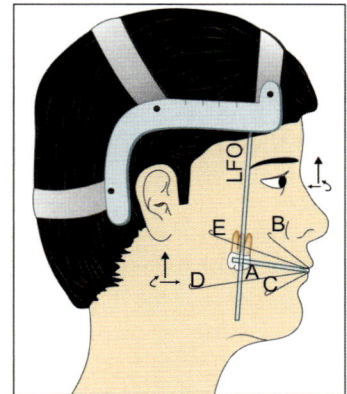

Fig. 15.175: Vertical pull headgear

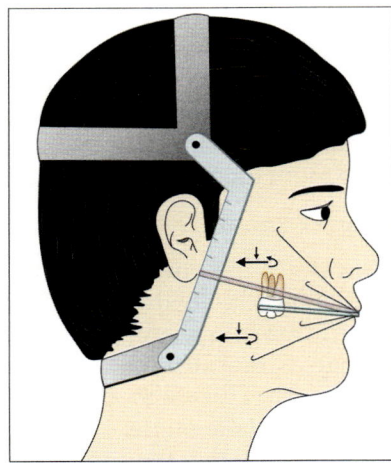

Fig. 15.176: Straight pull headger

is given to molars with expansion of inner bow. It is a combination of the high pull and cervical headgears with the advantages of increased versatility. Depending upon the force system desired, the orthodontist has the opportunities to change the location of the LFO.

HIGH PULL HEADGEAR

It always produces an intrusive and posterior direction of pull due to the position of the head cap. The direction of the moment that is produced is dependent on the position of the outer bow. If the outer bow is placed anterior to the line (angulated more than 45° to the occlusal plane) moment produced will be counter clockwise. On the other hand, if the outer bow is placed posterior to the line (angulated less than 45° to occlusal plane), the moment produced will be in a clockwise direction.

BIBLIOGRAPHY

1. Dentofacial orthopedics with functionl appliances. In: Graber TM, Rakosi T. Petrovic AG, editors. Principles of functional appliance. St Louis: Mosby; 1985.
2. Concepts of functional jaw orthopedics. In: Graber TM, Neumann B, editors. Removable orthodontic appliances. 2nd ed. Philadelphia Sauders: 1984.P-87.
3. Rakosi TR, Graber TM, Petrovic AG. Dentofacial orthopedics with functional appliances. St Louis: Mosby;1985.

PREVIOUS YEAR'S UNIVERSITY QUESTIONS

Essay

1. What are the different types of headgears, and describe and give their indications.
2. What is orthopedic force? Describe the various interceptive procedures of growth modulation for maxillary skeletal discrepancies.
3. Describe the principles of headgear and write about cervical headgear in detail

Short Questions

1. Chin cap
2. Face mask
3. Types of headgear
4. Uses of headgear
5. Combipull headgear
6. Center of resistance of maxilla

MCQs

1. *Which of the following are true of chin cap?*
   a. It has to exert 2–3 pounds, if worn for 10–2 hours
   b. It has to exert 1–2 pounds, if worn for 16–18 hours
   c. It has to be worn for 24 hours/day to correct severe prognathic mandible
   d. All of the above   **(Ans: d)**

2. *Main drawback of cervical headgear therapy:*
   a. Extrusion of upper molars
   b. Intrusion of upper molars
   c. Extrusion of lower molars
   d. Intrusion of lower molars   **(Ans: a)**

3. *Orthopedic force is:*
   a. Light force (50–100 gm)
   b. Heavy force (300–500 gm)
   c. Both A and B
   d. None of the above   **(Ans: b)**

4. *Face mask is also called:*
   a. Reverse pull headgear
   b. Protraction headgear
   c. Both a and b
   d. None of the above   **(Ans: c)**

5. *Which type of face mask has least patient acceptance?*
   a. Delarie type of face mask
   b. Tubinger type of face mask
   c. Petit type of face mask   **(Ans: a)**

6. *Outer bow of face bow can be:*
   a. Short   b.   Medium
   c. Long   d.   All of the above   **(Ans: d)**

7. *Where center of resistance of maxilla is located:*
   a. Between the roots of the premolar teeth
   b. Between the roots of the molar teeth
   c. Between the roots of the second molar teeth
   d. None of the above   **(Ans: a)**

8. *Cervical headgear is contraindicated in:*
   a. Open bite
   b. Occipital headgear
   c. High pull headgear
   d. All of the above   **(Ans: c)**

Methods of Gaining the Space

Chapter Outline

- Introduction
- Different methods of gaining space
- Proximal reduction

- Choice of teeth for extraction
- Molar distalization
- Uprighting of molars

INTRODUCTION

The correction of malocclusions requires space in order to move the teeth into more ideal locations. For achieving majority of the treatment objectives, space has to be created within the jaws.

DIFFERENT METHODS OF GAINING SPACE

- Reproximation
- Molar distalization
- Extraction
- Expansion of arches
- Derotation of posteriors
- Protracting anteriors/flaring
- Uprighting of molars
- Distraction osteogenesis

Synonyms

- Slenderization
- Proximal disking
- Interproximal reduction
- Reproximation
- Proximal slicing

Need for space in the clinical conditions like
- Crowding
- Proclination
- Deep bite

- Rotated anterior
- Constricted arches

Definition

The proximal stripping is a method by which the proximal surfaces of the teeth are sliced in order to reduce the mesiodistal width of the teeth

Indications

- Proximal stripping is usually indicated when the space required is minimal, i.e. 0–2.5 mm, according to Carey's analysis.
- If the Bolton's analysis shows mild tooth material excess in either of the arches, it is possible to reduce the tooth material.
- It can be undertaken in the lower anterior region as an aid to retention.
- According to Peck and Peck analysis, proximal stripping is indicated, if the mesiodistal dimension of tooth is less than labiolingual dimension.

Contraindications

- Proximal stripping is not carried out in young patients, as they possess large pulp chamber, which increases pulpal exposure.
- Patients who are susceptible to caries or those who have a high caries index.

Investigation

- Carey's arch perimeter analysis
- Bolton's analysis
- Diagnostic set up
- Intraoral periapical radiographs
- Peck and Peck ratio

PROXIMAL REDUCTION

There are two types of proximal reduction:

1. *Localized reduction:* Localized reduction is usually done on lower and upper anterior teeth.
2. *Generalized reduction:* Generalized interproximal reduction is carried out in moderate space discrepancy cases.

Proximal reduction is performed using abrasive strips (Fig. 16.1), safe-sided diamond disc, long thin tapered fissure bur (Fig. 16.2) and very thin and carborundum disk (Fig. 16.3). Care should be taken to establish proper contact between the teeth. Contact points are usually converted into contact area. Not more than 40% of the enamel thickness should be reduced.

Fluoride Application

Subsequent to interproximal reduction, topical fluoride application is recommended. This is done for twofold purpose:

- To reduce the postproximal slicing sensitivity
- To reduce caries attack

Advantages

- Extractions are avoided
- To establish normal interarch relation in patients with Bolton's discrepancy.

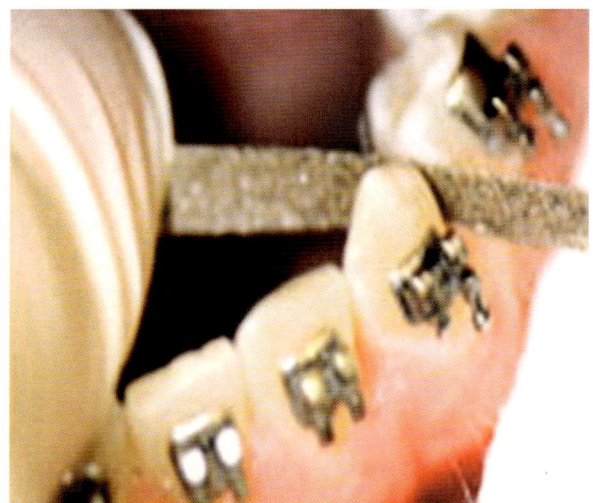

Fig. 16.1: Abrasive strips

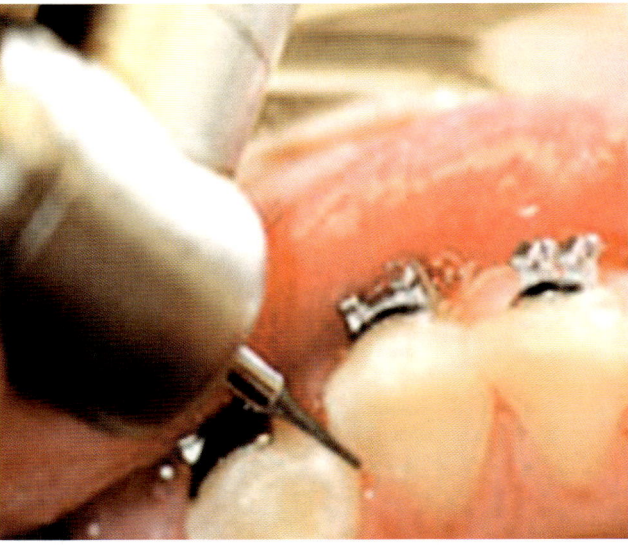

Fig. 16.2: Long thin tapered fissure bur

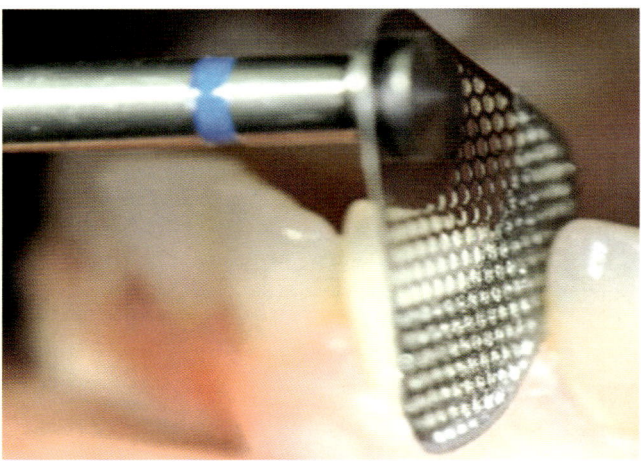

Fig. 16.3: Carborandum disk

- Minor interarch problems are corrected, e.g. single tooth crossbite.

Disadvantages

- Shape of the grossly altered gingivitis
- Loss of normal contact
- Altered esthetics
- Hypersensitivity
- Deposits of plaque and calculus leading to gingivitis
- More chances for proximal caries
- Unsightly appearance with enlarged embasures

According to Sheridan (Fig. 16.4)

- 0.4 mm reduction per each surface of posterior teeth.
- 0.25 mm reduction per each surface of anterior teeth.

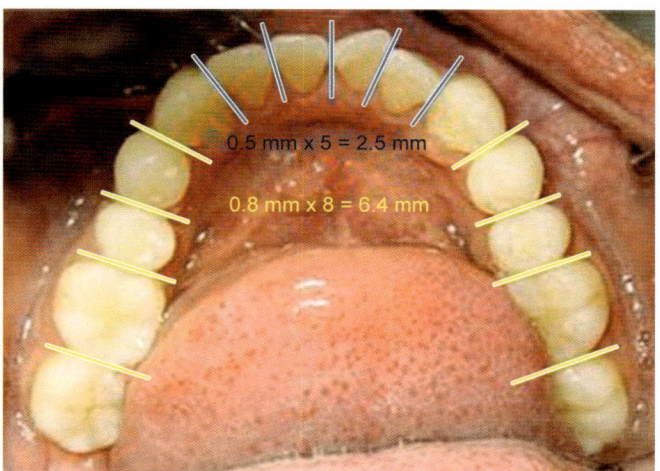

Fig. 16.4: Total space gaining is 8.9 mm

0.5 mm x 5 = 2.5 mm
0.8 mm x 8 = 6.4 mm

CHOICE OF TEETH FOR EXTRACTION

The following factors are considered to select the teeth for extraction:

- The amount of tooth material excess in relation to arch length and site of crowding
- The anteroposterior interarch relationship
- Profile of the patient
- Age of the patient and dental developmental status
- The direction of jaw growth
- Carious status of the teeth
- General health status of the dentition

Maxillary Central Incisors

Incisors are esthetically the most prominent teeth due to their position in the arches. So, it is rarely undertaken unless their condition necessitates their extraction.

Indications

- Unfavorably impacted maxillary central incisor which cannot be aligned properly.
- Severely fractured maxillary central incisor
- Grossly decayed tooth that cannot be conserved.
- Upper central incisor with severely dilacerated root, which cannot be moved orthodontically.

Maxillary Lateral Incisors

The teeth exhibit greatest variation in form, number and eruption pattern.

Indications

- When it is palatally blocked and good contact with central incisor and canine.

- When one upper lateral is congenitally missing, the other side of lateral may be the choice for extraction so as to balance the arch symmetry.
- Malformation of the tooth.

Mandibular Incisors

Lower incisor extraction is often followed by narrowing of intercanine width, lingual inclination of the remaining incisor teeth deepening of the bite and eventually leads to collapse of the lower arch.

Indications

- When a lower incisor is completely excluded from the arch with good alignment of the remaining teeth.
- Due to gingival recession and loss of periodontal support.
- In case of Class III malocclusion with lower incisor crowding, a central incisor can be removed to obtain normal overjet and relief of crowding.

Canines

Canines have the longest and strongest roots of all teeth that provide excellent anchorage in the alveolar bone. It gives high esthetic value because it occupies the corner of the mouth and also assists in guiding the teeth into intercuspal position by canine guidance. Due to all these reasons, the canine extraction should be avoided and should be attempted when it is absolutely necessary and completely justified.

Indications

- Ectopically erupted or unfavorably impacted canines
- When the canine is completely out of arch.

First Premolars

First premolars are routinely extracted as a part of orthodontic treatment.

- Since the first premolars are positioned immediately next to the anterior segment, their extraction provides maximum space which can be utilized for the retraction of proclined anteriors and thus maximum lip retraction is possible.
- Extraction of premolars is least likely to disturb molar intercuspation.
- First premolars are also extracted in the serial extraction procedure.

Extraction of Second Premolars

- In borderline cases
- Unfavorable impacted or rotated grossly in the arch

- It is preferred in open bite cases as it would encourage deepening of the arch

Extraction of First Molars

It is considered to play a key role in the establishment of occlusion by Angle. It is usually not extracted unless indicated. Extraction of fist permanent molar is not advisable due to the following reasons:
- It does not provide an adequate space for decrowding of anterior.
- Following first molar, the second premolar may tip into the extraction space.
- Masticatory function of the patient is affected.

Indications
- When it is grossly decayed.
- Extraction of first molar is advantageous in open bite cases as this may lead to deepening of the bite.

Benefits
- Prevention of impaction of third molars.
- It helps in relieving posterior crowding.

Limitations
- Extraction results in lack of anchorage for orthodontic therapy.
- Extraction of first permanent molar makes it difficulty to define the type of malocclusion according to Angle's classification.
- Mesial drifting of second molar into the first permanent molar extraction space.

Extraction of Second Permanent Molar

- To prevent third molar impaction
- For distalization of molars
- In open bite cases
- To relieve lower incisor crowding
- To relieve impaction of second premolar

Extraction of Third Molar

Although extraction of third molars may be beneficial in open bite cases as this encourages deepening of bite.

Indications
- Progressive crowding of lower anterior is observed in adolescence and early adult life. Some orthodontists advocate extraction of third molars to prevent such late crowding.
- Pericoronities

- Impacted third molars which are not likely to erupt into ideal position are frequently extracted.

Different Extraction Procedure

- Balanced extraction
- Compensatory extraction
- Phased extraction
- Enforced extraction
- Therapeutic extraction
- Wilkinson's extraction
- Serial extraction

Balanced Extraction

Balanced extraction is defined as the method of extraction where removal of another tooth on the opposite side of the same arch is done. The teeth distal to the extraction space move into the space while the teeth mesial to the extraction space can also move distally into the space. Thus, the midline of the arch may shift to the side of the extraction space, creating asymmetry in the arch.

Compensating Extraction

It refers to the extraction of a tooth in the opposite jaw of the same teeth group (antagonistic tooth). For example, if third molar is extracted in the right quadrant of the maxillary arch then the third molar in the right quadrant of the mandibular arch is also extracted. This type of extraction is called compensatory extraction. When a tooth is removed in one arch, the opposing tooth may supraerupt.

Phased Extraction

It may be advantageous to extract the indicated teeth in two phases, especially to affect a change in the molar occlusion. In this method, the tooth in one arch is extracted a few months earlier than in the other arch.

Enforced Extraction

Orthodontist is sometimes forced to extract the teeth in poor condition, e.g. grossly decayed, fractured, unfavorably impacted and periodontally compromised teeth. This is called enforced extraction.

Therapeutic Extraction

Certain healthy tooth may have to be sacrificed to facilitate proper alignment of other teeth in cases of severe arch length–tooth material discrepancy. This is called therapeutic extraction.

Wilkinson's Extraction

Reason for the extraction of first permanent molar by Wilkinson is that it is highly prone for dental caries.

Serial Extraction

This will be discussed in the Interceptive Procedures Chapter.

MOLAR DISTALIZATION

Correction of Class II malocclusion without extractions requires maxillary molar distalization by means of intraoral or extraoral forces. Headgears are quite successful except for its patient compliance.

Hilgers introduced the term non-compliance to orthodontics, where patient cooperation is minimally needed. Molar distalizer is a technique that has added a new column in the practice of every orthodontist to produce consistent, predictable and high quality results.

Since space is easier to gain in the maxillary arch than in the mandible because of increased trabecular structure of supporting bone and increased anchorage afforded by the palatal vault, the distalization of maxillary molar is of significant value for the treatment of cases with mild to moderate arch discrepancy and Class II molar relationship associated with a normal mandible.

Indications

- Mesial tipping or migration of maxillary first molars due to carious attack of primary molars, early extraction of primary molars.
- The discrepancy anterior to the first molars does not exceed 2–3 mm on either side or when there is no evidence of developing posterior crowding.
- An end-on Class II molar relationship due to the ectopic eruption of either the first or second bicuspid, impacted canine, unerupted and ectopic eruption of cuspids.
- Mild to moderate arch discrepancy.
- Incisors are retroclined or when the profile affords some proclination.

Molar Distalization in Lower Arch

- Lip bumper
- Modified lingual appliance
- Distal jet for lower
- Franzulum appliance

Limitations

- Unfavorable growth pattern
- TMJ problem

- Excessive proclination of anterior
- Posterior crowding

Distalization of maxillary first molars aids in increase in vertical height. This is due to that they move closer to the hinge axis of rotation of the TMJ and come into occlusal contact sooner with the opposing teeth during the act of closure thereby increasing the vertical dimension of occlusion.

Timing of Distalization

The patient should be treated before the age of 9 years as the roots of the molar have not completed their growth and the orthodontic distal tipping or distal bodily movement is easier. If the treatment is delayed too long and the second molar begins to erupt, then it requires vastly increased anchorage and a very efficient appliance approach in moving first and second molars distally.

Many clinicians suggest that molar distalization is very efficient, if it is carried out when the second molar crown is at the apical third of the first molar.

Maxillary Second Molar Extraction in Maxillary First Molar Distalization

Hilgers in 1992 suggested that when a great deal of distal movement is needed, it is preferable not to extract the upper first bicuspids; it is always beneficial to remove the upper second molars and let the third molars drift into place.

The extraction of second molar delivers almost double the space gained by bicuspid extraction. It offers relief of crowding in both the anterior and posterior segments, simultaneously.

The optimal time for extracting second molar is when the third molars have migrated sufficiently in the maxillary alveolar bone.

In this chapter, a few molar distalizers are described.

The Pendulum Appliance

Dr James J Hilgers in 1992 developed the pendulum appliance which is a hybrid that uses a large Nance acrylic button in the palate for anchorage, along with 0.032 TMA springs that deliver a light continuous force to the upper first molars without affecting the palatal button (Fig. 16.5). Thus, the appliance produces a broad, swinging arc or pendulum of force from the midline of the palate to the upper molars. The springs are extended close to center of palatal button to have a maximum range of motion, to have easier insertion and to reduce forces to an acceptable range. If the expansion of the upper arch is needed, a mid-palatal jack-screw can be

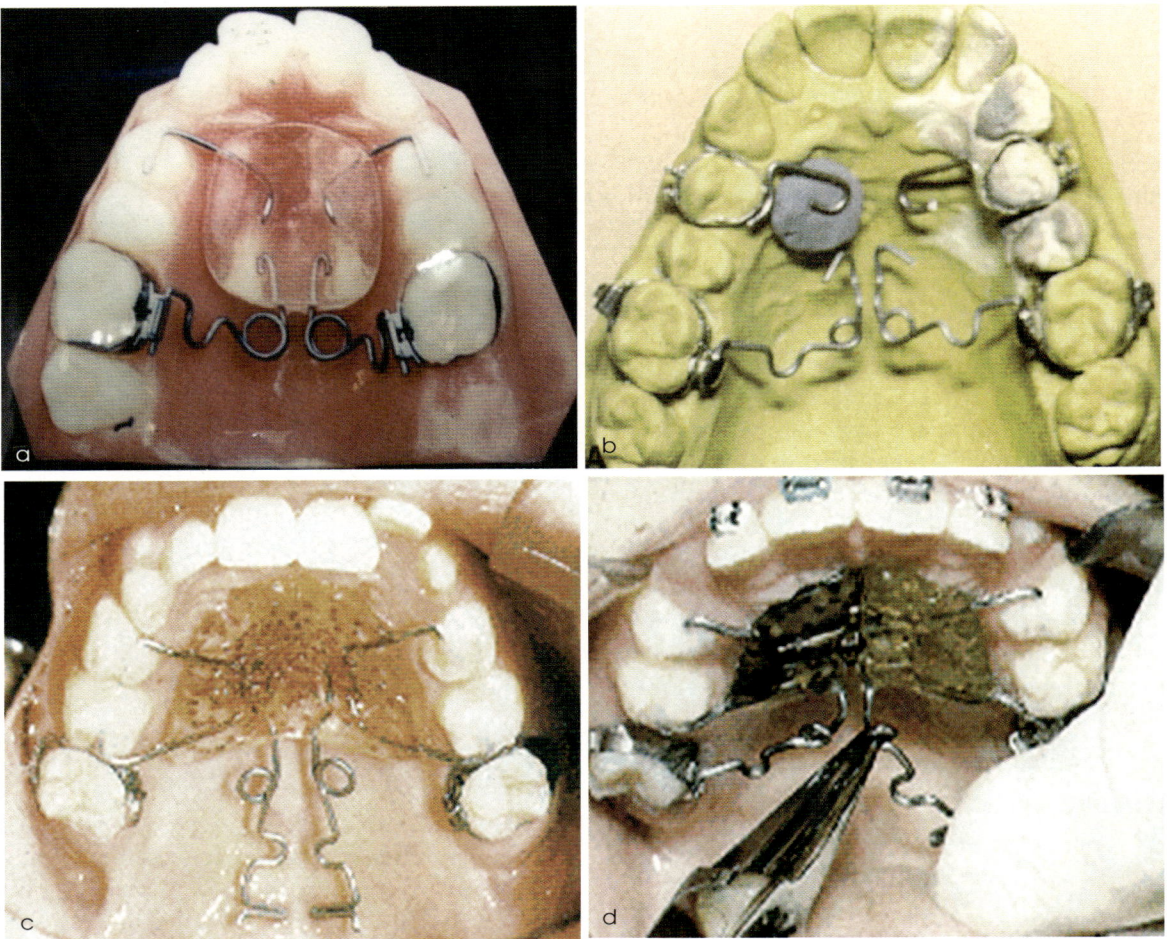

Fig. 16.5: (a) Pendulum appliance; (b) Wire fabrication; (c) Preactivation and placement; (d) Reactivation

incorporated into the center of Nance button and the screw is activated one-quarter turn every 3 days, after a week. This version is known as 'pend-X'.

It is better to preactivate the springs before appliance placement by bending them parallel to the midline of the palate or perpendicular to the body of the appliance. A 60° activation of the pendulum springs produces a force of 230 gm per side. Molar bands are cemented and adhesive is put over the occlusal rests and smoothened. Then, the spring is brought forward with finger pressure and mesial end of the recurved loop is grasped with Weingart plier and spring is seated in lingual sheath. Once the molar is distalized, it should be stabilized by either overcorrection or Nance button.

Lokar Distalizer

Scott in 1996 described the Lokar distalizer which utilizes continuous, ideal forces of NiTi springs. It is easy to insert, to ligate and use. Precise distalization

can be accomplished usually with one activation. It can be used unilaterally and is easy to adjust. It can be used in early treatment or with appliance in place. Anchorage can be achieved with Nance button or by employing full sized arch with fixed appliance. The appliance is placed in the buccal tubes distally and mesially ligating it to the premolar brackets and activates it.

After the distalization, Nance button is placed molar to molar for stabilization (Fig. 16.6).

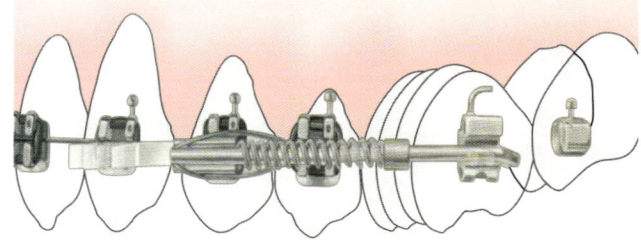

Fig. 16.6: Lokar distalizer

Magnets

Repelling Magnets

The repelling magnets are used for distalization of molars. The modified Nance appliance to the maxillary first premolars is fixed with a wire extending from the first premolars to the palatogingival surfaces of the incisors and soldered to the framework of the appliance. The acrylic button is placed anteriorly to contact the incisors. This reinforces the anchorage potential of the conventional Nance button by including the incisors in the system. The force exerted by the magnets begins at 200–225 gm, but drops substantially as space opens. With 1 mm of space between magnets, the appliance force is only 75 gm. Consequently, retying the ligature once a week to ensure at least 75 gm of force against the molars reactivates the magnets. The molars are distalized about 3 mm in seven weeks in those patients who do not have second molars. The rate of molar movement in patients with second molars is usually 0.75–1 mm per month (Fig. 16.7).

THE DISTAL JET/THE LINGUAL DISTALIZER SYSTEM

A distal jet appliance/lingual distalizer system was developed that can distalize maxillary molars without disadvantages.

Bilateral tubes of 0.36 mm internal diameters are attached to an acrylic Nance button. A coil spring and a screw-clamp are slide over each tube. Nickel titanium coil springs of 150 gm for children and 250 gm for adults of stainless steel springs can be used. The wire extends from the acrylic through each tube in a bayonet bend that is inserted into the lingual sheath of the first molar band. An anchor wire from the Nance button is soldered to bands on the second premolars.

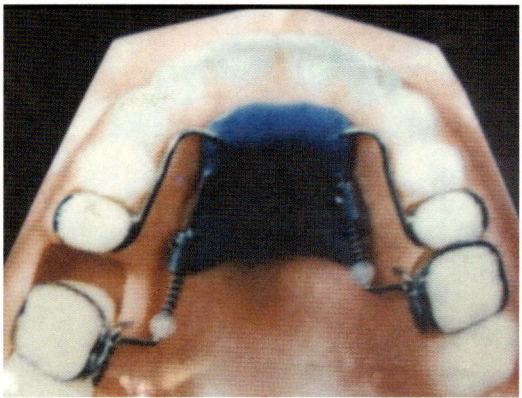

Fig. 16.8: Distal jet

Reactivation is done by sliding the clamp closer to the first molar once a month. Once distalization is complete, the appliance can be converted to a Nance retainer simply by replacing the clamp-spring assemblies with light-cured of cold-cured acrylic and cutting of the arms to the premolars. Maxillary molar distalization of 3 to 5 mm with presence of second molar takes approximately four months with a minimal anchorage loss. It is ideal for unilateral or bilateral molar distalization (Fig. 16.8).

Lip Bumper

It is also known as 'Plumpers'. The lip bumper is a heavy labial archwire, which is inserted into buccal molar tubes. The wire has a flange of plastic added anteriorly to engage the lip and is stopped anteriorly to the molar tubes with a vertical loop or compressed coil spring. Lip bumpers may be used to maintain the arch perimeter, position the molar distally, or permit changes in incisal portion. It can be fabricated or prefabricated which is available in the market (Figs 16.9 and 16.10).

Classification

Various classifications of lip bumpers have been given. According to Australian Orthodontic Journal, March 1990; classification of lip bumpers is as follows:
- Removable or non-removable

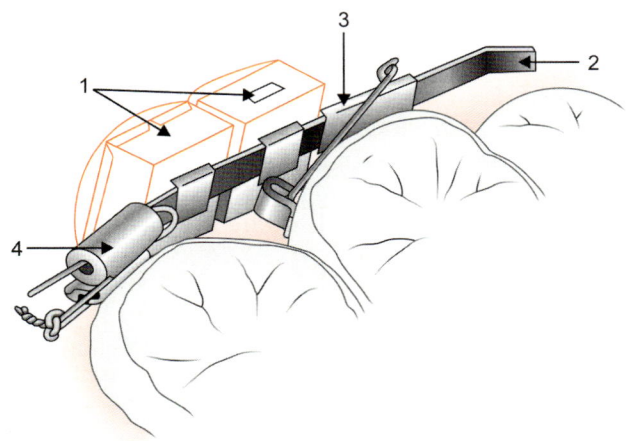

Fig. 16.7: Molar distalizer using repelling magnets

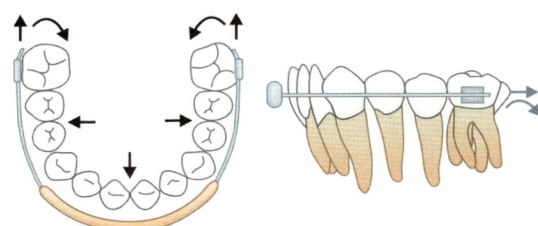

Fig. 16.9: Effect of lip bumper on the dentition

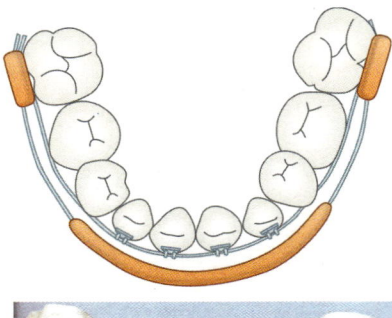

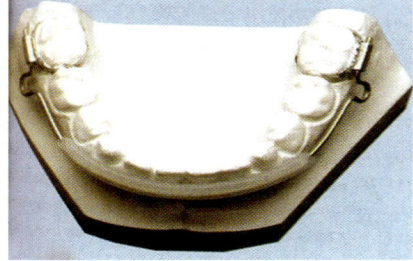

Fig. 16.10: Lip bumper with or without loop

- Running
- Stopped
  - Loops
  - Stops
  - Offsets
  - The covering material
- Covering the anterior part for lips
  - Prefabricated
  - Plastic tubing
  - Custom made with acrylic
- Various sizes and forms of wire

Another classification could be considered and that is whether a lip bumper is intended to be used for short term which is usually on a tooth moving basis, or if it is to be used on a longer term basis which is usually to try influence lip function and growth. Longer duration means longer than one year.

As with Frankle's buccal shields, mandibular flexible lip bumper minimizes restrictive cheek and lip pressures and allows arch development and relief of crowding, while promoting molar distalization and controlling molar rotations. The lip bumper is best in achieving patient's cooperation than with Frankle or headgear.

The Korn Lip Bumper

This is made up of 0.45 inch stainless steel with adjustment loops mesial to the mandibular first molars. The appliance is positioned 2 mm anterior to the mandibular incisors at the gingival margin and is inserted pssivlt into the molar tubes to reduce the

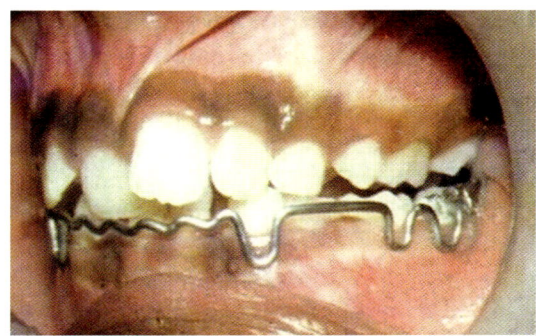

Fig. 16.11: The korn lip bumper

needs for patient compliance, the lip bumper is secured to the first molar band with ligature wire. The lip bumper is advanced as needed during the routine appointments (every 4 weeks) to maintain the initial position (Fig. 16.11).

Wide Lip Bumper

The hard plastic (polypropylene) pumper design provides the necessary surface area to transfer adequate pressure from the lip to the molars while preventing the lips and cheek from applying pressure to the teeth.

Bayne Lip Bumpers

Wire is encapsulated in polyethylene in the anterior portion to minimize abrasion, two types plain and looped lip bumpers are available.

Flexible Lip Bumpers

Korn and Shaprio (1994) described the flexible lip bumpers as an adjunct to molar distalization therapy. The lip bumpers are made of malleable, 0.040" stainless steel wire with preformed vertical loops and posterior adjustment bends. The vertical loops maximize lip contact in the maxilla and allow anteroposterior adjustments in both the arches. Fitting and insertion of the bumpers simply requires the placement of molar bayonet bends that act as posterior stops. About 3 mm of clearance is recommended between the bumper and the teeth to allow proper lip contact with minimum discomfort during treatment, the lip bumpers are activated so that one molar is rotated while the other is distalized.

New Molar Distalizers

- First class appliance
- Superspring
- Palatal orthodontist implants
- Franzulans appliance
- Klapper appliance

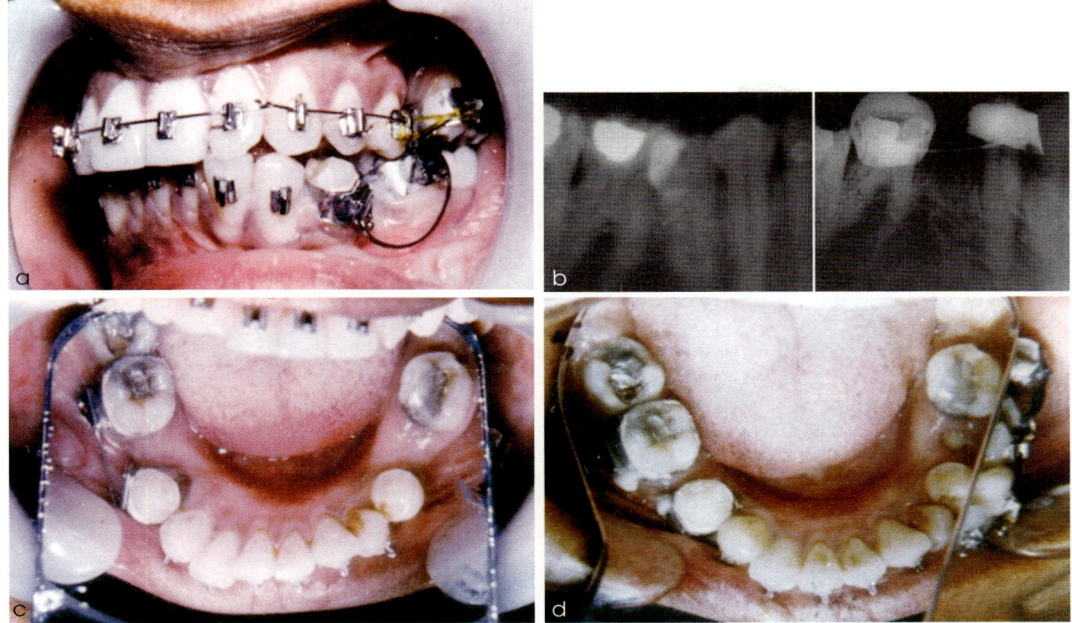

Fig. 16.12: MUST appliance: (a) Fixed appliance with MUST appliance in lower dentition; (b) IOPA X-ray depicting pre- and post-treatment results; (c) A photograph of post-treatment result; (d) Pre-treatment photograph

UPRIGHTING OF MOLARS

Tilted posterior teeth always occupy more space. Molars tend to tip mesially when the deciduous second molars are lost early or decay on the distal surface of this tooth is not restored at the appropriate time. A delayed eruption of the first or second molar may also cause the posterior teeth to tilt mesially.

Uprighting of molars can lead to the arch length gain of 1–1.5 mm. Fixed appliances using NiTi wires or implants, space regainers and lip bumper are giving good results.

Molar Uprighting Simple Technique (MUST)

In the MUST, a 0.018" × 0.025" tube is soldered cervically to the molar tube, parallel to the occlusal plane. A shorter 0.018" × 0.025" tube is soldered horizontally to the distocervical wing of the premolar bracket. The tubes should have 0° torque to avoid gingival interference. The active component of the uprighting spring is superelastic 0.016" × 0.022" NiTi wire which produces light and continuous force throughtout treatment. The wire extends from the mesial of the premolar tube to the distal of the molar tube. Once inserted into the tubes, the wire is activated by pulling it mesially out of the molar tube. Any excess wire is cut off and the ends are bent back and coated with glass ionomer cement to prevent irritation.

This activation augments the internal tension in the wire, thus increasing forces, couples and moments. It also generates a horizontal distalizing force against the molar as a reaction to the mesial pull of the wire. The premolar can be anchored by fixed appliances on the entire mandiular arch. In addition, lingual buttons may be bonded to the molar and premolar and connected by a passive elastic chain to help prevent unwanted distal movement or rotation (Fig. 16.12).

Derotation of Posteriors

The rotated posteriors occupy more space and space can be gained by derotation of posterior teeth. It can be achieved by using a force couple by using transpalatal arch, NiTi palatal expander and quad helix, etc. (Refer Expansion Appliance).

Proclination of Anterior

Incisors can be proclined so that they can be arranged along an increased arch circumference, thus providing the extra space. This is possible in case of retroclined incisors, Class II division 2 and in case of upright anterior and concave profile.

BIBLIOGRAPHY

1. Daugaard-Jensen I. Extraction of first molars in discrepancy cases 1973; 64:115–36.
2. Gianelly AA. Distal movement of the maxillary molars. Am J Orthod 1988; 114:66-72.
3. Sidan JJ, Air-rotar stripping and proximal sealants. J Clin Orthod 1989; 23:790–4.
4. Thampson FG. Second premolar extraction in Begg technique. J Clin Orthod 1977;11:610–3.

PREVIOUS YEAR'S UNIVERSITY QUESTIONS

Essay

1. Enumerate various methods of gaining space. Discuss in detail about extraction as a method of gaining space.
2. What is molar distalizer? Write in detail about pendulum appliance.

Short Questions

1. Reproximation
2. Lip bumper
3. Wilkinson's extraction
4. Therapeutic extraction

MCQs

1. *Synonyms of proximal stripping includes:*
   a. Proximal slicing of a tooth/teeth
   b. Reproximation
   c. Slenderization/disking of a tooth
   d. All of the above   **(Ans: d)**

2. *Uprighting of molars can be done using:*
   a. Uprighting spring
   b. Open coil spring
   c. Closed coil spring
   d. All of the above   **(Ans: a)**

3. *Correction of rotated teeth helps in:*
   a. Relieving crowding in the arches
   b. Prevention of dental caries
   c. Prevention of periodontal disease
   d. All of the above   **(Ans: d)**

4. *Correction of rotated posterior teeth is best done by:*
   a. Fixed appliance using couple of force
   b. Removable orthodontic appliance
   c. Myofunctional appliance
   d. All of the above   **(Ans: a)**

5. *Who introduced the pendulum appliance?*
   a. Hilgers
   b. Casino
   c. Testa
   d. None of the above   **(Ans: a)**

6. *How much force is produced from pendulum appliance?*
   a. 230 g/side
   b. 231 g/side
   c. 229 g/side
   c. 250 g/side   **(Ans: a)**

7. *How many activations pendulum appliance required?*
   a. It requires only a one time activation of 60–70°
   b. It requires only a one time activation of 40-60°
   c. It requires only a one time activation of 10–20°
   s. It requires only a one time activation of 90°
      (Ans: a)

8. *The major drawback of slenderization*
   a. Increased susceptibility to caries
   b. Sensibility
   c. Periodontal problem
   d. Tooth mobility   **(Ans: a)**

9. *Exraction undertaken as a part of orthodontic treatment is called:*
   a. Balanced extraction
   b. Serial extraction
   c. Therapeutic extraction
   d. Wilkinson's extraction   **(Ans: c)**

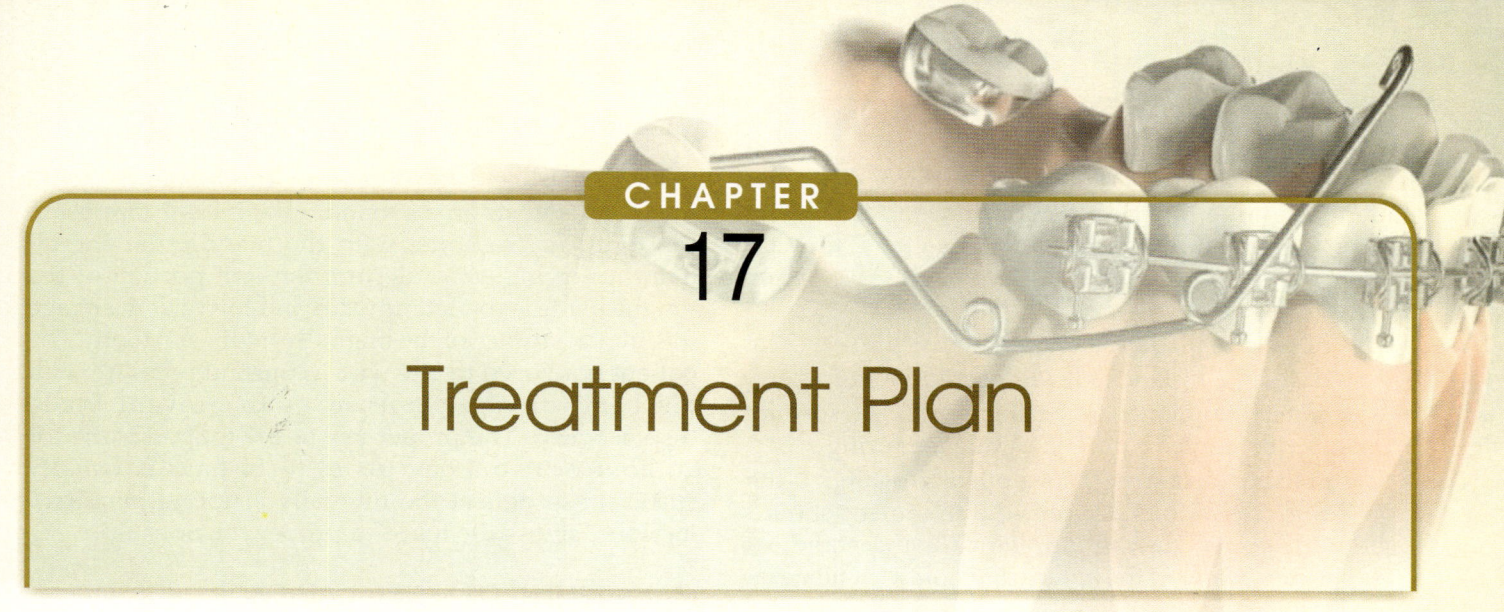

Treatment Plan

17.1 MANAGEMENT OF CLASS I MALOCCLUSION

Chapter Outline

- Causes for anterior crossbite
- Correction of anterior crossbite
- Developing anterior crossbite
- Management of skeletal anterior crossbite

Class I malalignment occlusion, as defined by Angle, incorporates a normal interarch relationship. Class I malocclusion exists when a harmonious relationship of the underlying skeletal structures and the malocclusion component is restricted to the dental malrelations only. Class I malocclusion includes individual tooth malalignments and/or malocclusions in the vertical or transverse planes. The most commonly encountered malocclusions are the bimaxillary protrusion/proclination cases and cases involving crowding in the maxillary and mandibular arches.

It can involve single tooth or two teeth or more than two teeth. It should be corrected as soon as detected in the arch because it can hamper the normal developmental process. There are two types of anterior crossbite:

1. *Developing crossbite:* It means that the crossbite occurs before the root completion.
2. *Developed crossbite:* It means that the anterior crossbite is developed after the root completion.

CAUSES FOR ANTERIOR CROSSBITE

The etiological factors are classified into:
- Dental
- Skeletal
- Functional

Dental factors:
- In adequate arch length
- Retained deciduous teeth
- Delayed eruption
- Traumatic injury to the tooth germ

Skeletal factors:
- Skeletal Class III malocclusion
- Deviation of mandible either due to trauma or to the condyle and fractured condyle.
- Maxillary defects as in cleft palate and syndromes associated with cleft palate.

Functional factors: Cuspal interference.

CORRECTION OF ANTERIOR CROSSBITE

- Lower inclined plane
- Modified inclined plane

For patients with an anterior dental crossbite, where the upper and lower incisors are lingually and labially inclined, respectively, an inclined plane is contraindicated. In these circumstances, a modified incline plane is the better choice. A modified incline plane is a removable appliance which structurally resembles a Hawley appliance with an inclined plane placed at the anterior portion. The incline plane portion covers the lower anterior teeth up to their incisal third. When the patient bites, the incline plane portion raises the bite and proclines the upper anteriors labially. The metal parts consist of a labial bow and occlusal rests or Adam's clasps.

- Use of tongue blade (developing crossbite)
- Use of fixed appliance (developed crossbite)
- Mechanical appliance using bilateral posterior bite plane with single or double cantilever spring
- Use of expansion screw (developed crossbite): If the anterior crossbite is noticed, the treatment should be with upper Hawley appliance using standard expansion screw in the anterior region with bilateral posterior plane.

  If the dental anterior crossbite is noticed along with bilateral posterior crossbite, the treatment is carried with three-dimensional screws.

- Stainless crown and cast metal guide plane (developing crossbite)
- Banded inclined (developing crossbite)
- 2 × 4 or 2 × 6 appliance (developed crossbite)

Basic configuration of the appliance is 2 bands on the molars and 4 incisors bonding and hence it is called 2 × 4 appliance. If the appliance is with 2 bands on the molars and 6 anteriors bonded, then it is called 2 × 6 appliances.

DEVELOPING ANTERIOR CROSSBITE

Several approaches are possible. If the dentist is fortunate enough to anticipate and intercept the developing crossbite as the permanent teeth, the use of a tongue blade may be quite sufficient. Let us make as an example the most common type of crossbite, the lingual malposition of a maxillary central incisor. The child is instructed to place a tongue blade in such a manner that rests on the mandibular incisors opposing the tooth in crossbite, with the mandibular incisal margin serving as a fulcrum, the oral portion of the tongue blade is rotated upward and forward to engage the lingual surface of the lingually malposed tooth. The patient is advised to bite with a constant pressure with his hand on the blade so as to prevent blade displacement. The proper use of the tongue blade for an hour or two a day for 10 to 14 days is usually sufficient to deflect the lingually erupting maxillary incisors "across the fence" a proper relationship.

MANAGEMENT OF SKELETAL ANTERIOR CROSSBITE

Mixed Dention Period

Anterior crossbite that occurs as a result of retrognathic maxilla should be treated with reverse pull headgear. If the anterior crossbite is due to prognathic mandible, it should be intercepted with chin cap.

Permanent Dentition

- Expansion appliance
- Surgical orthodontic procedure. It should be attempted after the growth period is ceased, may be after 14 years.

The *functional crossbite* can be relieved by grinding the teeth.

BIBLIOGRAPHY

1. Hammond BA. Treatment of a Class I crowded malocclusion. Am j Orthod 2002. pp. 411–8.
2. Rocke RA. Management of a severe Class I div 1 malocclusion. Begg J Orthod 1963;2:37–47.

17.2 MANAGEMENT OF CLASS II MALOCCLUSION

Chapter Outline
• Introduction
• Components of Class II malocclusion
• Etiological factors of Class II malocclusion
• Classification of Class II malocclusion
• Management of Class II malocclusion

INTRODUCTION

Angle defined Class II malocclusion as the condition in which "distobuccal cusp of the upper first permanent molar occludes in the mesiobuccal groove of the lower permanent first molar" (Fig. 17.1).

Class II malocclusion is not a single entity but results from numerous combinations of both skeletal and dental alveolar components. The earliest description, solely a dental description, was provided by Edward Hartley Angle. The Class II division 1 was later shown to also be characterized by a retrognathic mandible or a prognathic maxilla with variable vertical dimensions. The Class II division 2 patients is shown to exhibit an orthognathic maxilla, a short and retrognathic mandible, brachyfacial growth pattern, retroclined maxillary central incisors, and a relatively prominent chin, as well as dental deep bite. In later years, further assessment of the dental Class II provided information regarding the underlying skeletal components.

COMPONENTS OF CLASS II MALOCCLUSION

Class II is the most common and difficult to treat malocclusion as compared to other malocclusions, due to its wide ranging varieties and interplay of various types of etiological factors.

It is important for every orthodontist to have adequate knowledge and correct understanding of the various types of Class II malocclusions before instituting a treatment plan. There is no universal method of managing the condition. It is essential to have an adequate knowledge of normal growth pattern and various cephalometric analyses for proper diagnosis and treatment planning.

Classification

Flowchart 17.1 describes the classication of components of Class II malocclusion.

ETIOLOGICAL FACTORS OF CLASS II MALOCCLUSION

They are categorized into the following three factors:
• Prenatal factors
• Natal factors
• Postnatal factors

Prenatal Factors

• *Genetic and congenital:* The facial dimensions are principally determined by heredity through genes.
• *Teratogenesis:* Administration of certain drugs during pregnancy has a potential of yielding abnormal development of arches leading to Class II malocclusion. Such drugs are referred to as teratogens.

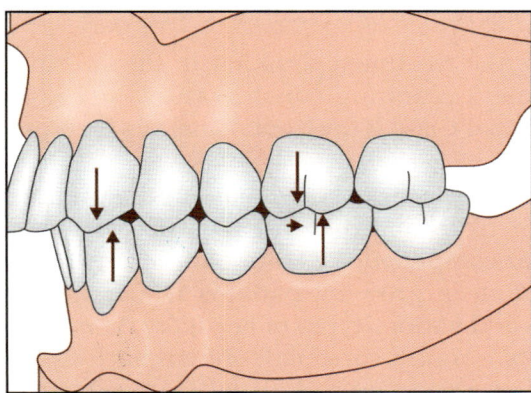

Fig. 17.1: Position of molar and canine in class III malocclusion

Flowchart 17.1: Classification of components of Class II malocclusion

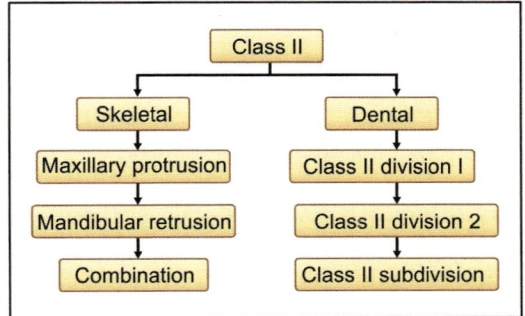

- *Irradiation:* Irradiation therapy during fetal life can also be a causative factor for Class II malocclusion.
- *Intrauterine fetal posture:* Abnormal posture of the fetus such as hands across the face is found to affect mandibular growth.

Natal Factors

Improper forceps application during delivery can lead to condylar damage/fracture causing internal hemorrhage into the joint area. TMJ can get ankylosed or fibrosed later leading to underdevelopment of the mandible.

Postnatal Factor

Certain conditions that can influence the normal development of the craniofacial skeleton are:
- Traumatic injuries
- Long-term irradiation therapy
- Oral habits such as thumb sucking
- Congenitally missing teeth
- Anomalies in the shape of teeth

CLASSIFICATION OF CLASS II MALOCCLUSION

- Angle's classification
- Moyers classification
- Classification based on abnormal skeletal pattern

Angle's Classification

- Angle Class II division 1
- Angle Class II division 2

Moyers Classification

- Six horizontal types (Fig. 17.2)
- Five vertical types (Fig. 17.3)

Six Horizontal Types

- Type A—normal skeletal, but Class II dental
- Type B ⎫
- Type C ⎪
- Type D ⎬ Syndromal types of Class II
- Type E ⎭
- Type F—mild skeletal features

Type F: It is a large heterogeneous group with mild skeletal Class II tendencies. It is a milder form of types B, C, D, E.

Moyers differential diagnosis of Class II malocclusions allows to more easily determine the components of the Class II malocclusion problem. It identifies the skeletal problem and the dentoalveolar problem and thus

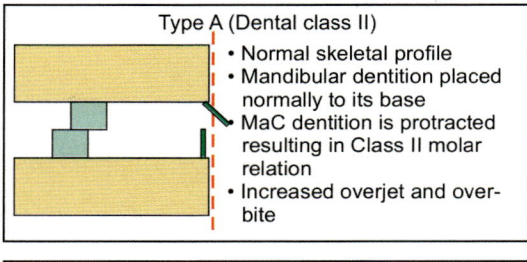

Type A (Dental class II)
- Normal skeletal profile
- Mandibular dentition placed normally to its base
- MaC dentition is protracted resulting in Class II molar relation
- Increased overjet and over-bite

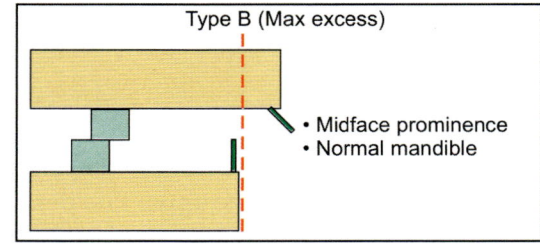

Type B (Max excess)
- Midface prominence
- Normal mandible

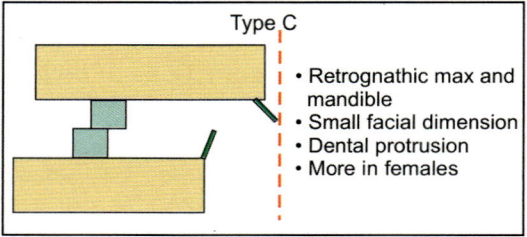

Type C
- Retrognathic max and mandible
- Small facial dimension
- Dental protrusion
- More in females

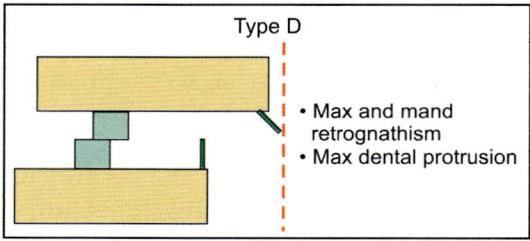

Type D
- Max and mand retrognathism
- Max dental protrusion

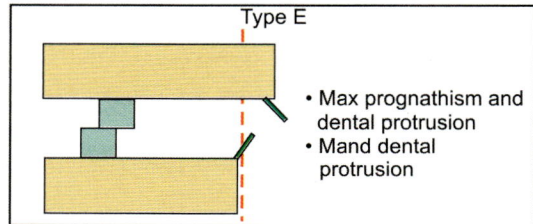

Type E
- Max prognathism and dental protrusion
- Mand dental protrusion

Fig. 17.2: Moyers classification—horizontal types

directs the treatment thinking to the specific areas. Treatment planning considerations using Moyers differential Class II horizontal analysis is summarized above.

In additions to the horizontal considerations, proper patient treatment also requires assessment of the vertical components. Treatment options for vertical correction in growing patients would include bite blocks and various types of headgear. In non-growing patients, surgical correction options such as Lafford I maxillary impaction and alveolar procedures may be required.

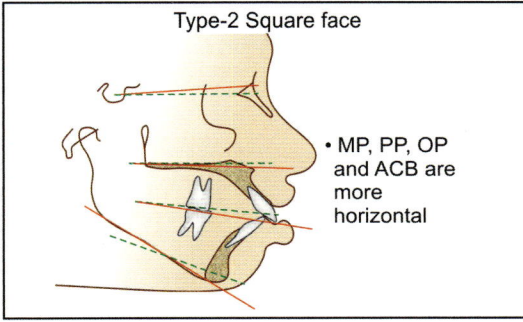

Type-1 Steep mandibular plane or high angle case

- Mand plane and occlusal plane are steeper than normal
- Palate tipped down
- ACB tipped up

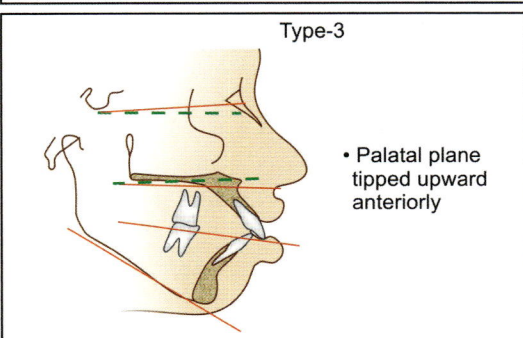

Type-2 Square face

- MP, PP, OP and ACB are more horizontal

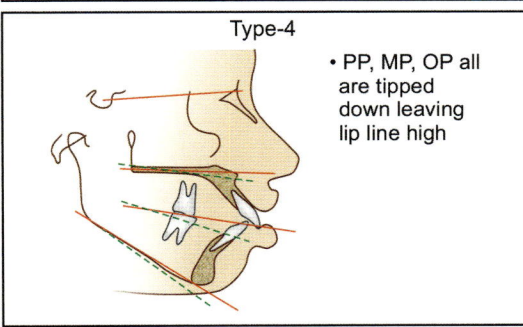

Type-3

- Palatal plane tipped upward anteriorly

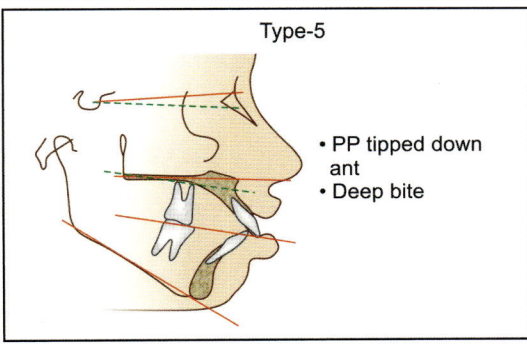

Type-4

- PP, MP, OP all are tipped down leaving lip line high

Type-5

- PP tipped down ant
- Deep bite

Fig. 17.3: Moyers classification—vertical types

Classification Based on Abnormal Skeletal Pattern
(Fig. 17.4)

- Maxillary prognathism
- Mandibular retrognathism
- Maxillary prognathism and mandibular retrognathism

MANAGEMENT OF CLASS II MALOCCLUSION
(Flowchart 17.2)

Treatment of Class II Malocclusion

- Primary dentition
- Preadolescents
- Adolescents
- Adults

Strategies of Class II Division 1 Malocclusion

- Two-phase treatment (early and late)
- One-phase treatment

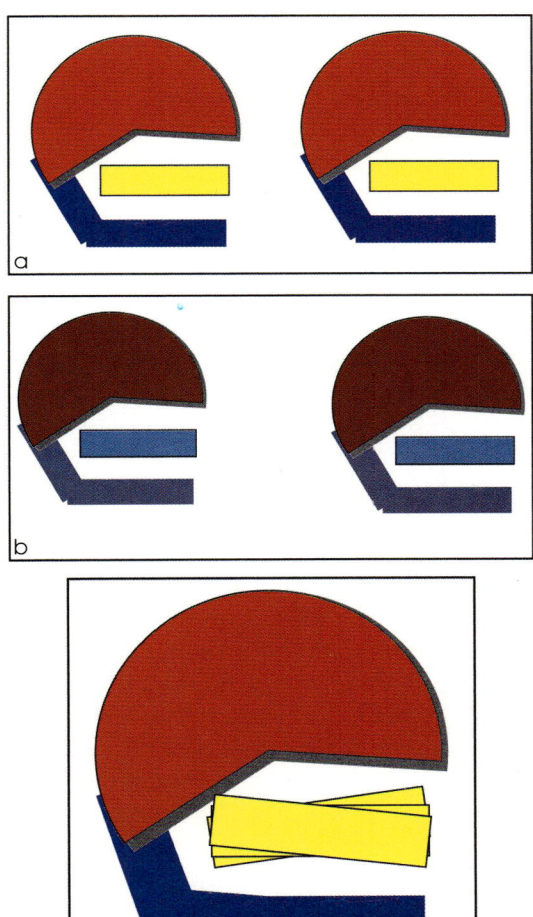

Fig. 17.4: (a) A skeletal Class II—fault with the maxilla; (b) A skeletal Class II—fault with the mandible; (c) A skeletal Class II—vertical

Flowchart 17.2: Management of Class Ii malocclusion

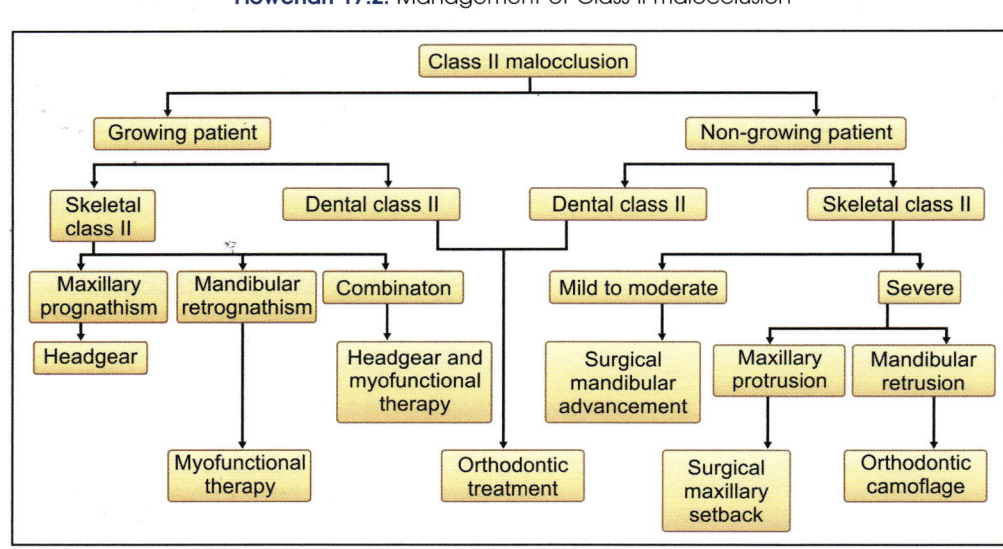

Two-phase treatment
- Early treatment at the age of 8–10 years
- Late treatment at the age of 11–14 years

One-phase treatment: The treatment will be finished in one phase.

The treatment principles depend on three important factors:
a. Age at which the patient is seen.
b. Nature and severity of the problem.
c. Etiological factors

So accordingly, there are three approaches:
  a. It intends to prevent the malocclusion from occurring
  b. Intercept the developing malocclusion
  c. Corrective orthodontics

Management by preventing the possible etiological factors like functional disturbances, abnormal habits, etc. that would have contributed or exaggerated the Class II malocclusion or by modifying the growth either by restricting the maxillary growth or enhancing the mandibular growth. If the patient is seen after the growth period, then camouflaging of skeletal jaw discrepancy by orthodontic tooth movement by fixed mechanotherapy is the treatment of choice. It is just a compromised treatment for mild to moderate skeletal discrepancy. But, if the skeletal discrepancy is severe, then surgical intervention is the only alternative choice and should be undertaken after the cessation of growth.

Management of Functional Disturbances
- *Mouth breathing:*
  – Any condition like chronic nasal infections, allergic rhinitis, cold, deviated nasal septum,

enlarged tonsils and adenoids should be looked for and managed.
  – Habit breaking appliances
- *Abnormal tongue position and swallowing patterns:*
  – Adequate motivation of the patient by explaining the deleterious effect is tried and if they fail, then
  – Any other secondary causes, leading to nasal airway obstruction, should be looked for and eliminated.
  – An abnormally large tongue should be considered for surgical reduction.
- *Management of abnormal habits like thumb sucking and finger sucking habits:*
  – No intervention is needed until deciduous teeth are erupted because they usually tend to stop by then.
  – Reward system and reminder systems are also suggested.
  – The offending digit can be painted with pungent substance. If all the above fails, then
  – Treatment by fixed or removable habit breaking appliances is the treatment of choice.

Management during Mixed Dentition
Before instituting a treatment, three important things should be considered.
- Age of the patient
- Location of the fault (maxilla, mandible or combination)
- Type of growth pattern (horizontal or vertical)
1. *Management of Class II malocclusion with maxillary prognathism with normal mandible:* Here the primary goal is mainly to restrict the excessively growing

maxilla. Management by extraoral force using headgears is the most effective approach. A maxillary splint can be used.

2. *Management of mandibular deficiency:* The primary goal is to enhance mandibular growth rather than restricting the maxillary growth.

   The various functional appliances used for the purpose are:
   1. Activator
   2. FR II—Frankel
   3. Twin block appliance
   4. Bionator
   5. Various other bite jumping devices

3. *Management of dentoalveolar Class II malocclusion with normal skeletal relationship:*
   - Space maintainer
   - In prematurely exfoliated cases or extracted cases where mesial drift has already occurred, space regaining devices are to be used. They fall under two category:
     – Intraoral distalization appliances which include pendulum appliances, distal slide or first class appliance, springs, screws and miniscrews.
     – Extraoral appliances for distalization of the upper buccal segment can be done using headgears.
     – Intraoral appliances using various methods of gaining space.

   Whenever there is space deficiency, the methods of gaining space that strikes are: Extraction, expansion and stripping.

Management of Class II Malocclusion in Adults

The dentoalveolar correction is brought about by various multibanded appliance therapies.

1. *Management by orthognathic surgery:* Any type of orthognathic surgery should be undertaken only after cessation of growth. This is especially true for boys, who tend to have their postpubertal growth extending up to 18 years. There are two surgical approaches for the correction of maxillary prognathism like Total maxillary repositioning and partial maxillary repositioning.

2. *Surgical approach for mandibular retrognathism:* Though there are several techniques that have been followed such as inverted L-osteotomy (intraoral approach), C-osteotomy (extraoral approach), subapical surgical procedure, and the procedure that is mostly frequently used currently is the intraoral bilateral sagittal split osteotomy.

Management of Class II Division 2 Malocclusion

In general, Class II division 2 malocclusions are easier to correct during the growth period than in adulthood, especially when favorable growth occurs during treatment.

A number of factors need to be considered for these patients:

1. *Correction of axial inclination of maxillary incisors:* It can be done by two approaches—palatal root torqueing of incisors and labial tipping of crowns of incisors. Excessive lingual inclination of maxillary incisors generally locks the mandible and lead to a functional mandibular retrusion. Mandible can be freed either by tipping the maxillary central incisors labially or by placing an anterior bite plate to disarticulate the anterior teeth and allowing the mandible to assume a position dictated by the musculature.

2. *Correction of deep bite and exaggerated curve of Spee:* To level the dental arches orthodontically, one must either extrude the molars and premolars or intrude the anterior teeth. It can be done by intrusion of upper incisors or extrusion of lower posterior teeth or a combination of both. Both plates, archwires with exaggerated COS and anchor bends, intrusion arches are used for this purpose.

3. *Extraction versus non-extraction:* Treatment of Class II division 2 malocclusions with a low mandibular plane angle and deep overbite is best managed with a non-extraction approach to avoid retraction of incisors and further labial movement of roots and protraction of the molars; these movements tend to further deepen the overbite. Due to horizontal growth pattern, the mandibular body is horizontal, the muscles are strong, the trabecular pattern of bone is almost perpendicular to long axis of teeth. In such cases, the mesial movement of buccal teeth to close the spaces is very difficult. Any attempt to close the extraction spaces leads to over retraction of incisors and torque loss.
   - Even the patient's profile does not allow extraction because these patients have relatively retrusive lips, but prominent chin and nose. Extraction of premolars followed by incisor retraction will further retrude the lips. It worsens the profile and results in an unacceptable "edentulous look".
   - Before considering the extraction of premolars, there is need to evaluate several factors including the prominence of the nose and chin, nasolabial angle, presence of a functional mandibular retrusion, growth potential and headgear cooperation, extent of tooth size–arch length

discrepancy and the periodontal condition of lower anterior teeth. As a rule, in borderline crowded Class II division 2 cases, it is best to start the treatment with a non-extraction approach. It has been seen that the relieving of anterior crowding, flaring of upper incisors unlocks the mandible, which can be redirected forward with the help of Class II elastics.

Timing of Treatment

Treatment of Class II division 2 malocclusion should be initiated in the late mixed dentition. During active growth periods, the functional appliances can be used to the skeletal relationship. The incisors are proclined so that overjet is created just like in Class II division 1 and then functional appliance can be given to bring mandible forwards. During late growth period, fixed functional appliances should be used to take full advantage of remaining growth.

Stability

It depends on:
- Correction of the interincisal angle to maintain stability of overbite correction by providing an occlusal stop for the mandibular incisors.
- Avoiding excessive lower incisor proclination.
- Favorable mandibular growth—an anticlockwise mandibular rotation can result in relapse of deep overbite correction.

Anterior Open Bite (Table 17.1)

Causes

Mechanical interference with eruption: Either before or after tooth emerges from alveolar bone. Mechanical interferference may be—ankylosis of tooth to the alveolar bone (trauma), e.g. trauma, supernumerary teeth, non-resorbing deciduous roots.

After the tooth emerges from the alveolar bone— pressure from the soft tissues (cheek, finger and tongue) can be obstacle to eruption.

Crowding

Hereditary Crowding

- Due to tooth size–arch length discrepancy
- The signs are:
  - Protrusion of incisors
  - Midline displacement of mandibular incisors with early exfoliation of deciduous canine or blocked lateral incisor on the affected side
  - Ectopic eruption of first molars

Table 17.1: Causes of anterior open bite	
• Skeletal pattern	• Increase in lower anterior facial height such that the compensatory ability of the incisors to erupt into contact is exceeded
	• This may be worsened by a downward and backward pattern of facial growth
• Soft tissues	• Rarely endogenous tongue thrust
• Habits	• Persistence of digit sucking, which often leads to an asymmetric anterior open bite
• Localized failure of alveolar development	• Occurs in cleft lip and palate

Environmental Crowding

- Trauma
- Discrepancy in individual tooth size
- Iatrogenic treatment
- Abnormal shape of tooth
- Abnormal eruption path
- Rotation of the tooth
- Transposition of tooth
- Ankylosed primary tooth
- Premature loss of primary tooth
- Prolonged retention of primary tooth
- Altered eruption sequence
- Proximal caries
- Supernumerary tooth
- Later lower incisor crowding

Etiology of Late Lower Incisor Crowding

- Late mandibular growth
- Reduction of intercanine width
- Gingival fibers and occlusal forces
- Lack of approximal attrition
- Role of mandibular third molars

Clinical Features

- Crowded mandibular incisor teeth
- Premature exfoliation of deciduous canine on the crowded side due to displacement of erupting tooth
- Splaying out of maxillary permanent lateral incisor
- Gingival recession on the labial surface of mandibular incisors
- Bulging of canines in the unerupted position
- Reduced leeway space
- Impaction of second permanent molar, if no treatment is given.
- Vertical pallisading of permanent maxillary first, second and third molars

Table 17.2: Treatment of crowding		
	Timing	*Treatment*
Slight crowding: Slight changes in the position of anterior	Wait and watch	No treatment
Moderate crowding: Lack of space by width of one lateral incisor	Can wait till or premolar eruption	Expansion guidance of eruption
Pronounced crowding	Immediate treatment	Expansion Guidance of eruption Serial extraction Extraction and orthodontic treatment

Factors to be Considered while Treatment Planning

- The patient's age and the likelihood of the crowding increasing or reducing with growth
- The position, presence and prognosis of remaining permanent teeth
- The location of the crowding
- The degree of crowding
- The patient's profile

Treatment (Table 17.2)

In mixed dentition

- Serial extraction
- 2 × 4 fixed appliance with utility arch design
- Driftodontics
- Proximal reproximation followed by removable or fixed appliance in case of borderline cases
- Active lingual arch in case of single lower incisor crowding which is lingually placed.
- Wilson arch appliance

In permanent dentition: Extraction cases: Fixed appliance utilizing aligning arch wires like coaxial wire, 0.014" stainless steel wire, NiTi wire

Posterior Crossbite

- *For bilateral posterior crossbite:* Upper Hawley's appliance with bilateral posterior bite plane and expansion screw in the midline for lateral expansion (Fig. 17.5).
- Expansion appliance for single or two teeth crossbite with unilateral posterior plane on the normal side (Fig. 17.6).
- NiTi expander
- Rapid expander
- Through the bite elastic
- Quad helix appliance

Treatment for Deep Bite

- Upper Hawley's appliance with anterior bite plane

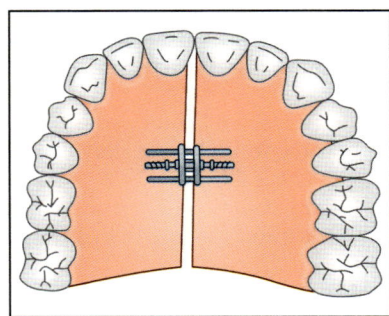

Fig. 17.5: Universal expansion appliance for bilateral posterior crossbite

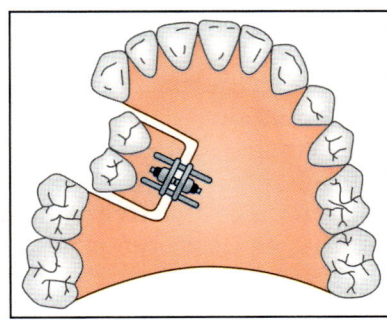

Fig. 17.6: Expansion appliance for two teeth posterior crossbite

- In the mixed dentition:
  a. Oral screen
  b. Activator
  c. Bionator
  d. Twin block appliance
- In the permanent dentition
  a. Upper Hawley's appliance with anterior bite plane (Fig. 17.7)
  b. Fixed appliance

BIBLIOGRAPHY

1. Bowman SJ. Class II combination therapy. J Clin Orthod 1998; 32:611–20.
2. Cetlin NM, Ten Hoeve A. Non-extraction treatment. J Clin Orthod 1983; 17:396–413.

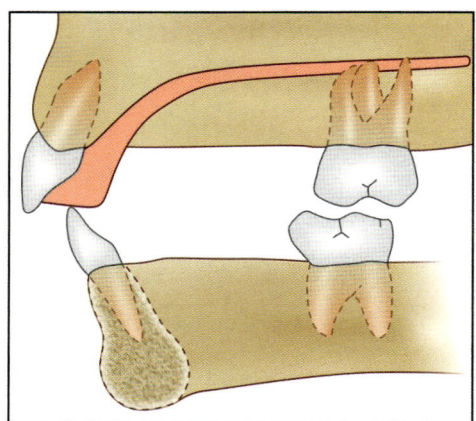

Fig. 17.7: Deep bite correction by supraeruption of molars

3. Firouz M, et al. Dental and orthopedic effects of high pull headgear in treatment of Class II division 1 malocclusion. Am J Orthod 1992; 104:277–84.
4. Selwyn-Barnett BJ. Class II division 2 malocclusion: A method of planning and treatment. Br J Orthod 1996;23:29–36.

PREVIOUS YEAR'S UNIVERSITY QUESTIONS

Essay

1. Define disto-occlusion. Describe the various growth modulation techniques to intercept Class II skeletal pattern.
2. Describe the different treatment modalities of a Class II skeletal malocclusion.
3. Discuss the management of Class II division 1 malocclusion.
4. How do you manage the treatment of Class II division 1 during mixed dentition?

Short Questions

1. Growth modification
2. Moyers classification of Class II malocclusion
3. Classification of Class II malocclusion

MCQs

1. *Most Class II division 1 malocclusion exhibit:*
   a. Bimaxillary protrusion
   b. Deep bite
   c. Abnormal muscle activity
   d. All of the above   **(Ans: c)**

2. *Which of the following may be used to correct anterior deep bite in Class II malocclusion?*
   a. Anterior bite plane
   b. Reverse curve of Spee wires.
   c. Anchor bends in arch wires
   d. All of the above   **(Ans: d)**

3. *Treatment of skeletal Class II malocclusion is done by:*
   a. Growth modification
   b. Camouflage
   c. Surgical correction
   d. All of the above   **(Ans: d)**

4. *Growth modification in Class II division 1 is undertaken during:*
   a. Mixed dentition period
   b. Early permanent dentition period prior to cessation of growth
   c. Both a and b
   d. None of the above   **(Ans: c)**

5. *Prenatal factors in etiology of Class II malocclusion include:*
   a. Heredity
   b. Teratogenesis
   c. Irradiation
   d. All of the above   **(Ans: d)**

6. *Post-natal factors in etiology of class II malocclusion is:*
   a. Traumatic injury to mandible and TMJ
   b. Long time radiation therapy
   c. Habits such as thumb sucking or mouth breathing
   d. All of the above   **(Ans: d)**

7. *The appliance which best treats Class II division 1 malocclusion at the end of growth period is:*
   a. Herbst appliance
   b. Jasper jumper
   c. Activator
   d. Both a and b   **(Ans: d)**

8. *The initial stage in correction of class II div 1 malocclusion should be focused on:*
   a. Management of functional disturbances
   b. Management of deep bite
   c. Management of bimaxillary protrusion
   d. None of the above   **(Ans: a)**

9. *Myofunctional appliances when given in class II division 1 malocclusion results in:*
   a. Correction of maxillary retrognathism
   b. Restriction of the growth of maxilla
   c. Correction of mandibular prognathism
   d. Correction of mandibular retrognathism
      (Ans: d)

10. *Distalization of maxillary molars as a part of orthodontic camouflage is done:*
    a. Prior to eruption of second molars
    b. In late mixed dentition period
    c. Mild Class II division 1 cases
    d. All of the above   **(Ans: d)**

17.3 MANAGEMENT OF CLASS III MALOCCLUSION

Chapter Outline

- Difinition
- Etiological factors of Angle Class III malocclusion

- Posterior crossbite
- Treatment plan for Class III malocclusion

Definition

Angle defined Class III malocclusion as the condition in which "the MB cusp of upper first permanent molar lies distal to MB groove of lower first permanent molar" (Fig. 17.8).

ETIOLOGICAL FACTORS OF ANGLE CLASS III MALOCCLUSION

- Heredity
- Unilateral/bilateral hyperplasia of mandibular condyle
- Occlusal prematurity
- Enlarged adenoids
- Habitual forward positioning of the mandible
- Premature loss of deciduous molars

POSTERIOR CROSSBITE

A posterior crossbite is an abnormal buccolingual relationship of a tooth or teeth in the maxilla or mandible or both when the two dental arches are brought into centric occlusion. Clinically, they may be expressed as a lingual crossbite, a complete lingual crossbite or a buccal crossbite. It may be unilateral or bilateral with one or more teeth involved.

Etiological factors that may give rise to a posterior crossbite condition are classified as either dental or skeletal or both.

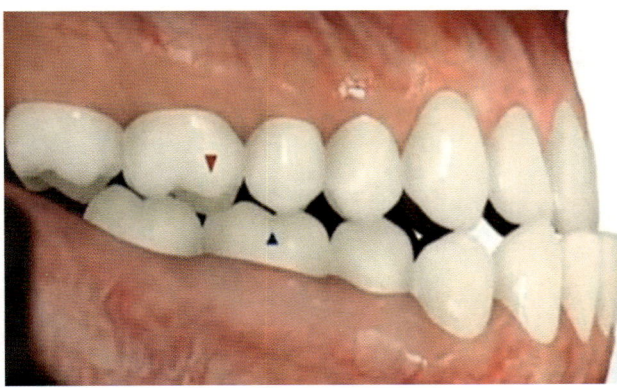

Fig. 17.8: Mesiocclusion

Dental Factors

- A faulty eruption pattern wherein a tooth erupts out of position.
- Insufficient arch length, which can result in a tooth or teeth deflected lingually or buccally during eruption.
- Prolonged retention of primary teeth.
- Sensitive and traumatized teeth or loose primary teeth that cause a lateral shift of the mandible during centric closure.
- Ectopic eruption of the permanent first molar, resulting in the premature loss of the second primary molar, subsequent loss of space and the eventual buccal or lingual eruption of the second bicuspid.
- Prolonged thumb or finger sucking, causing a narrowing of the maxillary arch and lingual tipping of posteriors.

Skeletal Factors

Those skeletal factors associated with posterior crossbite include:
- Cleft palate
- Microglossia
- Macroglossia
- Gross mediolateral disharmony of the craniofacial skeleton produced by aberrations in the bony growth of the maxilla or mandible in which there is either an asymmetrical growth of the two or a lack of agreement in widths caused by insufficient lateral growth of the maxilla or an overgrowth of mandible.

It is generally agreed that early treatment and correction of certain posterior crossbite conditions are desirable. Without treatment, the following undesirable sequelae have been observed.
- Abnormal wear of the dentition.
- Interference of normal development and growth of the dental arches and possible wraping of the alveolar ridges.
- Pain from adverse muscular spasms from an abnormal lateral shift of the mandible during centric closure.
- Possible destruction of the periodontium from abnormal occlusal forces.

MAXILLARY DEFICIENCY

Maxillary deficiency can involve all three planes of space. In-patient without cleft palates, it is more, common to observe deficiency in one of two patterns:

- A primarily transverse deficiency, with horizontal and particularly vertical dimensions less affected (or)
- A horizontal and vertical deficiency, with reasonably normal, transverse dimensions

Generally, a narrow palatal vault distinguishes skeletal maxillary constriction. It can be corrected by opening the mid-palatal suture which widens the roof of the mouth and the floor of the nose. Growth at this, suture is an important mechanism for normal widening of the arch, which continues in most children until the late teens, other ceases.

The age of the patient definitely is obtaining separation of the suture. Like all craniofacial sutures, the mid-palatal suture becomes more tortuous and interdigited with increasing age.

After mid-adolescence, there is a change that periosteal bridges will have formed across the suture, partially obliterating it and making skeletal expansion impossible.

Expansion across the suture can be done in two ways:
1. Rapid expansion
2. Slow expansion.

With both methods, the teeth are used as points, some tooth movement occurs but the two halves of the maxilla separate widening the midpatalal suture and leading to bone apposition.

Class III malocclusion can be (Flowchart 17.3):
- Skeletal
- Dental (Fig. 17.9)
- Pseudo

Skeletal Class III

It is due to discrepancy in the relation of upper and lower jaw bases, where mandible is related mesially/ anteriorly to maxilla as compared to normal Class I relation (Fig. 17.10).

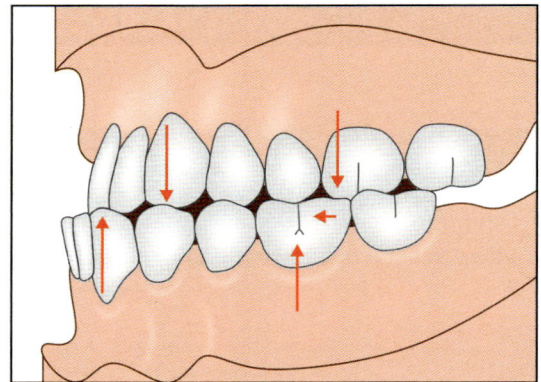

Fig. 17.9: Dental Class III

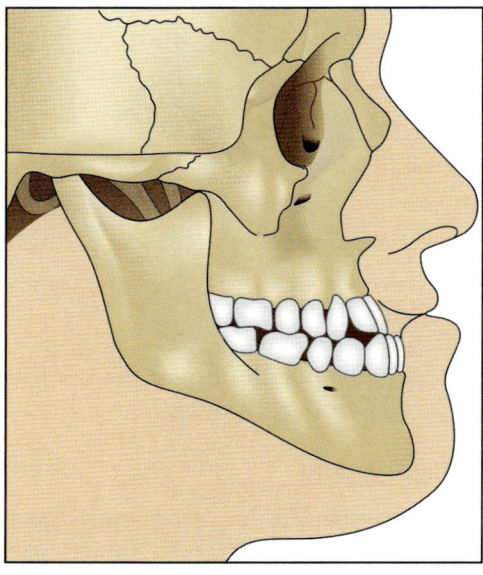

Fig. 17.10: Skeletal Class III

Pseudo Class III

The mandible shows a forward path of closure due to prematurities in incisal region and assumes a Class III molar and skeletal relation with maxilla (Fig. 17.11).

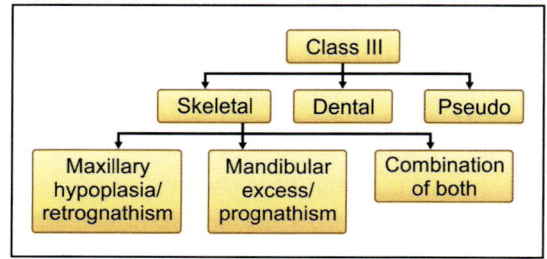

Flowchart 17.3: Classification of Class III malocclusion

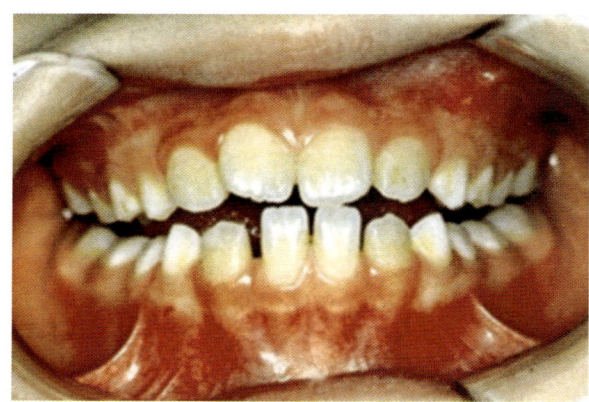

Fig. 17.11: Pseudo Class III

TREATMENT PLAN FOR CLASS III MALOCCLUSION
(Flowchart 17.4)

- Growing patient
  - Skeletal
  - Dental
- Non-growing patient
  - Skeletal
  - Dental

Treatment of Preadolescent Child

- Functional appliance like Class III Frankel, Class III activator, Class III bionator and twin block appliance (Fig. 17.12)
- Chin cap (growing child)
- Rapid maxillary expansion with face mask
- *3D expansion screws:* The three-dimensional expansion screws are capable of expanding the maxilla in all the three directions.
- Vesco protraction units for rapid skeletal protraction of the maxilla and midface
- Modified tandem appliance (MTA)

Vesco Protraction Units for Rapid Skeletal Protraction of Maxilla and Midface

Vesco protraction units are a set of lip–pad attachments and molar tubes, which are passed through the rectangular base archwire in maxillary fixed appliance. These maxillary lip pads relieve restrictive forces of upper lip on anterior maxilla.

The elastics are attached from these pads to the reverse face mask to apply a pulling force on the maxillary arch. Also, these reverse pull elastics create a labial root torque transmitted to maxillary incisors which prevents their proclination during maxillary protraction (Fig. 17.13).

Modified Tandem Appliance (MTA)

It is used for Class III patient with mild skeletal mid-facial deficiency for better patient cooperation (Fig. 17.14).

Treatment of Adolescent Child

Treatment in the adolescent phase is limited to orthodontic camouflage or orthodontic decompensation in an effort to prepare the patient for surgery.

Camouflage can be achieved by proclining the maxillary anterior and tipping the mandibular incisors lingually. Single arch extractions, extraction only in the mandibular arch, are frequently done to create space for the retraction of the mandibular anterior segment. Class III elastics are frequently used in an effort to tip/retract the mandibular incisors.

Treatment during Adulthood

Treatment during adulthood is similar to that during adolescent age group except that the emphasis is more on orthognathic surgery. Orthodontic camouflage is possible only within the range and over ambitious treatment plans should not be attempted.

The two commonly used procedures are the bilateral sagittal split osteotomy with retraction of the mandible. In cases with maxillary deficiency, a LeFort I down fracture may be attempted.

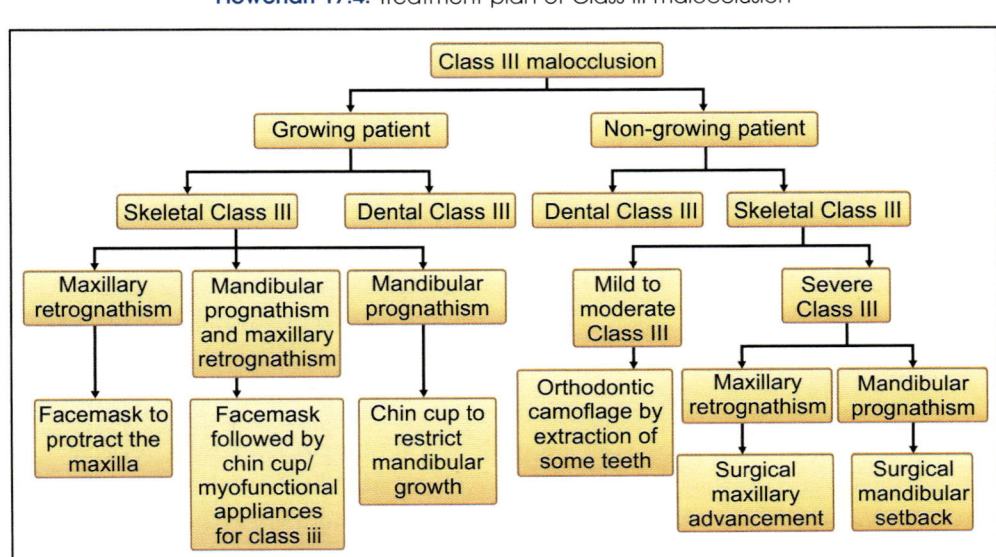

Flowchart 17.4: Treatment plan of Class III malocclusion

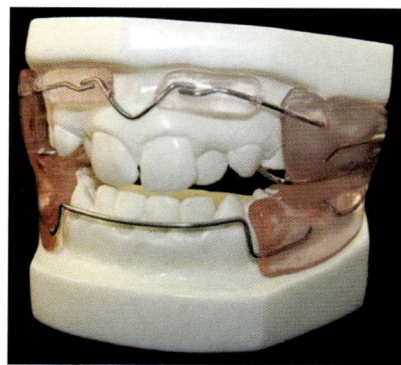

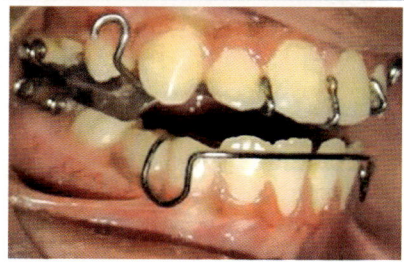

Fig. 17.12: (a) Class III FR; (b) Class III activator

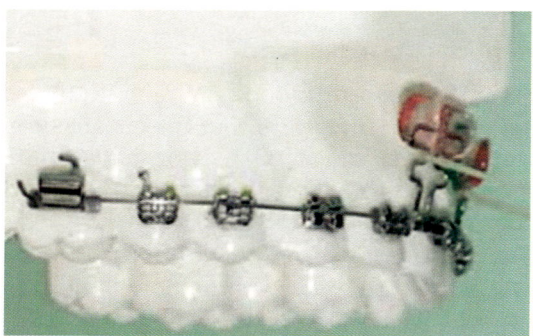

Fig. 17.13: Vasco protraction unit for rapid skeletal protraction of the maxilla and midface

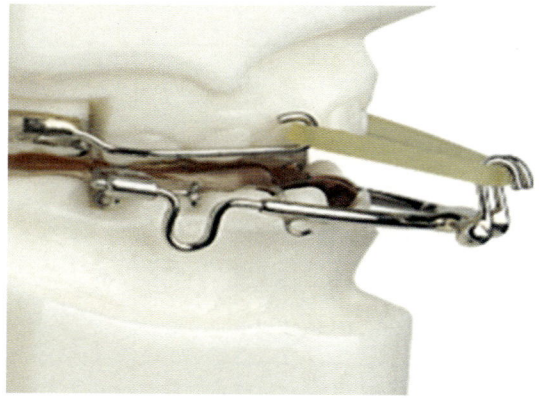

Fig. 17.14: Modified Tandem appliance

Stability of Class III Malocclusion

Relapse of Class III correction may be related to:
- An inadequate overbite to maintain the corrected incisor position.

- *Unfavorable growth in the AP and vertical skeletal dimension:* Unfavorable AP growth can result in a relapse of overjet correction whereas unfavorable vertical growth can result in a reduction of overbite.

BIBLIOGRAPHY

1. Baccetti T, et al. Skeletal effects of early treatment of Class III malocclusions with maxillary expansion and face mask therapy. Am J Orthod 1998;113:333–42.
2. Battagel JM. The aetiological factors in Class III malocclusion. Eur J Orthod 1993;15:347–70.
3. Grabber LW. Chin cup therapy for mandibular prognathism. Am J Orthod 1997;72:23–41.
4. Kondo E. Non surgical and nonextraction treatment of a skeletal Class III patient with severe prognathic mandible. World J Orthod 2001;2:115–26.

PREVIOUS YEAR'S UNIVERSITY QUESTIONS

Essay

1. How do you manage Class III patients in growing patients?
2. How do you treat Class III patients in non-growing patients?

MCQs

1. *Edge-to-edge relation is a feature of:*
   a. Class I malocclusion
   b. Class III malocclusion
   c. Class II division 1 malocclusion
   d. Class II division 2 malocclusion   **(Ans: b)**

2. *Crowded upper arch and spaced lower arch is usually found in:*
   a. Class I malocclusion
   b. Class III malocclusion
   c. Class II division 1 malocclusion
   d. Class II division 2 malocclusion   **(Ans: b)**

3. *Gonial angle in class III malocclusion is:*
   a. Acute
   b. Obtuse
   c. 90°
   d. None of the above   **(Ans: b)**

4. *Unfavorable incisal guidance leads to pseudo Class III, if unattended, can lead to true skeletal Class III:*
   a. Statement I is true
   b. Statement I is false
   c. Statement II is true
   d. Both statements are true   **(Ans: d)**

5. *3D expansion screws when used in Class III malocclusion brings about:*
   a. Forward placement of maxilla
   b. Lateral expansion of maxilla
   c. Expansion in all three directions
   d. All of the above **(Ans: c)**

6. *Vertical and anteroposterior deficiency of maxilla with normal mandible is seen in:*
   a. Pierre Robin syndrome
   b. Cleidocranial dystosis
   c. Cleft lip and palate
   d. All of the above **(Ans: c)**

7. *Pressure from chin cup tends to:*
   a. Tip the mandibular incisors lingually
   b. Tip the mandibular incisors labially
   c. Tip the maxillary incisors lingually
   d. Tip the mandibular incisors labially **(Ans: a)**

8. *Recent advancement in treating Class III malocclusion includes:*
   a. Chin cup
   b. Anterior face mask
   c. 3D screws
   d. RME with anterior face mask **(Ans: c)**

Early Orthodontic Treatment for Preadolescent Children

Chapter Outline

- Goals of early orthodontic treatment
- Phases of early orthodontic treatment
- Benefits of the early treatment approach
- Open bite
- Crossbite

- Deep bite
- Midline diastema
- Crowding
- Skeletal problems

In order to apply the proper treatment at the proper time, it is necessary to look first at the principles and strategy of early orthodontic intervention.

GOALS OF EARLY ORTHODONTIC TREATMENT

The strategy and major techniques intervention include the following important goals:
- Elimination of primary etiologic factors, if possible
- Correction of obvious problems
- Interception of developing problems
- Prevention of worsening of obvious problems
- Preparation of an environment for normal occlusal development and function
- Guidance of growth in a more favorable direction by unlocking occlusal interferences, which can have an adverse effect on occlusion.
- Management of arch size-tooth size discrepancy.
- Reduction in susceptibility to trauma and incisor fractures (increased overjet)
- Correction of skeletal dysplasia at an early stage of development.

PHASES OF EARLY ORTHODONTIC TREATMENT

Early orthodontic treatment protocols can be performed in two separate phases. Depending on the type of problem, the age of the patient, and the stage of dentition, this procedure can be accomplished in one phase and sometimes in two phases. Occasionally, a three-phase treatment plan might be implemented, if some correction of primary dentition is needed, such as elimination of posterior crossbite, and serial extractions in the mixed dentition must be followed by a final phase of treatment for the permanent dentition.

During each phase, the main objectives of intervention and treatment include reducing adverse growth, preventing dental and skeletal disharmonies, improving the esthetics of the smile, enhancing the patient's self-image, and improving the occlusion. First-phase early orthodontic treatment offer many advantages to both the doctor and the patient. These therapies should be part of every orthodontist's armamentarium.

One-phase Early Orthodontic Treatment

To clarify the different types of early intervention used in orthodontic practice and clearly distinguish between the meanings of these terms. It is necessary to explain them first:
- One-phase early treatment consists of a type of interceptive or corrective treatment that is performed during the primary or mixed dentition stage to eliminate the cause and to correct the present abnormality.

- One-phase early treatment of Class II malocclusion is a single phase of comprehensive treatment usually started around the end of mixed dentition, just before the growth spurt and ending after the completion of canine eruption. This usually takes about 2 to 3 years.
- The major goal of late mixed dentition treatment is growth modification to take advantage of growth potential during the growth spurt. This type of treatment involves orthopedic management such as extraoral traction, functional therapy and rapid maxillary expansion.

Two-phase Treatment

Two-phase treatment is advocated to address skeletal, dental and neuromuscular problems such as abnormal habits, hyperactive musculature, crowding, dental crossbites, hypodontia, supernumerary teeth and problems of tooth eruption in order to eliminate or reduce the severity of the problem and a short phase of treatment will be required to align the permanent occlusion.

An example of two-phase treatment is serial extraction, where preparation of anchorage, extractions and guidance of canine eruption are performed in phase 1. After canine eruption and completion of the permanent dentition, the second phase begins with full bonding of appliances for uprighting of teeth, correction of rotation, and minor space closure to finalize the treatment.

Another example of two-phase treatment is early intervention and control of abnormal habits which might be started during the primary or mixed dentition and followed by an interim phase of supervision during the transitional dentition, until eruption of the permanent dentition for phase 2 treatment.

BENEFITS OF THE EARLY TREATMENT APPROACH

The types of treatment and services that can be provided to young children during the developmental stages of the dentition and skeletal growth are tremendous. Many dental and skeletal anomalies can be prevented or intercepted during the primary or mixed dentition. Some might be treated in one phase and others in two phases, but proper intervention can definitely reduce the duration and complications of second phase treatment.

The following services can be provided to young patients, if treatment is initiated at the proper time.
- Space management.
- Management of incisor crowding.
- Management of deleterious oral habits.

- Orthodontic management of missing teeth
- Orthodontic management of supernumerary teeth
- Diagnosis and management of abnormal frenum attachments
- Early detection and treatment of eruption problems
- Management of sagittal, transeverse and vertical dentoskeletal problems in the primary and early mixed dentition stages.

Benefits to Patients

- Improvement of facial appearance and self-esteem.
- Easier resolution or interception of developing malocclusion.
- Early detection and interception will minimize the severity of problem.
- *Correction of functional problems:* Some tooth malalignments, such as prematurities and incorrect dental inclinations (anterior and posterior crossbites), can result in mandibular shift, functional discomfort and structural defect and have an adverse effect on normal growth patterns. Early correction can eliminate the patient's discomfort and prevent many complicated problems that can happen later.
- *Prevention of damage to teeth and dentoskeletal structures:* Some irregularities, such as severe dental protrusion and overjet, increase the risk of fracture of the maxillary incisors because of trauma. Early correction of these irregularities would prevent such problems.
- *Reduction in the need for extraction:* Much of the crowding that develops during the mixed dentition can be corrected by space regaining, expansion or growth modification. These corrections might not be possible after completion of the growth spurt and eruption of the permanent dentition.
- *Greater patient compliance:* Prior to their teen ages, most children are enthusiastic about getting brace and are more comfortable wearing appliances.
- *More stable results:* Young patients are more adaptive to the changes of orthodontic tooth movement, and the results are more stable.
- Less traumatic and, therefore, less painful, treatment procedures. Younger children seem to have a lower resistance to bone and tooth movement and tend to complain less.
- Prevention of psychological problems, which may occur in some children.
- *Lower treatment costs:* The total fee for early orthodontic treatment is less than that of comprehensive treatment of the permanent dentition because therapy is less extensive, there is less chair time per

visit, and appointment intervals are longer. Also, if a second phase of treatment is needed, it tends to be easier and for a shorter period of time.

Benefits to Practitioners

- *Availability of more treatment options:* Because of the patient's age, the possibility of guidance of eruption, and the growth potential, more options are available in treatment planning, especially because the abnormalities are still in developmental stages.
- *Better patient compliance:* A patient's compliance in orthodontic treatment is one of the most important factors in treatment success. Cooperation is much greater among children aged 7 to 10 years than among other patients. If an adolescent or adult insists on having the appliance removed before the proper results are obtained, the orthodontist might be forced to compromise treatment goals.
- *Better use of growth potential:* One of the most important benefits of early treatment is utilization of the growth potential to correct skeletal abnormalities and the potential to modify growth which is impossible to achieve after termination of growth. Proper orthopedic treatment during jaw growth can result in significant reduction of dentoskeletal deformities in three dimensions. These include early Class III correction involving overgrowth of the mandible or underdevelopment of the maxilla, correction of the constricted maxilla for better mandibular growth, or stimulation of mandibular growth in the retrognathic mandible.
- *Reduction in the need for extraction:* As mentioned earlier, the availability of more options for regaining lost space or creating new space in crowding situations has the potential to reduce the need for tooth extraction.
- *Easier control of habits:* Control of serious deleterious habits is easier to obtain in young children. Also, future skeletal damage to the dentition and alveolar skeletal structure can be prevented. If abnormal habits continue, there is more potential for damage and management of the problems will be more complicated.
- *Better management of problematic growth patterns:* Long-term observation facilitates control of abnormal, complex problems in the growth pattern, e.g. by guiding adjustments to the treatment plan when necessary.
- *Less need for mass tooth movement and complex therapy:* En masse tooth movements, such as torqueing movements, usually are not necessary in early treatment. Early treatment also reduces the need for second-phase treatment.

- *Shorter treatment time in the second phase:* Proper intervention at the proper time reduces the duration of the second phase and significantly reduces the severity of the problems treated in phase 2.
- *More stable results:* Relapse after the completion of treatment is one of the most disturbing events to confront an orthodontist. This failure happens more often after treatment initiated in the permanent dentition than it does after early-age treatment. Early-age treatments are usually performed during occlusal development, providing a normal environment for the dentition. Most tooth movements in early treatment are the result of natural eruption processes caused by guidance techniques. Therefore, the dentition has more potential to adapt to the changes, making post-treatment relapse less likely.

Possible Stages of Orthodontic Treatment Timing

- Preschool/primary dentition treatment typically age 3–6 years.
- Preadolescent/mixed dentition treatment: Early—6–9 years. Late: 9–12 years.
- Adolescent/early permanent dentition treatment 12–15 years.

DENTAL PROBLEMS

Open Bite

The glossary of orthodontic terms defines open bite as a developmental or acquired malocclusion whereby no vertical overlap exists between maxillary and mandibular anterior or posterior teeth.

Definition

Open bite is the failure of a tooth or teeth to meet their antagonist in the opposite arch.

- Open bite is descriptive of a condition where a space exists between occlusal or incisal surfaces of maxillary and mandibular teeth in the buccal or anterior segments when the mandible is brought into habitual or centric occlusion. (Graber)
- Open bite is a condition of malocclusion wherein there is an overlap between the maxillary and mandibular dentition.

Open bite is present when:
- There is less than an average overbite
- There is edge-to-edge relationship
- There is definite degree of openness

Open bite is a condition where there is localized or generalized absence of occlusion, while remaining teeth are in occlusion. It is one of the malocclusions found in vertical plane. It was verified and found that there is 12% prevalence of anterior open bite is more frequent in males, in patients with Class I in the age group of 7 years.

Open bite creates significant problems, such as:
- Difficulty in speech (dysphonia)
- TMJ disorders
- Functional imbalance
- Bad esthetics
- Alteration of incisor guidance
- Reduction of normal functional activity

Features of Open Bite

- Increase in the lower facial height
- Clockwise rotation of the mandible
- Extrusion of molars

Classification of Open Bite

Open bite is classified:
1. *On the basis of region involved:*
   - Anterior open bite
   - Posterior open bite
2. *On the basis of etiological factors:*
   - Skeletal open bite
   - Dental open bite
3. *On the basis of clinical evaluation:*
   - Simple (occurs between the incisors)
   - Complex (extends from premolars or deciduous molars from one side to the other)
   - Compound/infantile open bite (completely open including the molars)
   - Iatrogenic open bite (consequence of orthodontic or surgical therapy)
4. *On the basis of molar relationship:*
   - Class I open bite
   - Class II open bite
   - Class III open bite

Dentoalveolar Open Bite

The extent of the dentoalveolar open bite depends on the extent of the eruption of the teeth, e.g. supra-occlusion of the molars and infraocclusion of the incisors can be primary etiologic factors (Fig. 18.1).

In vertical growth patterns, the dentoalveolar symptoms include a protrusion in the upper anterior teeth with lingual inclination of the lower incisors (Fig. 18.2).

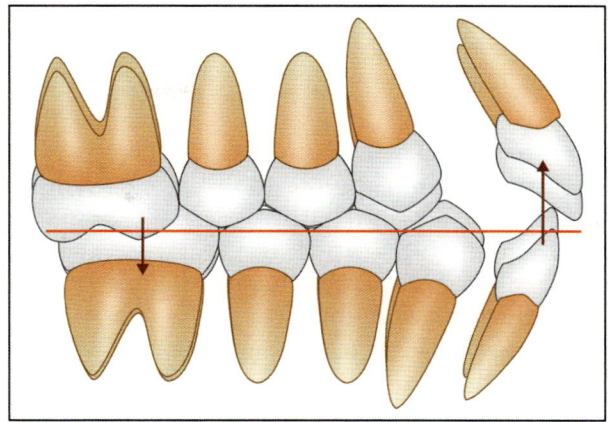

Fig. 18.1: Dentoalveolar open bite

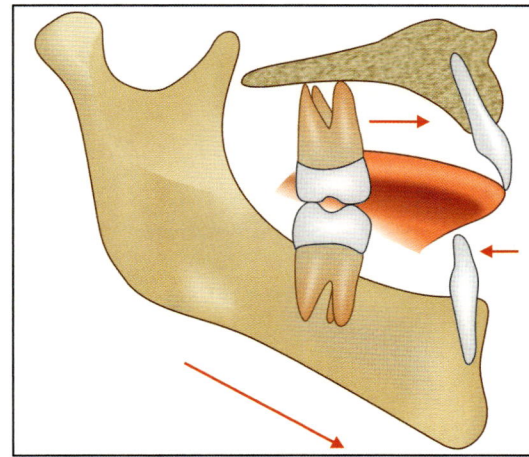

Fig. 18.2: Open bite in vertical grower

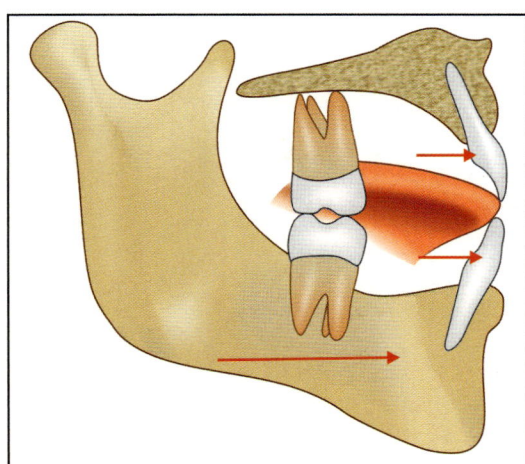

Fig. 18.3: Open bite in horizontal grower

In horizontal growth patterns, tongue posture and thrust may cause proclination of both upper and lower incisor (Fig. 18.3).

A lateral open bite may be considered as dento-alveolar in combination with infraocclusion of molar teeth (Fig. 18.4).

Anterior Open Bite

Anterior open bite is a condition where there is no vertical overlap between the upper and lower anteriors. Anterior open bites are esthetically unattractive particularly during speech when the tongue is pressed between the teeth and lips.

Anterior open bite can be present either as:
- Dental anterior open bite (Fig. 18.5)
- Skeletal anterior open bite (Fig. 18.6)

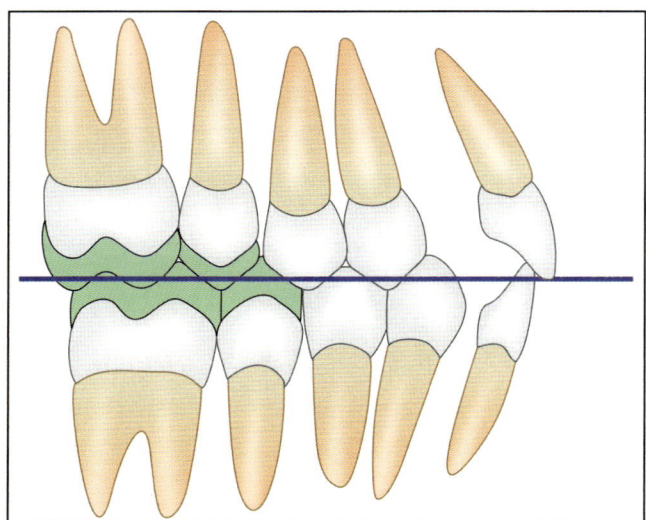

Fig. 18.4: Lateral open bite

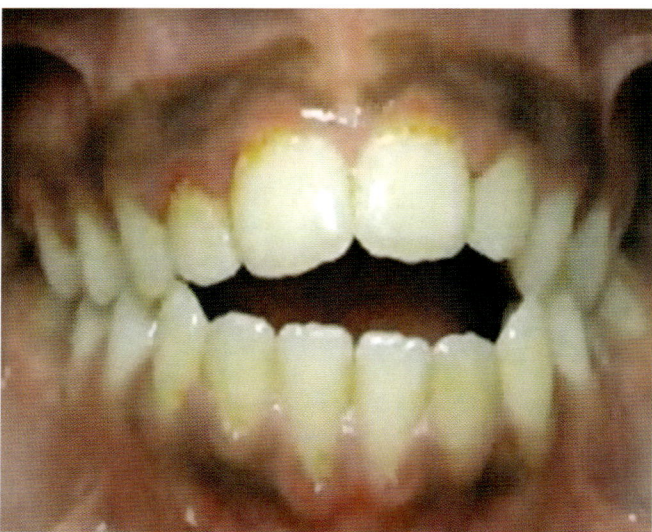

Fig. 18.5: Dental open bite

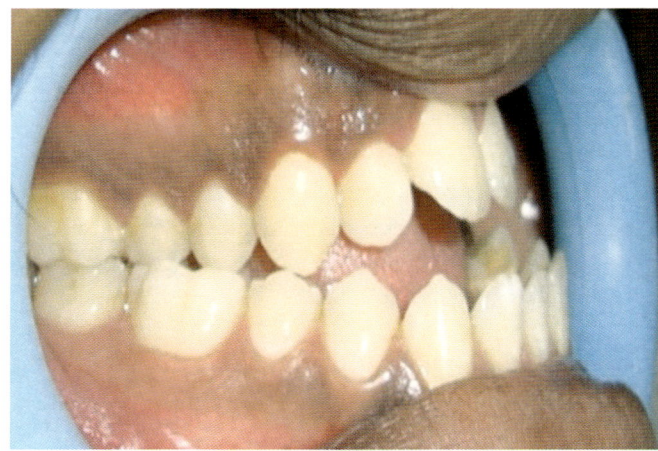

Fig. 18.6: Skeletal open bite with Class III malocclusion

Dental Open Bite

Dental open bite is seen between canine-to-canine whereas open bite is seen between premolar-to-premolar in skeletal open bite.

Dental open bite is associated with some of the following characteristics:
- Normal craniofacial pattern
- Upper incisors are proclined.
- Under erupted anterior teeth
- Normal or slightly excessive molar height
- Mesial inclination of posterior dentition
- Failure of eruption of teeth with unknown etiology
- Divergent of upper and lower occlusal plane
- No gummy smile
- No vertical maxillary excess
- Habits like thumb or finger sucking and tongue thrusting
- There may be spacing between anterior.
- Speech defects can be found with lisping of voice. There may be associated upper respiratory infections. Lisping associated with anterior open bite and spacing is called interdental stigmatism.

Diagnosis
Clinical
- Overjet combined with an openbite less than 1 mm—Pseudo open bite.
- Open bite with more than 1 mm space between opposing incisors and with posterior teeth in occlusion—simple open bite.
- Open bite extending from the premolar or deciduous molar on one side to the corresponding teeth on the other side—complex open bite.
- Compound or infantile open bite is completely open including molars.

- Iatrogenic open bite is the consequences of orthodontic/surgical therapy:
  - An open activator with a high construction bite causes tongue-thrusting habit and resultant open bite. Intrusion of posterior teeth creates a posterior open bite especially in the deciduous molar areas.
  - Expansion treatment: Buccal segments tip buccally along with elongation of the lingual cusp. This creates a prematurity and open the bite.
  - In distalization of the maxillary first molar with extraoral forces, the molars are often tipped downwards and back elongating the mesial cusp. This creates open bite and, therefore, excessive anterior facial height

Treatment

- *Removable of cause:* Removable or fixed habit breaking appliance.
- *Myofunctional appliances:* FR IV or modified activator or open bionator, fixed appliance therapy with Box elastic (Fig. 18.7)
- Removable or fixed appliance with fixed habit breaking cribs
- Reminder or blue grass appliance
- Tongue exercises

Skeletal Open Bite

Skeletal open bites are caused mainly by over eruption of the upper posterior teeth or vertical over growth of the posterior dentoalveolar complex. These could be due to posterior rotation of the mandible, superior repositioning of the glenoid fossa due to under-development of these effects. Skeletal open bite with a long face can be divided into two types—one caused by clockwise rotation of the mandible and the other by skeletal deformation such as tipping of the maxilla and diversion of the gonial angle of the mandible. Skeletal anterior open bite also called stigmata of malocclusion.

Etiology: Open bite develops as a result of the interaction of many etiological factors:

- In young children, digit habits and pacifiers are the most common etiologic agents.
- In the mixed dentition years other than normal transitional open bite, some open bites are probably attributable to lingering habits, where others are clearly skeletal in nature.
- In the adolescent and the adults, it is difficult to assign singular causation. The influence of the tongue, lip and airway on the development of malocclusion remains to be substantiated. Variations in growth intensity, the function of the soft tissues and the jaw musculature and the individual dentoalveolar development influence the evolution of open bite problems.
- Skeletal factors on development of open bite. The combination of:
  - Excessive development of the upper midface heights (cranial base to molars).
  - A lack of development of posterior facial height (S-Go) results in the downward and backward rotation of the mandible (Fig. 18.8).
  - The posterior half of the palate is tipped downward, carrying the molars further downward. This gives rise to a large palatomandibular plane angle (Fig. 18.9).
  - Because of the short ramus and the lower palate, the pharyngeal space is constricted. In order to breathe, these persons keep their tongues forward. Further enchanced by the dental open bite, there is a tongue-thrusting tendencies.

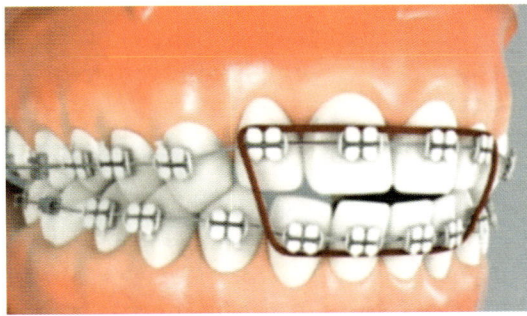

Fig. 18.7: Box elastic used to correct open bite

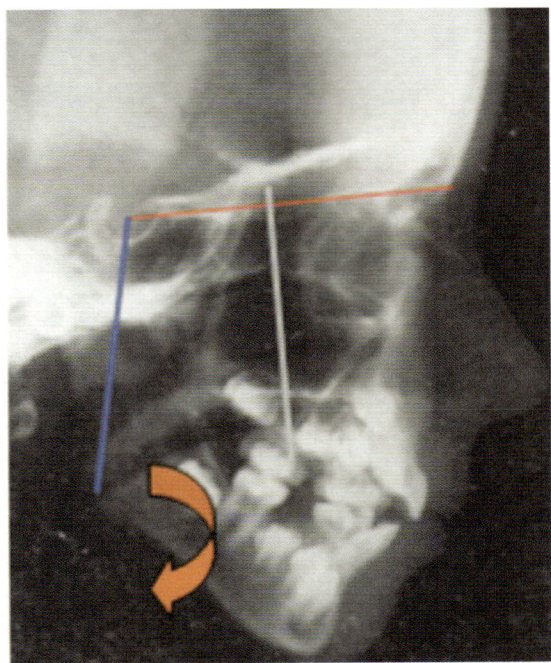

Fig. 18.8: Short facial height causing anterior open bite

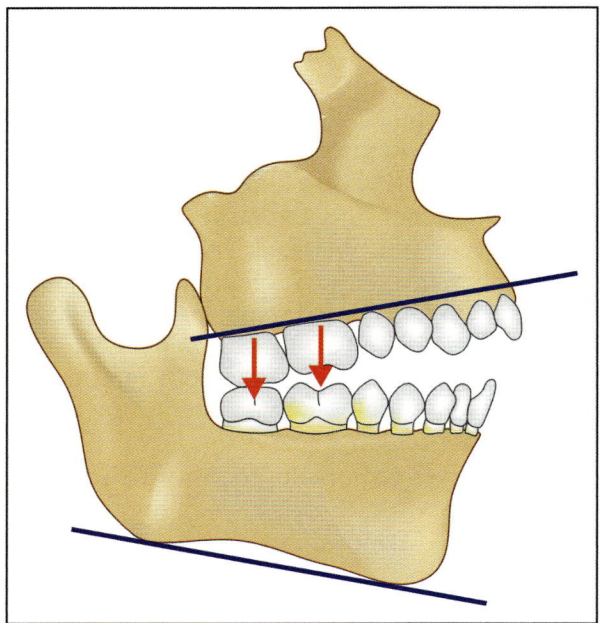

Fig. 18.9: Downward tilt of palate causing anterior open bite

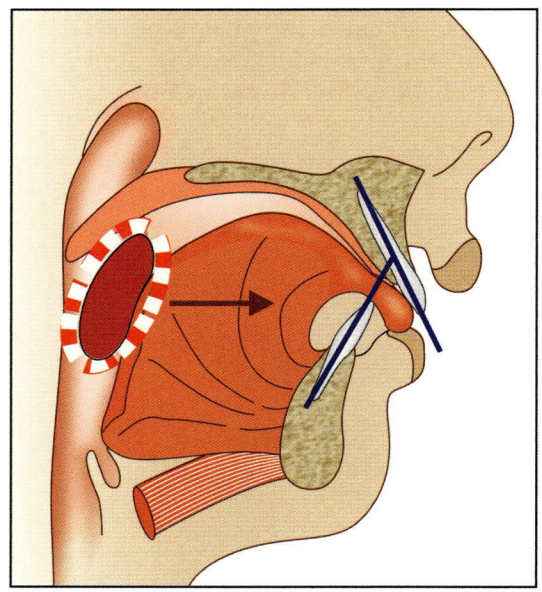

Fig. 18.10: Enlarged tonsils causing open bite

– When enlarged tonsils are present, the tongue is further confined anteriorly. As the narrow palatal vault reduces the necessary space, there is a tendency towards tongue protrusion. This, in turn, may be a factor in the creation of bidental protrusion (Fig. 18.10).
• It can be classified into:
 – Epigenetic
 – Environmental (or)
 – Disturbances in the eruption of teeth or alveolar growth (ankylosed teeth)

– Mechanical interference with eruption and alveolar growth (thumb of digit sucking)
– Vertical skeletal dysplasias

Epigenetic Factors
• Posture, morphology and size of the tongue
• Skeletal growth patterns of the maxilla and the mandible
• The vertical relationship of the jaw bases

Environmental Factors
• *Abnormal function*
 – Thumb- or digit-sucking habit
 – Tongue-thrusting habit
• *Improper respiration:* Mouth breathing

Thumb- or digit-sucking habit:
• This is one of the most common habits seen in children.
• The habit is quite reversible till the age of 3 or 4 years
• Beyond this age, this habit becomes the cause of many malocclusions
Causes of the habit: Sigmund Freud emotional security derived from the oral phase of psychological development of first 3 years of life

Tongue-thrusting habit: Infantile/visceral swallowing is the physiological basis for the neonate/infant to create a proper lip seal during sucking. When the deciduous teeth erupt, the pattern of swallowing changes to adult/mature swallow. If the visceral swallow persists after the 4th year of life, the habit is called retained infantile swallow or tongue thrust.

It may be:
• Skeletal Class I open bite
• Skeletal Class II open bite
• Skeletal Class III open bite

Skeletal Class I Open Bite (Positional deviations)
According to Sassouni, the four bony planes of the face are steep to each other bringing the center "0" close to the profile (Fig. 18.11).

Dimensional deviations
1. The total posterior facial height (S-Go) tends to be half the size of the anterior total facial height (N-Me) (Fig. 18.12a).

 The lower anterior facial height exceeds the upper anterior facial height (Fig. 18.12b).

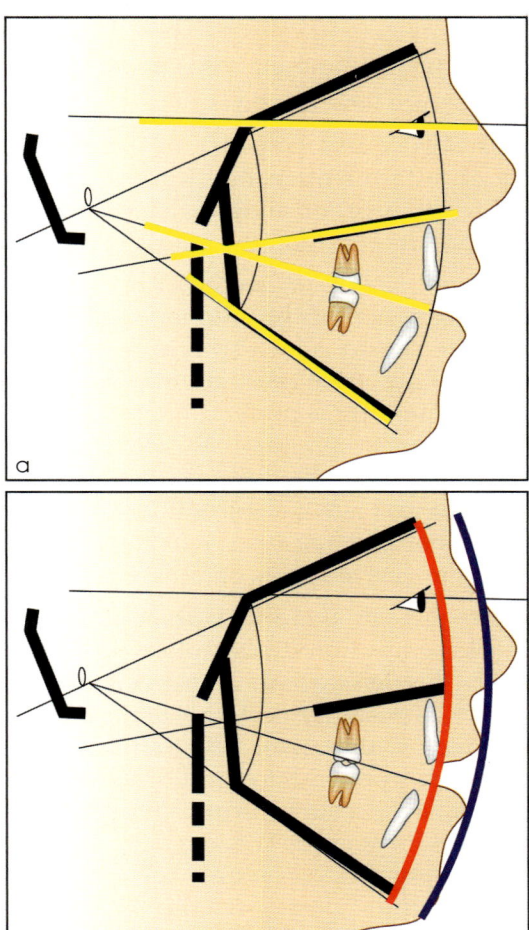

Fig. 18.11: The anterior arc, therefore, follows the convexity of the profile: (a) Decrease of posterior facial height; (b) Increase of lower anterior facial height

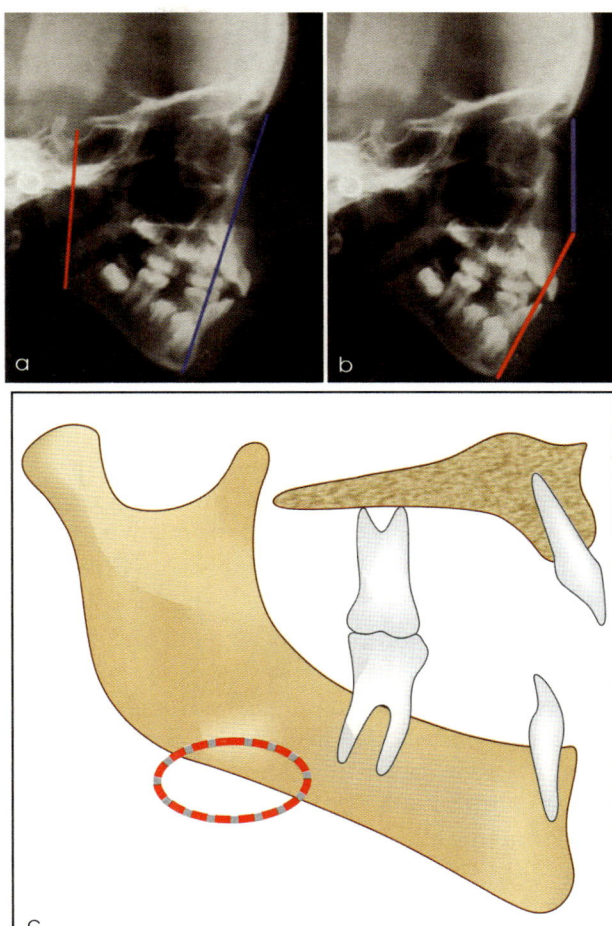

Fig. 18.12a to c: Short ramus and antigonial notch

2. The facial breadths tend to be narrow giving a long ovoid appearance in the frontal view.
3. The ramus is short with an antegonial notch at its lower border (Fig. 18.12c).
4. The mandibular symphysis is narrow antero-posteriorly and long vertically.
5. There is a lack of chin mental protuberance development.
6. According to Sheldon, the open bite type rates high in ectomorphs.
7. The palatal vault is high and narrow.

Skeletal Class II Open Bite

1. In this type, in some instances, the rotation of the mandible may be purely positional. Often this is due to a downward and backward rotation of the mandible (Fig. 18.13).
2. This rotation is associated with excessive extrusion of the molars. If these interferences are removed, the

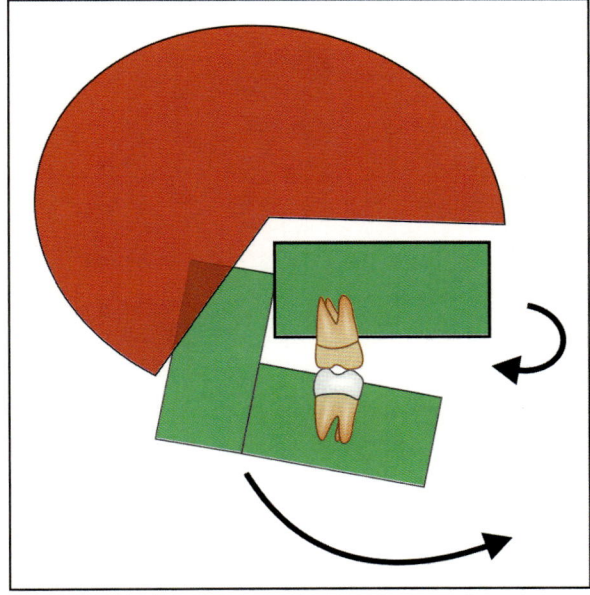

Fig. 18.13: Downward and backward rotation of the mandible causing skeletal II open bite

mandible can be permitted to rotate in a closing direction, improving the Class II and the open bite patterns simultaneously.

Skeletal Class III Open Bite

This combination consists primarily of an open bite with a palatal deficiency or a large mandible (Fig. 18.14).

Features of Skeletal Open Bite

The anterior skeletal open bite is called apertognathia. The problem is related to the skeletal bases. A patient having a skeletal anterior openbite is characterized by the following:

- The patient often has a long and narrow face with marked convex profile. A patient with underlying skeletal Class III bases may have concave profile.
- The patient may have a short upper lip with excessive maxillary incisor exposure.
- Increased lower anterior facial height and decreased upper anterior facial height.
- A steep mandibular plane angle (high angle). The angle FMA is increased and more than 30°. There is clockwise rotation or backward rotation of the mandible with increased lower anterior facial height.
- Small mandibular body and ramus.
- Divergent jaw bases as well as other horizontal cephalometric planes.
- There is upward rotation of maxillary jaw base (the ANS and PNS plane gives maxillary jaw base).

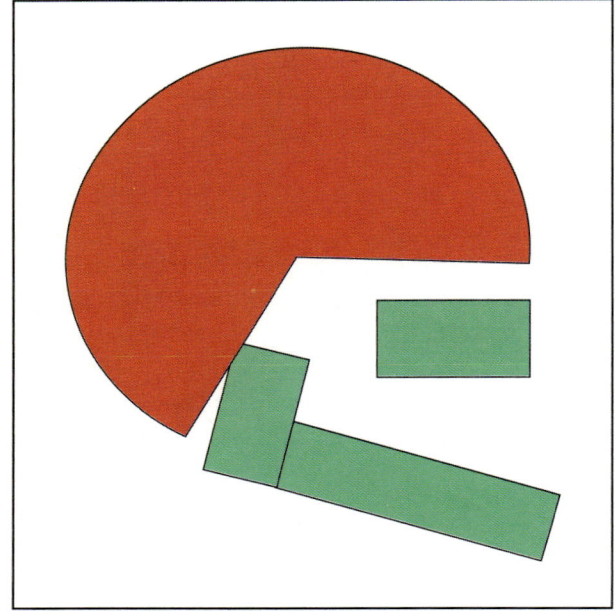

Fig. 18.14: Skeletal III open bite

Different Approaches to Correct Skeletal Open Bite

Surgical intervention such as LeFort I procedure is the treatment of choice for a severe skeletal open bite.

High-pull headgear is a popular approach to the correction of anterior open bite inhibiting vertical maxillary development and allow for a forward rotation of the mandible, thus closing the bite.

Bilateral posterior bite block: The anterior open bite is corrected by extrusion of the anterior, which is often unsatisfactory due to poor esthetic result. Hence, intrusion of the posterior resulting in autorotation of the mandible anteriorly is preferred (Fig. 18.15).

The correction is achieved by preventing the maxillary and mandibular posterior teeth from erupting and by opening the bite several millimeters so as to stretch the posterior muscles of mastication causing them to act as intrusive agents on the maxilla.

Active vertical corrector: It is an adaption of the present day bite block therapy introduced in 1986 by Dr. Eugene L Dellinger. It works as an energized bite block consisting of two posterior occlusal splints one for the upper and one for the lower jaw. Samarium cobalt magnets are incorporated into acrylic splints over the occlusal region of the teeth to be intruded. One magnet per distal quadrant is used. The magnets in the upper splints are incorporated in a mode to repel the magnets in the lower splints, therefore, the appliance is a combination of acrylic posterior bite blocks and repelling magnetic forces.

The magnets used are cylindrical in shape with a diameter of 10 mm. The magnets along with the bite blocks measured 12 mm in height. Because samarium Cobalt is a highly reactive, rare earth material, they are best isolated from the oral environment. Hence, they are hermetically sealed in stainless steel capsules. The magnets are also parylene coated to prevent leaching

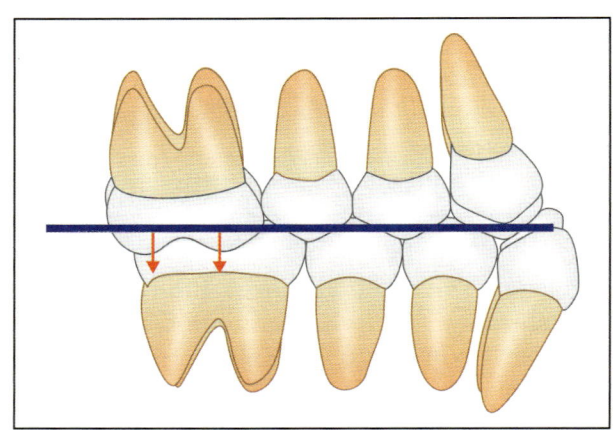

Fig. 18.15: Bilateral posterior bite block

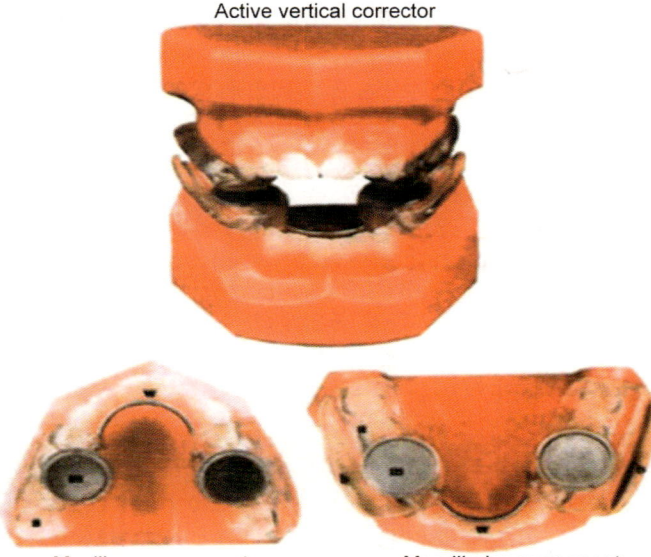

Active vertical corrector

Maxillary component   Mandibular component
Acrylic component samarium cobalt magnet
Buccal flange heavy gauge stainless steel wire

Fig. 18.16: Active vertical corrector

out of cytotoxic materials. The magnets generate a force of 700 gm per unit at zero air gaps in repulsion. The bite registration is done with 5 mm space in the posterior region to accommodate magnets, casings and acrylic splint (Fig. 18.16).

Posterior Open Bite

Posterior open bite is a condition characterized by lack of contact between the posteriors when the teeth are in centric occlusion. It may be present either unilaterally or bilaterally.

Iatrogenic Open Bite

- Iatrogenic open bite is due to failure of orthodontic treatment.
- It occurs as a result of poor mechanics during fixed appliance therapy.
- It leads to extrusion of posterior teeth especially molars or hanging palatal cusps which open the bite.

Treatment

- *Removal of cause:* Lateral tongue spikes for lateral tongue thrust.
- Due to infraocclusion of ankylosed teeth, it is best treated by crowns.

CROSSBITE

Dentoalveolar anterior crossbite represents a linguoversion of one or more maxillary anterior teeth with resultant locking behind the opposing mandibular teeth in full closure.

It is usually acquired malocclusion resulting from local etiological factors that interfere with normal eruptive positioning of the maxillary anterior teeth.

Crossbite is a type of malocclusion that is frequently encountered in the practice of orthodontics. This malocclusion is identified when the lower teeth are in a buccal or labial position with regard to the upper teeth, in a unilateral, bilateral, anterior or posterior manner. This malocclusion can have a skeletal or dental component or mix of both, they are relatively easy to intercept at an early age; so that surgical correction is not needed in future.

It is divided into two types:
- Sagittal type crossbite
- Transverse type crossbite

Sagittal Type Crossbite (Anterior Crossbite)

It is again subdivided into:
- Developing crossbite
- Developed crossbite

Developing Crossbite

One of the major responsibilities of the dental practitioner is to intercept adverse patterns of dental eruption in the child. Among the developmental problems, frequently seen in the mixed dentition, is the anterior crossbite. It is called developing crossbite because the roots are still growing.

The anterior dental crossbite may be the result of 1 or a combination of several etiologic factors:
1. Traumatic injuries to the primary dentition that cause a lingual displacement of the permanent tooth bud.
2. An over-retained primary tooth.
3. A labially situated supernumerary tooth.
4. A sclerosed bony or fibrous tissue barrier caused by losing a primary tooth prematurely.
5. An inadequacy of arch length causing the lingual deflection of the permanent tooth during eruption.
6. Detrimental habit patterns.
7. A repaired cleft lip.

A few factors to consider before selecting a treatment approach:
1. Adequate space in the arch to reposition the tooth.
2. Sufficient overbite to hold the tooth in position following correction.
3. An apical position of the tooth in crossbite that is the same as it would be in normal occlusion.
4. A Class I occlusion.

There are many possible approaches to the treatment of a simple anterior dental crossbite. The following treatment approaches have been recommended for simple anterior dental crossbite.

Tongue blade therapy: Opposing mandibular tooth acts as fulcrum and the patient is asked to rotate the oral part of the blade upward and forward. The proper use of tongue blade for an hour or two for 10 to 15 days is sufficient. It resembles a flat ice-cream stick. It is placed inside the mouth contacting the erupting tooth in crossbite on its palatal aspect (Figs 18.17 and 18.18). With lower incisor margin as a fulcrum, the oral portion of the tongue blade is rotated upwards and forward to engage the lingual surface of the upper incisors. The patient is advised to bite with a constant pressure on the wood and at the same time to exert a slight but constant pressure with his hand on the blade, so as to prevent tongue blade displacement. The tongue blade therapy is advised for an hour or two, in a day. 10–14 days of practice is usually sufficient to defect the lingually erupting maxillary incisors into proper relationship.

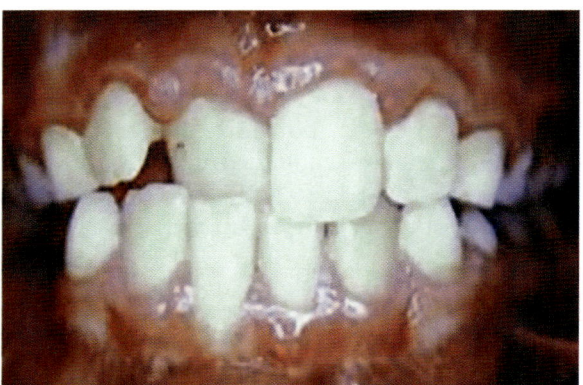

Fig. 18.17: Developing crossbite

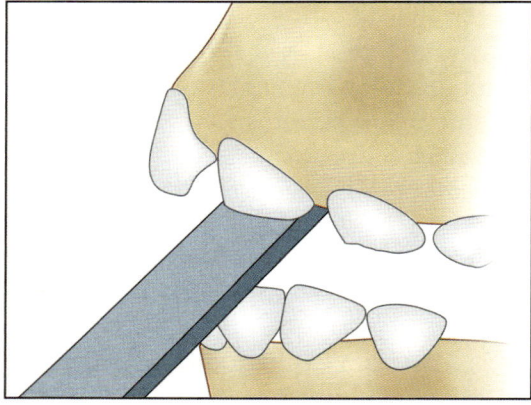

Fig. 18.18: Tongue blade therapy

Lower inclined plane: Treatment of anterior dental crossbite involving 1 or more teeth may be accomplished by using a cemented lower inclined acrylic plane. This technique has the possibility of opening the bite, if worn for more than 3 weeks. This is dealt in Removable Functional Appliance Chapter.

Three stainless steel or composite crowns: Another method is cementing a reverse anterior stainless steel crown on the lingually locked incisor at a 45° angle to the occlusal plane. This method is subject to all the disadvantages of the inclined plane method and is difficult to apply to partially erupted maxillary incisors.

Hawley retainer with auxiliary springs: This appliance is used frequently for minor tooth movement in pediatric dentistry. In this procedure the prognosis, depends on patient cooperation and parental supervision. Hawley's appliance with either single or double cantilevers or Z springs and bilateral posterior bite plane is given to correct anterior crossbite.

Labial and lingual archwires: The use of labial and/or lingual archwires has proven successful. The disadvantage of the use of these appliances is the expense and additional training required to use efficiently.

Skeletal anterior crossbite

- *Growing patients:* Myofunctional appliance, chin cup appliance
- *Non-growing patients:* Mandibular set back or maxillary advancement surgical procedures

Functional anterior crossbite: *For example pseudo Class III malocclusion:* The functional crossbite is treated by eliminating occlusal prematurities.

Developed anterior dental crossbite (Fig. 18.19a–d): It is called developed crossbite because the roots are fully completed.

Transverse Type Crossbite (Posterior Crossbite)

It is further classified into
- Dental posterior crossbite
- Skeletal posterior crossbite
- Functional posterior crossbite

Dental posterior crossbite: The anterior crossbite might involve either single or group of teeth. The posterior crossbite may be unilateral or bilateral or total crossbite.

Skeletal posterior crossbite: The entire lower anterior are labial to upper incisors (reversed overjet). It is usually associated with Class III (true) malocclusion.

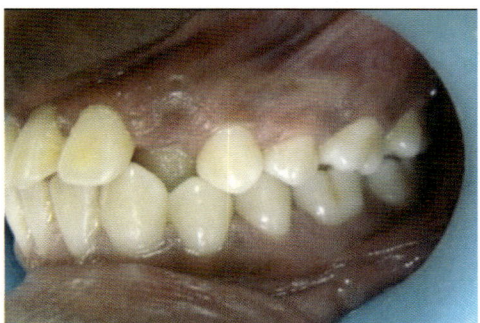

Fig. 18.19a: Developed anterior crossbite involving single tooth

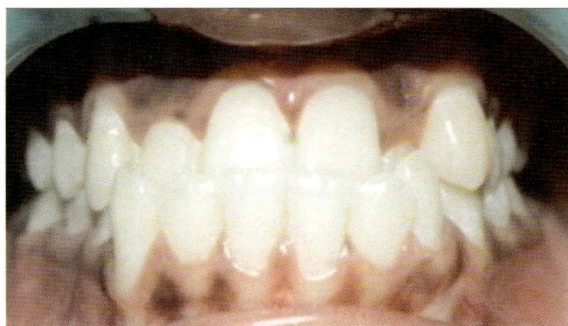

Fig. 18.19d: Dental anterior crossbite involving group of teeth

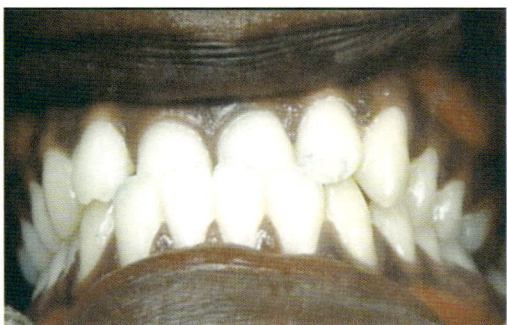

Fig. 18.19b: Developed anterior crossbite involving two teeth

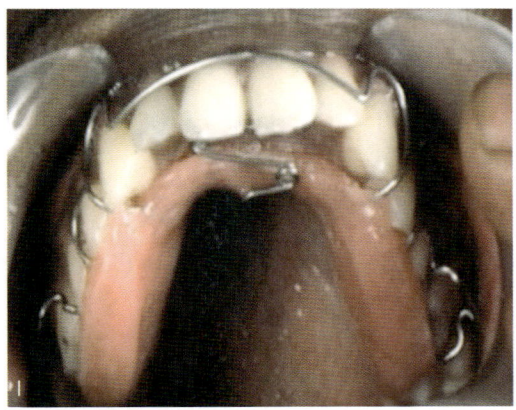

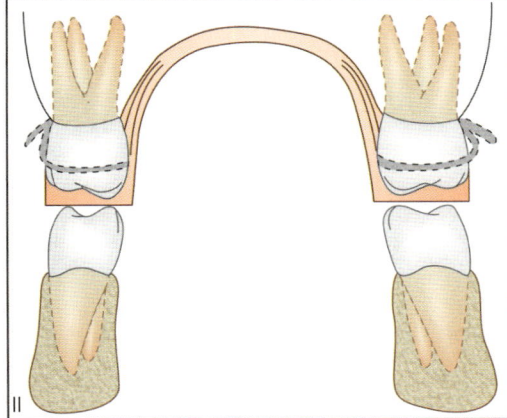

Fig. 18.19c: I. Upper Hawley's appliance with double cantilever spring; II. Bilateral posterior plane

Functional posterior crossbite: Due to cuspal interferences, the mandible during the path of closure slides in habitual occlusion.

Classification

The following classification was proposed by Moyers (1966).

Functional crossbite: There is occlusal interference that displaces the mandible to the left or the right during the last phase of closure.
- They are unilateral crossbite.
- There may be a chin deviation.
- Lower dental midline deviation as a consequence of the mandibular deviation.

Dental crossbite
- It can affect the tooth or a group of teeth (Fig. 18.20a and b)
- It may be unilateral or bilateral.

Skeletal crossbite: The most frequent alteration is the insufficient growth of maxilla.

Scissor bite: It is the one in which the palatal aspect of an upper premolar or molar contacts, the buccal aspect of the lower antagonist (Fig. 18.21).

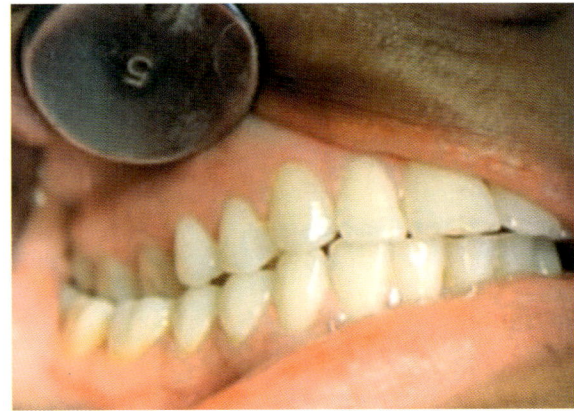

Fig. 18.20a: Dental posterior crossbite

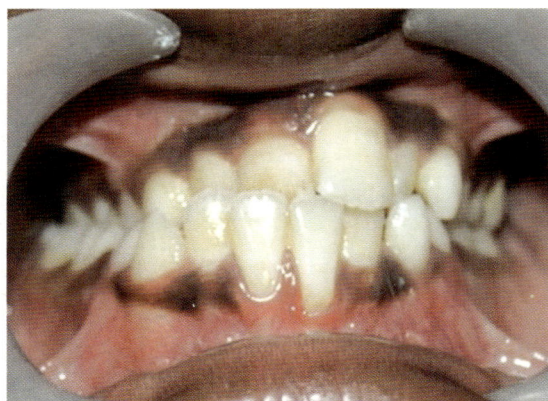

Fig. 18.20b: Dental unilateral anterior crossbite involving right incisors and posterior crossbite

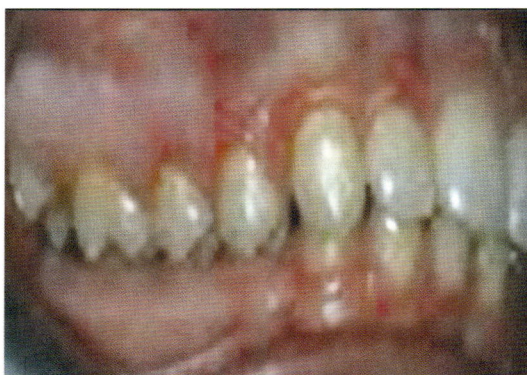

Fig. 18.21: Scissor bite

Treatment

Appliances and methods used in treatment of posterior dental crossbite are:

- Slow expansion appliance
- Rapid expansion appliance
- Through the bite elastics
- NiTi expander appliance

DEEP BITE

Dental deep bite: The deep overbite or deep bite can be defined by the excess amount or percentage of overlap of the lower incisors by the upper incisors.

Graber: It is defined as a condition of excessive overbite where the vertical measurement between the maxillary and mandibular incisal margins is excessive when the mandible is brought into habitual or centric occlusion.

Classification

- *According to its origin:*
  a. Dental deep bite
  b. Skeletal deep bite (Fig. 18.22)

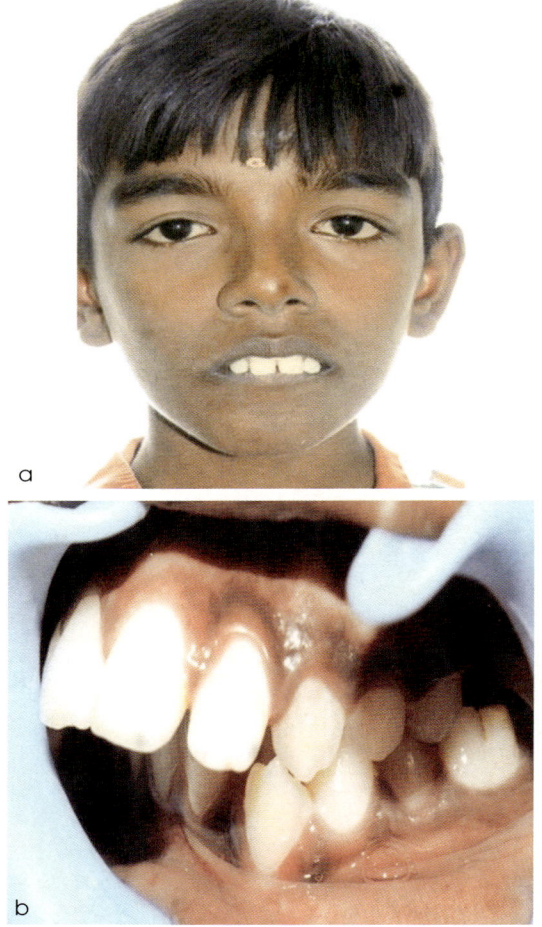

Fig. 18.22: (a) Extraoral photo—front view; (b) Intraoral photo

- *According to functional classification* (Table 18.1):
  a. True deep bite
  b. Pseudo deep bite
- *Depending on the extent of deep bite:*
  a. Incomplete overbite
  b. Complete overbite
- *According to dentition:*
  a. Primary dentition deep bite
  b. Mixed dentition deep bite
  c. Permanent dentition deep bite

Deep bite is again subclassified into mild, moderate and severe deep bite (Fig. 18.23).

Dental Deep Bite

Dental deep bite occurs due to overeruption of anterior or infraocclusion of molars. The result may be labial version of the upper incisors and impingement of the lowers into the palatal mucosa.

Table 18.1: True and Pseudo deep overbite	
True deep overbite	*Pseudo deep overbite*
It is caused by infraocclusion of molars	It is caused by overeruption of the anterior but with normal eruption of posterior segment teeth
It is seen in Class II division 2 malocclusion	It is seen in Class II division 1 malocclusion
There is a large interocclusal clearance and flat curve of Spee	These patients exhibit an excessive curve of Spee. The interocclusal clearance is usually normal or small as the molars are fully erupted.
Treatment in the mixed dentition period requires the elimination of environmental factors that are inhibiting eruption of the posterior teeth. It is ideal for functional appliance	Incisors cannot be intruded effectively using functional methods during mixed dentition
Extrusive mechanics of molars possible	All possible intrusive mechanics on the incisor teeth with fixed appliances are usually indicated. Extrusion of molars is possible only to a limited extent.

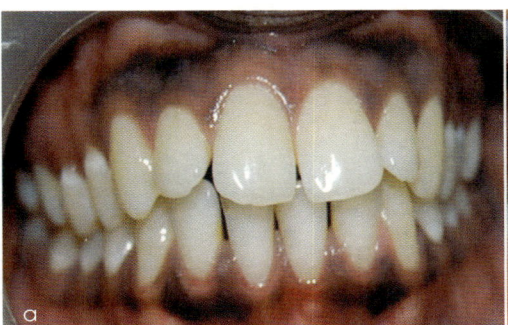 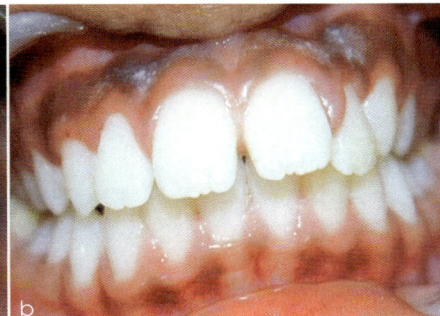 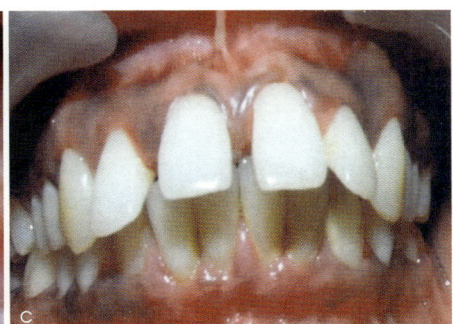

Fig. 18.23a to c: Mild, moderate and severe deep bite

Complex (Skeletal) Deep Bite

A skeletal type of overbite may be due either to mal relationship of alveolar bones and/or underlying mandibular or maxillary bones or to an overgrowth or undergrowth of one or more alveolar segments. The diminished anterior vertical height of the face is also an important criterion for diagnosis of skeletal deep bite.

Incomplete and Complete Deep Bite

Incomplete overbite is an incisor relationship in which the lower incisors fail to occlude with either the upper incisors or the mucosa of the palate when the teeth are occluded.

Complete overbite on the other hand is a relationship in which the lower incisors contact the palatal surface of the upper incisors or the palatal tissue when the teeth are in centric occlusion. This kind of deep bite often results in trauma of the mucosa palatal to the maxillary incisors.

Etiology of Deep Bite

- *Heredity*

- *Skeletal:*
  a. An overgrowth or undergrowth of one or more alveolar segments.
  b. An excess of growth of the ramus and posterior cranial base permits the mandible to rotate upward. Thus, long ramus and short body with decreased gonial angle is characteristic feature.
  c. Convergent upper and lower jaw bases.
  d. Horizontal growth pattern or forward rotation or anticlockwise rotation of the lower jaw.
  e. The four planes of the face—infraorbital, palatal, occlusal and mandibular as seen from lateral roentgenograms—are horizontal and nearly parallel to each other.
- *Dental:*
  a. Loss of mesial tipping of posterior teeth.
  b. Early loss of teeth and lingual collapse of the anterior.
  c. Overeruption of the incisor teeth, infraocclusion of the buccal segment or a combination of both.
  d. Overbite may be caused or accentuated by an aberration in the tooth morphology.
  e. Periodontal disease: Bite may deepen, if the posterior teeth drift mesially during the

pathological migration and worsen the existing condition.

f. When the teeth are reduced in size and number, the dental arches oppose less resistance against mandibular closure.

- *Muscular:* When the posterior vertical chain of muscles is strong and anteriorly positioned, a greater depressive action is transmitted to the dentition.
- *Habits:*
    a. Lateral tongue thrust swallow
    b. Finger sucking
    c. Lip sucking

Features and Effects of Deep Overbite

Extraoral Features

- Brachycephalic and europroscopic face
- Straight to mild convex profile
- Short anterior facial height
- Diminished anterior lower face height
- The lips are thin and with an excess of lip height relative to face height. This gives a curled appearance of the lips
- Deep mentolabial sulcus
- Mandibular deficiency characterized by long mandibular ramus and short body, square gonial angle, flat mandibular plane, prominent zygoma and prominent chin.

Intraoral Features

- May involve a group of teeth or whole dentition
- In skeletal deep bite, the patient may exhibit gummy smile, if there is clockwise rotation of maxilla
- The palatal vault is flat. A crowding of lower incisors may be present as a result of the deep bite. Deep curve of Spee in the lower arch or a reverse curve of Spee in the maxillary dentition.
- Occlusal functions become impaired.

Treatment Modalities in Growing and Non-Growing Patients

- *Natural bite opener:* After the first molar erupts into the oral cavity, the deep bite is reduced and bite opens.
- *In mixed dentition:* Orthodontic trainer
- *Removable appliance:* Upper Hawley's appliance with deep bite. This appliance should be passive in the beginning. This appliance works by supraeruption of posterior. The bite opening takes 3 to 4 months. After supraeruption, the bite opens up and the anterior part of anterior bite plane should be completely trimmed and then the labial bow should be activated.

- *Fixed appliance*
- *Skeletal deep bite in mixed dentition and early permanent dentition:* Activator, bionator, twin block appliance and fixed functional appliance.
- *Skeletal deep bite in permanent dentition:* Pre-orthodontic treatment with fixed appliance for aligning, leveling correction of rotation, orthognathic surgery and postsurgical orthodontic completion.

MIDLINE DIASTEMA

It is defined as space greater than 0.6 mm between the proximal surfaces of adjacent teeth (Fig. 18.24a–d).

The teeth on either side of a space are called "*dents du Bonheur*" or lucky teeth in France. True midline

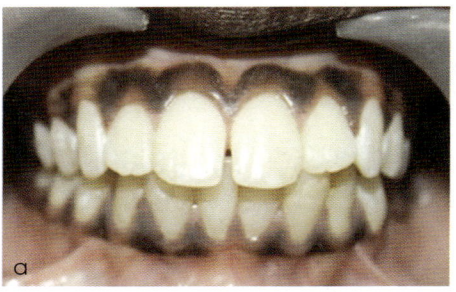

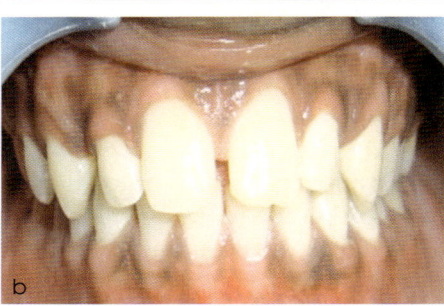

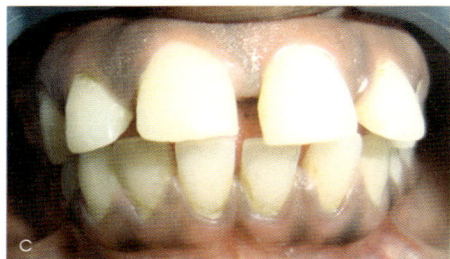

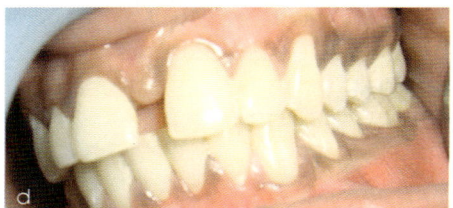

Fig. 18.24: Midline diastema: (a) 1 mm; (b) 2 mm; (c) Associated with localized spacing; (d) With 6 mm spacing

diastema is defined as one without periodontal/periapical involvement and with the presence of all anterior teeth in the arch.

Different Methods of Correction

- *Ugly duckling stage:* The space can be a normal growth characteristic during the primary and mixed dentition and generally is closed by the time the maxillary canines erupt. It is a self-correcting anomaly during the transition stage. It does not require any orthodontic therapy.
- Fixed appliances incorporating springs or elastics bring about the most rapid correction of midline diastema.
- Elastic thread or elastic chain can be used between the two central incisors for the same purposes.
- An alternative is to stretch a closed coil spring between the two central incisors.
- *Magnets:* Muller (1984) suggested midline diastema closure with small SmCo magnets. He recommended magnet size of 5 mm, 3 mm and 1 mm. For better control of tooth movement, a mesial bevel is given for both magnets. Attractive mode of magnets should be fixed to the labial surface of central incisors by indirect bonding (Fig. 18.25).
- *Removable appliances:* Upper Hawley's appliance with finger springs (Fig. 18.26) or split labial bow.
- M-spring (Fig. 18.27)

Etiology of Midline Diastema

- Normal developing dentition:
  a. Ugly duckling stage
  b. Imperfect fusion of midline of premaxilla: A "V" shaped or "W" shaped osseous septum may be associated with this condition.
  c. Ethinic and familial
- Tooth material deficiency:
  a. Microdontia

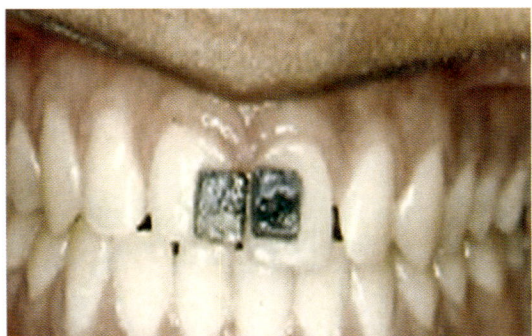

Fig. 18.25: Midline diastema closure with attractive pole of magnets

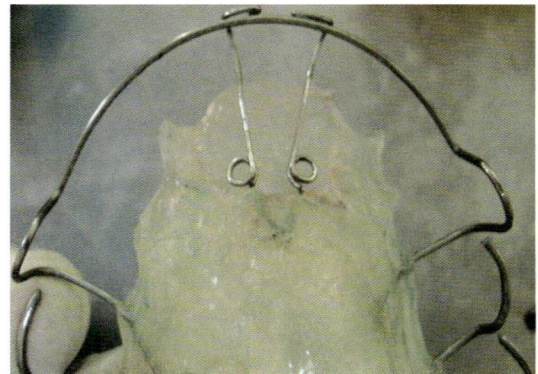

Fig. 18.26: Midline diastema closure with finger spring

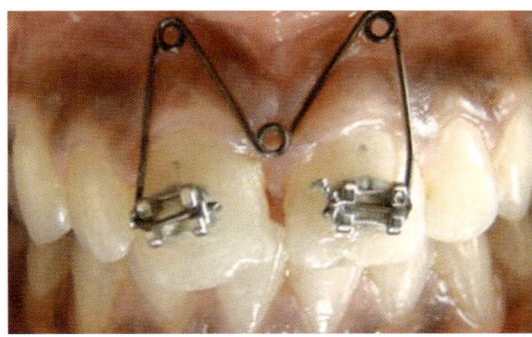

Fig. 18.27: M-spring

  b. Macrodontia
  c. Missing lateral peg-shaped laterals
  d. Extracted teeth
- Abnormal frenal attachment: 70% cases with a midline diastema associated with a large fleshy frenum attached to the incisive papilla. Collagenous fibers of a large frenum disrupt the normal transseptal fiber system between upper central incisors.
- Presence of supernumerary
- Abnormal pressure habits like thumb-sucking and tongue-thrusting
- Heredity
- Pathological migration of upper anterior
- Any radicular cyst in relation to lateral incisors

Diagnostic Feature for Midline Diastema

1. History
2. Clinical examination
3. Intraoral radiograph to check for any pathological lesions like midline cyst, odontomes, supernumerary tooth and radicular cyst. Radiologically, a 'V' shaped crestal notch between upper incisors.
4. Blanching in the region of the frenum can occur when tension is applied by lifting the upper lip.

Treatment of Midline Diastema

- *Diastema due to ugly duckling stage:* No treatment is required. It is self-correcting anomaly. During this transition period, the space gets closed spontaneously as the canine erupts into the oral cavity.
- *Diastema due to imperfect fusion at the midline:* Excision of included interdental tissue between the incisors. A flap is raised interdentally and fissure bur inserted gently into the cleft. With the bur, the included tissues are removed and flap sutured. An orthodontic appliance is given to close the midline during the healing process.
- *Iatrogenic cause:* Midline diastema can occur when certain therapeutic procedures are undertaken. The appearance of midline diastema is an important prognostic signs.

    During rapid maxillary expansion, it indicates the opening of intermaxillary suture at the rate of 0.5 mm to 1 mm/day, 1 mm or more of expansion is obtained in two to three weeks. A space is created at the mid-palatal suture which is filled initially by tissue fluid and hemorrhage.
- *Diastema due to microdontia and macrognathia:* It can be treated by orthodontic means or Jacket crown or composite build up.
- *Diastema due to missing teeth/extracted teeth:* Space can be consolidated and replaced with implant or bridge (Fig. 18.28).
- *High frenal attachment:* Frenectomy is done by laser treatment. Mild midline diastema is closed before frenectomy. Large midline diastema partially closed before frenectomy and completely closed after surgery. Delay in orthodontic treatment after surgery results in scar formation.
- Removable Hawley's appliance using split labial bow or finger springs.

Relapse

The relapse tendency following orthodontic therapy for midline diastema closure is more about 84%. In order to minimize the relapse , the patients need bonded retainer following transeptal fibrotomy, frenectomy and corticotomy in the midline as adjunct therapy.

Treatment of Congenitally Missing Lateral Incisors

The treatment of congenitally missing maxillary lateral incisors is very challenging and complex, requiring very careful case selection, treatment planning, and often the coordinated interdisciplinary efforts of the orthodontist, periodontist or oral surgeon, and restorative dentist. It is imperative that there is continuous communication among team members.

The two categories of treatment options include space closure with canine substitution and space opening with prosthetic replacement, each has its own separate criteria for tooth placement, and many times the final esthetics are determined by the initial evaluations and recommendations made by the orthodontist. The orthodontist is responsible for assessing facial types, growth patterns, tooth positions, occlusal schemes, but more importantly the orthodontist is responsible for putting the teeth in a position where the surgeon and the restorative dentist can execute a conservative and esthetic restoration.

At the current time, the two most commonly recommended ways to manage congenitally missing laterals are canine substitution and a single-tooth implant. The other prosthetic alternatives that include the resin-bonded, fixed partial denture, the conventional fixed partial denture, and removable partial denture can also be used with a high degree of success, if used in the correct situation (Fig. 18.29a to c).

In the realm of contemporary dentistry, implants are probably the most favored treatment modality for replacing missing anterior teeth. The implant approach in the anterior region, however, is a delicate situation, which can be challenging esthetically in the long term. In this scenario, it is necessary to work as a team in order to develop the ideal conditions before and after implant placement. In today's dentistry, where there is

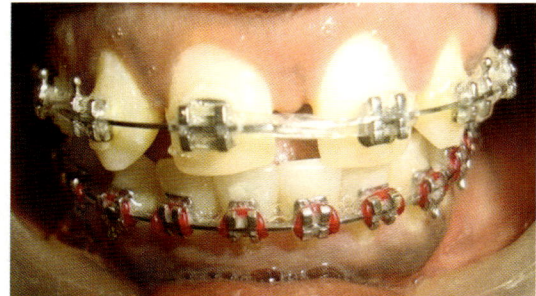

Fig. 18.28: Midline diastema closure with elastic chain in case of congenital missing lateral incisors

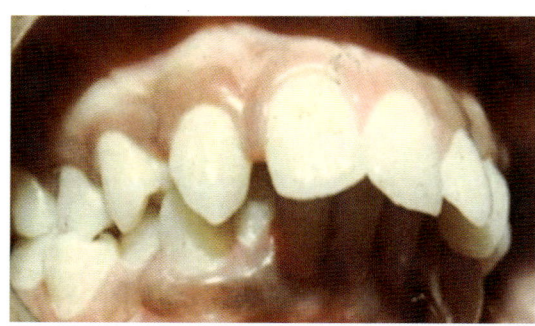

Fig. 18.29a: A case of congenitally missing laterals

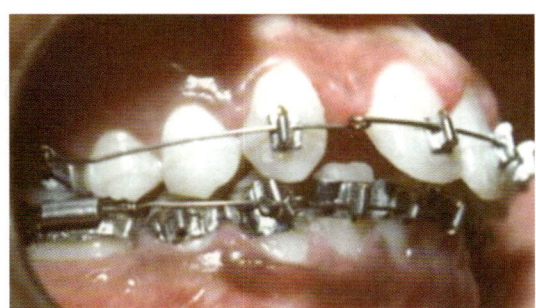

Fig. 18.29b: Fixed appliance for replacement of laterals

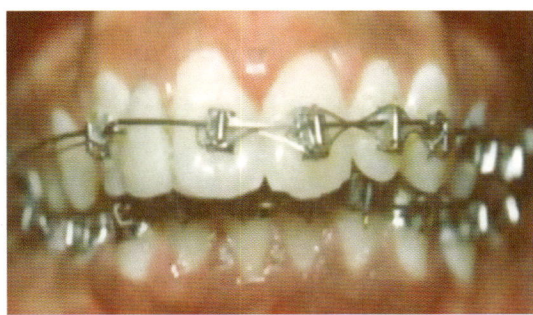

Fig. 18.29c: Semipermanent bonded replacement after fixed appliance correction

such a high degree of emphasis placed on esthetics, it is not possible for a dentist to work alone, especially when dealing with challenging situations like the congenitally missing lateral incisor.

CROWDING

Lower incisor crowding is the most common malocclusion condition.

- Dental crowding can be defined as a discrepancy between tooth size and jaw size that results in malalignment of the tooth row.
- Arch length is a measurement of space available in the dental arch for alignment of teeth.
- Arch length discrepancy is a difference between the space available in the dental arch and space required to align the teeth.

Clinical Features

- Crowding is present unilaterally or bilaterally
- Crowding is localized or generalized
- Poor oral hygiene due to inaccessibility of certain tooth surfaces in crowded areas to toothbrush.
- Halitosis
- Gingivitis and periodontitis may occur.

Planning space requirements: Most malocclusions require space to move teeth to more ideal positions

Correction of crowding:
- It requires space.
- Rule of thumb is that for every mm of crowding, 1 mm of arch length is required.

Rotations
- Rotated anterior teeth occupy lesser arch length.
- It is calculated by subtracting the distance between the proximal surfaces of adjacent teeth from total mesiodistal width of rotated teeth.

Leveling curve of Spee
- In skeletal malocclusion, there is increased curve of Spee.
- Some provision should be made to provide space for leveling.

Types of Crowding

Crowding is classified into (Fig. 18.30a–e):
1. *Depending on the amount of space deficiency*
   - Mild
   - Moderate
   - Severe crowding

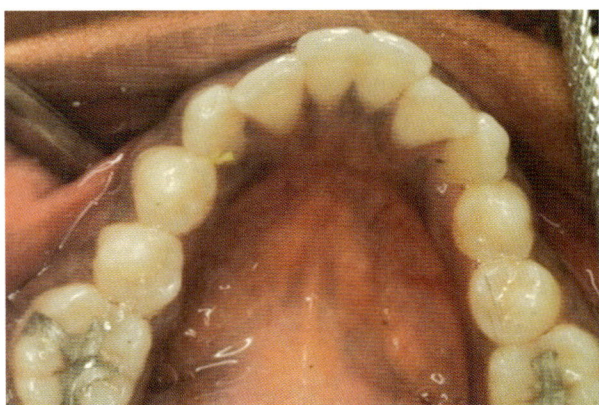

Fig. 18.30a: Mild crowding

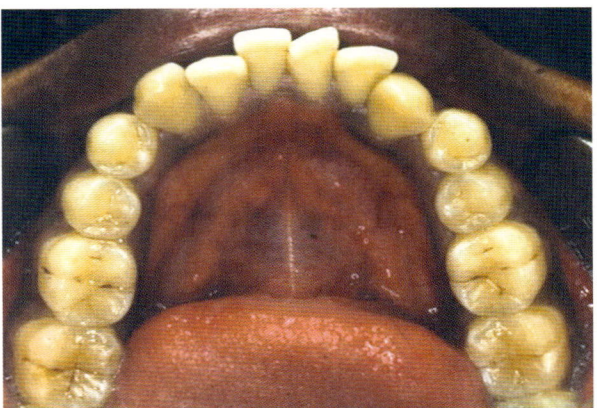

Fig. 18.30b: Moderate crowding

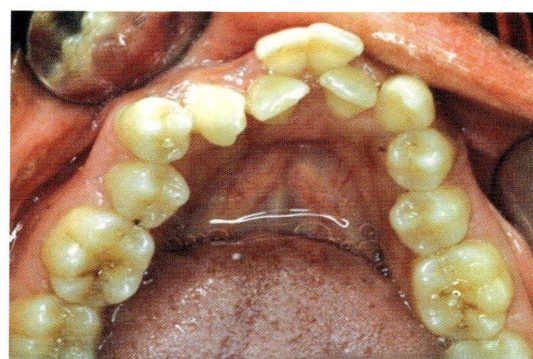

Fig. 18.30c: Severe crowding

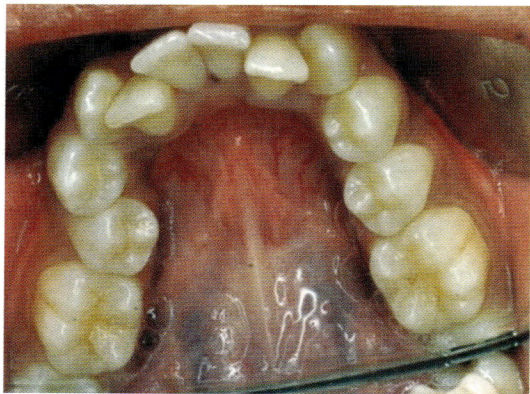

Fig. 18.30d: Posterior and anterior crowding

2. *According to Proffit*
   - *If TSALD is less than 5 mm:* This is mild crowding and it is a non-extraction case.
   - *If TSALD is more than 5 mm but less than 8 mm:* It is moderate crowding and it is a borderline case.
   - *If TSALD is more than 8 mm:* This is severe crowding.
3. *According to etiology of crowding:* It can be primary crowding, secondary crowding and tertiary crowding.
   a. *Primary crowding:* It is hereditary crowding and is determined genetically. It occurs due to disproportion in tooth size and jaw bases.
   b. *Secondary crowding:* It is an acquired crowding which occurs due to mesial drift of posterior permanent teeth due to premature loss of primary teeth in buccal segments and leading loss of arch length and thus deviated eruption or impaction of teeth.
   c. *Tertiary crowding:* It occurs due to natural phenomenon, especially jaws, at around 18–25 years age especially the terminal AP growth of mandible. It thrusts the mandible forward and upward lingual to the upper incisors. It leads to

either spacing in the upper teeth or crowding in lower incisors due to their lingual shifting. A small force from erupting mandibular third molars is also considered to be a factor in this crowding.

4. *According to the inclination of teeth to their apical bases:* Crowding can be:
   - *Coronal crowding:* It is the irregularity of crowns of teeth, which may be due to abnormal axial inclinations and also lack of space.
   - *Apical crowding:* It is the crowding of roots in the bone. It is due to the mesial inclination of long axes of roots of teeth reducing the inter-radicular bone.
5. *Another way of classifying crowding based on location of crowding:*
   - Anterior crowding
   - Posterior crowding (Fig. 18.30e)
   - Sometimes, Both anterior and posterior crowding (Fig. 18.30d)

Etiology of Crowding

There are many causes of development of crowding:
1. *Heredity:* For example, crowding, spacing, congenitally missing tooth
2. *TSALD:* It is a discrepancy between tooth size and jaw size that results in malalignment of the tooth.
3. *Abnormal size or shape of teeth:* For example, macrodontia, micrognathia or combination leads to crowding. It is mainly genetically controlled.
4. Presence of supernumerary
5. Prolonged retention of primary tooth
6. Premature loss of primary tooth.
7. Caries of primary teeth.
8. *Abnormal pressure habits:* They lead to disturbance in the force equilibrium around the dental arches. Lower lip trap is one of the causes leading to lingual tilting of lower incisors and their crowding.
9. Improper growth of jaws.

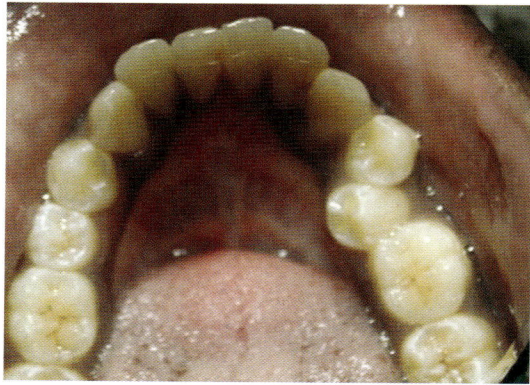

Fig. 18.30e: Posterior crowding

Treatment

Treatment of crowding is based on the diagnosis and model analysis.

Lower Anterior Crowding

- Serial extraction
- *Proximal reproximation:* The stripping technique involves three steps—reduction, recontouring and protection. With a micromotor and a high-speed handpiece, these three steps can be performed for one arch in one appointment. If the total amount of possible reduction in each quadrant is less than the amount of space needed, then another treatment must be chosen. The distal surface of first, the second and third molars should not be stripped, if possible to preserve anchorage.

  If crowding is moderate (2–6 mm), sequential slicing of posterior deciduous teeth can allow the spontaneous alignment of incisors, distal eruption of canines and premolars. The technique was proposed by Sheridan JJ in 1985.
- *Mandibular expansion:* The type of expansion produced can be arbitrarily divided into orthodontic expansion, passive expansion or orthopedic expansion.

- *Schwarz appliance* that incorporates one or more expansion screws is particularly effective in 6 to 9 years old age group. In case with manibular incisor crowding of 3 to 4 mm, a Schwarz appliance is indicated and the patient is instructed to activate the appliance once per week. About 1 mm of expansion is produced with every 5 turns and less than 1 mm of expansion occurs during each month of wear. The appliance is worn as an active appliance for 5 to 6 months. At the end of this time, a tendency toward a lingual crossbite is observed. Later, a lingual holding arch maintains the leeway space.
- *Lower incisor extraction:* If any one lateral incisor is placed completely out of arch, lateral incisor can be indicated for extraction.
- Dr HE Wilson is called the father of second molar extraction concepts. He observed that the posterior teeth could be distalized to relieve crowded anterior.
- *Active lingual arch* is indicated with loop mesial to lower molar for relieving one tooth which lingually placed.
- *Mandibular lip bumper:* The lip bumper can be used to gain an incredible amount of space in the lower arch, while maintaining a good control of the molars and incisors. It is an alternative for extraction therapy in mild to moderately crowded arches. It can gain and maintain arch length, width and perimeter.

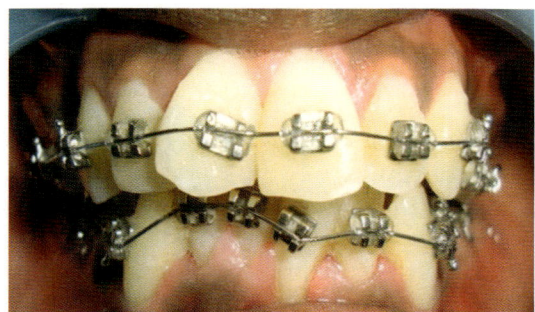

Fig. 18.31: Straight wire appliance with NiTi wire aligning archwire

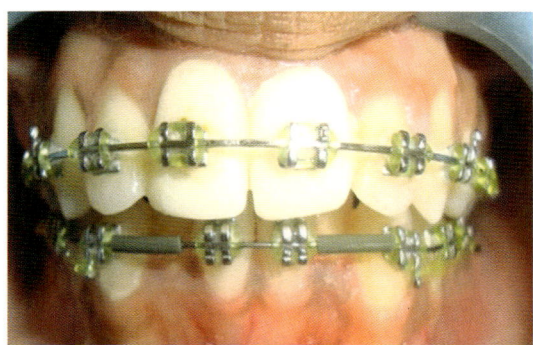

Fig.18.32: Straight wire appliance with open coil spring in the lower arch

Upper Arch Crowding

1. *In the mixed dentition*
   - 2 × 4 appliance with utility archwire
   - 2 × 6 appliance with aligning archwire
2. *In the permanent dentition*—Fixed appliance

Extraction: All first premolar extraction and fixed appliance (Figs 18.31 and 18.32).

Skeletal problems: Refer Surgical Orthodontics, Expansion Appliance and Funcional Appliance chapters.

BIBLIOGRAPHY

1. Olsen CB. Anterior crossbite correction in uncooperative or disabled children. Case reports. Aust Dent J 1996;41:304–309.
2. Deam JA. McDonald RE, Avery DR. Managing he developing occlusion. In: McDonald RE (ed). Dentistry for the child and adolescent. 7th ed London; Mosby, 2000:677–741.
3. Tse CS. Correction of single tooth anterior crossbite. J Clin Orthod 1997;31:188.
4. Justus R. Correction of Anterior open bite with spurs: Long term stability. World J Orthod. 2001;2:219–31.
5. Janson G, Crepaldi MV, de Freitas KM, de Freitas MR, Janson W. Evaluation of anterior open bite treatment with oclusal adjustment. Am J Orthod 2008 Jul;134(1):10-1.

PREVIOUS YEAR'S UNIVERSITY QUESTIONS

Essay

1. What are the benefits of the early treatment approach?
2. How do you manage the dental open bite problems orthodontically?
3. Define midline diastema. Discuss in detail about etiology, investigations and orthodontic management.
4. Write the differences between dental and skeletal open bite and discuss in detail the classification, etiology and orthodontic management.

Short Questions

1. Classification of crossbite
2. Crowding
3. Deep bite
4. Open bite
5. Tongue blade therapy

MCQs

1. *Secondary phase of treatment in midline diastema*:
   a. Elimination of habit
   b. Frenectomy
   c. Treatment of midline pathologies
   d. Active orthodontic therapy   **(Ans: d)**

2. *Split labial bow to treat midline diastema should extend up to:*
   a. Distal surface of canines on opposite sides
   b. Distal surface of lateral incisors on opposite sides
   c. Distal surface of central incisors on opposite sides
   d. Combination of the above   **(Ans: c)**

3. *The third phase of treatment of midline diastema includes:*
   a. Elimination of oral habits
   b. Removal of any midline pathologies
   c. Active orthodontic therapy
   d. Retaining the corrected midline diastema   **(Ans: d)**

4. *"M-spring" used in treatment of midline diastema is activated by:*
   a. Closing the three helicles of the spring
   b. Closing the two helicles of the spring
   c. Opening the three helicles of the spring
   d. Opening the two helicles of the spring   **(Ans: a)**

5. *Midline diastema needs:*
   a. Short-term retention
   b. No retention
   c. Long-term retention
   d. Any of the above   **(Ans: c)**

6. *Cephalometric analysis of anterior skeletal open bite reveals:*
   a. Downward and forward rotation of mandible
   b. Upward tipping of maxillary skeletal muscle
   c. Vertical maxillary increase
   d. All of the above   **(Ans: d)**

7. *Mild to moderate open bite can be treated by fixed orthodontics by using:*
   a. Class I elastics
   b. Class II elastics
   c. Class III elastics
   d. Box elastics   **(Ans: d)**

8. *Box elastics in treatment of open bite is:*
   a. Elastics stretched in upper anterior and lower anterior separately
   b. Stretched between upper and lower anteriors
   c. Stretched between upper and lower molars
   d. All of the above   **(Ans: b)**

9. *Posterior open bite is a condition characterized by lack of contact between posterior when:*
   a. Teeth are in centric occlusion
   b. Teeth are in centric relation
   c. Either of the above
   d. None of the above   **(Ans: a)**

10. *Fish mouth appearance is a characteristic feature of:*
    a. Anterior crossbite
    b. Anterior open bite
    c. Anterior deep bite
    d. All of the above   **(Ans: b)**

11. *Incomplete overbite is a condition characterized by:*
    a. Presence of overjet but not vertical overlap
    b. Confined to tooth and alveolar process
    c. More than 1 mm of space is seen between the incisors
    d. All of the above   **(Ans: a)**

12. *Cephalometric findings of deep bite is:*
    a. Increased interincisal angle
    b. Decreased interincisal angle
    c. Normal interincisal angle
    d. None of the above   **(Ans: a)**

13. *Cross-elastic is stretched from:*
    a. Palatal surface of maxillary posterior teeth to buccal surface of mandibular teeth
    b. Anterior teeth to posterior in the same arch
    c. Maxillary canine to mandibular molar
    d. Maxillary molar to mandibular canine   **(Ans: a)**

Cleft Lip and Palate

Chapter Outline

- Introduction
- Classification of cleft lip and palate
- Etiology of cleft lip and palate
- Embryological background
- Theories of cleft lip and palate

- Various problems
- Possible mechanism for formation of isolated cleft palate
- Management of cleft lip and palate
- Role of orthodontist in cleft lip and palate

INTRODUCTION

Cleft lip and palate is one of the most common congenital anomalies affecting humans in the craniofacial region. Cleft palate can be defined as "Breach in continuity of palate". Clefts of lip and palate can occur isolated or together in various combinations and/or along with other congenital deformities or syndromes.

The functional and esthetic problems associated with cleft lip and palate depend on the size of the cleft and whether it is unilateral or bilateral (Fig. 19.1).

It is managed by team work as shown in Fig. 19.2. It requires the expertise of various specialists at different milestones of life. Treatment of cleft lip and palate involves a multidisciplinary approach involving the following members from various specialties.

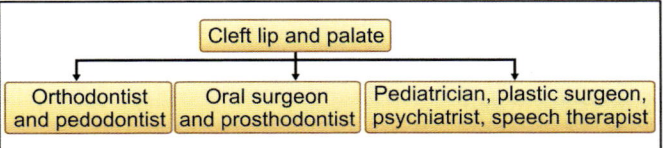

Fig. 19.2: Members of management team

Since the orthodontist is involved with the patient from immediately after birth till the permanent teeth have been brought into functional and esthetically acceptable position.

CLASSIFICATION OF CLEFT LIP AND PALATE

Davis and Ritchie Classification (1922)

They classified clefts based on their position in relation to the alveolar process.

Group I: Pre-alveolar clefts involve only the lips (Fig. 19.1):
- Unilateral
- Median
- Bilateral

Group II: Post-alveolar clefts that involve the soft palate only or clefts of soft and hard palate that extend up to the alveolar ridge, submucous clefts also included.

Group III: Alveolar clefts—complete clefts of palate, alveolar ridge and lip.

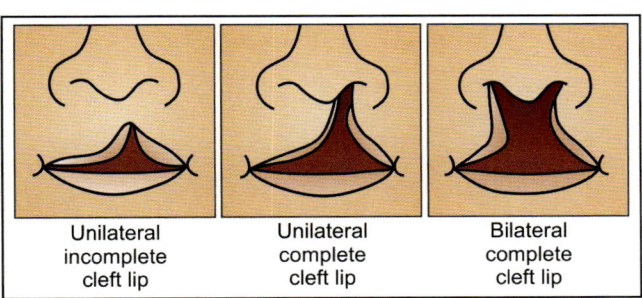

| Unilateral incomplete cleft lip | Unilateral complete cleft lip | Bilateral complete cleft lip |

Fig. 19.1: Extension of cleft lip

- Unilateral
- Median
- Bilateral

Veau's Classification (1931)

It is classified into four groups (Fig. 19.3):

Group I: Cleft of soft palate only.

Group II: Cleft of hard and soft palates extending no further than the incisive foramen, thus involving the secondary palate alone.

Group III: Complete unilateral cleft of soft and hard palates, lip and alveolar ridge.

Group IV: Complete bilateral cleft of soft and hard palates, lip and alveolar ridge on both sides.

Fogh Andersen (1942)

It is classified into three groups:

Group I
- Clefts of lip only
- Single (unilateral or median)
- Double (bilateral)

Group II
- Clefts of lip and palate
- Single (unilateral or median)
- Double (bilateral)

Group III: Clefts of the palate extending up to the incisive foramen.

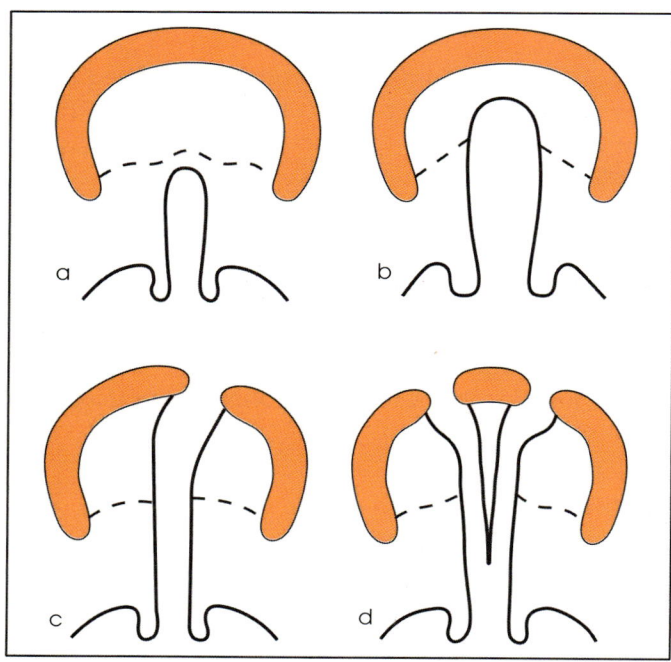

Fig. 19.3: Veau's classification

Kernahan's Striped 'Y' Classification (Fig. 19.4)

In this classification, the incisive foramen is taken as the reference point. The arms of 'Y' logo are arch divided into three sections, representing the lip, the alveolus and the hard palate as far back as the incisive foramen. The stem of the 'Y' is also divided into three parts, representing varying degrees of clefting of the hard and soft palates.

The classification uses a stripped 'Y' having numbered blocks to represent a specific area of the oral cavity.

- Blocks 1 and 4—lip
- Blocks 2 and 5—alveolus
- Blocks 3 and 6—hard palate anterior to the incisive foramen
- Blocks 7 and 8—hard palate posterior to incisive foramen
- Block 9—soft palate

The boxes are shaded in areas where the cleft has occurred.

Millard's Classification (1977) (Fig. 19.5)

It is a modification of Kernahan's 'Y' classification. He added two triangles inverted over one another which represent the nose and the upright triangles representing the nasal floor. This increased the number of boxes to 11 as:

- Blocks 1 and 5—nasal floor
- Blocks 2 and 6—lip
- Blocks 3 and 7—alveolus
- Blocks 4 and 8—hard palate anterior to incisive foramen
- Blocks 9 and 10—hard palate posterior to the incisive foramen
- Block 11—soft palate

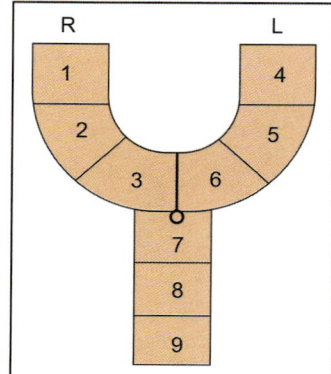

Fig. 19.4: Kernahan's striped Y classification

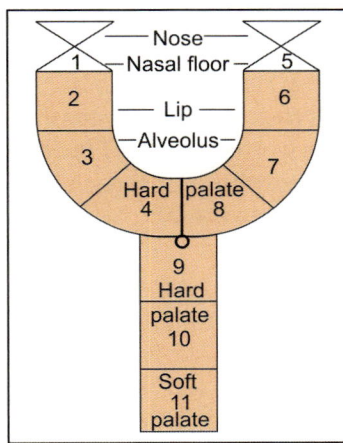

Fig. 19.5: Millard's classification

Lashal Classification

This classification was presented by Okreins in 1987. The term LASHAL is an anatomic paraphrase of lip, alveolus and palate. The classification is based on the fact that clefts of lip (L), alveolus (A) and hard palate (H) occur bilaterally and of soft palate (S) is usually unilateral. Areas involved in the cleft are denoted by specifically indicating the alphabet standing for it.

L: Lip
A: Alveolus
H: Hard palate
S: Soft palate
H: Hard palate
A: Alveolus
L: Lip

LAH-S-HAL

LAH represents the right lip, alveolus and hard palate LAHS-L stands for cleft of right lip, alveolus, hard palate and soft palate together with left cleft lip.

American Cleft Palate Association's Classification (1962)

Cleft Lip

a. Unilateral—right, left, extent in thirds
b. Bilateral—right, left, extent in thirds
c. Median—extend in thirds
d. Prolabium—small, medium, large
e. Congenital scar—right, left, medium, extent in thirds

Clefts of Alveolar Process

a. Unilateral—right, left, extent in thirds
b. Bilateral—right, left, extent in thirds
c. Median—extend in thirds, submucous right, left, median.

Cleft of Prepalate

Any combination of foregoing type:
a. Prepalate protrusion
b. Prepalate rotation
c. Prepalate arrest (median cleft)

Clefts of Palate

- *Cleft of soft palate:*
  a. Extent—posteroanterior in thirds.
  b. Width (maximum in mm)
  c. Palatal shortness—none, slight, moderate, marked.
  c. Submucous cleft—extent in thirds
- *Cleft of the hard palate:*
  a. Extent—posteroanterior in thirds
  b. Width (maximum in mm)
  c. Vomer attachment—right, left, absent
  d. Submucous cleft—extent in thirds
- Cleft of hard and soft palate
- Clefts of prepalate and palate

International Confederation for Plastic and Reconstructive Surgery Classification (1968)

Group I: Cleft of anterior primary palate
- Lip—right, left, both
- Alveolus—right, left, both.

Group II: Clefts of anterior and posterior palate
- Lip—right, left, both
- Alveolus—right, left, both
- Hard palate—right, left, both

Group III: Clefts of posterior secondary palate
- Hard palate—right, left
- Soft palate—median

Goslon Yardstick for UCLP (Mars et al. 1987)

The Goslon (Great Ormond Street, London and Oslo) Yardstick is a clinical tool that allows categorization of the dental relationships in the late mixed and/or early permanent dentition stage into five categories.

It was designed to categorize malocclusions in patients with unilateral clefts of lip and palate in a way that would represent the severity of the malocclusion and the difficulty of correcting it.

Group 1: Excellent growth (overjet more than 2 mm)

Group 2: Good growth (overjet less than 2 mm) requiring simple or no orthodontic treatment

Group 3: Adequate growth (edge-to-edge bite) requiring complex orthodontic treatment to correct the malocclusion.

Group 4: Poor growth (reverse overjet more than 2 mm) requiring orthognathic surgery.

Bauru Yardstick for BCLP (Ozawa et al. 2005)

Score 1 (excellent result)

Score 2 (good result) represents the most favorable dental arch relationships. The patients in this category would be treated by orthodontic treatment alone.

Score 3: Patients scoring 3 usually have an edge-to-edge apical base relationship and require more complex orthodontic treatment to correct the malocclusion.

Score 4 (poor result) represents the patients who require complex orthodontic treatment, probably in combination with orthognathic surgery.

A very poor dental arch relationship is scored as 5 which represents the patients who require orthognathic surgery.

ETIOLOGY OF CLEFT LIP AND PALATE

Cleft cases are divided into 2 forms:

1. Syndromic clefts which are associated with other congenital disorders.
2. Nonsyndromic clefts which are not associated with other congenital health disorders.

Syndromic Cleft

Associated Syndrome

Cleft lip may be associated with the following syndromes:

- Down syndrome (Fig. 19.6)
- Trisomy 21
- Wardenburg's syndrome: Abnormalities of pigmentation of hair, iris and skin, deafness
- Van der Woude syndrome
- Orofacial digital syndrome: Median cleft lip associated with post-axial hexadactyly and bilateral accessory toes are found only in Indians.

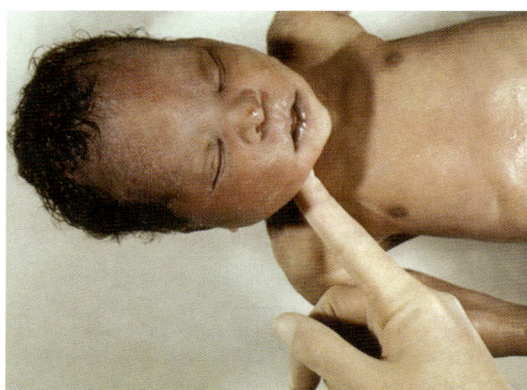

Fig. 19.6: Down syndrome newborn

- Treacher Collins syndrome: Hypoplastic zygoma, micrognathia, external and middle ear defects (Fig. 19.7).
- Pierre Robin syndrome: Micrognathia, glossoptosis with respiratory obstruction (Fig. 19.8)
- Klippel-Feil syndrome: Short neck with an abnormal or missing cervical vertebra.

Congenital

Congenital refers to an anomaly which must be present at birth. It can either be hereditary, genetically determined or induced (environmental teratogens).

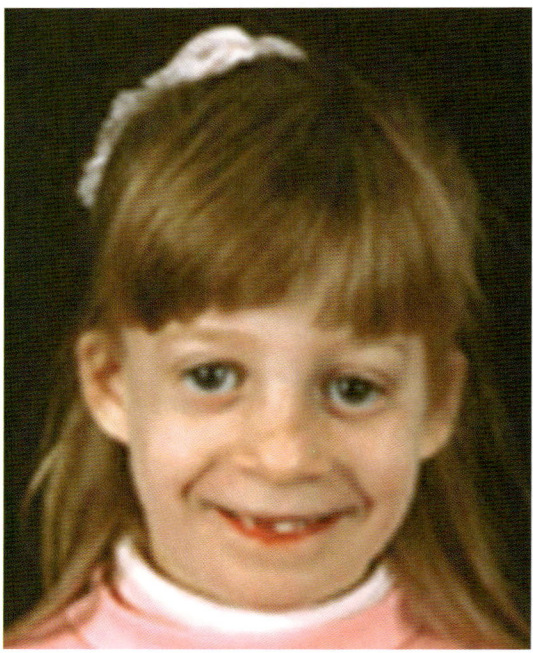

Fig. 19.7: Treacher Collins syndrome

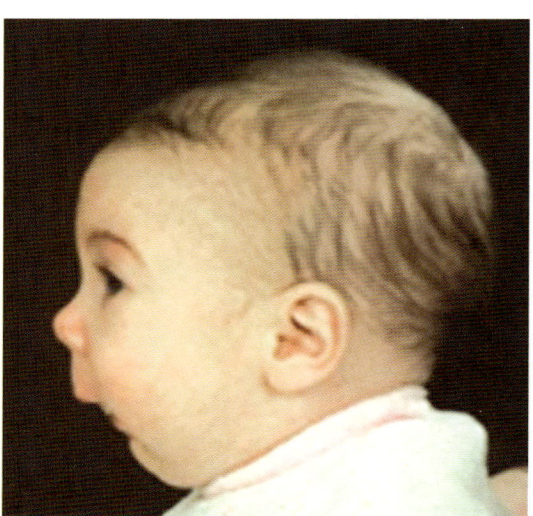

Fig. 19.8: Pierre Robin syndrome

Hereditary anomalies may or may not be present at birth and may appear in due course of time.

Congenital anomalies may be brought about by the following agents/teratogens:

Infections: Infections like rubella, influenza, toxoplasmosis, etc. to the mother during the first 3 months of pregnancy may cause formation of the cleft to the fetus.

Drugs: Cases have been reported in which acute hypoxia produced by carbon monoxide or morphine overdose was followed by a birth of a malformed child. Aminopterin, an antifolate drug, is occasionally used as an abortifacient. Surviving fetuses of such abortion attempts were grossly malformed. All cytotoxic anticancer drugs, such as alkylating agents, have been blamed for producing clefts. Cortisone is a suspected teratogen.

An alcoholic mother may give birth to a child with fetal alcoholic syndrome which may be associated with cleft plalate. Thalidomide may have a similar effect.

Radiation: Today, radiations such as X-rays, gamma rays, etc. are used widely in medicine for diagnosis and treatment. Theses are ionizing radiation and are capable of producing either somatic or genetic effects. Somatic effects are those which become manifested in the exposed individual. Genetic effects are those which are expressed in individual's descendents. The genetic effects include anomalies such as cleft palate, cleft lip, microcephaly and neonatal death. These radiation anomalies are due to the irradiation of the embryo/fetus during pregnancy.

Diet: Dietary deficiency of riboflavin, folic acid and hypervitaminosis A, may act as environmental teratogens.

Cigarette smoking: 30% increase in cleft lip and palate and 20% increase in cleft palate is observed due to smoking during pregnancy.

Parental age: Shaw et al presented evidence that women above the age of 35 had a doubled risk of having a child with CLCP and above 39 had a tripled risk of CLCP.

Consanguineous marriages: Marriages amongst the same community may lead to increased risk of CLCP in child.

EMBRYOLOGICAL BACKGROUND

The fusion of various embryonic processes around the stomodeum (the primitive oral cavity) leads to the formation of the nasomaxillary complex.

The mesoderm covering the forebrain proliferates and descends towards stomodeum. This process is called frontonasal process. As the nasal pits develop, the frontonasal process gets divided into the medial nasal process and two nasal processes.

The first branchial arch, called the mandibular arch, is placed lateral to the developing stomodeum. From its dorsal aspect, it gives rise to the maxillary process. The maxillary processes join the lateral and the medial nasal processes to form the future upper lip and maxilla.

THEORIES OF CLEFT LIP AND PALATE

Classical theory of His (1974): The maxillary processes give rise to the palatal shelves. The palatal shelves grow medially and as the developing tongue descends downward, the palatal shelves fuse with the frontonasal process at the end of 6th and 7th week of the intrauterine life to form the palate. Failure of fusion results in complete or incomplete cleft of lip, alveolus and palate.

The mandibular process gives rise to the lower lip and jaw. Defective fusion or incomplete fusion between the various processes leads to different types of cleft formations.

Mesodermal reinforcement theory—Victor Veau (1936): It suggests that the upper lip and jaw are formed by the penetration of the mesoderm between the layers of a pre-existing epithelial membrane. As the mesoderm penetrates, it gives rise to the surface swellings as median and lateral nasal processes. A congenital cleft of lip or palate is due to failure of penetration of mesoderm and subsequent breakdown of the epithelial membrane.

Possible Mechanism for Formation of Isolated Cleft Palate

- Agenesis or hypoplasia of the tissues involved.
- Palatal tissues may be obstructed from moving dorsal to the tongue by lack of intrinsic or extrinsic motivational force or by physical obstruction.
- Poor adherence of the medial edge epithelium of the palatal process to each other or a delay in transposition until fusion capacity is lost.
- Persistence of midline seam due to a failure of cellular degeneration might result in post-fusion breakdown in the midline.
- Lack of mesenchymal growth in the midline region may result in submucous cleft formation.

VARIOUS PROBLEMS

- Feeding problem
- Respiratory tract infection

- Airway obstruction
- Speech problems later
- Dental problems like malformed teeth, malocclusion and partial anodontia
- Middle ear infection
- Deficiency in maxillary and mandibular bone
- Eustachian tube malfunction and deafness

FEEDING PROBLEMS

The feeding problems vary with the degree of cleft.

Cleft lip: The infant takes a substantial part of the areola as well as the nipple into its mouth, sucking is not greatly hampered by cleft lip only.

Cleft palate with cleft lip: The infant has difficulty in obtaining adequate sucking and fluid regurgitates into the nasal cavity and nasopharynx and oozes out from the external nostrils. Hence, early placement of obturator is required (Fig. 19.9).

The cleft babies are usually brought to the outpatient department with a complaint of inability to suck mother's milk and nasal regurgitation of milk. Feeding the child is a major problem in this patient. Palate function is necessary for swallowing.

Feeding Advice

Babies with cleft palate are unable to suck mother's milk because intraoral negative pressure is not possible. Breastfeeding is allowed. It will take extra time and patience. Be open for alternatives, if this is not providing adequate nutrition for infant. Expressed mother's milk (manually or by breast pump) is given with the help of a spoon. Spoon feeding is easily learnt by the parents and maintaining hygiene is much easier. Second problem in these babies is nasal regurgitation of milk. This problem can be solved by raising the head end of

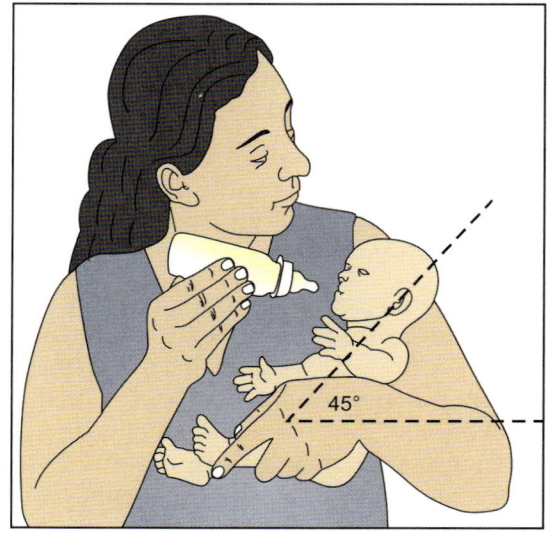

Fig. 19.10: Feeding a baby with cleft palate or cleft lip

the baby while feeding by approximately 45° (Fig. 19.10).

Third problem is of excessive air swallowing while feeding. For this, frequent burping is done during feeding (Fig. 19.11).

Burp your baby frequently. This helps expel swallowed air while the baby is upright. Otherwise the baby may spit-up while lying down, possibly resulting in bacteria entering the middle ear. Hold your baby sitting up, in your lap, facing you. Support the chest with one hand; use the other hand to pat the baby's back gently. If your baby seems fussy while feeding, stop the session, burp your baby, and then begin feeding again. Try burping your baby every 2 to 3 ounces when you bottle-feed. If your baby does not burp after a few minutes, try feeding again. Always burp when feeding time is over.

Cleft babies drool more often than normal, for obvious reasons. It is highly recommended to have an adequate supply of bibs available. One bib has about an hour before becoming thoroughly saturated in drool. The extra saliva can cause your baby to occasionally

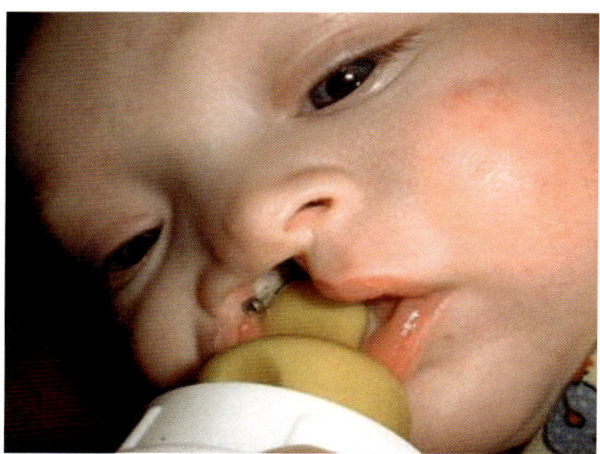

Fig. 19.9: Cleft palate with cleft lip

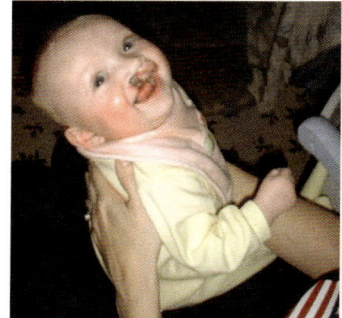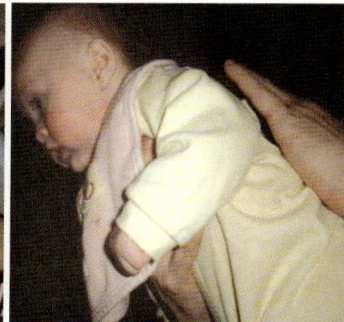

Fig. 19.11: Burping

cough or gag. This is usually nothing to worry about as long as your baby seems fine and shows no signs of a cold or flu and does not run a high fever. Keep your baby in an upright position for 10 to 15 minutes after feeding to help prevent the milk from coming back up. But do not worry, if your baby spits up a few times. It is probably more unpleasant for you than it is for your baby (Fig. 19.12).

Nipples

There are many types of bottles and nipples that can assist with feeding and infant with cleft palate (Fig. 19.13).

Feeding bottles:
- It is recommended by Pashyan and McNab to cross cut the bottle nipple. This enlarged cut provides improved ejection of milk into infant's mouth without any effort.
- Shirley (1971) devised a new technique—football pump system.
- When the nipple is pressed, the milk will go to the mouth. When the pressure is released over the nipple, the airway through the nipple's hole is blocked automatically and the milk will come to the nipple.
- Some authors recommend the use of a long spoon.

Nuk nipple: This nipple can be placed on regular bottles or on bottles with disposable bags. The hole can be made larger by making a criss-cross cut in the middle (Fig. 19.13).

Haberman feeder: This is a specially designed bottle system with a valve to help control the air the baby drinks and to prevent milk from going back into the bottle (Fig. 19.14).

Mead Johnson nurser: This is a soft, plastic bottle that is easy to squeeze and has a large crosscut nipple (Fig. 19.15).

Syringe

These may be used in hospitals following cleft surgery and may also be used at home. Typically, a soft rubber tube is attached on the end of the syringe, which is then placed in the infant's mouth. In some cases, supplements may be added to breast milk or formula to help infant meet his/her calorie need.

Respiratory Tract Infections

Frequent regurgitation of fluids and food into nasal cavity and nasopharynx often results in infection. This infection may spread to the other parts of the respiratory tract. Aspiration of ingested materials into lungs may be added problems.

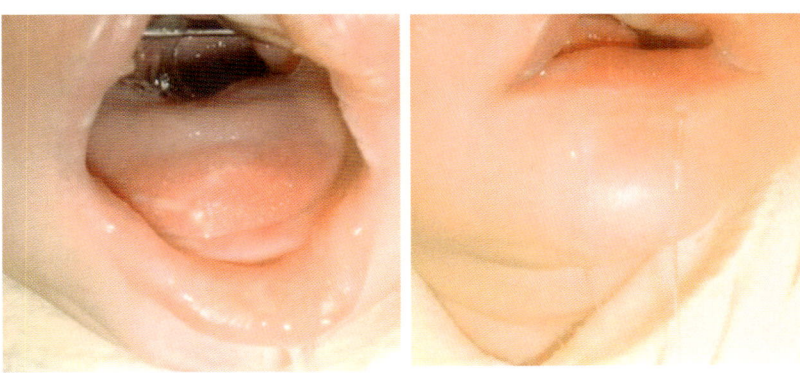

Fig. 19.12: Drooling

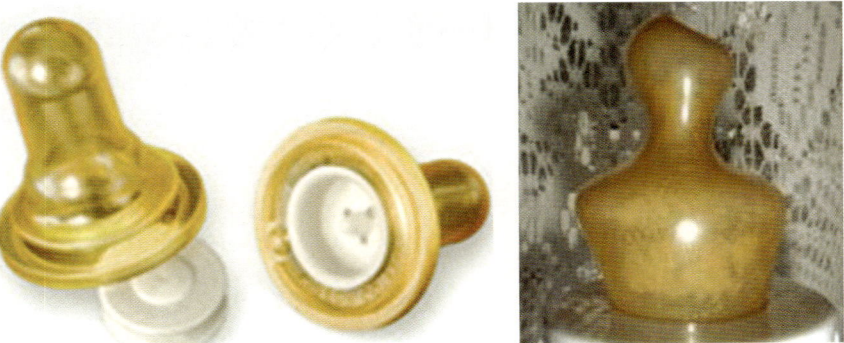

Fig. 19.13: Nipples

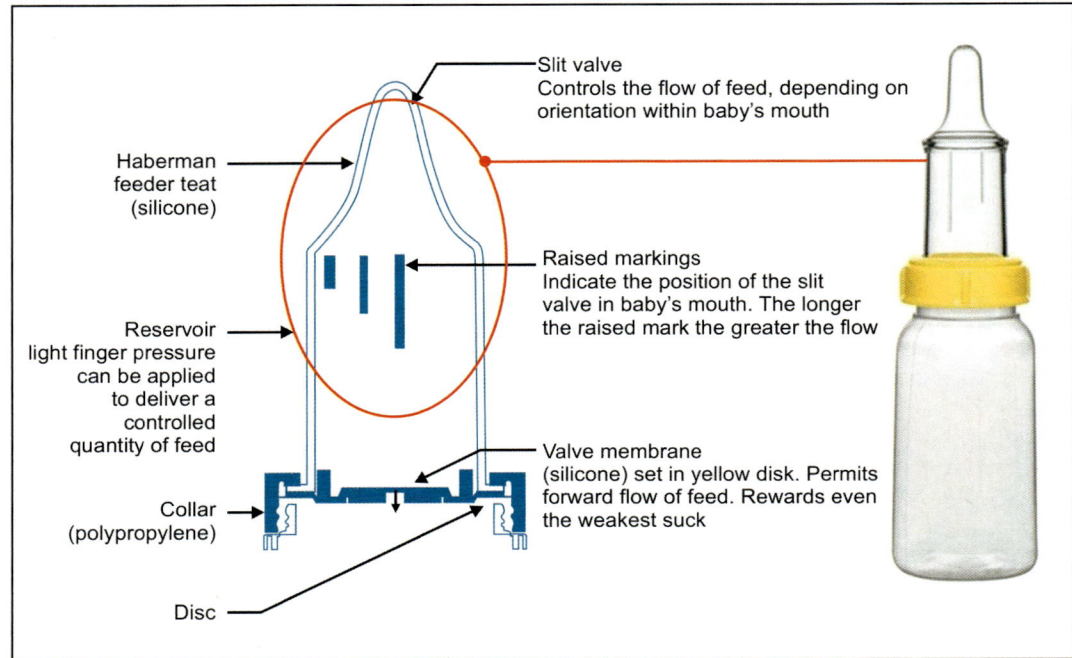

Slit valve
Controls the flow of feed, depending on orientation within baby's mouth

Haberman feeder teat (silicone)

Raised markings
Indicate the position of the slit valve in baby's mouth. The longer the raised mark the greater the flow

Reservoir light finger pressure can be applied to deliver a controlled quantity of feed

Valve membrane (silicone) set in yellow disk. Permits forward flow of feed. Rewards even the weakest suck

Collar (polypropylene)

Disc

Fig. 19.14: The Haberman feeder—how it works

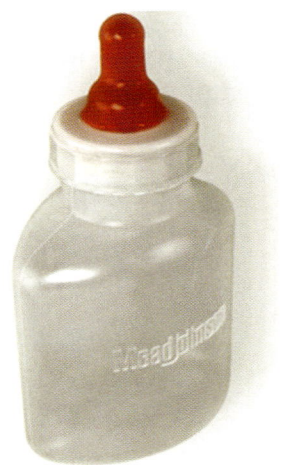

Fig. 19.15: Mead Johnson nurser

Airway Obstruction—Treatment

Clinical manifestations: A hoarse, croupy cough, an increased respiratory rate and a low grade fever. Increasing dyspnea and stridor are also signs of air hunger.

- The treatment should start as soon as the child starts to cough.
- Prevention includes placing the baby face down to clear the pharyngeal airway.
- Use of feeding appliance.
- Immediate oxygen, if air hunger develops.

- Clearing of the nasopharyngeal secretion.
- Sedatives and antihistamines

Speech Problem

Hard palate provides the partition between the oral and nasal cavities and soft palate functions with the pharynx is an important valve action referred to as velopharyngeal mechanism.

Velopharyngeal Mechanism

In normal speech, this valve action is intermittent, rapid and variable to affect normal sounds and pressures by deflecting the air stream with its sound waves out of the mouth. Without this valve, speech is hypernasal and deglution is impaired.

Most human speech and language require regulation of air flow through the nose and mouth. If air leaks out of the nose while we are speaking, many of the sounds we make do not sound right (Fig. 19.16).

When a lot of air leaks out of the nose, speech becomes almost intelligible. A child with an unrepaired cleft palate cannot step air from rusting out the nose during speech. This makes it very difficult for a child to learn how to speak correctly. It also makes it difficult for others to understand his/her speech.

Hearing Problem

The eustachian tube connects the throat to the middle ear and one of its jobs is to equalize the pressure in

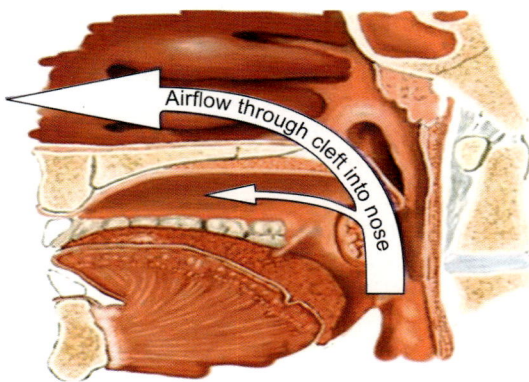

Fig. 19.16: Leakage of air through cleft into nose affects sound

front of and behind the eardrum. The eustachian tube is typically in a closed position and is opened by two muscles (tensor palatini and levator palatini) when pressure in front of and behind the eardrum is not same.

With the cleft patients, these muscles may not attach properly to the eustachian tube, making opening and closing of the eustachian tube difficult or impossible.

When the eustachian tube does not open effectively air is prevented from entering the middle ear. As a result, the middle ear may not be well ventilated and fluid may build up behind the eardrum causing a conductive hearing loss (Fig. 19.17).

A child has normal hearing when their hearing falls within 0 to 25 db HL range on the highest test form.

With conductive hearing loss, child's hearing may fall at the 30 to 50 db HL range on the audiogram. With this degree of hearing loss, conversational speech may be heard as a whisper. The hearing loss may affect both ears or just one.

Dental Problems

The hypoplastic maxilla will have common finding of pseudo prognathism or relative prognathism of the

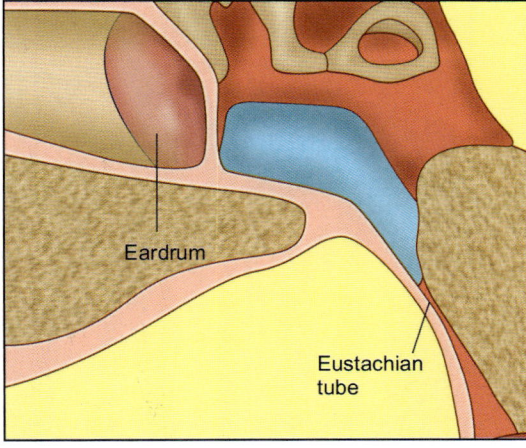

Fig. 19.17: Root cause for conductive hearing loss

mandible. Early palatal closures will bring about scar contraction and may severely limit the growth and development of maxilla, which will be deficient in all these planes. Constriction of the maxillary dental arch will be seen with narrowing of the palatal vault.

Tooth Defect In Cleft Lip and Palate

- Supernumerary teeth
- Congenitally missing teeth
- T-cingulum
- Peg-shaped teeth
- Thick curved hypoplastic incisors
- Normally formed lateral incisors usually absent and replaced by abnormally formed supernumerary teeth which can except at birth as 'natal' teeth.
- Gemination, fused supernumerary is frequently present.
- Geminated conical tooth may also be present in the region of lateral incisor.
- Delayed exception pattern of permanent teeth.
- High incidence of hypoplasia in the incisors next to alveolar defects.
- Isolated enamel developmental defects.
- Enamel defects can also occur in deciduous cuspids, molars and first permanent molars.
- Feeding difficulties.

Esthetic Problems

Examination of unilateral cleft lip and palate cases reveal nose deformity, lip deformity, cleft alveolus, hypoplastic and collapsed maxilla on the side of the cleft of the palate.

Bilateral cleft lip and palate cases, in addition to the features of unilateral cleft on either side, reveal a protruded premaxilla, small prolabium, absent or short columella and a shallow gingivolabial sulcus. Facial disfigurement varies from mild to severe. The orofacial structures may be malformed and congenitally missing. Thus esthetics is greatly affected.

Psychological Problems

Cleft lip and palate patients are under a lot of psychological stress. Due to their abnormal facial appearance, they have to put up with startling, curiosity, pity, etc. They also face problems in obtaining jobs and making friends. Studies have shown that these patients face badly in academics. This is usually as a result of hearing impairment, speech problems and frequent absence from school.

MANAGEMENT OF CLEFT LIP AND PALATE

The management of the patient can be divided into four distinct yet overlapping stages.

Stage I: Use of Presurgical Orthopedics

The first stage extends from birth to 24 months which helps:

- To facilitate feeding.
- To establish normal tongue posture.
- To provide psychological boost to the parents.
- To assist the surgeon in his initial repairs.
- To stimulate palate bone growth.
- To reestablish proper sutural growth patterns early, when the sutures are most responsive
- To restore the orofacial functional matrix.
- To expand or prevent collapsed segments.
- To reduce the need for later orthodontic treatment.
- To allow soft tissues to grow more before surgery.
- To improve esthetics.
- To guide tooth eruption

The orthodontist performs to fulfill the following two conditions:

1. Fabrication of a feeding plate or passive maxillary obturator.
2. Extraoral strapping of the premaxilla (Fig. 19.18) or other infant orthopedic procedures like nasoalveolar molding (NAM). It is important to note that both the procedures are optional and have inherent advantages and disadvantages. The procedures should be undertaken after evaluating the individual case.

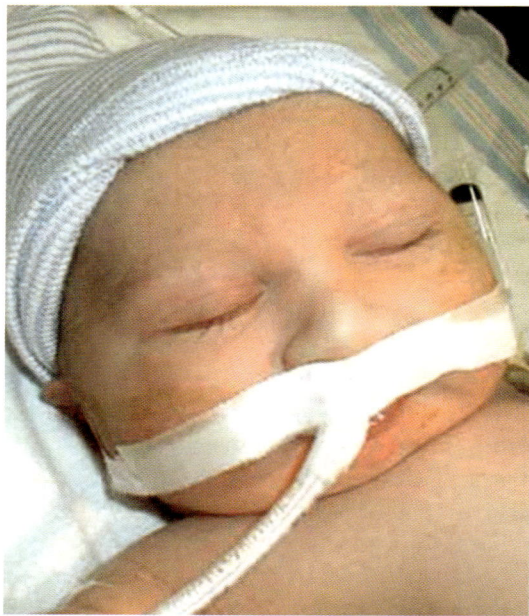

Fig. 19.18: Extraoral strapping of the premaxilla

Feeding Appliance (Fig. 19.19)

It should be started immediately after birth, latest by 6 weeks of age. To prevent the flow of alginate into the pharynx while impression taking, it was recommended by Pradhan et al to hold the infant upside down.

Infant orthopedic procedures were popular in late 1950s. They basically made use of removable orthodontic appliances to reposition the maxillary segments in early infancy, before the initial flap closure. In a unilateral cleft, the premaxillary segments are likely to be displaced facially adjacent to the cleft, whereas in bilateral clefts, the premaxilla is usually displaced significantly forward, with the posterior segments collapsed medially behind it. Repositioning the segments by nasoalveolar molding (NAM) before the initial lip surgery makes it easier to produce a more esthetic lip with the first operation. This made the patients look much better at an early stage.

Methods (Fig. 19.20a and b)

- *McNeil:* His goal was to control the dental arch in early infancy and prevent the high degree of arch collapse.
- *Burston:* Modified the original appliance of McNeil by incorporating the bite blocks.

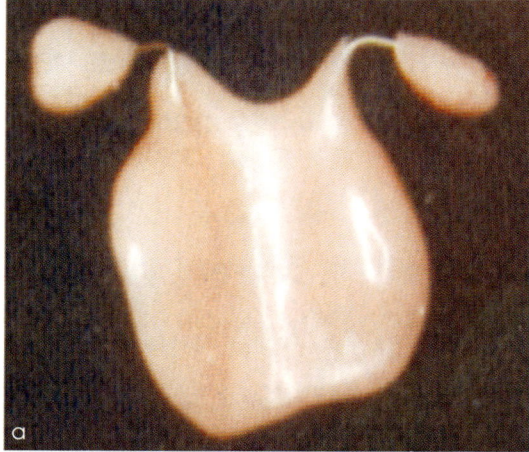

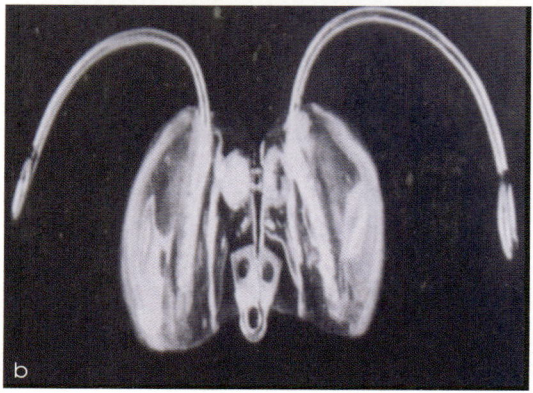

Fig. 19.19: Feeding appliance

- *Rosenstein:* Modified acrylic wings has two separate plates each covering the complete one segment. These plates are united by a reverse 'U' shaped wire of which ends are embedded in the acrylic. This wire can be activated by a loop causing expansion of the bony segments.

Nasoalveolar Molding

To eliminate the need for secondary alveolar bone grafting, to close the nasal floor and to achieve early esthetics, Millard in 1983 used Latham presurgical orthopedic appliances. These appliances help with alignment of alveolar segment within 2–3 mm so that mucoperiosteum creates a tunnel across the cleft allowing subsequent bone formation and eventual tooth eruption. These appliances help with the primary lip closure and palate repair.

- Simple to use, not-invasive and made of biofriendly, non-toxic, non-irritating dental resin.
- The plates prevent the tongue from pushing the cleft segments apart and allow them to move towards each other, thus reducing the width of the cleft.

- During the later stages of infant orthopedics, tape is often applied to gently mold the soft tissues of the lip and to close the defect.
- For unilateral cleft baby plates, stainless steel wires are provided for support. These are tapered to the baby's cheeks. The plates are discontinued once the lip is repaired.
- Presurgical NAM can rotate premaxilla, straighten the columella, lengthen the prolabium, lift the alar (nostril) and align the alveolar ridge (Figs 19.21 to 19.25).

Latham's Coaxial Pinned Screw Appliance

The use of such appliances has decreased over the years, because even though they improved the esthetics initially but the results over the years were not that encouraging.

Infants with bilateral cleft need two types of movements of maxillary segment; collapsed maxillary posterior segment must be laterally pushed and pressure exerted against the maxilla to reposition it, posteriorly. Repositioning can be done either by an appliance pinned to the segments, which applies a contracting force by the application of leucoplast over

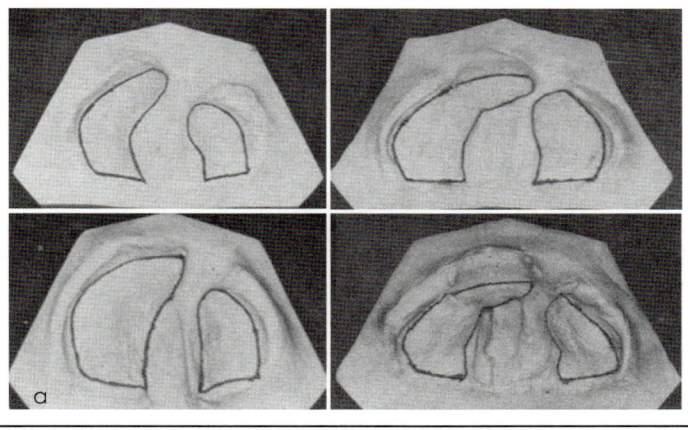

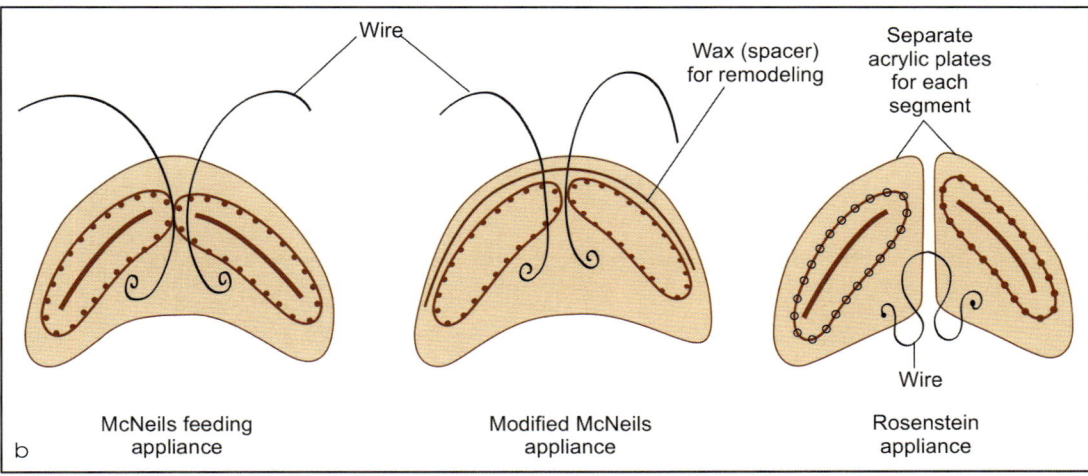

Fig. 19.20a and b: Nasoalveolar molding method

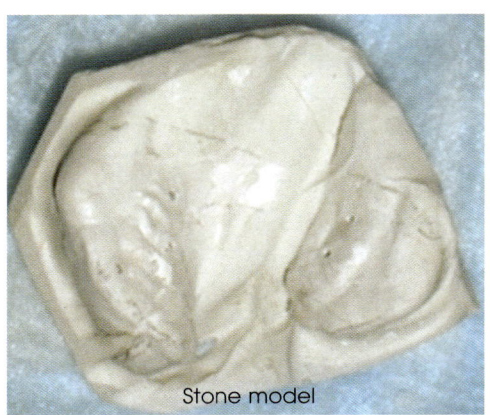
Stone model

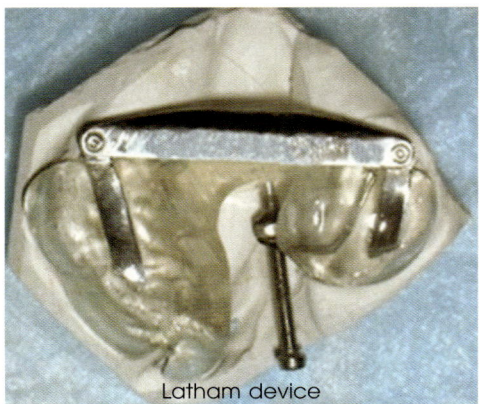
Latham device

Fig. 19.21: Working of the appliance

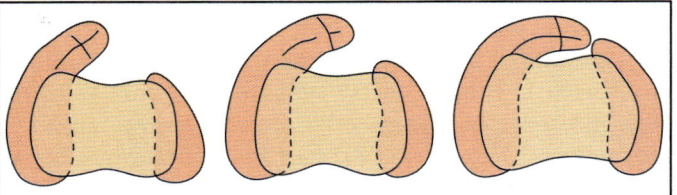

Fig. 19.22a: Unilateral case of cleft palate

the premaxillary segment. A similar force was also seen to have generated following an early lip repair.

Lip Closure

Surgical correction of lip is done in early infancy as it is compatible with a good long-term result. The common guidelines (as advocated by Millard) are age 10 weeks, weight 10 pounds and hemoglobin 10 gm%. Correcting the lip immediately after birth offer only psychological advantage to the parents and was popular in the 1960s. It involves a greater risk of surgical morbidity, and long-term esthetic results were found to be not as good.

Many surgical techniques have been developed for primary lip and nose closure. The rotation-advancement technique of Millard is commonly used.

Surgical Palate Repair

An intact plate aids the acquisition of normal speech, therefore, palate closure between the age of 12 and 24

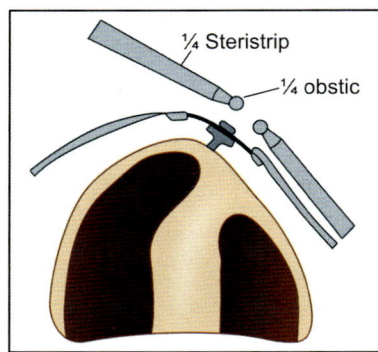
¼ Steristrip
¼ obstic

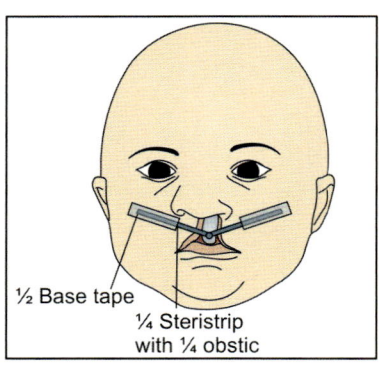
½ Base tape
¼ Steristrip
with ¼ obstic

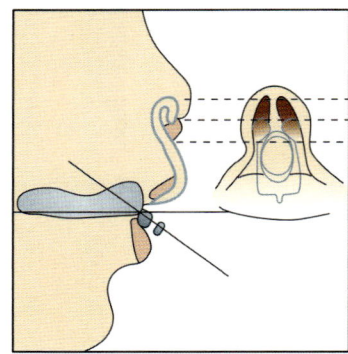

Fig. 19.22b: Unilateral case with appliance

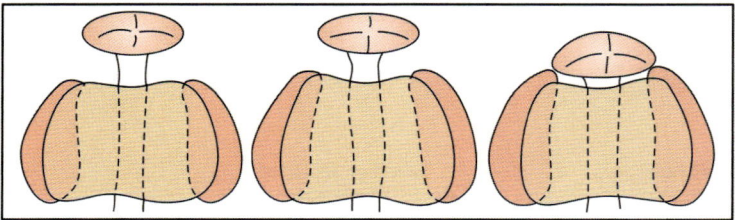

Fig. 19.23a: Bilateral case

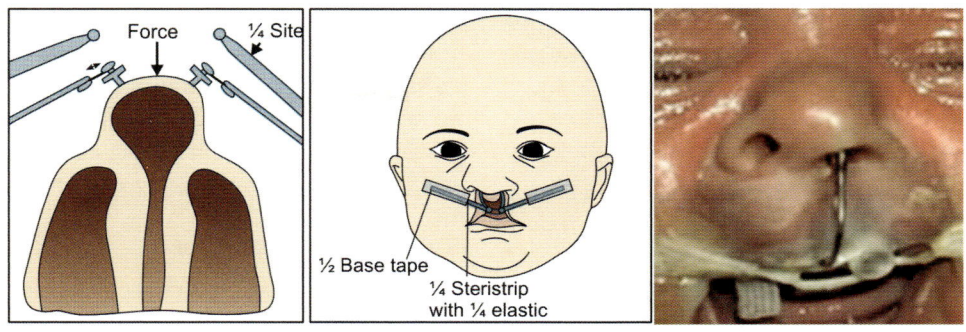

Fig. 19.23b: Bilateral case with appliance

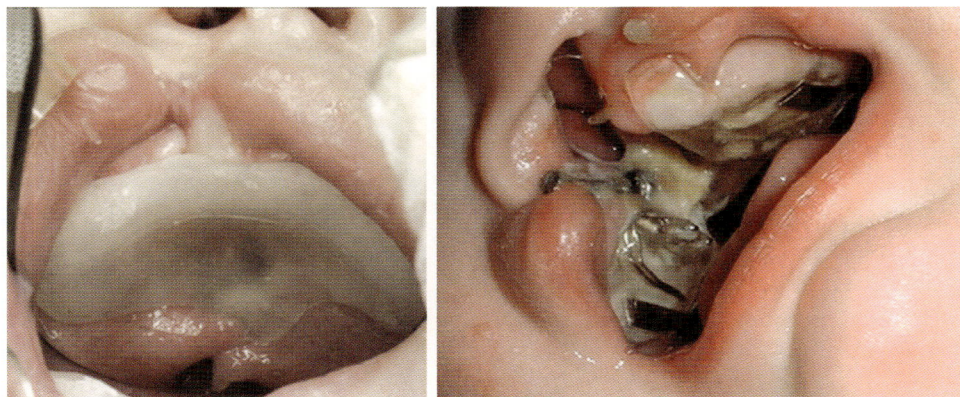

Fig. 19.24: Post-insertion

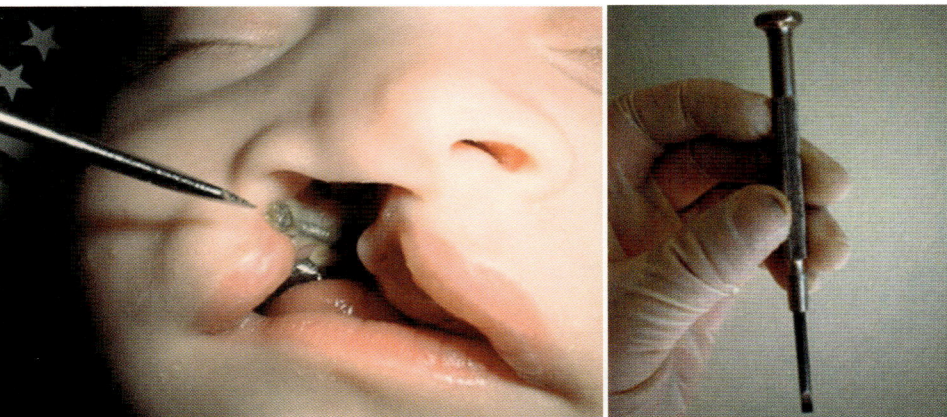

Fig. 19.25: Activation

months is recommended. Some authors prefer to wait and recommend palatal repair in the age group of 9 to 12 years.

The objectives of palatal surgery are to join the cleftal edges, lengthen the soft palate, and repair the levator palatini muscle.

Stage II: Treatment of CLCP in Deciduous Dentition

This stage extends from 24 months to 6 years of age. The period covers the primary dentition. The orthodontist palys the part of an observer and monitors the development of the dentition. Generally, no active orthodontic treatment is undertaken during this stage. Adjustments may be made in the obturator to accommodate the erupting deciduous teeth. Crossbites at this stage can be corrected with either removable (split palate) or fixed (lingual arch) appliances. The correction of crossbites at this stage is debatable, as crossbite problems tend to reappear and will require additional treatment in the mixed and permanent dentition period.

The oral-hygiene instruction may be emphasized upon and procedures undertaken to preserve the exisiting tooth structures.

Stage III: Treatment of CLCP in Mixed Dentition

This stage extends from 6 to 12 years of age, i.e. the mixed dentition stage. The orthodontist plays a major role during this stage.

- Arch expansion can be undertaken (Fig. 19.26)
- Maxillary protraction devices can be made use of.
- Fixed orthodontic treatment can be initiated, which will form the basis of the final alignment and position of the teeth. Arch expansion can be undertaken using appliances such as the NiTi expander or the quad helix. The NiTi molar rotator may be used prior to the use of expansion appliances to correct the rotated first permanent molars. A screw appliance can also be used.

Maxillary protraction appliances as in the reverse pull headgear is often used and has been found to be very effective in cooperative patients.

Alignment using fixed appliances can be initiated. The patient is referred for a secondary alveolar bone graft (ABG) in the palatal region before the eruption of the permanent maxillary canine (9–11 years). If the canine can be made to erupt through the graft, it adds to its stability. Cancellous bone from the iliac crest is the most preferred alveolar bone graft material used for cleft cases.

Stage IV: Treatment of CLCP in Permanent Dentition

This stage needs final correction. The arches are aligned the occlusion made to settle. Planning is done regarding the need for orthognathic surgery. Prosthetic rehabilitation should be done, if necessary. Lip revision, nasal correction and the restoration of the nasophiltral angle can be undertaken following the completion of all orthodontic treatment (Figs 19.26 and 19.27).

ROLE OF ORTHODONTIST IN CLEFT LIP AND PALATE

It extends from infancy to adulthood and during this long period of service, he/she actively participate by:
- Facilitating surgical repair of cleft lip and palate by aligning cleft segments
- Removing any interference to normal growth
- Preparing cleft sites for grafting

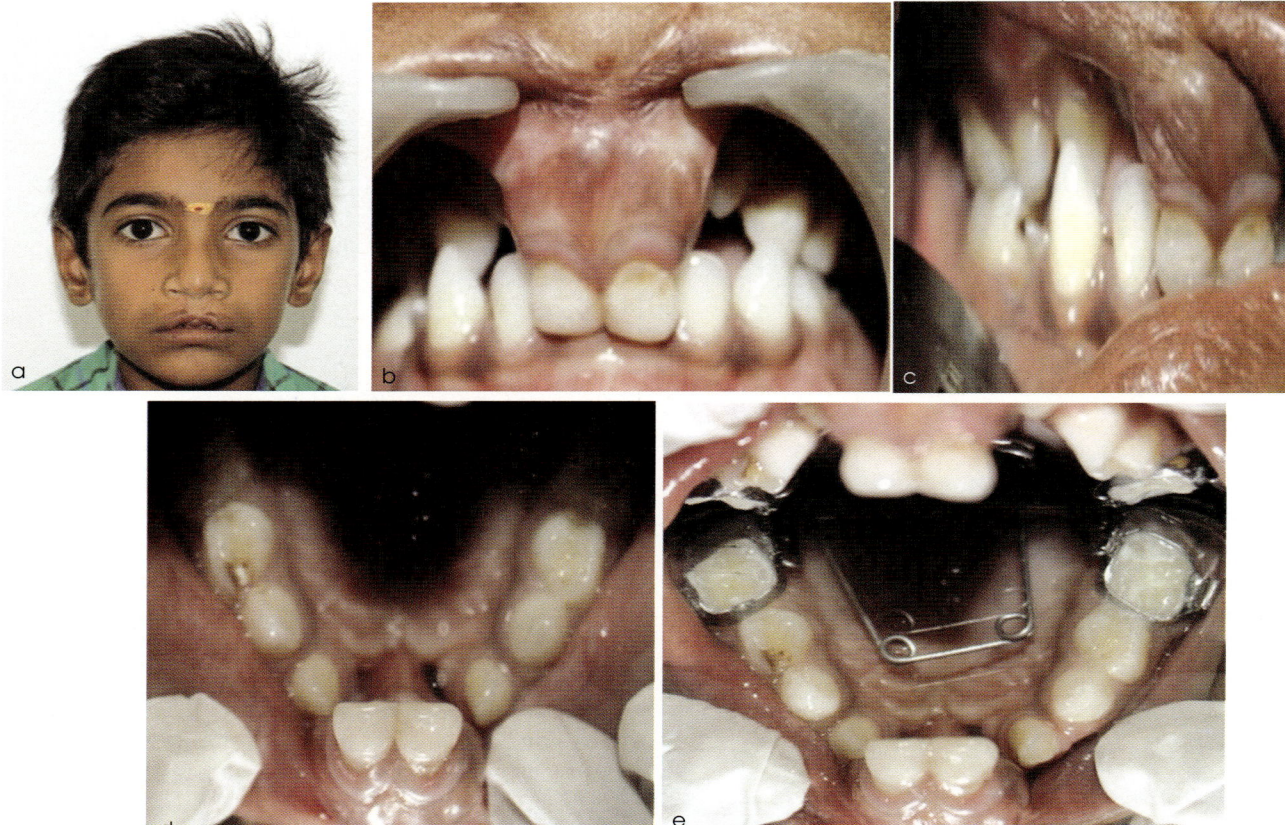

Fig. 19.26a to e: Quad helix appliance in mixed dentition

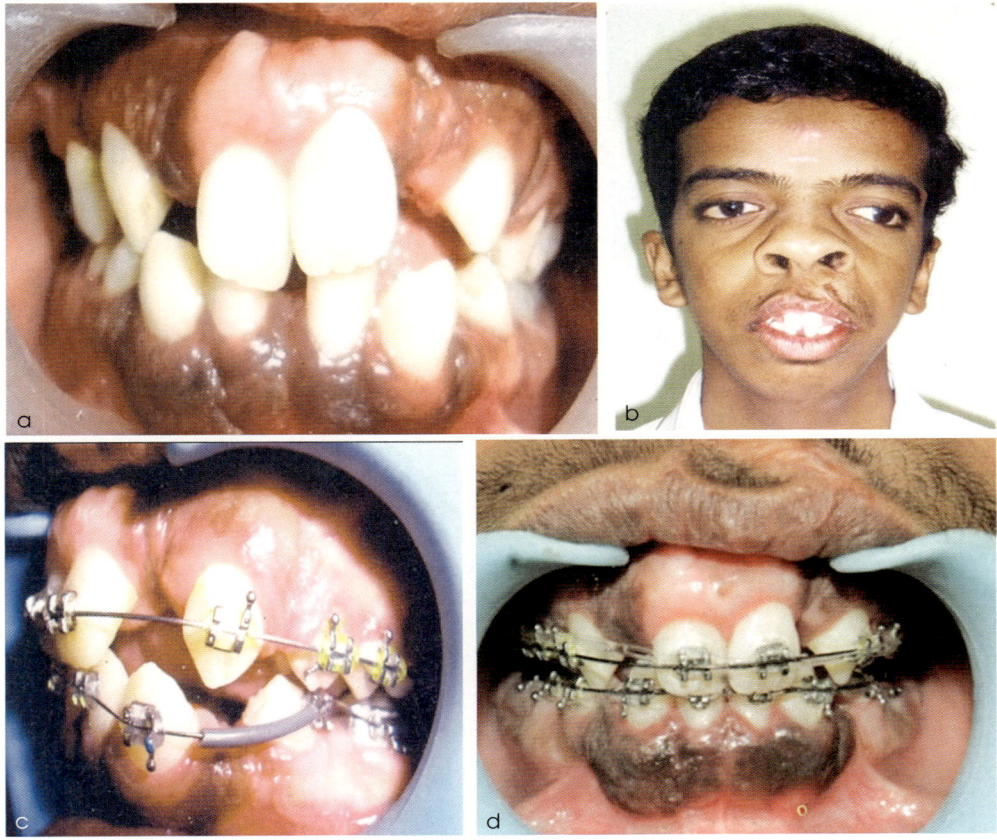

Fig. 19.27a to d: Patient-1 fixed appliance in permanent dentition

- Helping the child in feeding
- Helping to arch expansion

Surgical correction of the problem at this early age would allow normal function and development theoretically. Early surgery with its concomitant increased scarring has deleterious effect on future growth and development.

Excessive maxillary distortion at the time of the initial surgical-procedure may result difficult and less ideal lip repair. To optimize the surgical result, orthopedic appliances can be used to expand the posterior segments or reposition the premaxillary segments.

Expansion can be achieved by a jackscrew type or spring-loaded appliance. This appliance can also retract the premaxilla using a screw component, elastic bands between the premaxillary segment and the posterior portion or extraoral elastic traction across the premaxilla. Alternatively, preliminary surgical procedure, such as lip adhesion, can be carried out following the expansion.

These intraoral appliances also may be modified by the addition of acrylic or wire and acrylic stents that project into deformed nasal cavity. When combined with extraoral traction, these appliances can reshape nasal cartilages and increase columella length presurgically (Table 19.1).

Submucous Cleft

The term 'submucous' refers to the fact that the cleft is covered over by the lining mucous membrane of the roof of the mouth. This covering of the mucosa makes the cleft difficult to see when looking in the mouth.

A submucous cleft of the soft palate is characterized by a midline deficiency or lack of muscular tissue and incorrect positioning of the muscles. A submucous cleft can be felt as a notch or depression in the bony palate when the palate is palpated with a finger. Submucous cleft is often associated with a bifid or cleft uvula (Fig. 19.28).

Effect of Submucous Cleft

- Speech problem
- Middle ear disease
- Swallowing difficulties
- Bifid uvula
- Notching in the palate
- Very thin translucent strip of lining mucosa in the middle of the roof of the mouth.

Table 19.1: Treatment of CLCP: A brief overview

Stage	Age	Comment
Presurgical infant orthopedics	1 to 4 weeks	Repositioning palatal segments can facilitate lip repair, done less frequently now
Lip closure	8 to 12 weeks	May be preceded by preliminary lip adhesion as an alternative to presurgical orthopedics
Palate closure	18–24 months	Closing only the soft palate initially is an alternative but one stage closure of the hard and soft palate is the usual procedure
Speech therapy	6–11 years	Articulation errors often develop and child tries to compensate for cleft
Early orthodontics	7–8 years	Usually incisor alignment and maxillary transverse expansion
Alveolar grafting	6–10 years	Needed before permanent canines erupt, timing determined by stage and sequences of dental development
Comprehensive orthodontics	11–14 years	Class III elastics often useful
Pharyngeal flap surgery	9–19 years	Only if required to overcome nasal air leakage during speech; sometimes needed after loss of lymphoid tissue in the nasopharynx at adolescence or following maxillary advancement
Orthognathic surgery	17–19 years	Maxillary advancement perhaps combined with mandibular set-back; not done until growth completed except in rare instances of severe psychosocial impact; needed frequently
Fixed orthodontics	17–19 years	Replacement of missing laterals; consider temporary bonded bridge when fixed orthodontic appliance removed, comprehensive treatment only after growth completed

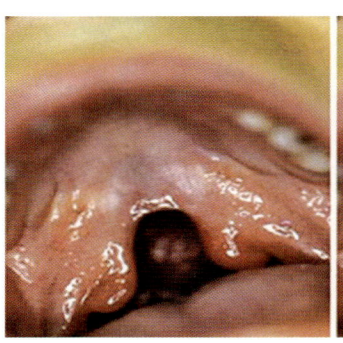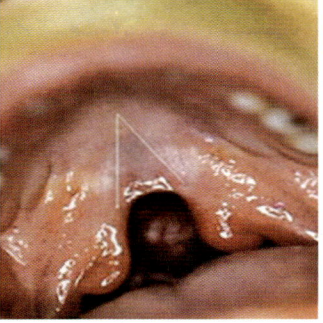

Fig. 19.28: Submucous cleft palate

Test to Detect Submucous Cleft

- X-ray examination
- Nasopharyngoscopy

Treatment of Submucous Cleft

- In case of velopharyngeal incompetence, surgical repair has to be done. The surgery consists of reconstruction of the abnormal tissues with a palatal repair with or without pharyngeal flap.
- In case of ear problems, antibiotics, surgical insertion of ventilating tubes in eardrum.

Parents Counseling at Birth

Parents are usually not prepared to face this problem. Sometimes they have a feeling of guilt that they had done something wrong during pregnancy.

They should be clearly informed that there is nothing known which definitely results in the cleft and there is nothing known which they could have done earlier to prevent its occurrence.

The management plan regarding surgery, dentistry and speech therapy should be explained properly. The nature and outcome of surgery is explained and they are informed how they can help in the outcome by co-operating during the course of treatment.

Speech Prosthesis

Some speech problems linked with VPI can be treated by speech therapy. Treatment focuses on teaching the child the correct manner and palate of articulation. In most cases, VPI speech symptoms cannot be decreased solely by speech treatment.

Velopharyngeal speech prosthesis can elevate the velum (lift), fill the residual velopharyngeal gap (obturator) or both (lift-orator).

Obturator (Fig. 19.29)

- It is like a modified dental retainer.
- Shaped uniquely to fit patient's muscle movement.

Palatal Obturator

Steps

- Alginate impression made—stone model produced.
- Block out excessive undercuts.
- Apply tin foil substitute over model and dry it.

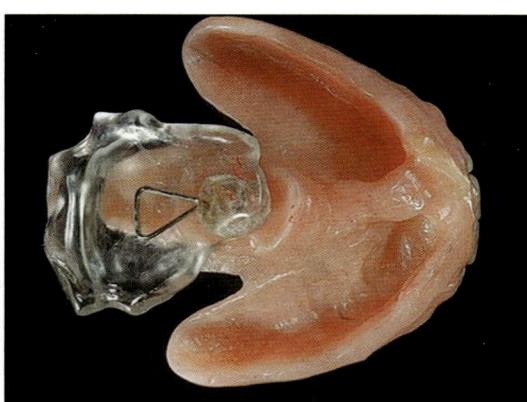

Fig. 19.29: Obturator

- Pour a mixture of soft autopolymerizing resin into cleft to the level of the palate.
- Place the model in a warm moist environment to cure for 20 minutes.
- Add autopolymerizing acrylic resin to the palate using 'salt and pepper method'.
- Remove appliance from mode, rinse wax and modeling dough off with hot water.
- Then trim and polish the appliance.

Advantages
- Provide false palate against which infant can suck.
- Provides maxillary cross-arch stability and prevent arch collapses.
- Provides maxillary orthopedic molding of the cleft segments into approximation before primary alveolar cleft bone grafting.
- Infants with airway obstruction secondary to Pierre Robin sequence may require intervention to aid breathing. An obturator with a posterior palatal extension should be used in an attempt to reposition the tongue downward and forward out of the cleft side.
- This palatal lift appliance acts by lifting the soft palate upwards and backwards which may help to encourage movements of the soft palate and the back of throat (Fig. 19.30).

Bulb Prosthesis

In case of a laterally deviated premaxilla in an infant with a bilateral cleft lip and palate, a straight extraoral force would not place the premaxilla in the facial midline. Therefore, the premaxilla must be positioned in the midline before premaxillary retraction.

An impression is made for construction of bulb prosthesis. This appliance is fitted over the protruding and laterally displaced premaxilla and anchored to infants head with a bonnet anchored to infants head with a bonnet appliance.

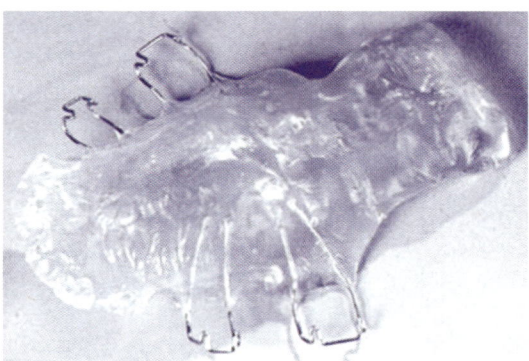

Fig. 19.30: Palatal lift appliance

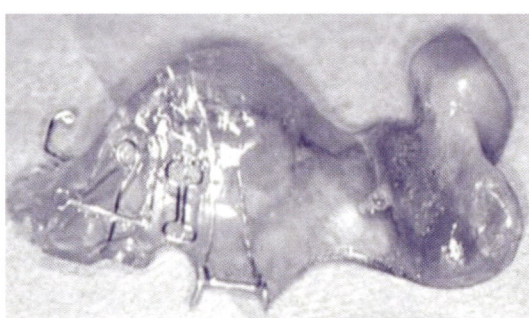

Fig. 19.31: Bulb prosthesis

By application of sequentially increasing differential forces to premaxilla with elastic straps attached to bulb prosthesis, the premaxilla is brought into the facial midline (Fig. 19.31).

Rationale for use of Bulb Prosthesis
- Affords greater control over differential forces applied to premaxilla.
- Movement of premaxilla into facial midline before retropositioning decreases the rise of distorting a vomer stalk.
- Need for a surgical premaxillary set back is eliminated.
- Optimum premaxillary positioning may eliminate the need for a staged lip closure.
- Appearance of nose and lip improved.

Bibliography

1. Graber TM. Craniofacial morphology in cleft palate and cleft lip deformities. Surg Gynec Obstet 1949;88:359–69.
2. Rosenstein SW. New concept in early orthopedic treatment of cleft lip and palate. Am J Orthod 1969;55:765–74.
3. Shaw WC, Semb G. Current approaches to the orthodontic management of cleft lip and palate. J R Soc Med 1990;83:30–3.
4. Thom AR. Modern management of the cleft lip and palate patient. Dent Update 1990;17:402–8.

PREVIOUS YEAR'S UNIVERSITY QUESTIONS

Essay

1. What are the causes for cleft lip and palate? How will you manage the problems associated with them?
2. Classify cleft lip and palate. Discuss the line of treatment of cleft lip and palate.
3. Discuss the various problems that the cleft lip and palate patients face.

Short Questions

1. Role of orthodontist in cleft lip and palate
2. American Cleft Palate Association's classification
3. Use of pre-surgical orthopedics
4. Etiology of cleft lip and palate
5. Feeding appliance
6. Theories of cleft lip and cleft palate

MCQs

1. *Cleft lip is also known as:*
   a. Lip of camel
   b. Harelip
   c. Sorcerer's lip
   d. None of the above   **(Ans: b)**

2. *What is the structure that is least affected by clefts?*
   a. Upper lip
   b. Lower lip
   c. Alveolar ridge
   d. Hard and soft palate   **(Ans: b)**

3. *Mildest form of cleft palate is:*
   a. Cleft of soft palate
   b. Cleft of hard palate
   c. Bifid uvula
   d. Cleft of incisive foramen   **(Ans: c)**

4. *Most clefts of alveolus and palate show:*
   a. Class I malocclusion
   b. Class II division 1 malocclusion
   c. Class II division 2 malocclusion
   d. Class III malocclusion   **(Ans: d)**

5. *Which of the following statements is true?*
   a. Babies with cleft lip and plate cannot swallow normally, if led towards the hypopharynx
   b. Structural defects of cleft lip and palate prevent positive oral pressure
   c. Cleft palate patients are predisposed to middle ear infection
   d. Babies should only be breastfed   **(Ans: c)**

6. *The management of cleft lip and cleft palate:*
   a. Starts at birth till 18 years of age
   b. Starts at 4 months till 16 years of age
   c. Starts at 5 years till 18 years of age
   d. Starts at 6 years till 11 years of age   **(Ans: b)**

7. *When is the first stage of management of cleft lip and palate?*
   a. From birth to 18 months
   b. From 18 months to 5 years
   c. From 6 years to 11 years
   d. As from 4 weeks   **(Ans: a)**

8. *At what age is lip repair carried out?*
   a. At birth
   b. At 3 months
   c. At 9–18 months
   d. At 9–10 years   **(Ans: b)**

9. *At what age is secondary alveolar bone graft usually carried out?*
   a. At birth
   b. At 3 months
   c. At 9–18 months
   d. At 9–10 years   **(Ans: d)**

10. *At what age is the repair of cleft palate started?*
    a. At birth
    b. At 3 months
    c. At 9–18 months
    d. At 9–10 years   **(Ans: c)**

11. *Who suggested the rule of 10?*
    a. Veau
    b. Millard
    c. Kernahan
    d. Davis and Rithcie   **(Ans: b)**

12. *What is the chance of having a child with a cleft, if parents have a cleft?*
    a. 2.5%
    b. 4–10%
    c. 15–20%
    d. 20–30%   **(Ans: a)**

13. *What percentage of cleft lip with or without cleft palate is genetic in origin?*
    a. 80%
    b. 60%
    c. 50%
    d. 40%   **(Ans: d)**

14. *Increased maternal age:*
    a. Increases the risk of clefting
    b. Decreases the risk of clefting
    c. Has no effect on clefting
    d. Is directly proportional to the risk of cleft palate only   **(Ans: a)**

Implants in Orthodontics

Chapter Outline

- Introduction
- History
- Common indications for placement of implants
- Classification of implants for orthodontic anchorage
- Sites of placement

- Methods of placement
- Use of orthodontic implants
- Implant material
- Parts of implant

INTRODUCTION

Successful orthodontic treatment is always required intraoral anchorage with a high resistance to displacement. Extraoral traction can be an effective reinforcement such as headgears require full patient co-operation. The size, bulk, cost and invasiveness of prosthetic osseointegrated implants have limited their orthodontic application. Introduction of implants in orthodontics has solved this problem.

The use of implants as the best source of anchorage has number of advantages as compared to traditional anchorage such as no patient cooperation required, easy to use, short treatment time and control on tooth movements (Table 20.1).

HISTORY

- Gainforth and Higley (1945) first published the use of subperiosteal vitallium implant to retract the maxillary canines in dogs.
- Linkow (1969) described endosseous blade implants with perforation for orthodontic anchorage.
- Kawahara (1975) developed bioglass-coated ceramic implant for orthodontic anchorage.

Table 20.1: Differences between conventional anchorage and implant anchorage		
Character	*Traditional orthodontic treatment*	*Orthodontic treatment using implants*
Anchorage source	Teeth and extraoral bony structure	Implants
Stability of anchorage	Position of anchor teeth is not stable during treatment	Position is stable during treatment
Number of anchor teeth	In order to get sufficient anchorage, maximum number of teeth must be included	For direct anchorage, teeth are not necessary; minimal number of teeth are needed for indirect force on implant anchorage
Treatment of efficiency	Applying force on teeth, part of it is wasted	More efficient as force is transmitted directly to the implant
Duration of treatment	Treatment time is prolonged	Shortened treatment time
Patient's cooperation	Obligatory	Minimal
Treatment acceptability	Most of treatment devices restrict patient's motion, do not meet esthetical requirements	Discomfort for patient is minimal

- The Brane Mark (1964, 1977), mentor for modern implant surgery, described the high compatibility and strong anchorage of titanium in human tissue.

COMMON INDICATIONS FOR PLACEMENT OF IMPLANTS

- In maximum anchorage case
- Patients with several missing teeth making it difficult to engage posterior units
- For difficult tooth movements, e.g. intrusion of anterior and posterior segments and distalization
- Where asymmetrical tooth movement is needed.
- To treat borderline cases with non-extraction method.
- Doing extreme orthodontics when patient is not willing to undergo orthognathic surgery.

CLASSIFICATION OF IMPLANTS FOR ORTHODONTIC ANCHORAGE

1. *According to the shape and size*
   a. Conical (cylindrical)
      - Miniscrew implants
      - Palatal implants
      - Prosthodontic implants
   b. Miniplate implants
   c. Onplant
2. *According to implant–bone contact*
   a. Osteointegrated
   b. Non-osteointegrated
3. *According to the application*
   a. It is used only for orthodontic purposes or TAD (temporary anchorage devices)
   b. It is used for prosthodontic and orthodontic purposes

Mini-Screws

Of all orthodontic implants, mini-screws have gained importance due to less surgical procedure and easy installation. The mini-screw can be loaded with forces in the range of 50 to 300 g. Common sizes of mini-implants often used are 1.2–2 mm in diameter and 6–10 mm in length in various combinations.

- Mini-screw placed high in maxilla must be more perpendicular to bone to avoid damaging maxillary sinus.
- If screw head is at mucogingival level, it should be inclined a 30–45° to inter-radicular bone.
- Mini-screw must be centered between roots of teeth to be intruded to avoid interference between teeth and screw.

Miniplates

The miniplate implants are comprised of bone plates and fixation screws. The plates and screws are made of commercially pure titanium that is biocompatible and suitable for osseointegration.

The miniplates consist of three components:
- Head
- Arm
- Body

a. The *head component* is exposed intraorally and positioned outside of the dentition so that it does not interfere with tooth movement. The head component has three continuous hooks for attachment of orthodontic forces. There are two different types of head components based on the direction of the hooks.
b. The *arm component* is transmucosal and is available in three different lengths:
   – Short—10.5 mm
   – Medium—13.5 mm
   – Long—16.5 mm
   The short, medium and long lengths are available to accommodate individual morphological differences.
c. The *body component* is positioned subperiosteally and is available in three different configurations—the T-plate, Y-plate and L-plate.

Onplants

These are button type implants used in the palatal region. They serve as anchorage source for expansion as well as maxillary protraction.

SITES OF PLACEMENT

Maxilla

- Infrazygomatic crest area
- Tuberosity area
- Between canine and premolar buccally
- Between incisors facially
- Mid-palatal area

Mandible

- Retromolar area
- Between 1st and 2nd molars buccally
- Between 1st molar and 2nd premolar buccally
- Between canine and premolar buccally

METHODS OF PLACEMENT

- *Pretapping method:* In this method, the mini-screw is driven into the tunnel of bone formed by drilling (making it tap during implant driving). This method is used when the small diameter mini-screws are used.
- *Self-tapping:* Here a slight notch is made and then the screw is tapped in bone. The pure titanium mini-

screw can be immediately loaded with forces in the range of 50 to 300 g available in either 1.5 mm or 2 mm diameter. The 1.5 mm comes as 6, 8 mm. The 2 mm comes as 7, 9 or 11 mm lengths. The placement of screw requires sufficient bone depth of at least 2.5 mm to protect the anatomic structures.

- *Self-drilling method:* Here the mini-screw is driven directly into bone without drilling.

USES OF ORTHODONTIC IMPLANTS

- Used for retraction of anterior (Fig. 20.1)
- Uprighting of molars
- Mesiodistal tooth movement
- Open bite correction
- Molar mesialization
- Distalization of 1st and 2nd molars
- Intrusion of anterior as well as molars (Figs 20.2 and 20.3)
- Onplants for expansion and protraction of maxilla
- Closing edentulous spaces in first molar extraction sites (Fig. 20.4)
- Orthopedic traction

Indications for Placement of Implants

Mini-implants are used where three-dimensional stable anchorages is needed in the following situations:

- It is used in the cases where it cannot afford any movement of reactive units.
- Patients with mutilated condition where the posteriors are missing.
- For difficult tooth movements, e.g. intrusion of anterior and posterior segments and distalization.
- It is indicated where asymmetrical tooth movement is needed.

IMPLANT MATERIAL

Material must be: Nontoxic, biocompatible, possess excellent mechanical properties, and provide resistance

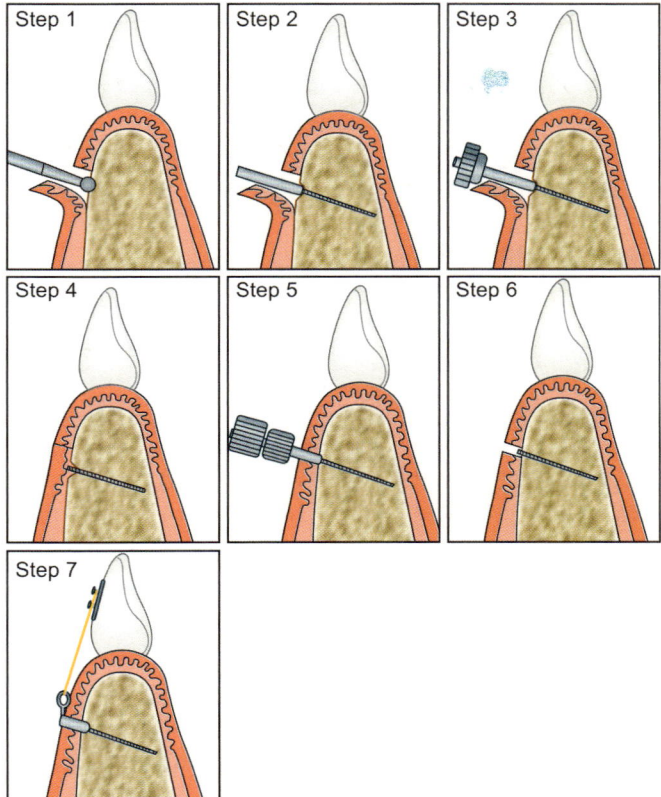

Fig. 20.2: Incisor intrusion

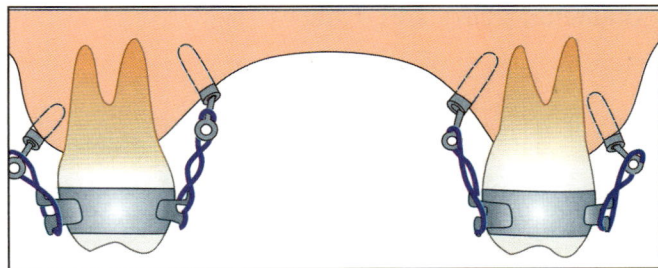

Fig. 20.3: Molar intrusion

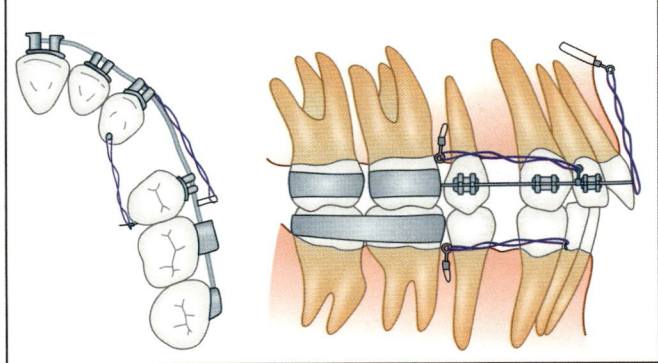

Fig. 20.1: Cuspid retraction

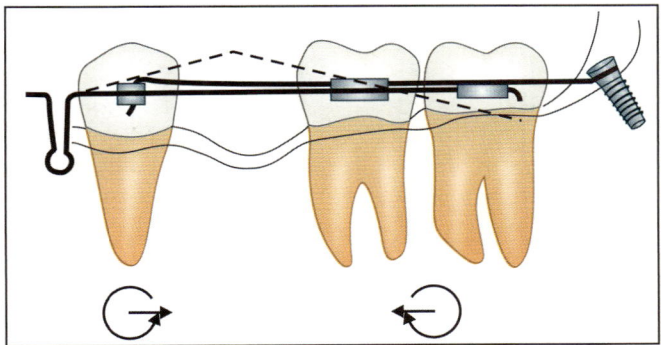

Fig. 20-4: Space closure

to stress, strain, and corrosion. Three categories of material are:

1. Biotolerant (stainless steel, chromium cobalt alloys)
2. Bioinert (titanium, carbon)
3. Bioactive (hydroxylapatite, ceramic oxidized aluminium)

PARTS OF IMPLANT (Fig. 20.5)

Implant head: It serves as the abutment and in the case of an orthodontic implant, could be the source of attachment for elastics/coil springs.

Implant body: It is the part embedded inside the bone. This may be a screw type or a plate type. The screw and plate design that has been used in orthodontics as the skeletal anchorage system varies from these conventional plate implants.

Implant neck: It is the part of the implant which connects the head and the body.

Implant Sizes

Various sizes of implants:

- Mini-implants—6 mm long, 1.2 mm in diameter
- Standard implants—6–15 mm long, 3–5 mm in diameter
- Maximal load is proportional to the bone–implant contact surface.
- Factors determining the contact area are length, diameter, shape, and surface design.

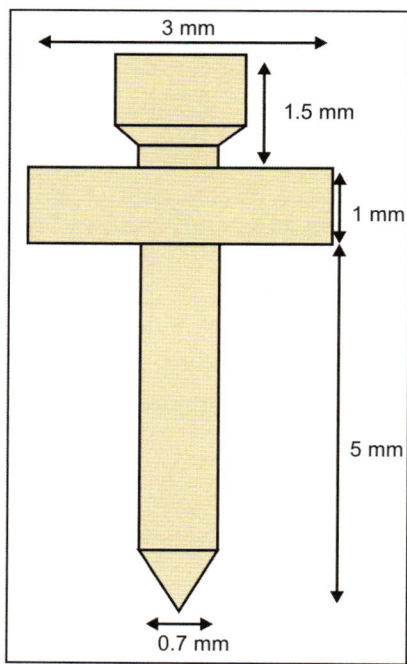

3 mm

1.5 mm

1 mm

5 mm

0.7 mm

Fig. 20.5: Parts of implant

Bone Implant Interaction

- Endosseous implantation into cortical bone elicits a unique sequence of modeling and remodeling events that are critical to healing, adaptation, and long-term maintenance of the bone implant interface.
- Callus formed at the endosteal and periosteal surfaces is the first vital bone to contact the implant.
- Initial healing response is driven by release of local chemical factors such as PDGF, TGF-β and PGs.
- Remodeling of bone–implant interface is of importance because it is the mechanism for forming a vital interface between the implant and host bone.

Bibliography

1. Contemporary Implant Dentistry—Carl E Misch.
2. Endosseous Implants for Maxillofacial Reconstruction, Block and Kent.
3. Dental Clinic of North America, Implantology, July 2006;50:3.
4. Dental implants—the art and science—Charles A Babbush.

PREVIOUS YEAR'S UNIVERSITY QUESTIONS

MCQs

1. *Which material has best osseointegration properties?*
   a. Pure titanium
   b. Pure gold
   c. Pure stainless steel
   d. Pure nickel   **(Ans: a)**

2. *What implants have the highest success rates?*
   a. Maxillary implants
   b. Mandibular implants
   c. Anterior maxillary implants
   d. Upper canine implants   **(Ans: b)**

3. *What age is considered safer for implant?*
   a. 6 years
   b. 10–12 years
   c. 16 years
   d. 18 years   **(Ans: d)**

4. *Which of the following statements is not true?*
   a. Implants can be used to study bone growth
   b. Endosseous implants are ankylosed in alveolar bone
   c. Implants cannot be used for orthodontic treatment
   d. Combination of implant placement and orthodontic therapy gives a better result   **(Ans: c)**

5. *What are the requirements to implant bone?*
   a. Good periodontal health
   b. Adequate bone volume
   c. Adequate oral hygiene
   d. All of the above   **(Ans: d)**

Laser in Orthodontics

Chapter Outline

- Principle of laser
- Laser tissue interaction
- Types of laser

- Advantages of laser
- Application of laser in orthodontics

Laser is the acronym for "Light Amplification by Stimulated Emission of Radiation". A laser produces a monochromatic collimated coherent beam of light energy.

Evolution of lasers: In 1960, research physicist Theodore H. Maiman built the first ruby laser at Hughes Laboratory in Malibu, California (Fig. 21.1).

Laser physics: Photon-smallest unit of energy which is released after an atom that has absorbed energy releases it. This is called Spontaneous emission. This concept was further theorized by Einstein (Fig. 21.2).

PRINCIPLE OF LASER (Fig. 21.3; Table 21.1)

- Light energy is converted to heat energy.
- The lasers work by their property of thermoablation.
- Laser beam is applied to skin—the striking energy is absorbed by the water molecules in the tissues.
- Raises the temperature within cells of the tissue.

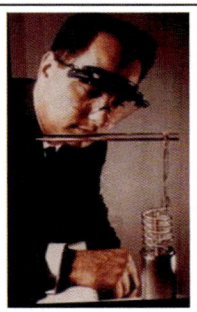

- Einstein's article on stimulated emission of radiant energy–1917.
- First working laser built by Maiman of Hughes research lab–1960.

Fig. 21.1: Spontaneous emission

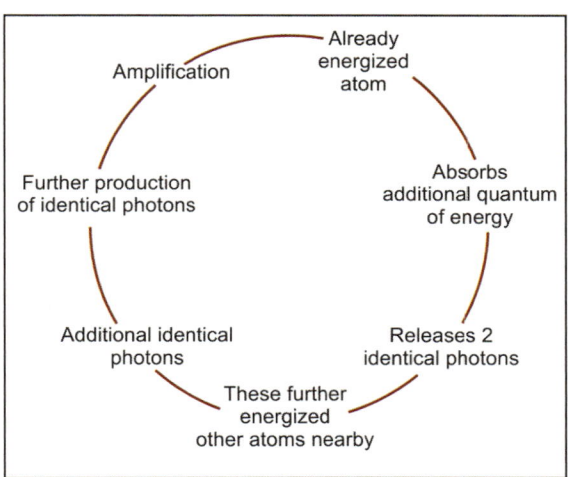

Fig. 21.2: Laser physics

- Sufficient energy gets deposited and the water molecules rapidly evaporate.
- Creates pressure—eventually helps in various therapeutic effects of lasers (Table 21.1).

Table 21.1: Differences between conventional and laser

Conventional light cure	Curing with lasers
Emits light over a broad range of wavelength (400–520 nm)	Emits light of low range of wavelength (457.9–14.7 nm)
Energy density of emitted light is not consistent	Consistent emission of light with substantial energy density
Wasted and unusable emission	Specific and efficient emission

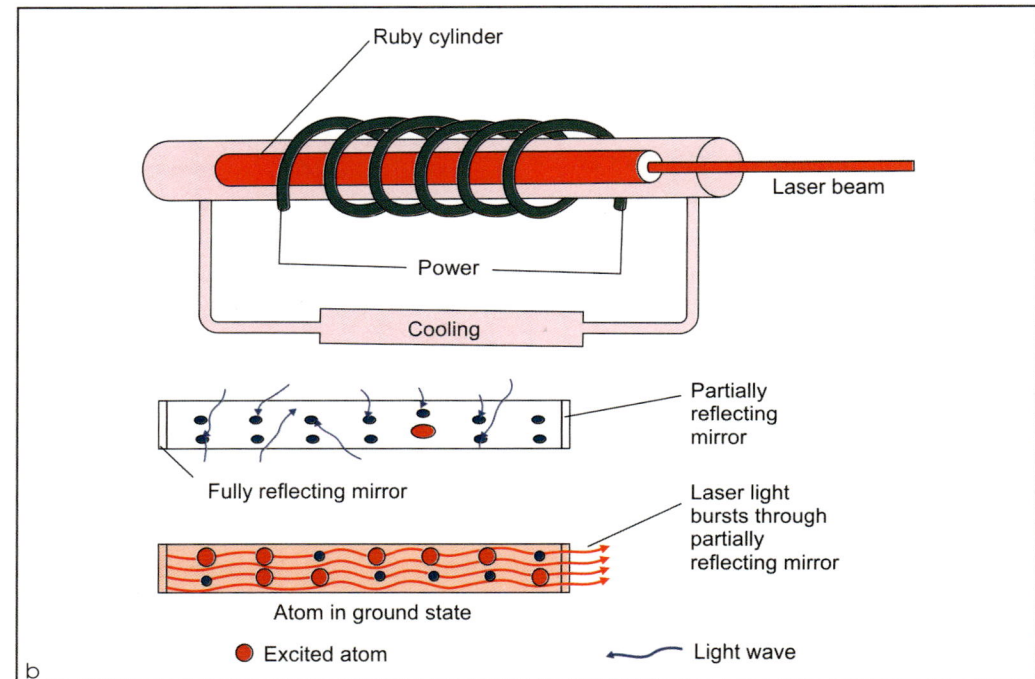

Fig. 21.3: Components of laser device

LASER TISSUE INTERACTION

When laser light emerges from a laser, it usually does in the form of pencil thin beam of laser energy travelling at the speed of light. This beam travels in a straight line until it hits something that reflects or refracts it or until it hits something that stops it and absorbs its energy. The laser beam diverges gradually as it travels away from laser, which means that the beams diameter increases with the distance between the headpiece and target tissue.

Laser light has either of four different interactions with the target tissue, depending on the optical properties of that tissue.

1. *Absorption:* Laser light is converted into effective thermal energy. The amount of energy that is absorbed by the tissue depends on the tissue characteristics, such as pigmentation and water content, and on the laser wavelength and emission mode. In general, the shorter wavelengths are readily absorbed in pigmented tissue and blood elements. Longer wavelengths are more interactive with water and hydroxyapatite.
2. *Transmission:* Light energy passes freely through the tissue, without interaction of any kind and has little or no effect. It is an inverse of absorption.
3. *Reflection:* Light energy reflects off tissue surface with little or no absorption and consequently has no effect on tissue. The laser beam generally becomes more divergent as the distance from the headpiece increases, which become dangerous because the energy is directed to an unintentional target, such as eye. This is a major safety concern for laser operation.
4. *Scattering:* Light energy is re-emitted in a random direction and ultimately observed over a greater surface area which produces less intense and less precisely distributed thermal effect. When laser light emerges from a laser it usually does in the form of pencil thin beam of laser energy travelling at the speed of light. This beam travels in a straight line until it hits something that stops it and absorbs its energy. The laser beam diverges gradually as it travels away from laser, which means that the beam's diameter increases with the distance between the headpiece and target tissue.

TYPES OF LASER

Lasers are mainly of two types: Hard tissue lasers and soft tissue lasers (Table 21.2).

CO$_2$

The CO$_2$ is a non-contact mode laser. The beam does not contact the tissue during the cutting phase; thus there is no tactile feedback during the surgical incision. CO$_2$ laser is well absorbed by water, and has fast thermal reaction. It operates with the wavelength of 10600 nm. It has an advantage of rapid soft tissue removal and shallow depth of penetration. It is useful in cutting dense fibrous tissue. New technology enables us to give precise cut in super-pulse mode making it extremely less traumatic and efficient soft tissue surgeries (Table 21.2).

Disadvantages: Less hemostasis compared to Nd: YAG/diode.

Erbium Laser

The erbium laser has a wavelength of 2790 to 2940 nm, which makes ideal for absorption by both hydroxy-apatite and water. It is used for caries removal, tooth preparation, soft tissue surgeries and bone ablation. New technology is slowly making the erbium family into all tissue lasers where it can effectively perform soft tissue surgeries (Table 21.2).

Disadvantages: Less hemostasis compared to Nd: YAG/diode.

Diode Laser

Diode laser is a solid active semiconductor. It has a wavelength of 812 to 980 nm. The laser energy is absorbed by pigmentation in the soft tissues and this makes the diode laser an excellent hemostatic agent. Diode laser is used in contact mode and it also provides tactile feedback during the surgical procedure.

It can often be used without anesthesia to perform very precise anterior soft tissue esthetic surgery or surgery in other areas of mouth without bleeding or discomfort. It is an excellent all purpose laser in dentistry. It can be used in bleaching, endodontics, soft tissue surgeries and periodontics. Good hemostasis can be achieved but it has to be judiciously used as it may cause damage to adjacent tissues due to rapid absorption.

Argon Laser

It has two wavelengths of 488 nm blue color and 514 nm blue green. It delivers the energy in either continuous or gated pulse mode. It is well absorbed in pigmented tissue and hemoglobin. It is useful as good hemostat and in acute inflammatory soft tissue lesions and it is also useful in vascular lesions (Table 21.2).

Nd:YAG Laser

It has a wavelength of 1064 nm and it can be easily absorbed by pigmented tissues. It delivers the energy

Table 21.2: Types of lasers		
State	Soft tissue lasers	Hard tissue lasers
Gas state	• CO$_2$ • He-Ne • Argon • Krypton	
Solid state	• Nd:YAG • Ruby • KTP • Diode • Ho:YAG	• Er:YAG • Cr:YSGG
Liquid state	• Rhodium	

in free running pulse mode. It is useful in periodontal surgery, sulcular debridement, cutting and coagulation, root canal sterilization (Table 21.2).

ADVANTAGES OF LASER

- No pain
- No bleeding
- Better visualization
- Less/no scarring
- Facilitates healing
- Laser cut is more precise than that of a scalpel.
- Minimum postoperative pain
- Laser application reduces the risk of postoperative infections.
- The laser sterilizes as it cuts.
- Laser application reduces the risk of blood-borne transmission of diseases.
- Less damage occurs to adjacent tissue following the use of lasers.

APPLICATION OF LASER IN ORTHODONTICS

Lasers have wide range of applications in dentistry. In this chapter, only a few important applications in orthodontics are discussed.

Exposure of impacted tooth by laser: Canine is the most commonly impacted tooth in the anterior segment of the dental arches due to arch length–tooth material discrepancy, this may delay the progress of orthodontic treatment. Exposure of impacted tooth by laser facilitates accessibility and decreases the risk of bond failure.

Frenectomy by laser: As permanent maxillary central incisors erupt in the oral cavity, the labial frenum shifts apically, in some instances frenum may persist even after complete eruption of permanent maxillary central incisors termed as high labial frenum attachment. Abnormal frenum attachment prevents approximation of maxillary central incisors resulting in midline diastema. Frencetomy by laser prevents recurrence and facilitates diastema closure. Patient acceptance with laser application is very high even in condition like tongue tie, as it facilitates healing, reduces the discomfort and no sutures are required.

Reduction of pain in orthodontic patient by application of laser: Procedures like separators placement and banding procedures are considered to be painful in the whole course of orthodontic treatment. Studies proved that the application of laser in patient with separators reduces the level of pain threshold (Fig. 21.4).

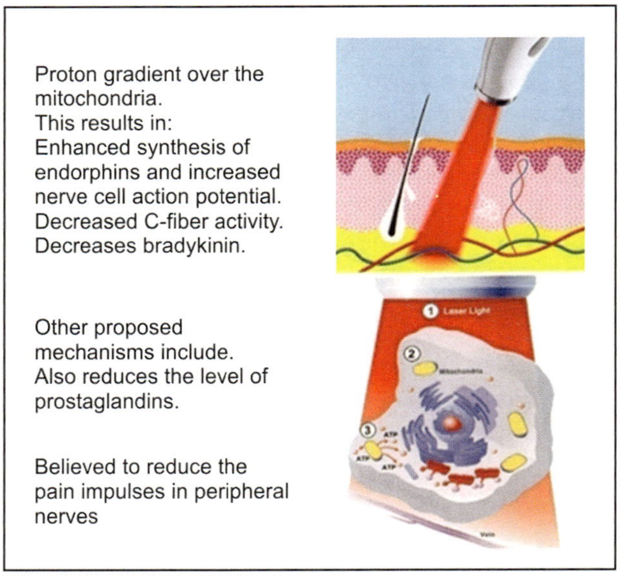

Proton gradient over the mitochondria.
This results in:
Enhanced synthesis of endorphins and increased nerve cell action potential.
Decreased C-fiber activity.
Decreases bradykinin.

Other proposed mechanisms include.
Also reduces the level of prostaglandins.

Believed to reduce the pain impulses in peripheral nerves

Fig. 21.4: Pain relief

Application of laser in bonding orthodontic bracket: Nowadays, laser is used in curing of orthodontic bracket in orthodontic procedure. Curing of orthodontic bracket by laser takes approximately 3–5 seconds. It reduces the chair time and increases the efficiency of bonding especially in uncooperative and very apprehensive patients (Fig. 21.5).

Laser ablation of surface enamel for orthodontic bracket placement: Laser ablation has been proposed as an alternative method to acid etching. Common problems during orthodontic treatment after acid etching the enamel are demineralization and

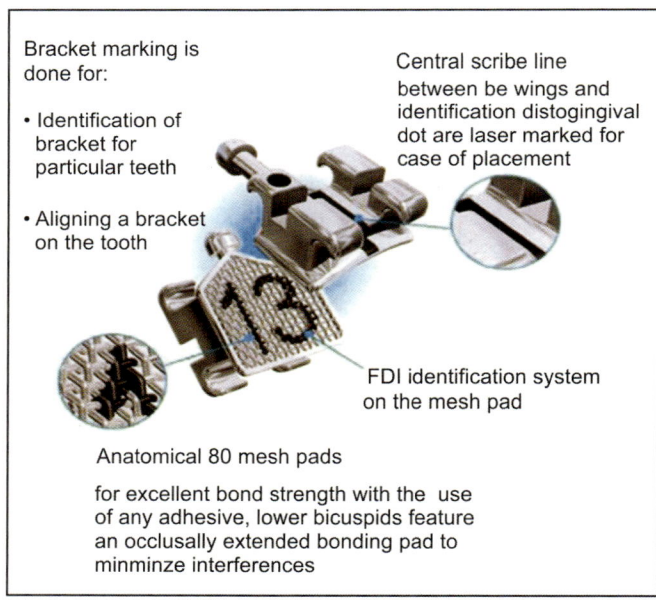

Bracket marking is done for:

• Identification of bracket for particular teeth

• Aligning a bracket on the tooth

Central scribe line between be wings and identification distogingival dot are laser marked for case of placement

FDI identification system on the mesh pad

Anatomical 80 mesh pads for excellent bond strength with the use of any adhesive, lower bicuspids feature an occlusally extended bonding pad to minminze interferences

Fig. 21.5: Bracket marking

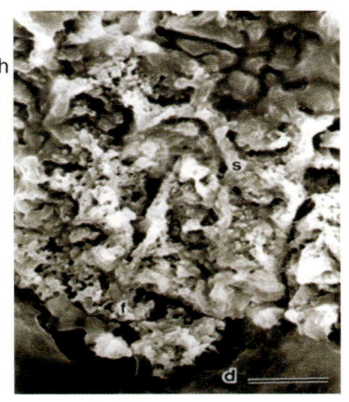

Etching: Process by which the surface of the tooth is made porous to increase the surface area for good bonding.

Lasers—act by localized melting and ablation of enamel surface.

Continuous vaporization and microexplosions—surface roughness.

Fig. 21.6: Etching

susceptibility to caries around brackets. Er:YAG laser ablation might overcome this drawback while offering other benefits like reduction in clinical time, good moisture control during bonding and bond strength similar to that of acid etching (Fig. 21.6).

Gaining access for bracket placement on partially erupted teeth: In certain cases, the orthodontic treatment is often prolonged due to incomplete or delayed eruption of the tooth, because the labial surface is covered by the gingiva, which hinders the bracket placement. In such cases, either we have to wait until tooth erupts completely till the occlusal plane or refer the patient to periodontist for removal of tissue to gain access for bracket placement. Either choice could add significant time to the overall treatment.

Removal of redundant gingival tissue by laser during orthodontic treatment: Poor oral hygiene in orthodontic patient results in swollen gingival tissue, which delays the orthodontic treatment. Laser can be used in the removal of redundant tissue, which fastens the progress of orthodontic treatment.

Management of aphthous ulcer by laser during orthodontic treatment: One of the most uncomfortable experiences for orthodontic patients is the formation of aphthous ulcer. Application of laser for aphthous ulcer helps in reducing the pain and also promotes healing. Healing usually takes place in a day. Laser irradiates the surface nerve ending and eliminates the painful stimuli.

Removal of operculae on second molar by laser: In some cases, second permanent molar is also bonded to provide additional anchorage and to avoid excessive repair visits. If second permanent molar is the last tooth in the arch, it is often associated with operculum.

Presence of operculum hinders the band placement. Removal of operculum by soft tissue laser facilitates the exposure of tooth, later providing accessibility for band placement.

Use of laser in controlling the growth of facial structure: Orthodontics is one of the important domains with interests in human growth and development. With the advent of 'high energy lasers' it may prove that research could lead to the use of lasers in the practice of orthodontics. 'High energy lasers' might be applied to manipulation of human facial growth leading to new methods to cope with problems either overgrowth or undergrowth.

Caries control during orthodontic treatment: Development/occurrence of dental caries is not an uncommon complication in orthodontic patient especially around brackets and in interproximal area after proximal stripping of teeth to gain space. Studies have demonstrated that Nd:YAG laser irradiation with fluoride application acts as an effective method of caires control during orthodontic treatment.

Tooth whitening by laser: Laser can be used for removal of intrinsic stains and/or postoperative tooth whitening to brighten the smile.

Depigmentation of gingiva by laser: Gingival pigmentation gives unesthetic appearance, especially during smiling and seen more commonly in black race groups. Lasers can be used to remove gingival pigmentation and helps in restoring the lost esthetics.

Crown lenthening procedure by laser: An excellent application of crown lengthening is when a canine is substituted for a congenitally missing lateral incisor. When the first premolar is in the canine position; its crown height looks too short. Some clinicians recommend intrusion of the premolar and placement of a laminate veneer to restore length. Another option; however, is to lengthen the premolar crown by laser gingivectomy.

Debonding of brackets by laser: Debonding of brackets is one of the most important procedures carried out after the active fixed mechanotherapy. Debonding of ceramic bracket is difficult and often results in fracture of brackets. Studies proved that application of lasers in debonding of metal brackets but also makes easy of ceramic bracket debonding and prevents fracture of enamel.

Holography

Holography is the science and practice of making holograms. Normally, a hologram is a photographic

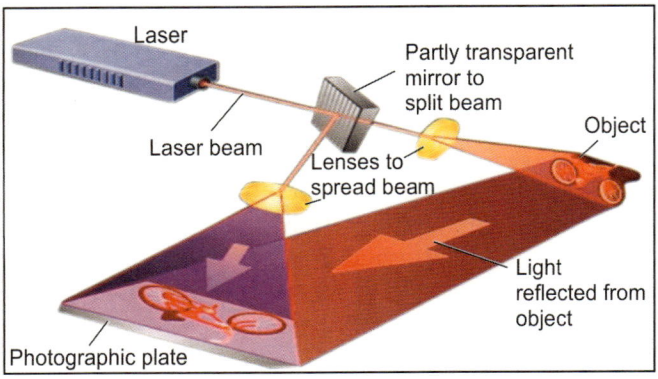

Fig. 21.7: Holographic studies

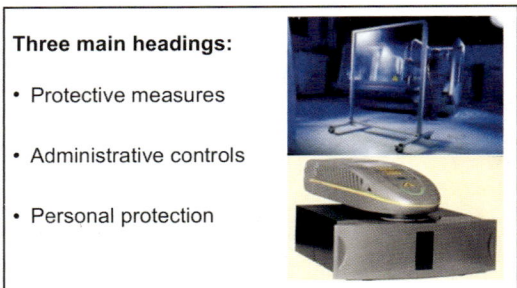

Fig. 21.8: Laser safty controls

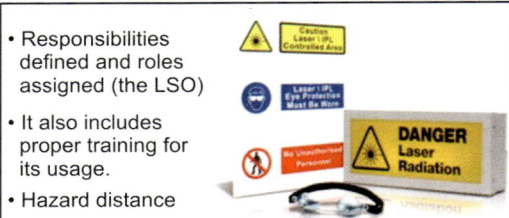

Fig. 21.9: Administrative controls

recording of a light field, rather than of an image formed by a lens, and it is used to display a fully three-dimensional image of the holographed subject, which is seen without the aid of special glasses or other intermediate optics.

Hologram is recorded using a flash of light that illuminates a scene and then imprints on a recording medium, much in the way a photograph is recorded. In addition, however, part of the light beam must be shone directly onto the recording medium—this second light beam is known as the reference beam. A hologram requires a laser as the sole light source. Lasers can be precisely controlled and have a fixed wavelength, unlike sunlight or light from conventional sources, which contain many different wavelengths. To prevent external light from interfering, holograms are usually taken in darkness, or in low level light of a different color from the laser light used in making the hologram. Holography requires a specific exposure time (just like photography), which can be controlled using a shutter, or by electronically timing the laser (Fig. 21.7).

Laser Safety (Figs 21.8–21.10)

Lasers are excellent tools, but they also bear a very high risk for severe injury and damage. Laser radiation mainly endangers eyes; the retina, cornea and the lens are concerned. Damage of the retina usually is permanent. Thus just a slight carelessness can impair your vision.

The second affected organ is although it is much less sensitive than eyes and damage occurs only at high energies. Hence, the high risks require suitable protective measures; their strict observation is the responsibility of the clinician and management.

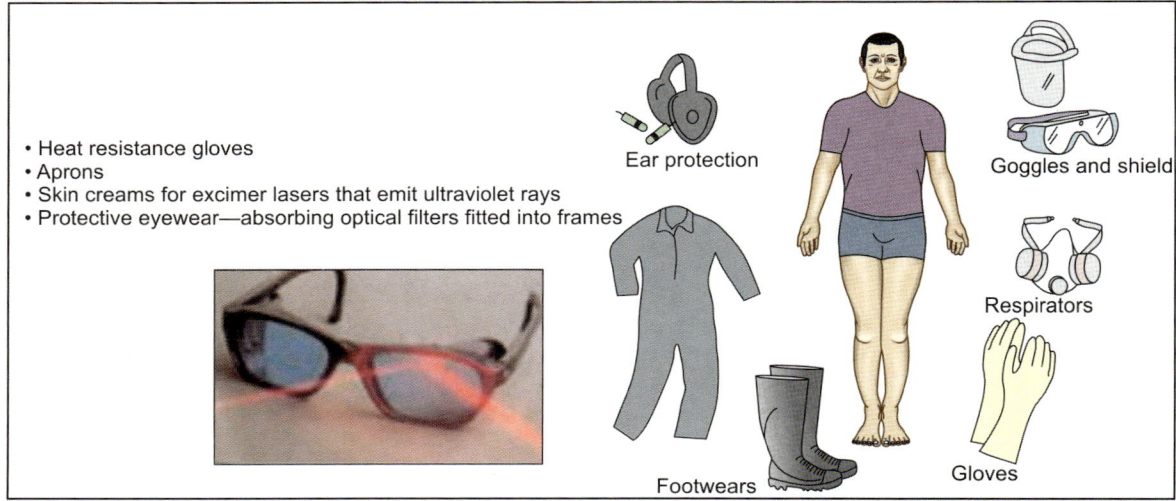

Fig. 21.10: Personal protection

Precautionary Measures

Following are the important precautionary measures prior to the handling and clinical applications of lasers (Fig. 21.10):

1. Always put on the protective eye glasses prior to the application of lasers. It is recommended to use only laser-specific protective eye glasses.
2. Make sure the door of the operatory room should always be closed.
3. Use of nonreflective instrument is recommended to avoid indirect hazard.
4. Cover the endotracheal tube with wet gauge piece or use special stainless steel tube to avoid combustion of anesthetic gases by laser beam.
5. Use of high vaccum suction or smoke evacuator for evacuation of toxic gases.

Laser Doppler Flowmetry (LDF)

It helps in assessing the vitality of the tooth during or prior to undergoing orthodontic treatment. It is a non-invasive electro-optical technique which measures the velocity of red cells.

Mode of action: Light emitted from the laser beam is scattered by the moving red cells within the pulp and the scattered light undergoes a frequency shift. The frequency shift is detected and processed to produce a signal that is a function of red cell influx therapy reflecting the vascular response.

Advantages: Non-invasive. It is valid as they reflect rather than nervous responsiveness.

Applications:
- Pulpal responses to orthodontic forces or orthopedic forces created by rapid maxillary expansion can be accurately assessed with LDF.
- It assesses the blood flow measurements after orthognathic surgery.

Growth Modfication

Low level laser (LLL) therapy is used in the growth modification procedure. It accelerates the process of bone regeneration during the consolidation phase after distraction osteogenesis. LLL associated with RME provides efficient opening of the midpalatal suture and influence the bone regeneration process of the suture accelerating healing.

Mode of action: It stimulates the mandibular growth by increasing the vascular endothelial growth factor (VEGF) and RUNX 2 in bone healing. RUNX 2 is involved in chondrocyte differentiation whereas VEGF and collagen type X are involved in endochondral ossification.

Influence of low level laser therapy on orthodontic tooth movement: Laser therapy causes the increase of receptor activator of nuclear factor Kappa-B ligand on periodontal ligament therapy increasing the rate of tooth movement during orthodontic treatment.

LLL therapy can increase macrophage colony-stimulating factor on the compressed side and may also increase osteoclastogenesis leading to tooth movement.

It increases osteoblastic cell proliferation and can, therefore, stimulate osteogenesis and increase bone density on the traction side.

Bibliography

1. Pick RM, Pecaro BC, Silberman CJ. The laser gingivectomy. The use of the CO_2 laser for removal of phytoin hyperplasia.
2. Sarver DM, Yanosky M. Principles of cosmetic dentistry in orthodontic part; part 3. Laser treatment for tooth eruption and soft tissue problems. Am J Orthod Dentofacial Orthop 2005; in press.
3. Midda M. The use of laser in periodontology. Curr Opin Dent 1992;2;104–8.
4. Von Fraunhofer JA, Allen DJ, Allen DJ, Orbell GM. Laser etching of enamel for firect bonding. Angle Orthod 1993; 63:73–6.

PREVIOUS YEAR'S UNIVERSITY QUESTIONS

MCQs

1. *Which of the following is not a soft tissue laser?*
   a. CO_2
   b. He-Ne
   C. Nd:YAG
   D. Er:YAG   **(Ans: d)**

2. *Which of the following is a hard tissue laser?*
   a. Cr:YSGG
   b. Ruby
   c. Argon
   d. Rhodium **(Ans: a)**

3. *An example of soft tissue laser in gas state:*
   a. Nd:YAG
   b. Ruby
   c. Rhodium
   d. CO_2 **(Ans: d)**

4. *Which of the following soft tissue lasers are in solid state?*
   a. He-Ne
   b. Argon
   c. Nd:YAG
   d. Rhodium   **(Ans: c)**

5. *Rhodium is an soft tissue laser and is in:*
   a. Solid state
   b. Liquid state
   c. Gas state
   d. All of the above   **(Ans: b)**

6. *Diode laser has a wavelength of:*
   a. 812 to 980 nm
   b. 10600 nm
   c. 2790 to 2940 nm
   d. 5000 to 8000 nm   **(Ans: a)**

7. *CO_2 laser operates with:*
   a. 10600 nm wavelength
   b. 20000 nm wavelength
   c. 1830 nm wavelength
   d. 2560 nm wavelength   **(Ans: a)**

8. *Frenectomy by laser has the following advantages, except:*
   a. Painless and bloodless procedure
   b. Recurrence can be prevented
   c. Facilitates the diastema closure
   d. Moves the maxillary permanent central incisors and thereby closes the midline diastema **(Ans: d)**

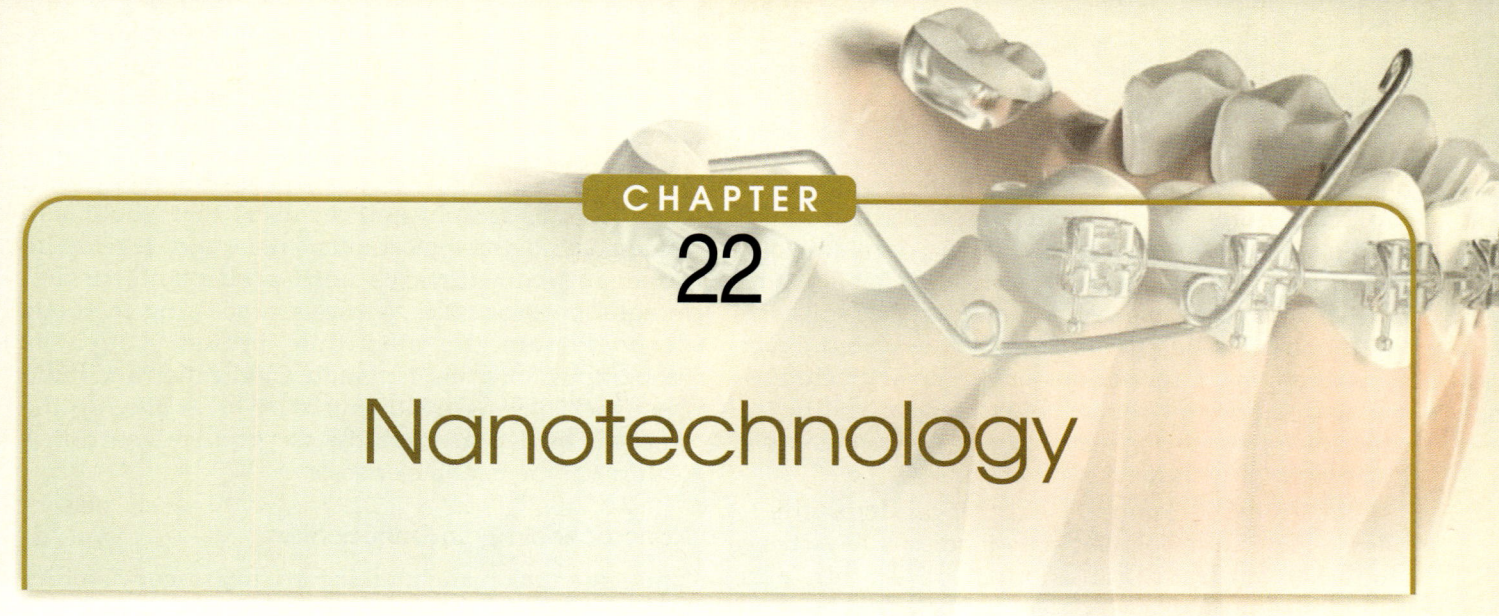

Nanotechnology

Chapter Outline

- Introduction
- Nanotechnology for craniofacial bone and cartilage tissue engineering
- Impact of nanotechnology on dental implants
- Nanotechnology in orthodontics
- Nanocoatings in archwires
- Nanoparticle in orthodontic adhesive
- Nanoparticle delivery from elastomeric ligature
- Shape memory polymers in orthodontics
- Control of biofilms during orthodontic treatment
- Smart brackets with nanomechanical sensors

INTRODUCTION

The term 'Nanotechnology' was coined by Prof. Kerie E Drexler. Nano is derived from the Greek word for 'Dwarf'. Nanotechnology is described as science and techniques which control and manipulate matter measured in the nanometer at a nanometric level, roughly the size of 2–3 atoms. A nanometer is one billionth of a meter or three to five atoms in width. It would take approximately 40,000 nanometers lined up in a row to equal the width of a human hair.

It has progressed tremendously in the last a few decades. Nanomaterials are materials with basic structural units, grains, particles, fibers or other constituent components smaller than 100 nm in at least one dimension and have great potential in disease prevention, diagnosis and treatment. To date, advances in this field have led to significant progress in tissue repair and regeneration. With the help of nanotechnology, it is possible to interact with cell components, to manipulate cell proliferation and differentiation and in the production and organization of extracellular matrices. New nanomaterials are leading to a range of emerging dental treatments that utilize more biometric materials that closely duplicate natural tooth structure.

The basic idea of this nanotechnology used in the narrow sense of the world is to employ individual atoms and molecules to construct functional structures. Minute particles with diameters of just million of a millimeter are the building blocks of new products known as nanoparticles. It deals with structures at sub-microscopic level.

The various nanoparticles are:
- Nanopores
- Nanotubes
- Quantum dots
- Nanoshells
- Fullerenas
- Nanospheres
- Nanowires
- Nanobelts
- Denfrimers
- Liposomes
- Nanorod
- Nanorings
- Nanocapsules

Nanotechnology for Craniofacial Bone and Cartilage Tissue Engineering

Craniofacial bone defects secondary to trauma, infection, cancer and congenital disorders represent major health problems. Current strategies aimed at replacing bony defects include the utilization of autografts, allografts and synthetic biomaterials. Despite the fact these substitutes restore stability and function to a reasonable degree, however, they still have limitations. Tissue engineering is considered as an optimal approach for various tissue repairs including craniofacial defect repair. Biomaterials, acting as scaffolds for tissue engineering, play an essential role in the process of tissue regeneration.

Due to the biometric features and excellent physiochemical properties, nanomaterials have been shown to improve adhesion, proliferation and differentiation of cells which would finally guide tissue regeneration.

Within the craniofacial tissue engineering field, the major types of materials used are natural and synthetic polymers, ceramics, composite materials and electrospun nanofibers. Synthetic and natural polymers are excellent candidates for bone/cartilage tissue engineering application due to their biodegradability and ease of fabrication. Nanophase ceramics are popular as bone substitutes, coatings and filler materials due to their dimensional similarity to bone/cartilage tissue and unique surface properties including surface topography, surface chemistry, surface wettability and surface energy.

Impact of Nanotechnology on Dental Implants

One of the challenges in implantology is to achieve and maintain the osseointegration as well as the epithelial junction of the gingiva with implants. An intimate junction of the gingival tissue with the neck of dental implants may prevent bacterial colonizations leading to peri-implantitis while direct bone bonding may ensure a biomechanical anchoring of the artificial dental root.

The first step of the osseointegration of implants is called primary stability and is related to the mechanical anchorage, design of implants and bone structure. This primary interlock decreases with time at the benefit of the secondary anchorage, which is characterized by a biological bonding at the interface between bone tissues and implant surface.

Many studies have attempted to enhance the osseointegration of implants by various surface modifications. The aim is to produce metal implants with surface biological properties for the adsorption of proteins, the adhesion and differentiation of cells and tissue integration. These biological properties are related to chemical composition, wettability and roughness of metal implant surfaces.

Nanotechnologies may produce surfaces with controlled topography and chemistry that would help understanding biological interactions and developing novel implant surfaces with predictable tissue-integrative properties. Various processing methods derived from the electronic industry such as lithography, ionic implantation, anodization and radio frequency plasma treatments may be applied to the surfaces of dental implants to produce controlled features at the nanometer scale.

Nanotechnology in Orthodontics

Nanoindentation and atomic force microscopy studies on orthodontic brackets and archwires the surface characteristics, i.e. roughness and surface-free energy (SFE) of the brackets play a significant role in reducing friction and plaque formation. A nanoindenter coupled with atomic force microscope (AFM) is used to evaluate surface characteristics of biomaterials. They have also been used to evaluate mechanical properties such as hardness, elastic modules, yield strength, fracture toughness, scratch hardness and wear properties by nanoindentation.

Nanocoatings in Archwires

Minimizing the frictional forces between the orthodontic wire and brackets has the potential to increase the desired tooth movement and, therefore, result in less treatment time. Nanoparticles have been used as a component of dry lubricants in recent years. Dry lubricants are solid phase materials capable to reduce friction between two surfaces sliding against each other without the need for a liquid media, inorganic fullerence like nanoparticles of tungsten sulfide (IF-WS2), which are potent dry lubricants, have been used as self-lubricating coatings for orthodontic stainless steel wires.

Nanoparticle in Orthodontic Adhesive

Polymer nanocomposites are a new class of materials containing nanofillers that are 0.005–0.01 µ in size. To make filler particles of the mechanically strong composites of today (such as macrofills, hybrids and microhybrids), one starts from dense, large particles like mine quartz, melt glasses, ceramics and comminute them to small particle size. Due to the reduced dimension of the particles and a wide size distribution, an increased filler load can be achieved that reduces polymerization shrinkage and also increases mechanical properties such as tensile and compressive strength and resistance to fracture. Geradeli and Perdiago reported that nanocomposites had a good marginal seal to enamel and dentin as compared with total arch etch adhesives. The advantages of the nano-composite materials include excellent optical properties, easy handling characteristics and superior polishability. Also, nanofillers can decrease surface roughness of orthodontic adhesives which is one of the most significant factors for bacterial adhesion.

In recent times, a nanoionomer which is resin-modified GIC (Ketac N 100 light-curing nanoionomer) has been introduced to operative dentistry. This light curing glass and nanofiller cluster combined to improve mechanical properties and high fluoride release.

Nanoparticle Delivery from Elastomeric Ligature

Elastomeric ligatures can serve as a carrier scaffold for delivery of nanoparticles that can be anticariogenic, anti-inflammatory and antibiotic drug molecules embedded in the elastomeric matrix. The release of anticariogenic fluoride from elastomeric ligatures has been reported in the literature previously. The studies conclude that the fluoride release is characterized by an initial Burt of fluoride during the first a few days followed by a logarithmic decrease. For optimum clinical benefit, the fluoride ties should be replaced monthly.

Shape Memory Polymers in Orthodontics

Over the last decade, there has been an increased interest in manufacturing esthetic orthodontic wires to complement tooth-colored brackets. Shape memory esthetic polymer is an area of potential research. Shape memory polymers are materials that have the ability to memorize a macroscopic or equilibrium shape under specific conditions of temperature and stress.

Once placed in the mouth, these polmers can be activated by the body temperature or photoactive nanoparticles activated by light and thus bring about tooth movement. The SMP orthodontic wires can provide improvements over traditional orthodontic materials as they will provide lighter, more constant forces which in turn may cause less pain for the patients. In addition, the SMP materials are clear, colorable and stain resistant, providing the patient a more esthetically appealing appliance during treatment. The high percent elongations of the SMP appliance (up to about 300%) allows for the application of the continuous forces over a long range of tooth movement and hence, result in fewer visits for the patient.

Control of Biofilms during Orthodontic Treatment

NPs present a greater surface to volume ratio (per unit mass) when compared with non-nanoscale particles, interesting more closely with microbial membranes and provide considerably larger surface area for antimicrobial activity. Metal NPS in the size range of 1–10 nm have particularly shown the greatest biocidal activity against bacteria. Silver has a long history of use in medicine as an antimicrobial agent. The mechanism of combining dental materials with NPs or coating surface with NPs is to prevent microbial adhesion with the aim of reducing biofilm formation. Resin composites containing silver ion implanted fillers that release silver ions have been found to have antibacterial effects on oral streptococci.

Smart Brackets with Nanomechanical Sensors

Nanomechanical sensors can be fabricated and be incorporated into the base of orthodontic brackets in order to provide real-time feedback about the applied orthodontic forces. This real-time feedback allows the orthodontist to adjust the applied force to be within a biological range to efficiently move teeth with minimal side effects.

BIBLIOGRAPHY

1. Warren SM, Fong KD, Chen CM, Loboa EG, Cowan CM, Lorenz HP, et al. Tools and techniques for craniofacial tissue engineering. Tissue Eng 2003;9:187–200.
2. Zhang LJ, Webster TJ. Nanotechnology and nanomaterial: promises for improved tissue regeneration. Nano Today 2009;4:66–80.
3. Gupte MJ, Ma PX. Nanofibrous scaffolds for dental and craniofacial applications. J Dent Res 2012;91:227–234.
4. Lavenus S, Louarn G, Layrolle P. Nanotechnology and dental implants. Int J Biomater 2010 (2010) 915327.

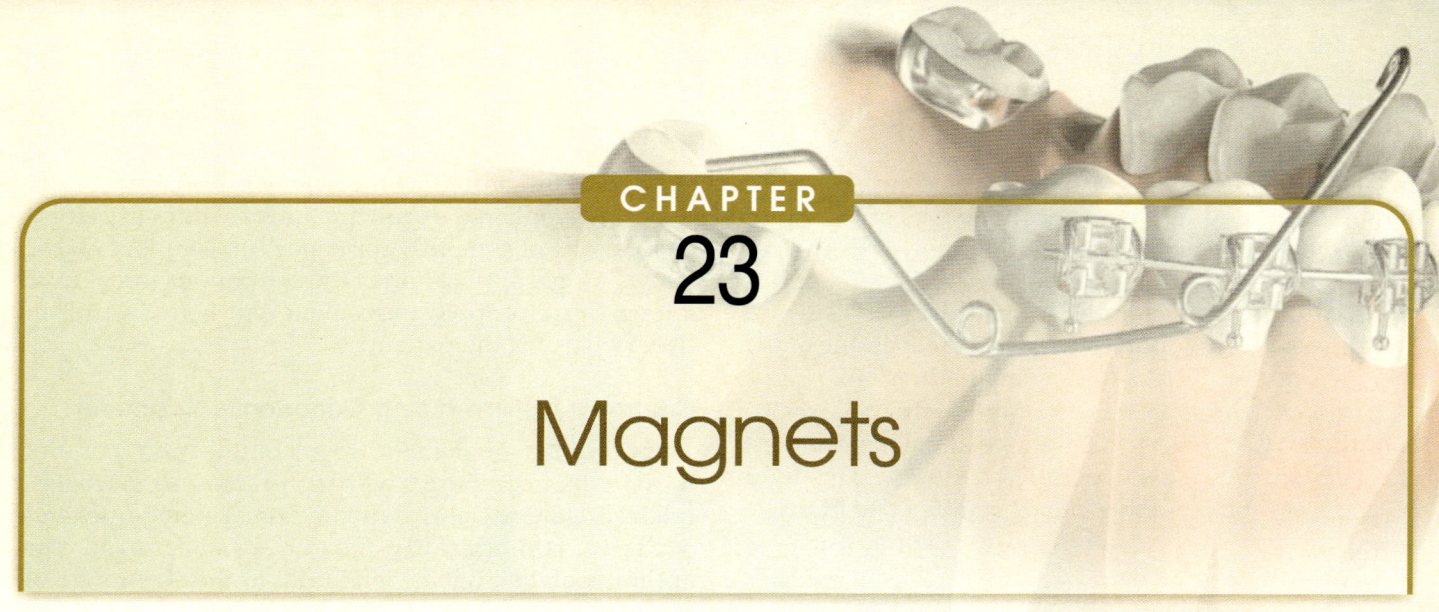

Magnets

Chapter Outline

- Introduction
- Properties of magnets
- Types of magnetic materials
- Biologic concept of magnetic force and histologic changes
- Magnetic force systems in orthodontics
- Recycling

INTRODUCTION

Magnets have been used in orthodontics since last a few years. Magnets have tendency of getting oxidized in the oral cavity and formation of corrosive products, leading to deterioration of magnetic properties. It can be overcome by coating magnets.

Magnetite is an iron ore discovered in Magnesia—a town in Asia Minor.

Chinese discovered that a free magnet always points in a North–South direction.

History

- The first use of magnets in dentistry was by Behran and Egan in the year 1953. They used it as implants for denture retention.
- First use of magnets for tooth movement was described by Blechman and Smiley by experimenting on cats.
- Becker in 1970 introduced rare earth magnets having properties superior to previously used magnetic alloys.
- 1978—in orthodontics, Blecham and Smily used aluminum, nickel.
- Cobalt magnets (Animal study)
- 1985—Abraham Blechman first used in human beings.

- 1970—Becker introduced the samarium cobalt magnets.
- Later, neodymium-iron-boron magnets were introduced.

Magnetic Substances

Iron, cobalt, nickel alloys are attracted by magnets—Ferromagnetic material. Artificial magnets are obtained by rubbing these alloys with natural magnetite. This process is called magnetization.

PROPERTIES OF MAGNETS

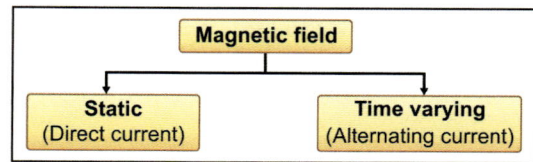

Hard Magnets—Resistant to Demagnetization

- Keeps its magnetic qualities in the presence of a higher magnetic field, an increase in temperature, a decrease in its size to 1 mm or less.
- Soft magnets: Opposite properties.
- Coulomb's law: The force between two magnetic poles is proportional to their magnitude and

inversely proportional to the square of the distance between them.
- Curie point: Magnets tend to lose their properties, if subjected to a specific temperature which causes their domain to return to random distribution. This point of temperature is called Curie point.
- Lines of forces

Characteristics of Lines of Forces (Fig. 23.1)

- Magnetic lines of force are closed curves starting from the north pole and ending on the south pole of the magnet. Within the magnet, they run from south to north.
- They are in a state of tension which causes them to shorten longitudinally.
- They repel each other sideways.
- They do not intersect each other.
- The density of lines is more where the field is stronger and less where the field is weak.

Other Characteristic Features of Magnets

- When a magnet is broken into two pieces, each portion behaves like a magnet with two poles. Opposite poles appear at the point of the break. This is due to the fact that the south poles are exposed at one side of the bar and free north poles at the other.

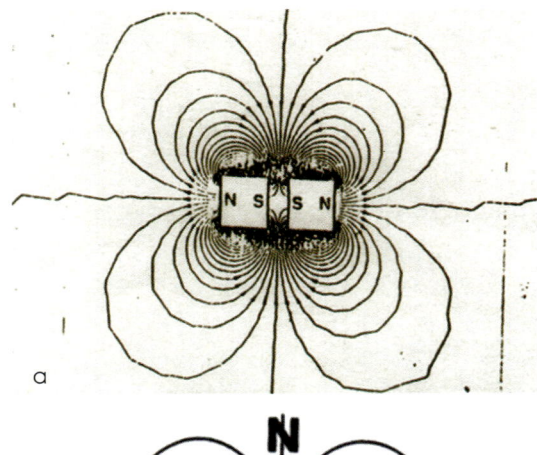

a

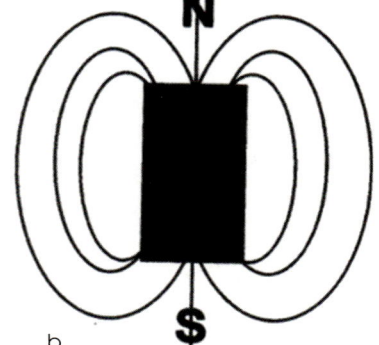

b

Fig. 23.1a and b: Lines of forces—Vean's classification

- A magnet cannot be magnetized beyond a certain limit. This is because once the orientation of the molecular magnets in the direction of the magnetizing field has taken place, the saturation point is reached. It cannot be magnetized further.
- When the magnet is heated or hammered, it loses its magnetism. The alignment of molecular magnets is disturbed due to heating or hammering and hence the magnetism is lost.
- When an iron bar is magnetized along its length, its length slightly increases. This is due to the alignment of molecular magnets parallel to its length. The increase in length is called magnetic traction.
- The two poles of a bar magnet are of equal strength because the number of free north poles is equal to the number of free south poles at the other end.
- If a steel bar is heated to redness and allowed to cool in N-S direction, it becomes a weak magnet.
- A bar magnet tends to become weaker with age owing to self-demagnetization.

Magnetic Induction

Non-magnetized steel, when kept near to, or in contact with a pole of magnet and then removed shows magnetic properties. This is called induced magnetism and the process—magnetic induction.

Magnetic Moment

The magnetic moment of a magnet is the moment of the couple acting on the magnet when placed at right angles to the direction of a uniform magnetic field of unit strength.

Energy Product

The energy product of a magnet indicates the stored energy.
- Calculated by multiplying the field flux density and the magnets motive force.
- Value is expressed in Gauss oersted.

Magnetic Properties Relevant

1. *High force to volume ratio:* In rare earth magnets, if we compare $SmCo_5$ magnet and $Nd_2Fe_{14}B$ magnets, it is found that $SmCo_5$ magnets are:
   - 20 times stronger
   - 20 times smaller (Fig. 23.2)
   - High magnetic induction
   - 240 times less susceptible to corrosion
2. *Maximum force at short distance:* All magnets follow Coulomb's law.

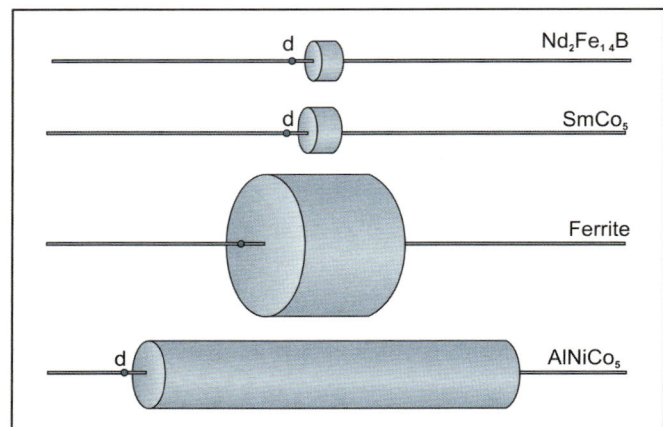

Fig. 23.2: Different magnetic size

3. *Three-dimensional centripetal orientation of attractive magnetic force:* When two magnets are displaced in all three places, they attract to complete overlap.
4. *No interruption of magnetic force lines by intermittent media:* Any media interposed between two magnets cannot bar the passage of magnetic force lines.
5. *No friction in attractive force configuration:* Frictional forces are excluded in attracting magnets (Darendililer). In repulsive magnets, Muller prongs guiding elements are used. They induce friction.
6. *No energy loss:*
   • High coercive force
   • Can maintain energy for years provided it is protected against corrosion, temperature and other biologic pertuberance.

TYPES OF MAGNETIC MATERIALS

In various dental applications of magnets, the following materials have been used.

Conventional magnets:
• Platinum-cobalt (Pt-Co)
• Aluminum-nickel-cobalt (AlNiCo)
• Ferrite
• Chromium-cobalt-iron

Rare earth magnets:
• Samarium-cobalt (SmCo)
• Neodymium-iron-boron ($Nd_2Fe_{14}B$)

Samarium-Cobalt Magnets ($SmCo_5$ and Sm_2Co_{17})

Becker in 1970 brought these into clinical application. It is a powdered metallurgically processed inter-metallic alloy of cobalt and rare earth metals and its main components can be expressed as $SmCo_5$.
• Superior magnetic properties when compared to other rare earth magnets except neodymium-iron-boron magnets.

• Even with a flat shape, there is hardly any demagnetization making it ideal and small for orthodontic use.
• The force necessary in orthodontics can be obtained from a small sized magnet (measurable in millimeters)
• Magnetic properties are invariable in course of time, i.e. high resistance to demagnetization with time.
• High Curie point of 680°C allowing heat sterilization and manipulation with heat up to 200°C without demagnetization.
• Corrosion resistance is high comparatively since they are parylene-coated to prevent leaking of toxic substances. They can also be encased in stainless steel jackets.
• They should be handled with care as they are brittle but are stronger than neodymium-iron-boron magnets. Hence they are difficult to process but can be filed slightly with dental tools.

Other properties:
• Density—8.1 g/cm³
• Coefficient of thermal expansion: Similar to chromium-cobalt casting alloy.
• Hardness is very high and elongation is nearly zero resulting in a slightly brittle and liable to cleave material.
• *Fabrication:* The magnet is difficult to process, though possible to file it with dental tools. Since it is impossible to cast it clinically, it is necessary to prepare standardized magnets which are designed commercially for specific applications.

Neodymium-Iron-Boron ($Nd_2Fe_{14}B$) Magnets

It was introduced by Robinson in 1984, an alloy of neodymium, iron and boron has been available in:
1. Various sizes and shapes suitable for intraoral use. They are produced by powder metallurgy.
2. Provide the highest energy per unit volume of any commercially available magnetic material.
3. They are 70% more powerful than a same size Sm-Co magnet and are supplied in a magnetized condition with a tin protective finish. Their disadvantage is that they are brittle and have to be handled carefully. But their added advantage is that they are reasonably priced.

BIOLOGIC CONCEPT OF MAGNETIC FORCE AND HISTOLOGIC CHANGES

Orthodontic tooth movement produces stress that induces various biochemical changes.

Magnets

- Magnetic forces inflicted a minimum of such stresses.
- No subcutaneous changes as inflammation.
- Reduced thickness of epithelium.
- Resorption of bone under magnets after 3–4 weeks.
- Erythrocytes become thinner and longer enhancing the movement in compressed periodontal ligament-reducing bone necrosis.

McDonald (1993)—increased proliferation and systemic activity in fibroblasts in presence of static magnetic field.

Lars Bondemark and Kurol—no difference in clinical gingival condition.

Nanda and Woods—biologically optimum intrusive force is 450 gm.

Sandler—found no biohazardous effects with rare earth magnets.

Cytotoxicity

Bondemark and Kurol-Cermy conducted studies on the cytotoxic effects of magnets. There are two methods—millipore filter method and extraction method.

Results

- Uncoated $SmCo_5$ showed high cytotoxicity.
- Uncoated $SmCo_{17}$ showed moderate cytotoxicity.
- Uncoated $Nd_2Fe_{14}B$ showed negligible cytotoxicity.
- Parylene-coated magnets showed negligible cytotoxcity.

Advantages

- It eliminates patient cooperation as it is totally operator controlled.
- It produces less pain and discomfort.
- Continuous force is exerted by magnets.
- Treatment time is reduced.
- Magnetic tooth movement is biologically more acceptable with reduced periodontal disturbance, root resorption and caries.
- No friction
- Appliance adjustments are minimal; therefore, it takes less chair time.
- Letter force, working range control is achieved by maintaining the distance between magnets. Better directional force control.

Disadvantages

1. They suffer significantly from tarnish and corrosion.
2. Tarnish and corrosion products are cytotoxic.
3. Concerns have been expressed on the bioeffects of static magnetic fields.
4. Bulk of magnets is still a concern in space limiting applications.
5. Cost is also an unfavorable factor.
6. Bitterness.

MAGNETIC FORCE SYSTEMS IN ORTHODONTICS

Magnetic force delivery systems are now popularly used for:

1. Relocating impacted teeth (Vardimon et al, 1991)
2. Expansion of arch (Alexander in 1987)
3. Distalization/mesialization of teeth (Anatomy Gianelly and others, 1988)
4. Intrusion of posterior teeth in open bite cases (Delligner, 1986)
5. Class II correction with functional appliance (Ali Darendeliler, 1993)
6. Skeletal correction with functional appliance (FOMA)
7. Closure of diastema (Muller, 1984)
8. Uprighting and derotation of teeth
9. Retainers (Springate, 1991)
10. Magnetic brackets (Terushige Kawate, 1987)
11. PUMA: Hemifacial microsomia (Chate, 1995)
12. Class II correction with magnetic twin block (Clark)
13. Non-extraction and extraction cases
14. Magnetic appliance for treatment of snoring patients with and without obstructive sleep apnea.
15. Extrusion of fractured teeth (Bondemark and Kurol 1997)

Magnets with Fixed Appliances (Abraham Blechman, 1985)

It is used for upper canine retraction. Magnetic assembly on upper and lower sectional arches which are free to slide. Retraction enhanced by three magnet assembly. Anterior magnets in repulsive mode whereas posterior magnets in attractive mode (Fig. 23.3).

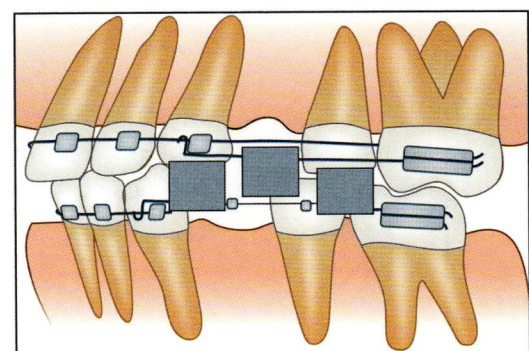

Fig. 23.3: Canine retraction using magnets

Premolar space closures in both upper and lower: Three magnetic assembly all in attractive mode are fixed with fixed appliance 2 mm air gap extraction cases: Class II mechanics produced by magnets in repulsion with zero air gap.

Magnetic Twin Blocks

It was introduced by WJ Clark. Addition of magnets on occlusal planes maximizes the orthopedic response to treatment. Attracting/repelling magnets can be used. Repelling magnets can also be used but attracting magnets are found to be advantageous (Fig. 23.4).

Magnetic Brackets (Alex D. Vardimon and Graber)

$Nd_2Fe_{14}B$ magnetic alloy is affixed between two machined down tie wings of a twin bracket and coated with parylene. Brackets are classified as vertical and horizontal according to the magnetic axis. A newly modified version developed by Kawata has a slot incorporated in the magnet. It allows simultaneous edgewise archwire mechanics with an attractive magnetic force system.

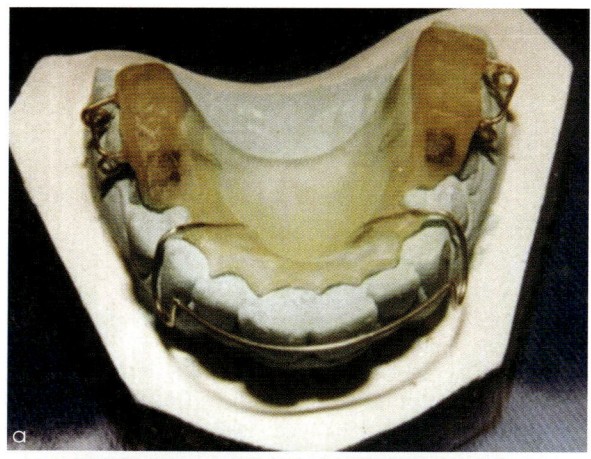

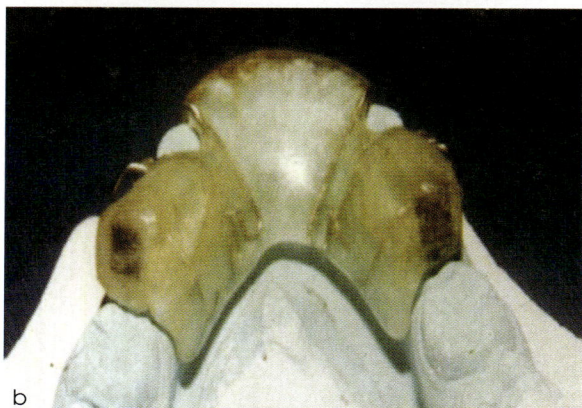

Fig. 23.4: (a) Upper bite block with magnet; (b) Lower bite block with magnet

Molar Distalization

The repelling mode works between upper premolar and molars. The activation is done once a week since force drops 200 to 75 gm on 1 mm movement. It should prevent untreated lateral shifts (Fig. 23.5).

Propellant Unilateral Magnetic Appliance (PUMA)

It is used by Chate. It stimulates autogenous costochondral graft in hemifacial microsomia using samarium magnet. Magnetic appliance is used for treatment of snoring patients with or without obstructive sleep apnea (Bennhold and Bondemark). It consists of two intraoral occlusal splints U and L and four parylene-coated neodymium-iron-boron magnets. It prevents backward movement of mandibular complex. It covers full tooth coverage to prevent unwanted tooth movements.

Rare Earth Magnets and Impaction (Vardimon, Darendililer and Sandler)

Magnetic bracket in an intraoral magnet is used to guide erupting teeth. It is used in impacted incisors and canines. Small bonded magnet is attached coronal to a larger magnet in a removable appliance. Small magnet is bonded on unerupted tooth coronal to a larger magnet in a removable appliance in case of molar impaction (Fig. 23.6).

Functional Orthopaedic Magnetic Appliances (FOMA) (Vardimon)

Functional appliance with magnets is incorporated in upper and lower plates. It corrects Class II (FOMA II) and Class III (FOMA III) malocclusion.

FOMA II: For Class II with upper magnet anterior to lower magnet

FOMA III: For Class III with magnets placed to stimulate maxilla and retard mandibular growth.

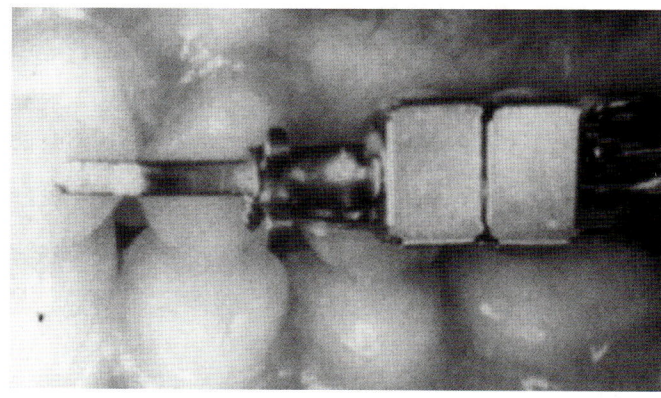

Fig. 23.5: Molar distalizer using repelling magnets

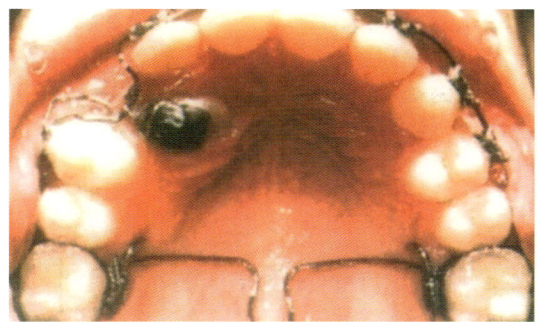
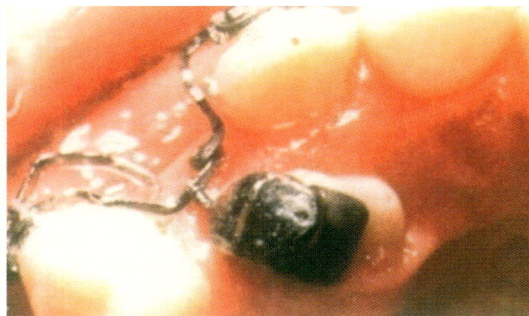

Fig. 23.6: Magnets in palatal impaction

Closing Diastemas (Fig. 23.7)

It was reported by Muller (1984). SmCo magnets (117.5 gm) are bonded on each central incisor labially or palatally in attracting mode. No friction and no reactivation are necessary.

Extrusion of Fractured Teeth (Fig. 23.8)

It was reported by Bondemark and Kurol (1997) for subgingival fractures $Nd_2Fe_{14}B$ magnets are placed coronal to remaining tooth. Larger attracting magnet is placed axially over it in a removable appliance. Magnets work in attractive mode with a gap of 2 mm.

Autonomous Fixed Appliance (Fig. 23.9) (Darendilier and Joho (1992)

They used full bonded upper and lower magnets of $SmCo_5$ on individual tooth. The individual magnets deliver a force of 20–30 gm. The magnets were coated with composite resin to prevent corrosion. It was also coated to prevent toxic leakage.

Magnetic Retainer (Fig. 23.10) (Springate (1991)

It is used $Nd_2Fe_{14}B$ magnets fixed palatally as a retainer in a case with persistant midline spacing.

Active Vertical Corrector by Eugene Dellinger (1986)

Skeletal open bites are caused mainly by over eruption of the upper posterior teeth or vertical over growth of

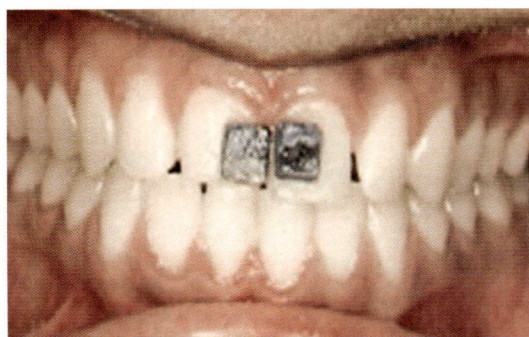

Fig. 23.7: Midline diastema using magnets. This picture shows post treatment

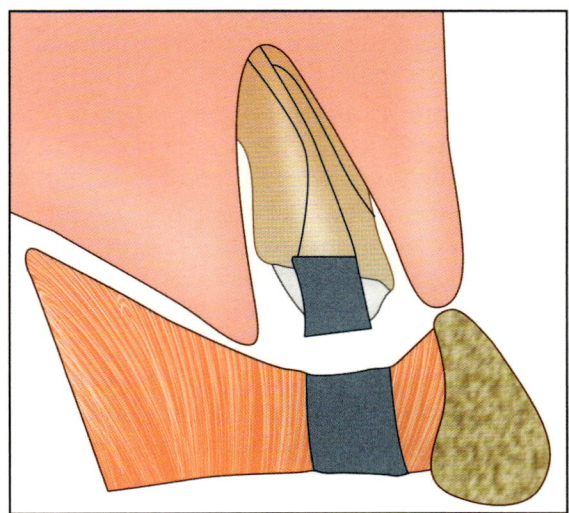

Fig. 23.8: Extrusion of fractured tooth

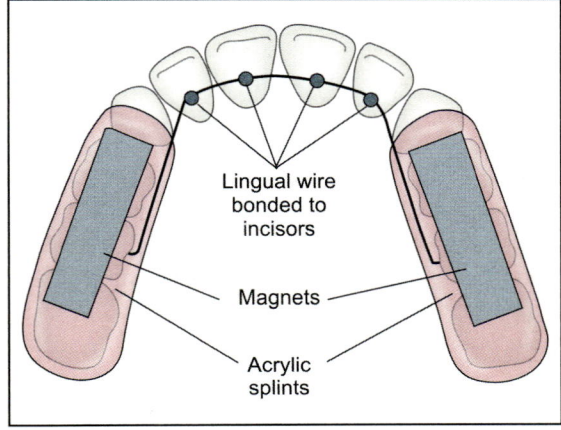

Lingual wire bonded to incisors

Magnets

Acrylic splints

Fig. 23.9: Fixed appliance

the posterior dentoalveolar complex. These could be due to posterior rotation of the mandible, superior repositioning of the glenoid fossa due to under development of the anterior portion of the maxilla or a combination of these effects.

Surgical intervention such as LeFort I procedure is the treatment of choice for a severe skeletal open bite.

Orthodontically, early correction can be achieved through high-pull headgears, activator, combined headgear and upper plate, open bite bionator and activator headgear combinations.

These are two treatment approaches available:

1. Orthodontically, early correction can be achieved through high-pull headgears, activator, combined headgear and upper plate, open bite bionator, activator headgear combinations, active and passive bite blocks and vertical chin cups. High-pull headgear is a popular approach to the correction of anterior open bite inhibiting vertical maxillary development and allow for a forward rotation of the mandible, thus closing the bite.

2. An alternative approach to open bite correction is posterior bite blocks to achieve inhibiton of maxillary posterior dentoalveolar development and autorotation.

This is achieved by preventing the maxillary and mandibular posterior teeth from erupting and by opening the bite several millimeters so as to stretch the posterior muscles of mastication causing them to act as intrusive agents on the maxilla.

The active vertical corrector (AVC) is an adaptation of the present day bite block therapy introduced in 1986 by Dr. Eugene L. Dellinger. The active vertical corrector is a patented appliance of Allessee Orthodontic Appliances (AOA) a subsidiary of ORMCO. In this article, a case report is presented treated with AVC.

Design of the Appliance

It works as an energized bite block consisting of two posterior occlusal splints, one for the upper and one for the lower jaw. Samarium-cobalt magnets are incorporated into the acrylic splints over the occlusal region of the teeth to be intruded. One magnet per distal quadrant is used. The magnets in the upper splints are incorporated in a mode to repel the magnets in the lower splints, therefore, the appliance is a combination of acrylic posterior bite blocks and repelling magnetic forces.

The magnets used are cylindrical in shape with a diameter of 10 mm. The magnets along with the bite blocks measured 12 mm in height. Because Samarium-cobalt is a highly reactive, rare earth material, they are best isolated from the oral environment. Hence, they are hermetically sealed in stainless steel capsules. The magnets are also parylene coated to prevent leaching out of cytotoxic materials. The magnets generate a force of 700 gm per unit at zero air gaps in repulsion (Fig. 23.11).

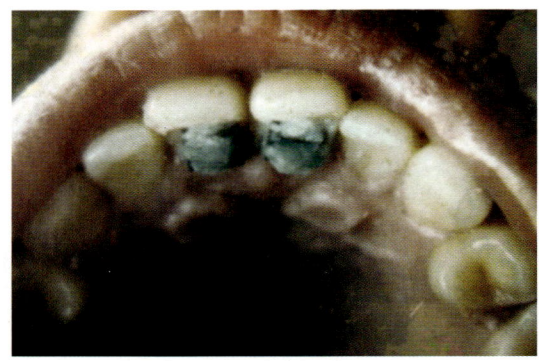

Fig. 23.10: Magnetic retainer

Bite Registration

The appropriate vertical height is established giving 5 mm space in the posterior region to accommodate magnets, casings and acrylic splints (4 mm plus 1 mm safety factor equals 5 mm).

Magnetic Activator Device (MAD)

Darendilier (1993) developed a series of magnetically active functional appliance of different varieties to be used in different conditions.

Types

- MAD I is used to treat mandibular deviations.
- MAD II for correction of Class II division 1 malocclusions. Sm_2Co_{17} magnets deliver forces ranging from 150 to 600 gm per side.
- MAD III for correction of Class III malocclusions. Upper MAD III can be used for magnetic expansion also.
- MAD IV for correction of open bite.

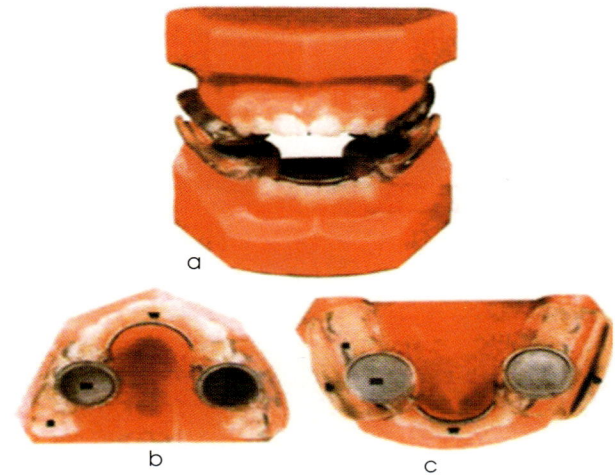

Fig. 23.11: (a) Active vertical corrector; (b) Maxillary component; (c) Mandibular component

RECYCLING

Recycling does not affect the biocompatibility and force stability of the magnets even though the recycling process involved autoclaving since it has a high Curie point of 680°C. New partially encased samarium-cobalt magnets can be stored in water for 24 hours before use to reduce the release of cytotoxic components.

Bibliography

1. Ali Darendeliler M, et al. Clinical application of magnets in orthodontics and biological implications: A review. The European Journal of Orthodontics 1997; 19(4) (Oxford University Press Permissions).
2. Martinette Muller. The use of magnets in orthodontics: an alternative means to produce tooth movement. The European Journal of Orthodontics 1984; 6(1) (Oxford University Press Permissions).

PREVIOUS YEAR'S UNIVERSITY QUESTIONS

Essay

1. What are the properties of magnets?
2. Write a brief note about Samavium Cobalt magnets.

Short Notes

1. What are the application of magnets in orthodontics?

2. Write the types of magnetic material.
3. Magnetic twin block
4. Active vertical corrector (AVC)
5. Coulomb's Law
6. Neodymium-iron-boron magnets
7. Cytotoxicity

MCQs

1. *Who introduced magnetic twin block?*
   a. William clark
   b. Eugene Dellinger
   c. Chate
   d. Springate   **(Ans: a)**

2. *Which material passes superior magnetic properties?*
   a. Samarium cobalt magnets
   b. Neodymium-iron-boron
   c. Chromium cobalt iron
   d. Platinum cobalt   **(Ans: a)**

3. *Who introduced neodymium-cobalt magnets?*
   a. Robinson
   b. Becker
   c. Alexander
   d. Vardimon   **(Ans: a)**

Radiography in Orthodontics

Chapter Outline

- History
- Role of radiography in orthodontics
- Intraoral radiographs
- Extraoral radiograph
- Computerized cephalometrics
- Hand wrist radiograph
- Xeroradiography

- Digital radiography
- MRI
- Conventional tomography
- CBCT
- Cinefluororadiography
- Photocephalometry
- Occlusogram

HISTORY

On November 8th, 1895, a Bavarian physicist Wilhelm Conrad Roentgen discovered X-rays. Dr. Otto Walkhoff developed the first original dental 'roentgenogram' from a portion of a glass imaging plate.

- In1904—introduction of bisecting technique by WA Price.
- In 1920—concept of paralleling technique by McCormack
- In 1923—first dental X-ray machine by Victor.
- In 1925—introduction of bitewing technique by R. Raper.
- In 1933—concept of rotational panoramic proposed by Numata.
- In 1948—introduction of panoramic radiography by Paatero.
- In 1955—introduction of d-speed films.
- In 1969—prototype scanner developed.
- In 1978—dental xeroradiography is introduced.
- In 1981—speed films are introduced.
- In 1987—intraoral digital radiography is introduced.
- In 1987—denta scan design is introduced.
- In 2000—speed films are introduced.

ROLE OF RADIOGRAPHY IN ORTHODONTICS

- Diagnosis (confirm/exclude) and treatment planning.
- During treatment and follow-up visits.
- For further investigations.
- To study the character of alveolar bone.
- Valuable aid in craniodentofacial analysis.
- For the calculation of the total tooth material (mesio-distal dimension of the permanent teeth)
- To confirm the axial inclination of roots of the teeth.

Intraoral radiographs:
- Intraoral periapical (IOPA) radiographs.
- Bitewing radiographs.
- Occlusal radiographs.

Extraoral radiographs:
- Orthopentemograph
- Cephalometric radiograph
- Hand-wrist radiographs
- Xeroradiography
- Digital radiography
- Tomography
- Cone beam computed tomography

- Occlusograms
- Digital subtraction radiography
- Photocephalometry
- MRI (magnetic resonance imaging)
- Laser holography
- Cinefluororadiography

INTRAORAL RADIOGRAPHS (Fig. 24.1)

Intraoral Periapical (IOPA) Radiograph

Most commonly used radiograph in dentistry. It is used to visualize the teeth and the supporting alveolar bone. Adult size IOPA film measures 32 × 41 mm. In this technique, the X-ray film is placed in the mouth lingual to the teeth to be examined. There are two methods of obtaining IOPA radiographs:

1. Paralleling technique
2. Bisecting angle technique

Paralleling Technique

X-film is placed parallel to the long axis of the teeth. Central ray of the collimated X-ray beam is perpendicular to the long axis of the tooth and the film.

Advantage: Reduced geometric distortion.

Disadvantage: Morphological limitations imposed by oral cavity in the correct placement of the film.

Bisecting Angle Technique

This technique is based on the principle of Cieszynski's rule of isometry, which is a geometric theorem. According to this principle, two triangles are equal when they share a common side and two equal angles. The central X-ray beams is perpendicular to the line formed by bisecting the long axis of the teeth and the long axis of the film.

Advantage: Convenient to the operator. The film is placed close to lingual surface of the tooth.

Disadvantage: Faulty X-ray beam angulation results in the foreshortening or elongation of the image.

Object Localization Technique (Tube Shift Technique)

This technique is done by comparing two periapical radiographs taken at different beam angles to determine the facial/lingual position of the impacted canine. This same lingual, opposite buccal rule (SLOB) is helpful in determining whether the impacted canine is labial or lingual to the incisor roots; however, the degree of displacement is difficult to determine.

Bitewing Radiograph (Fig. 24.2)

Bitewing radiographs take their name from the original technique which required the patient to bite on a small wing attached to an intraoral film packet. Modern film holders, have eliminated the need for the wing (now termed a tab), but the terminology and clinical indications have remained the same. An individual film is designed to show the crowns of the premolar and molar teeth on one side of the jaws. The central beam of the X-ray is perpendicular to the film.

Uses

- It records the coronal part of upper and lower dentition along with their supporting structures.
- Used to detect proximal caries
- Height and contour of interalveolar bone
- To detect periodontal changes
- To detect secondary caries below restorations
- To determine interproximal calculus
- Assessment of occlusal pattern.

Advantages

1. No geometric distortions.
2. No magnification.
3. Convenient to the patient and operator.
4. Can be taken for the children with ease when compared to periapical film

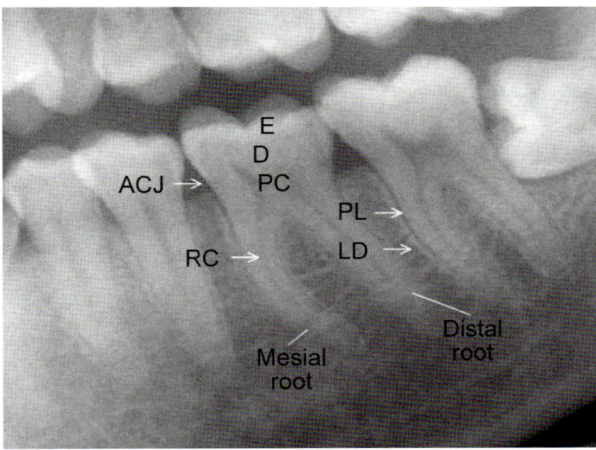

Fig. 24.1: Periapical radiograph

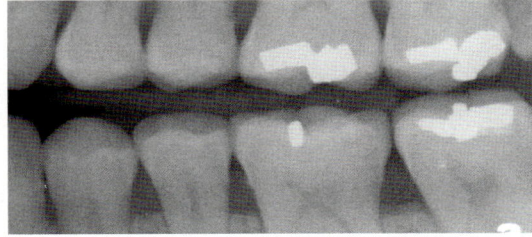

Fig. 24.2: Bitewing radiograph

Occlusal Radiograph

Occlusal radiography is defined as those intraoral radiographic techniques taken using a dental X-ray set where the film packet (5.7 × 7.6 cm) or a small intraoral cassette is placed in the occlusal plane (Fig. 24.3).

Classification

Maxillary occlusal radiograph (Fig. 24.3)
1. Topographic maxillary occlusal projection.
2. Cross-sectional maxillary occlusal projection.
3. Lateral topographic maxillary occlusal projection.

Mandibular occlusal radiograph
1. Topographical mandibular occlusal projection.
2. Cross-sectional mandibular occlusal projection.
3. Lateral cross-sectional mandibular occlusal projection.
4. Mental spine view.

Uses
- Enable to check for supernumerary and missing teeth.
- Used to observe abnormal eruption pattern of the canines.
- To analyse treatment effects after rapid expansion of maxillary arch.
- To differentiate buccal or lingual positioning of tooth.
- Buccal expansion of bony lesion can be studied clearly.
- In patients with limited mouth opening.

EXTRAORAL RADIOGRAPH

OPG

Panoramic radiography was introduced by Dickson and Copola (Fig. 24.4a and b). Panoramic radiography is a radiographic procedure used to record a single image of maxillary and mandibular arches and their supporting structures. It plays a role in support of orthodontic assessment both in pre-treatment planning and also in post-treatment evaluation of success or

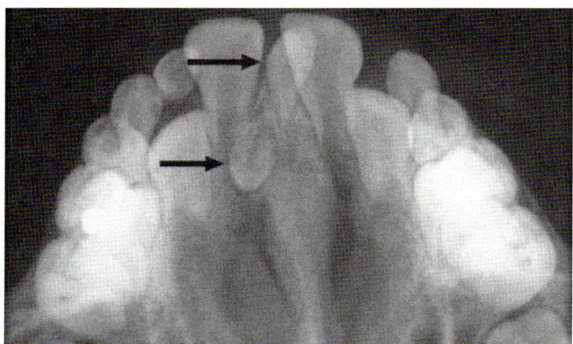

Fig. 24.3: Occlusal radiograph

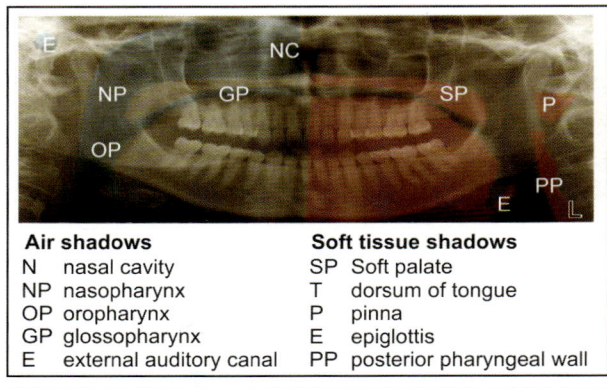

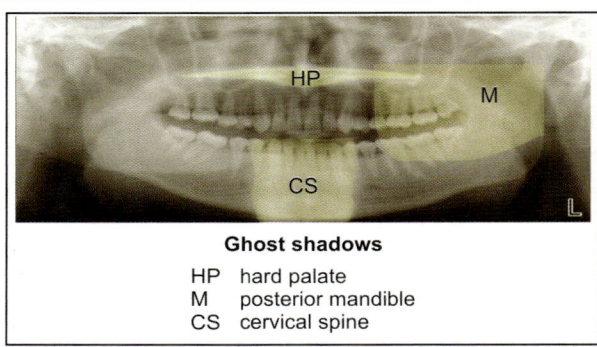

Air shadows
N   nasal cavity
NP nasopharynx
OP oropharynx
GP glossopharynx
E   external auditory canal

Soft tissue shadows
SP Soft palate
T   dorsum of tongue
P   pinna
E   epiglottis
PP posterior pharyngeal wall

Ghost shadows
HP hard palate
M   posterior mandible
CS cervical spine

Fig. 24.4a and b: OPG

failure. It is also known as 'pantomography', 'Rotational panoramic radiography'.

Uses
- Evaluation of dental development in the mixed dentition by assessing the root resorption in the deciduous teeth and amount of root development in the permanent teeth (Fig. 24.4c)
- To locate the supernumerary tooth or congenitally missing tooth.
- It is used to locate the impacted tooth.
- It is used to assess the development of third molar.
- Evaluation of mesiodistal angulation of permanent tooth and their relation to the resorbing deciduous root.
- It is used to locate the caries, bone loss secondary to periodontal disease, retained deciduous tooth, etc.

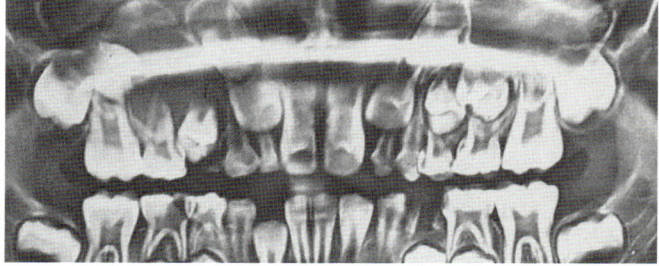

Fig. 24.4c: OPG in mixed dentition case

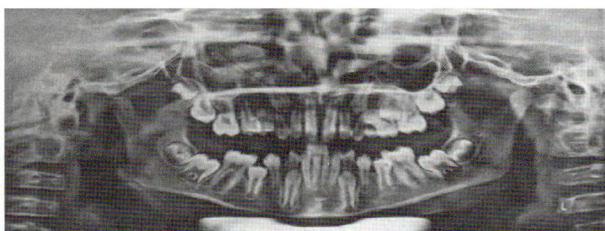

Fig. 24.4d: OPG in deep bite case

- To detect the pathological lesion of jaw bones and jaw bone fracture.
- To detect deep bite case (Fig. 24.4d)

Advantages

- Broad anatomic area can be visualized.
- Radiation exposure is low.
- Can be used in patient who are unable to tolerate intraoral films or unable to open the mouth, trismus.

Disadvantages

- Expensive equipment
- Inclination of anterior teeth cannot be visualized
- Less clear images as in periapical films
- Distortion, magnification and overlapping of the structures occur.

Cephalometric Radiograph

'Cephalo' means head and 'metric' means measurement. Cephalometric radiography is a standardized and reproducible form of skull radiography used extensively in orthodontics to assess the relationships of the teeth to the jaws and the jaws to the rest of the facial skeleton. Standardization was essential for the development of cephalometry—the measurement and comparison of specific points, distances and lines within the facial skeleton, which is now an integral part of orthodontic assessment (Fig. 24.5).

The greatest value is probably obtained from these radiographs, if they are traced or digitized and this is essential when they are being used for the monitoring of treatment progress.

Broadbent developed a head positioning device called cephalostat which he used to obtain lateral and anteroposterior views of patient's skull (Fig. 24.6). It became an integral part of orthodontic practice since then. It enables the clinicians to quantify facial and dental relationship. It gives information about the spatial relationship of superficial and deep structures. These techniques imply that the film is placed outside the oral cavity, against the side of the face to be radiographed and the X-ray beam is directed towards it.

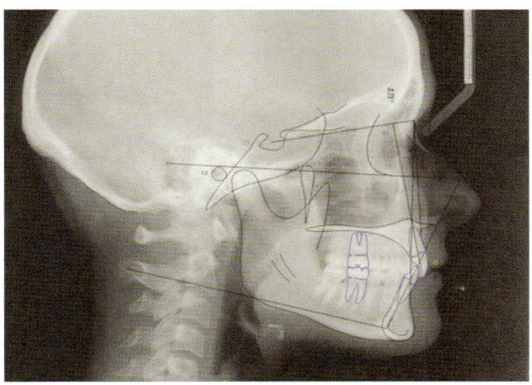

Fig. 24.5: Cephalometric radiograph

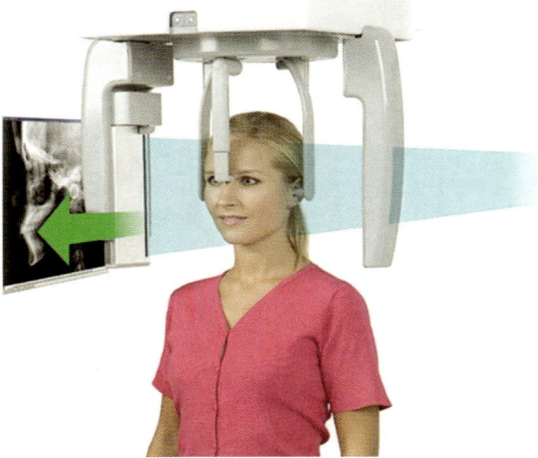

Fig. 24.6: Cephalostat

Indications

- When it is not possible to place the film intraorally as during trismus
- To examine the extent of large lesions, especially when the area of pathology is greater than which can be covered by an intraoral periapical film
- When jaws or other facial bones have to be examined for evidence of lesions and other pathological conditions
- To evaluate skeletal growth and development
- To evaluate the status of impacted teeth
- To evaluate TMJ area
- To evaluate trauma

Lateral Cephalometric Radiographs

In this technique, the X-ray source is placed 5 feet or 60 inches away from the patient's mid-sagittal plane. This is done to reduce the magnification. The film is placed 18 cm away from the mid-sagittal plane. Patient's Frankfort horizontal plane is oriented parallel to the floor by means of ear-rod inserted to the external acoustic meatuses and the orbital pointer. Mid-sagittal plane is parallel to the cassette for the lateral cephalogram. It is perpendicular to the cassette for posteroanterior cephalogram. The upper part of the face is supported by the forehead clamp positioned at the nasion.

Lateral cephalometric radiograph is a radiograph of the head taken with the X-ray beam perpendicular to the patient's sagittal plane. Natural head position is a standardized orientation of the head that is reproducible for each individual and is used as a means of standardization during analysis of dentofacial morphology both for photos and radiographs. The concept of natural head position was introduced by Moorrees and Kean in 1958 and now is a common method of head orientation for cephalometric radiography.

Registration of the head in its natural position while obtaining a cephalogram has the advantage that an extracranial line (the true vertical or a line perpendicular to that) can be used as a reference line for cephalometric analysis, thus bypassing the difficulties imposed by the biologic variation of intracranial reference lines. True vertical is an external reference line, commonly provided by the image of a free-hanging metal chain on the cephalostat registering on the film or digital cassette during exposure. The true vertical line offers the advantage of no variation (since it is generated by gravity) and is used with radiographs obtained in natural head position.

- With medium speed film and intensifying screens, the exposure time is 0.6–1.2 seconds. It is shorter when high speed films are used.
- Current technical specification is 80 kVp; 8 mA, and 0.8 second exposure time.
- Some amount of magnification invariably occurs with this technique. Acceptable magnification of the cephalogram is in the range of 5–7%.
- By convention, cephalograms are taken of the left side of skull.
- The film size is 8 × 10 inches and the film is placed in the cassette along side of the intensifying screen.

Indications

- Initial diagnosis
- Confirmation of the underlying skeletal and/or soft tissue abnormalities
- Treatment planning
- Monitoring treatment progress, e.g. to assess anchorage requirements and incisor inclination
- Appraisal of treatment results, e.g. 1 or 2 months before the completion of active treatment.
- To ensure that treatment targets have been met and to allow planning of retention.

Posteroanterior (PA) Cephalometric Radiograph (Fig. 24.7)

A radiograph of the head is taken with the X-ray beam perpendicular to the patient's coronal plane with the X-ray source behind the head and the film cassette in front of the patient's face.

PA cephalograms are usually taken for evaluation and treatment planning of patients with facial asymmetry. The head is rotated by 90° so that the central ray perpendicularly bisects the transmeatal axis. It is crucial that the Frankfort plane be accurately horizontal, because when the head is tilted, all vertical displacements measured are altered.

Anteroposterior (AP) Cephalogram

- It is also called frontal cephalogram (Fig. 24.8).
- The X-ray beam passes perpendicular to the patient's coronal plane.
- To evaluate the facial asymmetry.
- To diagnose malocclusion in the transverse plane.

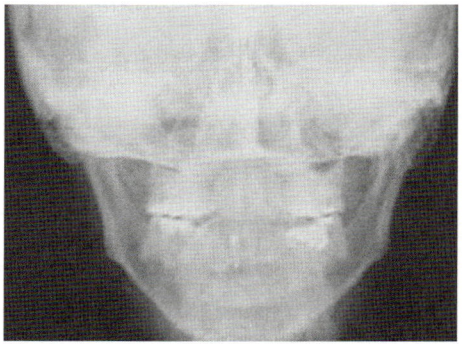

Fig. 24.7: Posteroanterior (PA) cephalogram

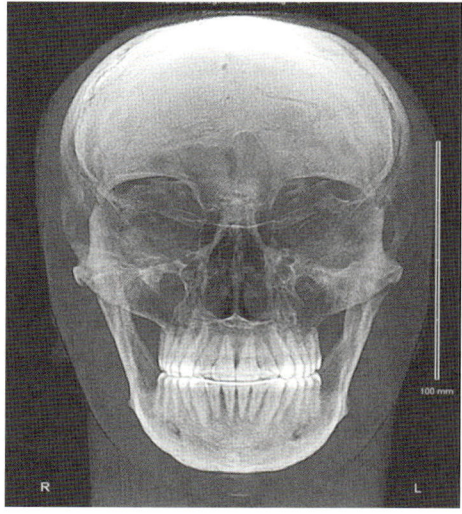

Fig. 24.8: Anteroposterior (AP) cephalogram

- It is used in two analyses:
  - Grummon's analysis.
  - Rocky mountain analysis.

Oblique Cephalogram

The right and left oblique cephalograms are taken at 45° to the lateral cephalogram, the central ray entering behind one ramus to obviate superimposition of the halves of the mandible. The Frankfort plane must stay horizontal; any tipping will alter the measurements. The oblique cephalogram is particularly useful for patients in the mixed dentition.But they are rarely prescribed by clinicians (Fig. 24.9).

Computerized Cephalometrics

It is the recently followed cephalogram in dental practice. This technique is useful for automatic measurement of landmark relationships. Depending on

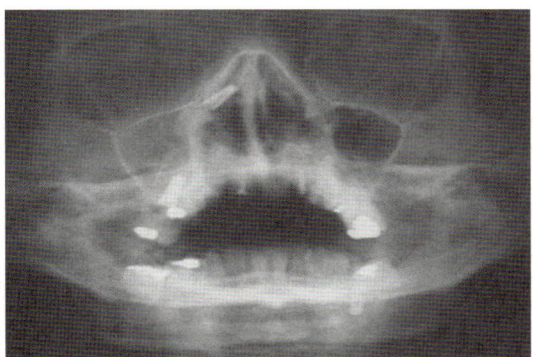

Fig. 24.9: Oblique cephalogram

the software and hardware available, the incorporation of data can be performed by digitizing points on a tracing. But it requires much amount of skills and difficult in performing and understanding (Fig. 24.10).

Drawbacks

- Patient is exposed to ionizing radiation which is harmful. Hence, it is used only when it is diagnostically and therapeutically desirable.
- The absence of anatomic references which remain constant with time is a serious disadvantage when clinicians wish to compare cephalogram taken at different time points.
- The process of image acquisition as well as measurement procedures is not well standardized.
- There is much more errors in identification.
- The difficulty in locating landmarks and surfaces on the X-ray image as the image lacks hard edges and well-defined outline.
- The structure being imaged is three-dimensional whereas the radiographic image is two-dimensional.
- Anatomic structures lying at different planes within the head undergo projective displacement.
- Some reference landmarks and planes do not agree with the anatomical landmarks.
- Patient is positioned with ear rods in the external acoustic meatus. The operator assumes that the meatus are symmetrical. It need not be so.
- Patient is made to bite in maximum intercuspation while taking the cephalogram. There could be a mandibular shift from centric relation.

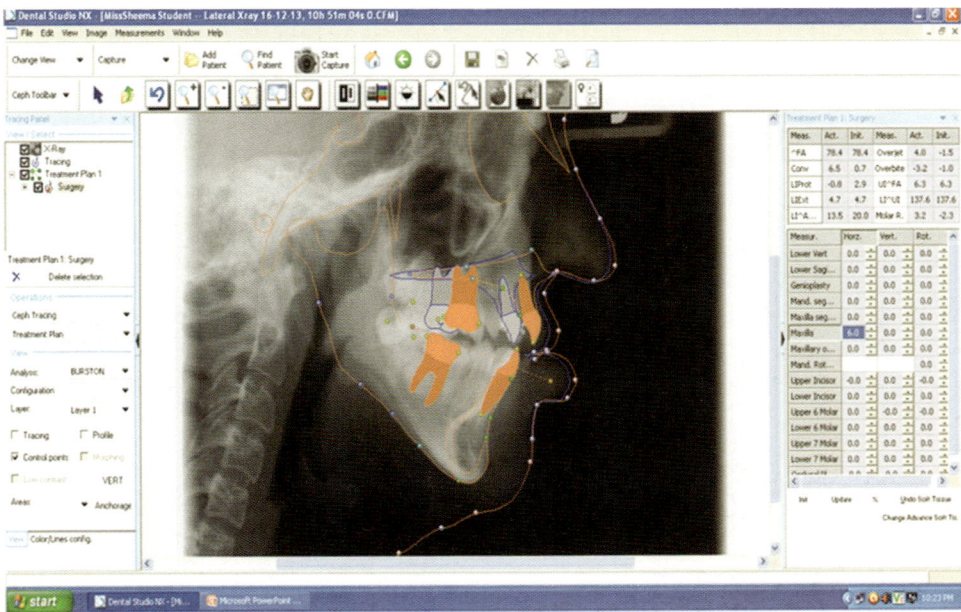

Fig. 24.10: Comuterized cephalometrics

- A cephalometric analysis makes use of means obtained from different population samples. They have only limited relevance when applied to individual patient.
- The composite of line and angles used in the cephalometric analysis yields limited information about the patient's dentoskeletal patterns.
- An orthodontic diagnosis cannot be made solely on the basis of cephalometric analysis.

Hand Wrist Radiograph

Carpal bones were first named by Lyser in 1683. Hand-wrist radiographic assessment of skeletal maturity is a valuable tool in orthodontics. Skeletal maturation staging from radiographic analysis is a widely used approach to predict timing of pubertal growth, to estimate growth velocity, and to estimate the proportion of growth remaining. There are numerous small bones in the hand-wrist region. They follow a pattern in the ossification and union of epiphysis with diaphysis. The left hand-wrist is used by convention and a PA view is taken to register the region and study growth (Fig. 24.11).

Indications

- To assess the potential for growth before treating the patient with skeletal Class II or Class III malocclusion.
- It is indicated when there is a major discrepancy between the dental age and the chronological age.
- To predict the pubertal growth spurt.
- To assess the skeletal age in a patient whose growth is retarded by infections or neoplasm.

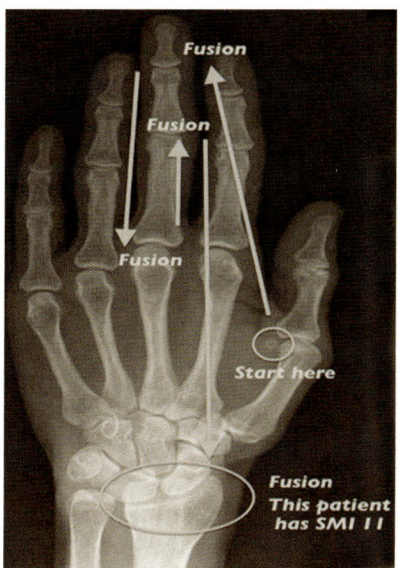

Fig. 24.11: Hand wrist radiograph

- To evaluate whether any growth is left prior to orthognathic surgery such that the chances of relapse linked to post-surgical growth can be minimized.
- Serial assessment of skeletal age is used in studying growth of an individual.
- It is used in research to elucidate the effect of heredity and enviornment on dentofacial growth.

Xeroradiography

Xeroradiography is the science of recording radiographic images electronically on a selenium plate (Fig. 24.12). The principal element in xeroradiography is a reusable photoreceptor plate, measuring approximately 24 × 36 cm. Consists of a thin photo-conductive layer of selenium adhering to an aluminum backing. The selenium semiconductor is given a uniform positive charge by an ionizing device, consisting of a number of electrodes and a grid, called a scorotron. When the selenium plate is exposed to light or to radiation (X-rays), the semiconductor layer increases its electrical conductivity and allows the positive charge on the plate to discharge. Since the discharge of the plate varies according to the quantity of X-ray energy reaching it, an electric charge pattern, which corresponds to the density of the object being X-rayed, is left on the plate. This resultant charge pattern is the latent image. The image thus formed is made permanent by transferring and fixing it by heat on a special paper. This is the xerogram (XR).

Advantages

- High edge enhancement
- Choice of positive and negative displays
- Wide exposure latitude
- Good detail
- Requires only about one-third of the radiation dose required for conventional radiograph

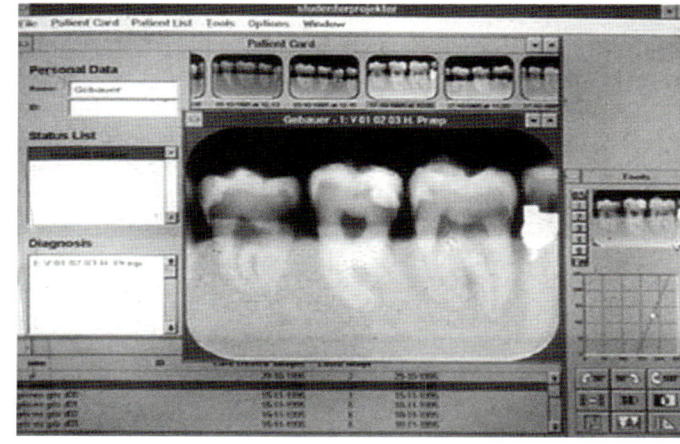

Fig. 24.12: Xeroradiography

Digital Radiography

Digital or electronic imaging has been available for more than a decade (Fig. 24.13). The first direct digital imaging system, radiovisiography (RVG), was invented by Dr. Frances Mouyens and manufactured by Trophy Radiologie [Vincennes, France] in 1984.

A filmless imaging system: It is a method of capturing a radiographic image using sensor, breaking it into electronic pieces and presenting and storing the image using a computer. The X-ray beam strikes the sensor. An electronic charge is produced on the surface of the sensor, and this electronic signal is digitized. The digital sensor transmits this information to the computer. Software on the computer stores the image electronically.

Computers operate on the binary number system in which two digits (0 and 1) are used to represent data. These two characters are called bits (binary digit), and they form words eight or more bits in length called bytes. The total number of the possible bytes for 8-bit language is $2^8 = 256$. The analogue-to-digital converter transforms analogue data into numerical data based on the binary number system.

Advantages

- Direct digital imaging systems produce a dynamic image that permits immediate display; image enhancement, storage, retrieval and transmission.
- Digital sensors are more sensitive than film and require significantly lower radiation exposure.

Magnetic Resonance Imaging (MRI)

MRI technique is based on two fundamental properties of proton that spin and small magnetic movement (Fig. 24.14). The proton of hydrogen ion which is in water is utilized in MRI. Each proton behaves like small spinning magnet and when placed in a magnetic field they tend to move parallel to the field. Because of the spin, the proton differently rotates within their axis

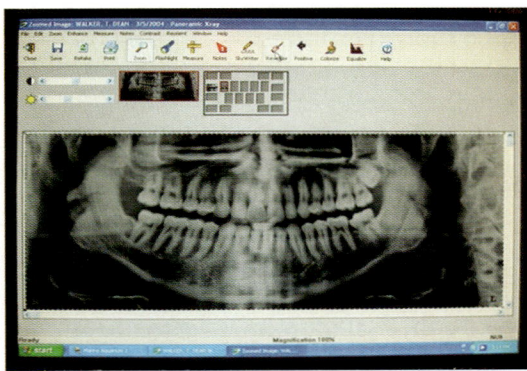

Fig. 24.13: Digital radiography

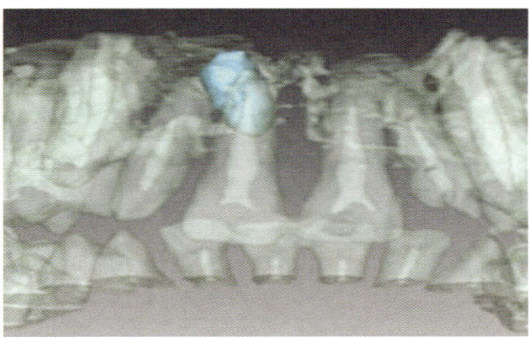

Fig. 24.14: Magnetic resonance imaging (MRI)

progressing about the direction of the magnetic field. If a coil is now wound around a volume of protons, they now progress at 90° around the magnetic field at the same frequency and induce a minute current in the coil which when amplified can be displayed over an oscilloscope this energy is utilized in scanning procedure.

Uses

- Evaluation of the position, mobility, and morphology of the articular disc of TMJ.
- Used to study internal derangements of disc.
- Used to evaluate the position of the articular disc after treatment with functional and orthopedic appliances.
- Examination of tongue movements during deglutition.

Advantages

- MRI does not have hazards as it uses non-ionizing electromagnetic radiation.
- Anatomical details are as good as in CT scan.
- Greater tissue characterization is possible.
- Imaging of blood vessel, blood flow, visualization of thrombus is possible.
- It is possible to get a better spatial resolution.
- No radiation exposure.

Disadvantages

- Time taken is more
- Not used in patients with cardiac pacemaker
- Non-visualization of bone makes it useless in bony lesions
- More expensive than CT scanning.

Tomography

Tomography can be used to visualize a section or a slice of the object and thereby eliminate undesirable overlap.

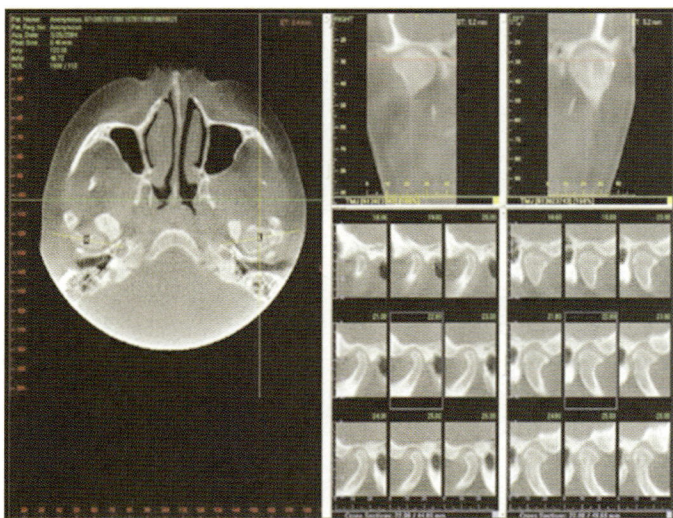

Fig. 24.15: Computed tomography

Tomography can be:
1. Conventional tomography
2. Computed tomography (Fig. 24.15)
3. Cone-beam computed tomography (Fig. 24.16)

Conventional Tomography or Plain Tomography

Focal plane tomography, which historically was the main tomography method in radiography nowadays mostly obsolete.

Computed Tomography

It produces two-dimensional projections of a three-dimensional object. Basic concept is the reconstruction of the internal structure of an object through multiple projections.

It is a method of imaging in which a thin X-ray beam rotates around the patient. Small detectors measure the amount of X-rays that pass through the particular area of interest. A computer analyses the data to construct a cross-sectional image. These images can be stored, viewed on a monitor, or printed on film. In addition, stacking the individual images or slices can create three-dimensional models of patient anatomy. As the CT scanning takes place, the table will advance the horizontally lying patient at small intervals through the scanner. Modern spiral CT scanners can perform the examination in one continuous motion.

This is a process by which a layer of an image within the body is produced while the images of structure above and below that layer are made invisible by blurring. Blurring of the image outside the plane of interest is accomplished by simultaneous movement of X-ray tube and film during the exposure. The tube and the film are connected so that movements occur around a point or fulcrum. As the distance from the point of rotation increases, amount of image blurring also increases. As the angle between the source/film and tissue increases, thickness of the image is reduced.

Principles of tomography can be mechanically implemented in two ways:
1. The X-ray tube and film can move synchronously in opposite direction in parallel planes.
2. The X-ray tube and film can move synchronously and in opposite direction in parallel planes but with motions other than straight lines that is circular spiral CT. This is also called CT or CAT (computed axial tomography).

CT systems are mainly complex imaging systems which use thin beams of X-ray that moves in asynchronous manner with an array of detectors which calculates and attenuate the X-ray beam at different angles and in different planes. This data is spread into computer which performs numerous calculations as per the program and constructs accurate image in the coronal axial plane.

Cone-Beam Computed Tomography

Cone-beam computed tomography (CBCT) is also referred to as c-arm CT, cone beam volume CT, or flat panel CT) is a medical imaging technique consisting or X-ray computed tomography where the X-rays are divergent, forming a cone.

It has become increasingly important in treatment planning and diagnosis in implant dentistry, oral surgery, endodontics and orthodontics.

During dental/orthodontic imaging, the CBCT scanner rotates around the patient's head, obtaining up to nearly 600 distinct images.

Uses

- Used in radiographic examination of TMJ.

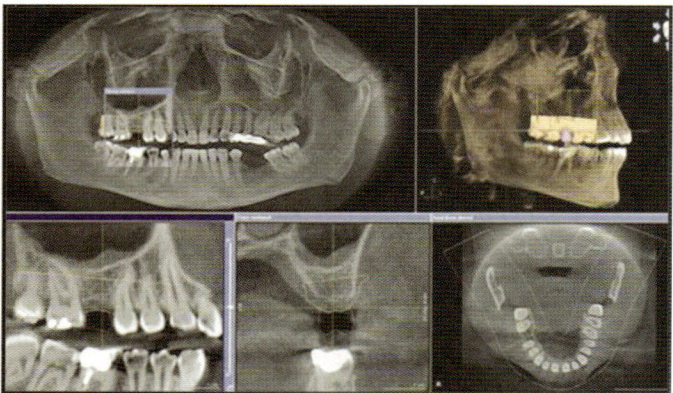

Fig. 24.16: Cone-beam computed tomography (CBCT)

- Analyze effects of rapid maxillary expansion.
- Evaluation of cortical bone thickness for orthodontic implants.
- Diagnosis and treatment planning for maxillary canine impaction.
- Study the effect of distraction osteogenesis devices.
- Assessment of patients with syndromes and clefts.
- Facial analysis
- Tongue posture and size
- Airway assessment
- Root resorption
- Cephalometric analysis

Advantages

- High geometric precision.
- Ability to discriminate between objects with minor difference in dentistry.
- Images can be manipulated by changing the contrast to highlight or accentuate areas of interest.
- Large amount of information secured in short period.
- Accurate visualization
- Computer programming makes to view images in different shapes and densities.

Disadvantages

- Radiation exposure is more in CT.
- High cost
- Need high equipment which is too costly.
- Slices of relatively thick tissue detail in vertically oriented teeth are quiet poor.
- Distortions are produced, if CT scans are done with orthodontic appliances in place.

Application of 3D Imaging to Modern Orthodontic (Fig. 24.17)

The 3D technique goes beyond the limitations of 2D analysis in many ways:

- Effective representation of true 3D morphology of the cranial structures without distortion, avoiding projection and identification errors.
- Reduced operator bias because the measurements are performed automatically.
- Ability to obtain CA using the three dimensions.
- The 3D imaging can be useful in evaluating treatment responses to functional orthopedics, orthognathic surgery and growth of the face.

Methods of 3D Craniofacial Skeletal Imaging

Within the next one or two years, the orthodontist will have available to them three or four methods to obtain 3D radiographic image of patients, namely:

1. Tomosynthesis
2. Tuned aperture CT (TACT)

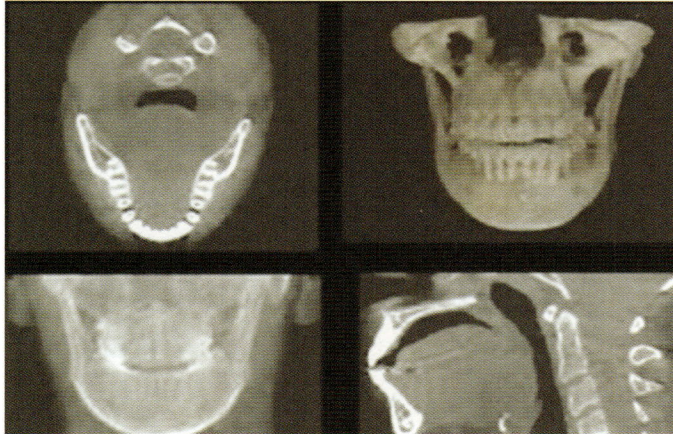

Fig. 24.17: Application of 3D imaging in modern orthodontics

3. Anatomic reconstruction
4. Cone beam CT

Methods of 3D Intraoral Dental Imaging

- The technology of laser scanning and SL can be miniaturized to image the dentition. A system that incorporates SL has been introduced Oramatrix Sure Smile—orascanner.
- A video camera records SL distortion on dental crowns as it passes over the dentition over the time period of one minute.
- A stream of images is fedback to a computer and proceeds are used to switch together a complete dental arch.

Photocephalometry

This technique is discovered by Thomas Hohl, et al in 1978 (Fig. 24.18). It involves taking the photograph and lateral cephalogram from the same distance and position. The photograph is enlarged in accordance with the cephalogram and it is superimposed.

Method

- Patient is made to assume natural head position with relaxed lips.
- 4 × 4 mm-sized radiopaque metallic markers are placed on the patients face and the anteroposterior cephalograms are taken.
- Lateral and frontal photographs are taken maintaining same distance and position.
- The photographic negatives are enlarged allowing the photographic images of the metal markers to be superimposed on the radiographic image on the cephalogram.
- The projection of enlarged negative is put in transparent photographic film which is superimposed on the cephalogram.

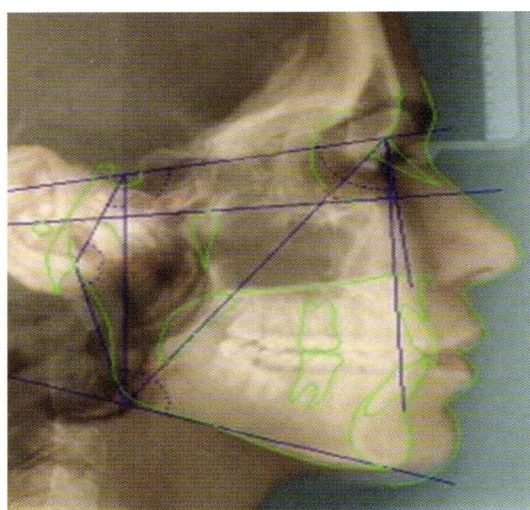

Fig. 24.18: Photocephalometry

Advantages

- Valuable quantitative information on soft tissue can be easily obtained.
- Permits direct measurement between skeletal and soft tissue landmarks.
- Changes in the soft tissue of the face can be compared pre- and post-orthognathic surgery.
- Useful in serial growth studies.

Disadvantages

- It is a complex procedure.
- Expensive when compared to conventional cephalometry.
- Accurate comparisons between the soft tissue and hard tissue anatomies by simply superimposing the images are not feasible because of the difference in the enlargement factors between the photographs and the X-ray films.

Cinefluororadiography (Fig. 24.19)

This is the technique of studying moving body structures—similar to X-ray 'movie'. A continuous X-ray beam is passed through the body part being examined, and is transmitted to a TV like monitor so that body part and its motion can be seen in detail. Used in barium X-rays, cardiac catheterization and placement of IV catheters.It may be a part of examination or procedure that is done either on out patient or in patient basis.

Method

The radiologist uses a switch to control an X-ray beam that is transmitted through the patient. The X-rays then

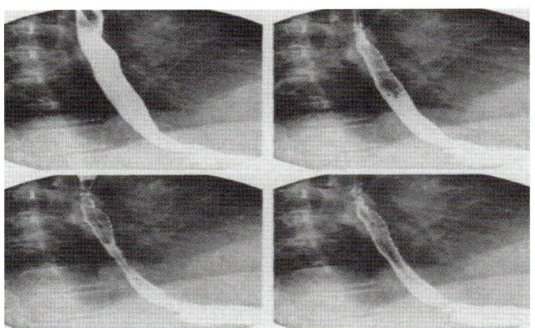

Fig. 24.19: Cinefluororadiography

strike a fluorescent plate that is coupled to an 'image intensifier' that is coupled to a television camera.The radiologist can then watch the images 'live' on a TV monitor.

Uses

- To evaluate swallowing patterns.
- To examine the upper airway in obstructive sleep apnea.
- Useful to evaluate the morphology of TMJ and its function.

Laser Holography

Holography is a visual recording and playback process that can record our 3D image on a 2D image record medium. The recorded image is called a hologram. Holography uses 2 coherent beams which converge to produce a constructive and destructive interference pattern which is recorded in a film. Pulse laser or gas laser beams are used for holographic set up (Fig. 24.20).

Uses

- Holographic images of study casts are more convenient in terms of storage and retrieval.
- To study the effect of rapid expansion on the maxilla.
- To study the effect of face mask protraction on the maxilla.
- To study bone deformities resulting from headgear forces in human skull.

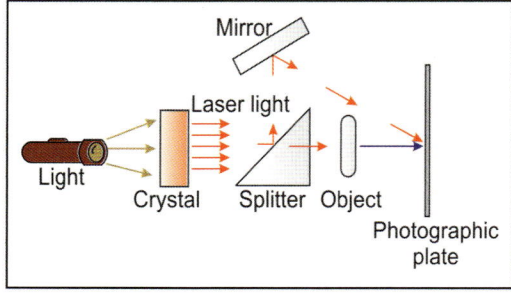

Fig. 24.20: Laser holography

- To measure incisor extrusion during orthodontic therapy.
- Locate the centre of resistance of the upper dentition and the nasomaxillary complex.
- To locate the centre of resistance of anterior teeth during intrusion.
- It is used to locate the centre of rotation of tooth undergoing orthodontic tooth movement.

Occlusograms

An occlusogram is a 1:1 reproduction of occlusal surfaces of plaster models on a tracing paper. The upper tracing is oriented to the lower tracing grooves cut in the back of plaster model. It is a tracing of photograph or a photocopy of a dental arch (Fig. 24.21).

Technique

For the occlusogram, photostatic or photographic copies of the maxillary and mandibular study models are made. Copies are taken parallel to the occlusal plane. Tracing of the teeth of the both the arches can be superimposed to match the occlusion.

Occlusogram Norms

- Biting edge of upper anterior lies in front of biting edge of lower anterior by 0.7 mm.
- Upper bicuspids are wider than the lower bicuspids by 1.9 mm each side.
- Upper posterior teeth extend beyond lower posterior teeth by 2.3 mm.
- Upper molars are wider than the lower molars by 1.4 mm each side.
- Each upper tooth touches 2 teeth below it except last molar.
- Key to firm static occlusion is the width and position of lateral incisors.

Uses

- It can be used to develop ideal natural individualized arch form.
- It permits the clinician to make accurate and reliable arch length discrepancy measurements.
- It is possible to identify problems in the transverse plane.
- It is possible to do occlusal stimulation.
- Anticipated movements can be simulated to determine the further position of teeth.
- It is useful for predicting occlusal relationship.

Disadvantages

- Occlusograms are two-dimensional records.
- They are inferior to study casts which permit a three-dimensionsal evalution of patient's occlusion.

Digital Subtraction Radiography

Radiographic assessment provides the only viable noninvasive method for evaluating the changes in hard tissue, but conventional radiography does not register alveolar bone loss or gain until 30 to 50% of the bone mineral has changed. On the other hand, the use of the diagnostic subtraction radiography technique in clinical radiographic image acquisition and subsequent subtraction analysis clearly enhanced the accuracy of alveolar bone loss detection when compared with conventional film viewing. It is suitable method for analyzing the healing process. An evaluation of the healing process can be obtained by calculating the regenerated bone area in the subtracted images (Fig. 24.22).

- Comparatively this decreases the amount of distracting background information and by allowing the eye to focus on the actual change that has occurred between two images.
- Technically, this is an image enhancement method that removes the structured noise from the images.

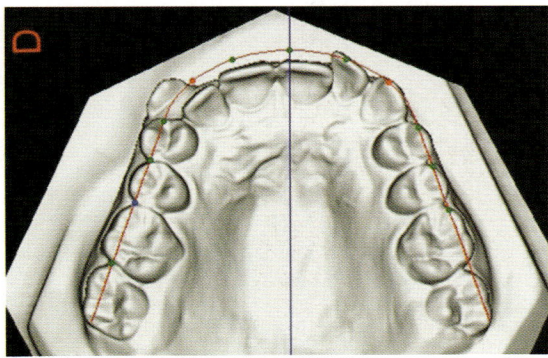

Fig. 24.21: Occlusogram

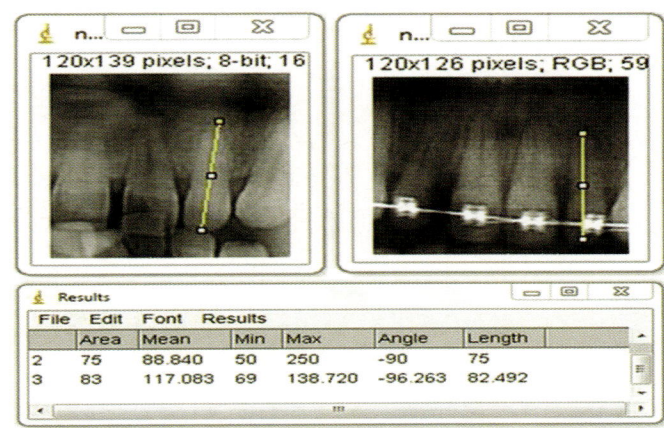

Fig. 24.22: Digital subtraction radiography

Bibliography

1. White and Pharoah. Principles and interpretation. 4th edition, pg 281–296.
2. W&P. Ch.14. Oral and Maxillofacial Imaging. Farman and NortjeNeill Serman, 2000.
3. Dr. Parish P. Sedghizadeh. Radiographic Pathology of the Head and Neck.
4. Brocklebank L. Dental Radiology, Oxford University Press 1997.
5. Deforge DH, Colmery BH. An Atlas of Dental Radiology, Iowa State University Press 2000.
6. Dental Radiographic Examination. HHS publicationFDA 88-8273 1987.
7. Radiographic Cephalometric by Alexander Jacobson
8. Van der Linden FPGM, Duterloo HS. Development of Human Dentitin. Hagerstown md 1976; 14, 26,27.
9. Textbook of Orthodontics: Gurkeerat Singh and Sridhar Premkumar.

PREVIOUS YEAR'S UNIVERSITY QUESTIONS

Essay

1. Discuss the role of radiography in orthodontics.
2. Discuss the various methods of obtaining intraoral radiograph.
3. Write in detail about cephalometric radiograph.

Short Notes

1. Bite wing radiograph
2. OPG
3. Computerized cephalometrics
4. Xeroradiogrpahy
5. Digital radigraphy
6. CBCT
7. Photocephalometry
8. Cinefluororadiography
9. Laser holography
10. Occlusograms

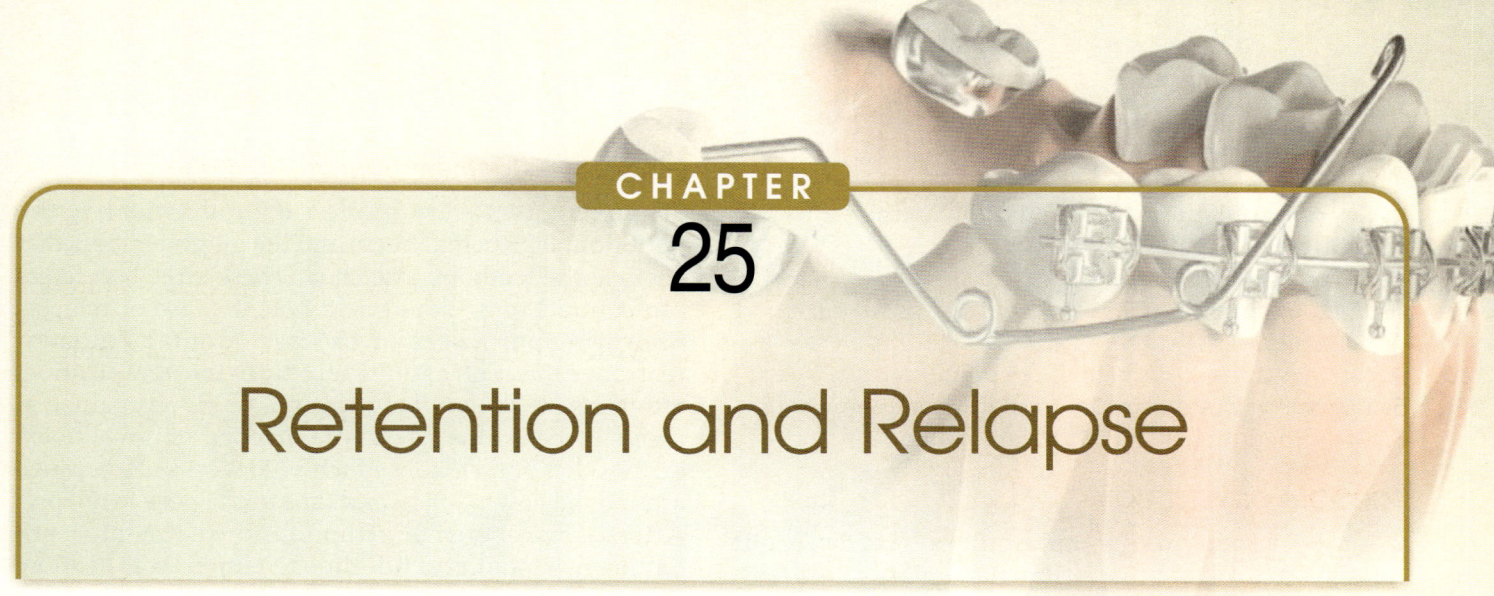

Retention and Relapse

Chapter Outline

- Introduction
- Schools of retention
- Causes of relapse
- Basic theorems of retention

- Retainers
- Bonded retainers
- Raleigh Williams six keys to eliminate lower retention
- Twelve keys to stability of lower incisors

INTRODUCTION

Retention is the phase of orthodontic treatment, which maintains the teeth in their orthodontically corrected positions following the cessation of active orthodontic tooth movement. Orthodontic retainer resists the tendency of teeth to return to their original position under the influence of periodontal, occlusal and soft tissue forces and continuing dentofacial growth.

Why Retention Necessary?

Retention is necessary for the following reasons:
- The gingival and periodontal tissues are affected by orthodontic tooth movement and require time for reorganization when the appliances are removed.
- The teeth may be in an inherently unstable position after the treatment so that soft tissue pressure constantly produces a relapse tendency.
- Changes produced by growth may alter the orthodontic treatment result.

Principles of Retention

- Relapse potential may be predicted by evaluation of initial occlusion; teeth usually want to return to their original position; this is due to gingival fibers and unbalanced lip-tongue forces.
- Full-time retention is required for 3–4 months to allow for reorganization of PDL.

- Retention should continue for at least 12 months in non-growing patients or until growth has ceased in growing patients.

Types of Retention

Retention can be of three types:
- Natural or no retention
- Limited or short-term retention
- Prolonged or permanent retention

Natural or No Retention

Conditions that do not require retention:
1. Anterior crossbite
2. Serial extraction procedures
3. Posterior crossbite in patients having steep cusps.
4. Highly placed canines in Class I extraction cases.

Limited or Short-term Retention

Most cases routinely treated fall in this category. Retention is given to allow bone in PDL tissues to adapt in their new location.
1. Class I, Class II division 1 and division 2 cases treated by extractions.
2. Deep bites
3. Class I non-extraction with dental arches showing proclination and spacing.

Prolonged or Permanent Retention

Cases requiring permanent retention are:
1. Midline diastema
2. Severe rotations
3. Arch expansion achieved without ensuring good occlusion
4. Certain Class II division 2 deep bite cases.
5. Patients with abnormal musculature or tongue habits.
6. Expanded arches in cleft palate patients.

SCHOOLS OF RETENTION

Over the years, various philosophies have been put forward to explain post-treatment stability.

These are referred to as schools of retention.

The Occlusion School

According to Kingsley, proper occlusion is a key factor in determining the stability of the newly moved teeth. The importance of this factor in safeguarding the stability in the new position has been agreed upon by several other authors and research workers.

The Apical base Method

- The apical base school has been formulated around the writings of several authors including Alex, Lundstorm, McCauley and Nance.
- Alex Lundstorm suggested that the apical base is an important factor in the correction of malocclusion and maintenance of the stability of treated cases.
- McCauley added that the interacanine and intermolar widths should maintain during orthodontic treatment to minimize retention problems.
- Nance noted that the arch length cannot be permanently increased to a major extent.

The Mandibular Incisor School

Grieves and Tweed have suggested that post-treatment stability was increased when the mandibular incisors were placed upright or slightly retroclined over the basal bone.

The Musculature School

The dentition is encapsulated from outside and inside by muscles. According to Rojers, functional muscle balance is necessary in order to ensure post-treatment stability.

CAUSES OF RELAPSE

Numerous are the causes attributed to relapse. No single factor can be said the sole cause of relapse. In most cases, relapse occurs due to a combination of causes.

Periodontal Ligament Traction

Whenever teeth are moved orthodontically, the periodontal principal fibers and the gingival fibers that encircle the teeth are stretched. These stretched fibers can contract and should be a potent cause of relapse. The principal fibers of the periodontal ligament rearrange themselves quite rapidly to the new position. Studies have shown that principal fibers reorganize in about 4 weeks time. The supra-alveolar gingival fibers on the other hand take as much as 40 weeks to rearrange around the new position and thus predispose to relapse. After comprehensive orthodontic treatment, teeth require 4–5 months of full-time retention so as to allow the reorganization of periodontal ligament fibers. After this period, retention should be continued on a reduced basis for a further 7–8 months so as to allow the more sluggish gingival fibers to readapt to the new tooth positions.

Relapse due to Growth Related Changes

Patients with skeletal problems associated with Class II, Class III, open bite malocclusion may exhibit response due to continuation of the abnormal growth that the original growth pattern resurfaces or dominates, if the orthodontic treatment is completed prior to the completion of growth. Hence, prolonged retention is indicated until active growth is completed.

Bone Adaptation

Teeth that have been moved recently are surrounded by lightly calcified osteoid bone. Thus, the teeth are not adequately stabilized and have a tendency to move to their original position. The bony trabeculae are normally arranged perpendicular to the long axes of the teeth. However, during orthodontic treatment, they get aligned parallel to the direction of force. During the retention phase, they revert back to their normal arrangement.

Muscular Forces

Teeth are encapsulated in all directions by a blanket of muscles. Muscle imbalance at the end of the orthodontic therapy can result in the reappearance of malocclusion. The orthodontist should aim at harmonising the muscles at the conclusion of the orthodontic treatment so as to increase the stability of the treatment results achieved.

Failure to Eliminate the Original Cause

The cause of the malocclusion should be determined at the time of diagnosis and adequate treatment steps should be planned to eliminate the same or reduce its severity. Failure to remove the etiology can result in relapse.

Role of Third Molars

The third molars erupt very late in the development of dentition. They erupt in most cases between the ages 18–21 years. By this time, most patients would have completed their orthodontic treatment. The pressure exerted by the erupting third molars is believed to cause late anterior crowding, predisposing to relapse.

Role of Occlusion

Good intercuspation of upper and lower teeth is an important factor in maintaining the stability of treated cases. The centric relation and centric occlusion should coincide or the slide from centric should be more than 1.5–2 mm in order to have greater stability of the treatment results. Presence of certain occlusal mannerisms, such as clenching, grinding, nail biting, lip biting, etc. is important causes of relapse.

BASIC THEOREMS OF RETENTION

Riedel summarized the philosophies regarding retention into the following nine theorems. Moyers has included the tenth theorem.

Theorem 1

"Teeth that have been moved tend to return to their former position".

It is proved beyond doubt that orthodontically moved teeth have a tendency to return to their original position. Factors, such as muscular forces, bone morphology and periodontal ligament and gingival fibers contribute to this tendency.

Theorem 2

"Elimination of the causes of malocclusion will prevent relapse".

All the possible causes of existing malocclusion should be identified at the time of diagnosis and all efforts should be made to eliminate them whenever possible. It is especially true for abnormal muscle forces aggravating the existing malocclusion, e.g. thumb sucking, tongue thrusting and other abnormal pressure habits.

Theorem 3

"Malocclusion should be overcorrected as a safety factor."

Although there is little evidence about its effectiveness, overcorrection appears to be helpful in the management of certain conditions, such as rotations, Class II and Class III malocclusions.

It is a common practice to overcorrect Class II malocclusion into edge-to-edge incisor relationship and to overcorrect rotations by slightly rotating the tooth in an opposite direction.

In this way, overcorrection allows some amount of relapse without deleteriously affecting function and esthetics.

Theorem 4

"Proper occlusion is a potent factor in holding teeth in their corrected positions".

Orthodontic treatment should aim at achieving harmonious centric, as well as functional occlusions of mandible. Proper intercuspation of teeth may aid in retention as one tooth in the arch is related to two teeth of the opposing arch.

Theorem 5

"Bone and adjacent tissues must be allowed to reorganize around newly positioned teeth".

During orthodontic tooth movement, there occurs bone remodeling, as well as reorganization of periodontal ligament fibers.

Considerable time is needed for the maturation of the newly deposited osteoid bone and reorganization of the fibers of the periodontal ligament. Retention appliances are aimed at providing sufficient time for this reorganization.

Theorem 6

"If the lower incisors are placed upright over basal bone, they are more likely to remain in good alignment".

It has been observed that post-treatment stability increases when the mandibular incisors are placed upright over the basal bone (perpendicular to the mandibular plane) or slightly inclined in a lingual direction.

Theorem 7

"Correction carried out during periods of growth is less likely to relapse".

Orthodontic treatment should be initiated at the earliest possible age so that the changes occurring during active growth periods can be positively influenced by the treatment.

By initiating the treatment early during periods of growth, orthodontist can retard or change the direction

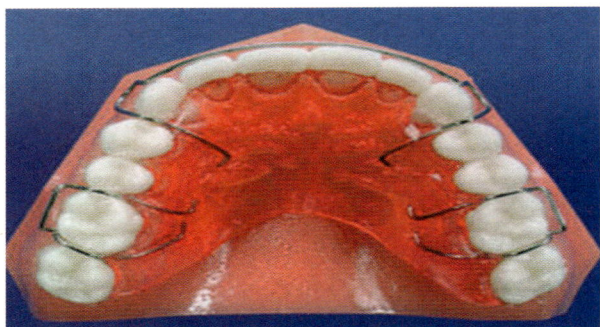

Fig. 25.1: Hawley's retainer

of growth of maxilla/mandible when indicated (indicated by using headgear/functional appliances). Hence, institution of early treatment allows growth modulations, interception of developing malocclusion and correction of skeletal malrelationships.

Treatment carried out during active growth periods is more stable because the tissue systems are adapted well.

Theorem 8

"The farther the teeth have been moved the less likelihood of relapse".

Although it is logical to think that the teeth moved farther away are less likely to return to their original position, such a measure may not always be justified and may even cause root resorption. It is more desirable to guide the proper eruption of teeth and intercept developing skeletal discrepancies rather than carrying out extensive tooth movement at a later stage.

Theorem 9

"Arch form, particularly in the mandibular arch, cannot be altered permanently by appliance therapy".

Studies have shown that the alteration of mandibular arch form carry an increased risk for relapse.

Theorem 10

"Many treated malocclusions require permanent retaining devices".

Some type of malocclusions require very long period of retention.

RETAINERS

Retainers are passive orthodontic appliances that help in maintaining and stabilizing the position of teeth long enough to permit reorganization of supporting structures after the active phase of orthodontic therapy. There are three types of retainers:
1. Removable retainers

2. Fixed retainers
3. Active retainers

Criteria for a Good Retainer
- Should retain all teeth that have been moved into desired positions.
- Should permit normal functional forces to act on the dentition.
- Should be self-cleansing and should permit oral hygiene maintenance.
- Should be as inconspicuous as possible.

Classification of Retainers

Removable Retainers

Hawley's retainer: Modifications of Hawley's retainer:
- Hawley's retainer with Adam's clasp on molar teeth (Fig. 25.1)
- Hawley's retainer with long labial bow
- Hawley's retainer with contoured labial bow
- Hawley's retainer with light elastic across the incisor teeth
- Hawley's retainer with labial bow soldered to bridge of Adams clasp (Fig. 25.2b)
- Hawley's retainer with bite plane
- Hawley's retainer with lingual extension clasps on molar (Fig. 25.2a)
- Hawley's retainer with occlusal rest
- Begg's retainer
- Clip-on retainer/spring aligner
- Wrap around retainer
- Kesling's tooth positioner
- Invisible retainer
- Kansal's retainer

Fixed Retainers
- Band and spur fixed retainer
- Banded canine-to-canine fixed retainer
- Bonded canine-to-canine fixed retainer

Active Retainers

If there is any residual space in the anterior after post treatment results, the labial bow in the retainer can be until it the space close activated.

Hawley's Appliance

It was designed in 1920 by Charles Hawley. It is most frequently used retainer. It consists of claps on molars and a short labial bow extending from canine to canine having adjustment loops.

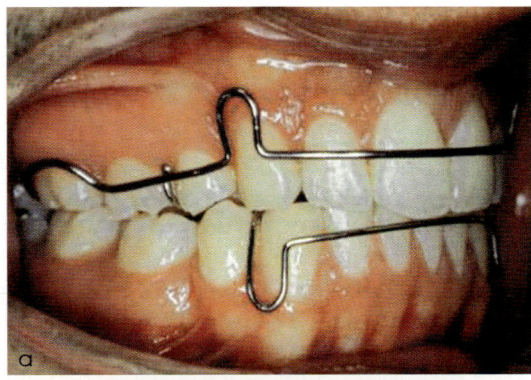

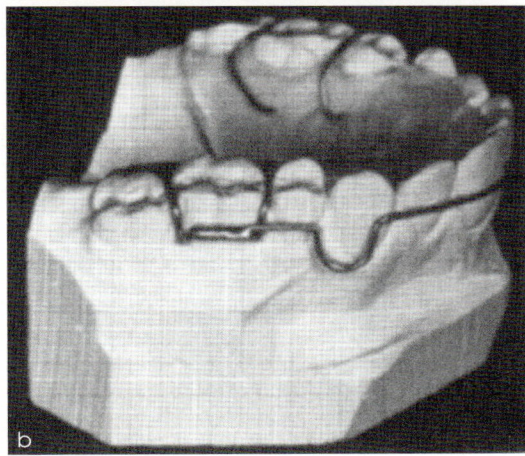

Fig. 25.2: (a) Hawley's retainer with molar extension; (b) Hawley's retainer soldered on the molar bridge

Hawley retainer's modification
1. Bow can be soldered to clasps on 1st molars.
2. Place C-clasps on second molars and allow bow to run around entire arch

Begg's Retainer (Fig. 25.3)

It consists of a labial wire that extends till the last erupted molar and curves around it to get embedded in acrylic that spans the palate.

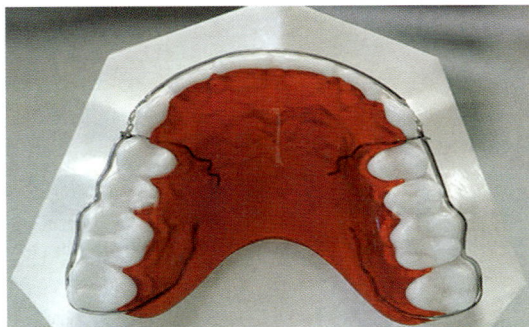

Fig. 25.3: Begg retainer

Advantage: There is no crossover wire that extends between the canine and premolar thereby eliminating the risk of space opening.

Clip-on Retainer or Spring Realigner (Fig. 25.4)

- Appliance made of wire framework that runs labially over the incisors and then passes between canine and premolar and is recurved to lie over lingual surface.
- Both the labial as well as lingual segments are embedded in a strip of clear acrylic.
- Less comfortable than Hawley's appliance.
- Not as good in overbite maintenance.
- Indicated in periodontal cases where splinting is needed.

Wrap Around Retainer (Fig. 25.5)

- Extended version of spring aligner that covers all the teeth.
- Consists of wire that passes along the labial as well as lingual surfaces of all erupted teeth which is embedded in a strip of acrylic.

Use: In stabilizing a periodontally weak dentition.

Kesling Tooth Positioner (Fig. 25.6)

It is described by HD Kesling in 1945. It is made of thermoplastic rubber-like material that spans the inter-

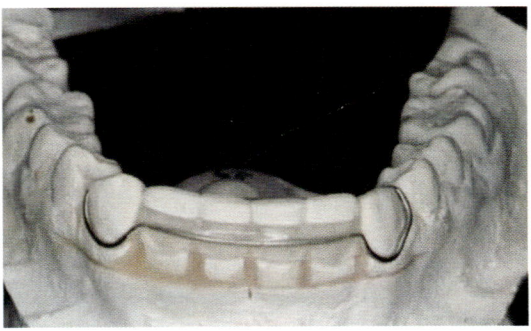

Fig. 25.4: Spring retainer

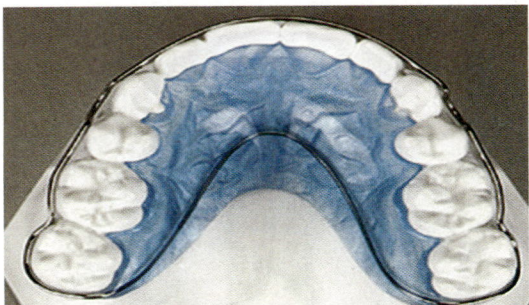

Fig. 25.5: Wrap around retainer

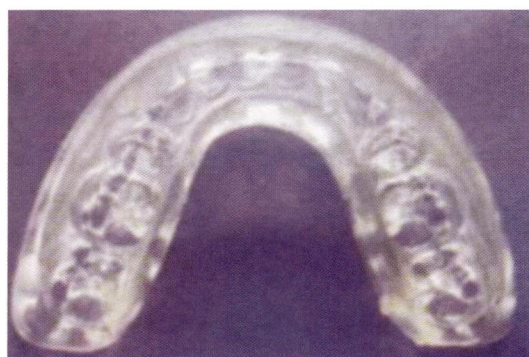

Fig. 25.6: Kesling tooth positioned

occlusal space and covers the clinical crowns of the U/L portion of teeth and a small portion of the gingiva. It needs no activation at regular intervals and is durable.

Disadvantages
- Bulky and difficult to wear full-time.
- Difficulty in speech and risk of TMJ problems.
- Do not retain incisor position as well as a conventional retainer b/c patients usually wear full-time.
- Overbite increases due to limited patient wear

Vacuum-formed (Essix) Retainer (Fig. 25.7)

It is developed in 1993. This is a polypropylene or polyvinylchloride (PVC) material, typically .020" or .030" thick, plastic removable appliance.

Advantages
- Esthetic
- Patient is more likely to wear
- Inexpensive
- Quick fabrication
- Minimal bulk
- High strength
- No adjustments
- Usually does not interfere with speech or function
- Studies have determined that Essix retainers are as efficient as Hawley-type or bonded wire retainers

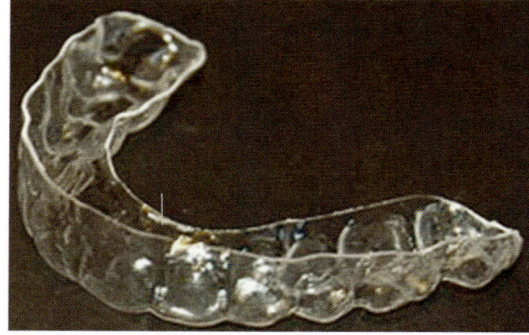

Fig. 25.7: Vacuum-formed retainer

Kansal's Retainer

Kansal's retainer is a removable, tooth-borne orthodontic retainer consisting of wire components and acrylic. The wire components include modified labial bow, Kansal's bow and pinhead clasps.

It has minimal acrylic which rests only on teeth and does not take the support of tissues for its retention, therefore, it is less bulky, has low food accumulation and it is easy to clean. Mini-U loops because no gingival impingement and also they are less visible, hence more comfortable and esthetic (Fig. 25.8a to d)

Types of Spring Retainer
- Modified spring retainer
- Mushroom type spring retainer (Fig. 25.9)
- Spring retainer with coils incorporated (Fig. 25.10)
  Modified spring retainer as shown in Fig. 25.9.

Spring retainer has mushroom type spring behind the central and lateral incisors. It is also used to adjust rotations in the anterior teeth and gives extra forces in the facial (Fig. 25.9).

BONDED RETAINERS

The term 'retention' itself implies that the teeth tend to revert, however, the orthodontic correction is carried out successfully especially in adults.

A special attention should be given towards the most predilection site for relapse. The adult patients are not willing to wear removable retainer for longer time. Hence a permanent retainer is inevitable.

Fixed Retainers—Types
- The fixed appliance
- Banded canine-to-canine retainer
- Bonded lingual retainers
- Band and spur retainers

Bonded retainer is a fixed permanent retainer to hold the corrected teeth in an ideal esthetic and functional position.

Fixed retainer can be usually given on 3–3 (canine-to-canine) (Fig. 25.11 or 4–4 premolar-to-premolar). After orthodontic correction with conventional fixed appliance, the canines are banded and 0.032" round arch wire is soldered to the lingual surface of the 3–3 band.

Now with the advent of the new bonding materials and new approaches, many orthodontists prefer to use bonded lingual retainer.

- 0.032 to 0.036" wire with loops at the terminal ends and terminal loops alone are bonded.

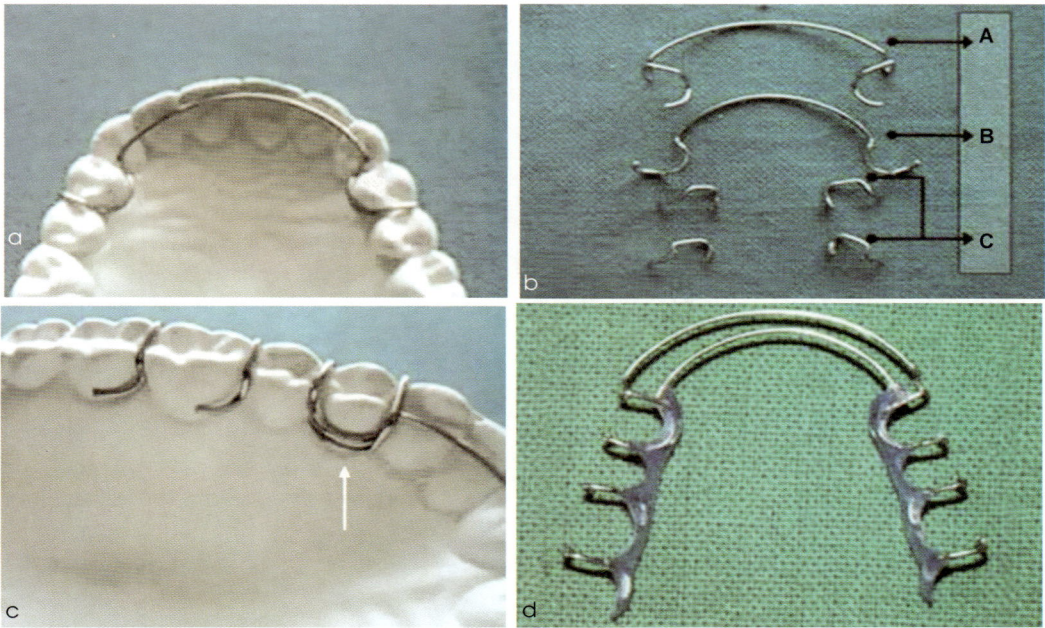

Fig. 25.8: (a) Kansal's retainer; (b) Wire components of Kansal's appliance (A. Modified labial bow, B. Kansal's bow, C. Pinhead clasps); and (c, d) Finished Kansal's appliance

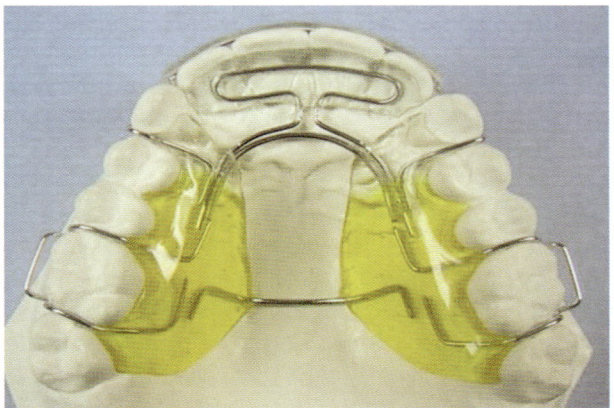

Fig. 25.9: Mushroom type spring retainer

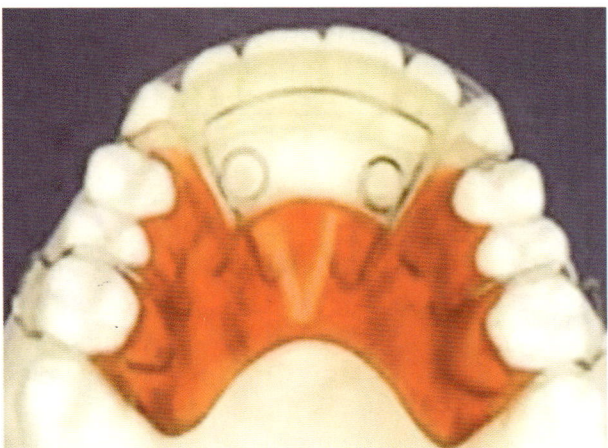

Fig. 25.10: Spring retainer with coils incorporated

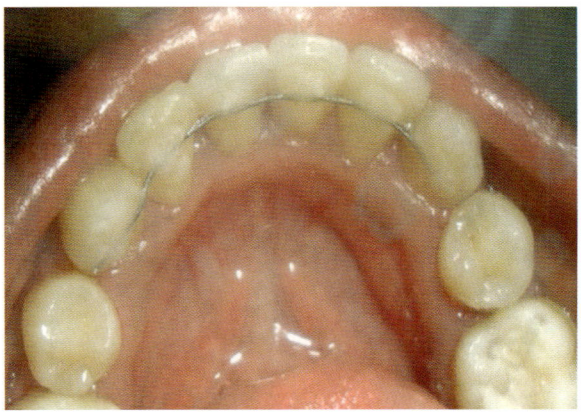

Fig. 25.11: 3–3 bonded retainer

- Readymade 3–3 retainers with bonding mesh pads are also available.
- Using flexible spiral wire.

Bonded Retainer with Multistranded Wire

Advantages

- It may allow safe retention of treatment.
- They allow physiologic tooth movement of all bonded teeth.
- It is invisible.
- It gives neat and clean appearance.
- It can be placed out of occlusion in most instance.
- It can be used alone or in combination with removable retainer.

Indications

- Midline diastema (Fig. 25.12)
- Spacing in the anterior
- Adult patients with periodontal involvement
- Accidental loss of maxillary incisors
- Moderate to severe crowding cases
- Severe rotation of upper incisors (Fig. 25.13)
- Palatally impacted canine
- Extraction of mandibular incisors

4–4 Bonded Retainer

Indications

- Deep overbite cases in which incisors are supraerupted. It helps to maintain lower intrusion
- It prevents the space from reopening of 1st premolar extraction site.

Bonding Procedure

It can be done indirectly as well as directly.

Direct approach

- After orthodontic correction, it is mandatory to use the working model as a guide in order to adjust the retainer wire closely on the lingual surface of anterior.
- Cut the flexible spiral wire (FSW) to the required length and check it in the mouth for good fit.
- Etch the enamel after polishing, then wash and dry it up.
- *Fixing of FSW:* The wire should be closely adapted on the lingual surface. Otherwise there will be two types of bond failures:
  - Separation at tooth adhesive interface is due to moisture contamination or movement of lingual wire during initial polymerization.
  - Separation at adhesive retainer wire interface is due to inadequate bulk of adhesive for sufficient strength. For this reason, many techniques have been described and adopted to place such retainers closely on the lingual surface
  - *Techniques are:* Dental floss, elastic thread ligature wire, etc.
- Sealant application and fix it with adhesive.

Banded Canine-to-Canine Retainer (Fig. 25.14)

- Commonly used in lower anterior region.
- Canines are banded and a thick wire is contoured over the lingual aspects and soldered to the canine bands.
- The bands predispose to poor oral hygiene and are unesthetic.

Band and Spur Retainer

It is used in cases where single tooth has been orthodontically treated for rotation correction or labio-lingual displacement. The tooth that has been moved is banded and spurs are soldered onto the bands so as to overlap the adjacent teeth (Fig. 25.15).

Maintaining Lower Incisor Position during Late Mandibular Growth (Fig. 25.16)

- Even mild mandibular growth between the ages of 16–20 years can cause lower incisor relapse.

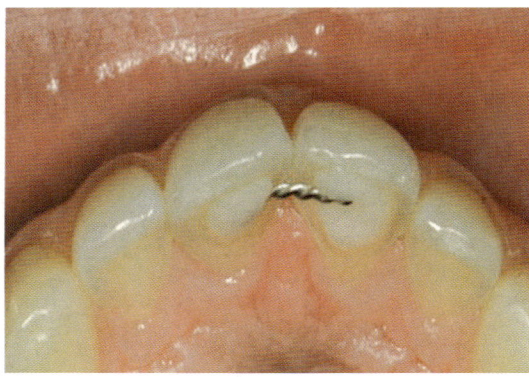

Fig. 25.12: After correction of midline diastema

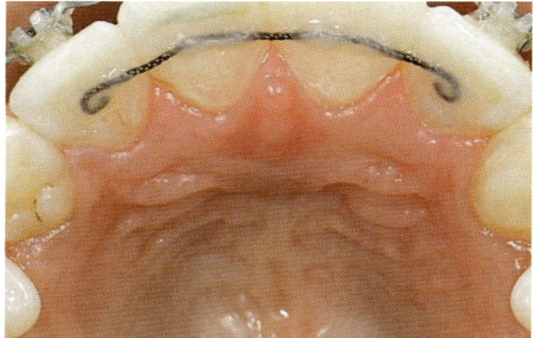

Fig. 25.13: Bonded retainer involving 4 incisors

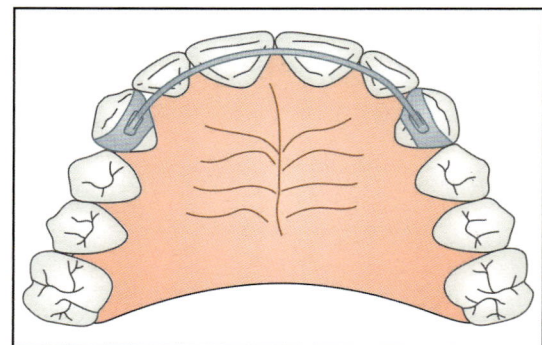

Fig. 25.14: Banded canine-to-canine retainer

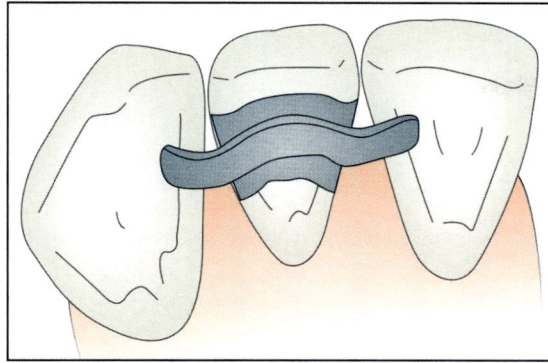

Fig. 25.15: Band and spur retainer

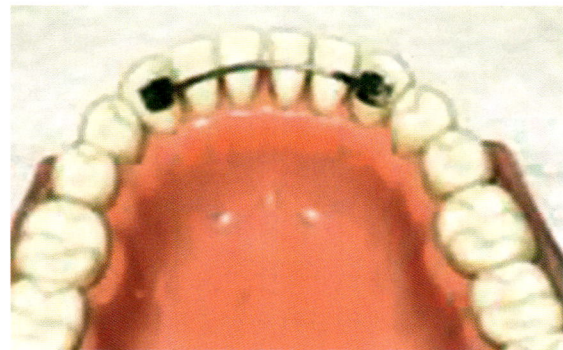

Fig. 25.16: Lower bonded retainer using mesh pad

- A fixed lingual bar bonded only to canines can prevent distal tipping of lower incisors.
- A heavy wire, 28 or 30 mm, should be used due to long span.
- Studies indicate that placing retention loops on canines will decrease breakage.

Retention: Class II

Relapse in these patients are most likely due to a combination of dental and skeletal changes.

Dental Changes (Short-Term Relapse)

- 1–2 mm of AP change tends to occur immediately following treatment, especially when Class II elastics are used.
- Overcorrection is important in preventing relapse.
- Forward movement of lower incisors more than 2 mm will require permanent retention, as lip pressure tends to upright these teeth, leading to an increase in crowding, overbite, and overjet

Skeletal Changes (Long-Term Relapse)

- Depends on age, sex, and maturity

- If original growth pattern continues, treatment that involved growth modification will most likely result in loss of at least some correction:
  1. Continue headgear at night along with retainer
  2. Use a "passive" functional appliance (activator/bionator) to hold position at night and conventional retainers during day (continue for 12–24 months).

  Patients most likely to require these treatments:
  - The younger the patient at the end of treatment
  - The greater the initial Class II problem
  - Much easier to prevent relapse than to correct later

Retention is brought by bionator/activator (Fig. 25.17):
- Maintain occlusal relationship
- Bite registration is taken in CR, so appliance is 'passive'.
- Not edge-to-edge like when used for "active" Class II correction.

Retention: Class III

- Relapse occurs mainly from mandibular growth.
- Use of chin cups to restrict mandibular growth has been recommended by some authors to counter the continued growth tendency of mandible.
- But chin cups and functional appliances rotate mandible downward causing more vertical growth. Not as effective as maintaining Class II.
- If relapse occurs in normal or excessive face height patients, may need surgical correction after growth.
- In less severe Class III cases: Utilize functional appliances such as reverse activator, FR 3 or Class III bionator or positioner.
- Will maintain occlusal relationship in these cases.
- May position jaws down and back to prevent relapse.

Retention: Deep Bite (Fig. 25.18)

- Must control overbite during retention period.

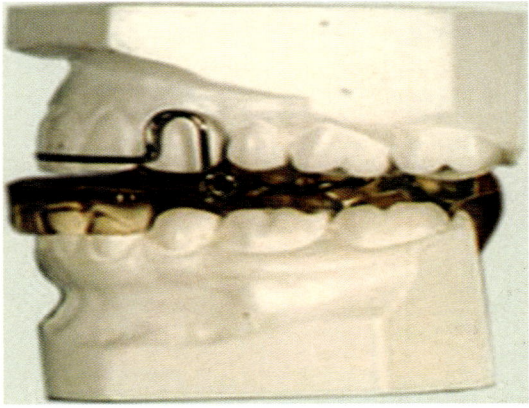

Fig. 25.17: Retention after functional appliance

- Construct upper removable retainer with a baseplate to prevent lower incisors from over-erupting; posterior occlusion is maintained.
- After stability is achieved, worn at night only.
- Nanda and Nanda found that the pubertal growth spurt in deep bite patients is 1.5–2 years later than that of open bite cases; therefore, longer retention period is required for deep bite cases.

Retention: Anterior Open Bite

Patients with habit (thumb or tongue):
- Relapse occurs due to incisor intrusion.
- Important to control the habit.

Patients without habit:
- Relapse is due to excessive growth tendencies and continued eruption of posteriors mainly upper molars (extrusion).
- Important to control eruption of upper molars.

RALEIGH WILLIAMS' SIX KEYS TO ELIMINATE LOWER RETENTION

First key: Incisal edges of the lower incisors should be placed on the AP line or 1 mm in front of it. This has been described as the optimum position for stability. It also creates optimum soft tissue balance in lower third of the face. Here, it is pertinent to add, incisor angulation of 90° to mandibular plane or 65° to FH plane is only esthetically appropriate and stable for those who have optimal north European skeletal configurations, but not for patients of other ethinic region (Fig. 25.19).

Second key: Lower incisors apices should be spread distally to the crowns, more than is generally considered appropriate. The apices of the lower lateral incisors must be spread more than centrals. When the lower roots are left convergent or even parallel, crowns

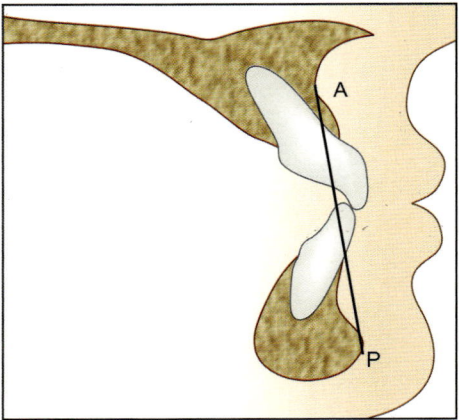

Fig. 25.19: Position of incisal edges of lower incisors should be 0-1 mm A-Pog line according to Raleigh Williams' rules

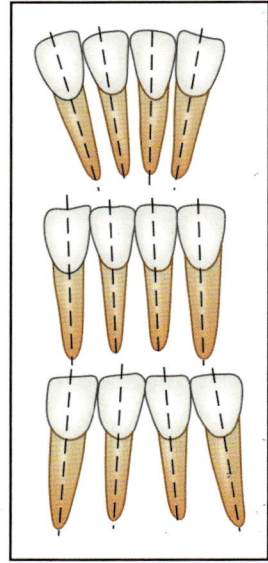

Fig. 25.20: Root position of lower incisors for stability according to Raleigh Williams' rules

tend to bunch up and a fixed retainer has to be used (Fig. 25.20).

Third key: Apex of lower cuspid should be positioned distal of the crown. This angulation of lower cuspid is important in creating post-treatment incisor stability, as it reduces the tendency of the cuspid crown to tip forward into the incisor area.

Fourth key: All four lower incisor, apices must be in the same labiolingual plane. Spreading roots distally causes strong reciprocal tendency for crowns to move mesially.

Fifth key: Lower cuspid root apex must be positioned slightly buccal to the crown apex. The old concept that lower intercanine width cannot be permanently

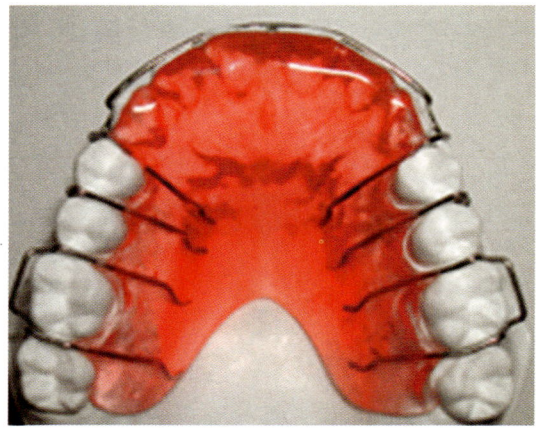

Fig. 25.18: Retainer with anterior bite plane in case of deep bite

increased is true only for some of the cases. After treatment, if lower cuspids are moved distally over wider arch and roots apex more buccal to crown, stability will be maintained.

Sixth key: The lower incisors should be slenderized as needed. Lower incisors which have had no proximal wear have round, small contact points that are accentuated, if the apices have been spread for stability. Subsequently, slightest amount of continuous mesial pressure can cause variable degrees of collapse. Flattening lower incisor contact points by stripping creates flat contact surfaces that help resist labiolingual crown displacement.

TWELVE KEYS TO STABILITY OF LOWER INCISORS (MARIELLE BLAKE, NANDA AND BURSTONE)

1. Whenever possible allow the lower incisors to align themselves either through serial extraction or the use of lip bumper in early mixed dentition.
2. Over correct lower incisor rotations as early in treatment as possible.
3. Reproximation of incisors early in treatment and again at retention enhances stability.
4. Avoid increasing the inter-canine width during active treatment.
5. Extract bicuspids in cases where mandibular arch discrepancy is 4 mm or greater, except where facial esthetics dictate otherwise.
6. Recognize that the more the tooth is moved, the more likely it is to relapse, and over correct accordingly.
7. Upright lower incisors to at least 90° whenever the profile permits.
8. Create a flat occlusal plane during treatment and overcorrect the overbite.
9. Prescribe supracrestal fibrotomy for severely rotated teeth.
10. Retain the lower arch until all growth is completed.
11. Place the retainers the same day, the appliances are removed.
12. Recognize that, compromise is often necessary in the interest of facial esthetics and that sometimes lifetime retention is necessary.

BIBLIOGRAPHY

1. Contemporary Orthodontics, William R. Proffit (5th. Edition).
2. Graber TM. Orthodontics: Principles and Practice, 3rd Ed. WB Sounders. 1988.
3. Henry Kaplan WJB. The logic of modern retention procedures. American Journal of Orthodontics and Dentofacial Orthopedics 1988;93($):325–340.
4. Williams R. "Eliminating Lower Retention". Journal of Clinical Orthodontics, May 1985;342–349.

PREVIOUS YEAR'S UNIVERSITY QUESTIONS

Essay

1. What is retention? What are the different causes of relapse? Describe the measures taken to prevent relapse.
2. Describe the various theorems of retention.
3. Classify retainer. Describe the procedure of fixing bonded retainer.

Short Questions

1. Apical base school of thought
2. Essex retainer
3. Invisible retainer
4. Band and spur retainer

MCQs

1. *Purpose of the post-treatment retention of an orthodontic case is:*
   a. To allow bony changes
   b. To prevent tongue thrusting
   c. To encourage the space closure
   d. To let the patient get used to the new functional position of the teeth.   **(Ans: d)**

2. *Relapse after orthodontic treatment can be totally prevented by:*
   a. Inactive fixed appliance
   b. Hawley's retainer worn for 1 year
   c. Wearing activator for 3 months
   d. None of the above   **(Ans: d)**

3. *Relapse after orthodontic tooth movement is due to:*
   a. Supracrestal gingival fibers
   b. Abnormal pressure habits
   c. Improper angulation of the teeth
   d. All of the above   **(Ans: d)**

4. *Best retainer advised after the closure of midline diastema is:*
   a. Hawley's retainer
   b. Hawley's retainer with finger spring
   c. Positioner
   d. Bonded retainer   **(Ans: d)**

5. *A corrected anterior crossbite is retained by:*
   a. Over-correction
   b. Normal incisor correction
   c. Hawley's retentive appliance
   d. Palatal acrylic appliance with no labial archwire.   **(Ans: b)**

6. *Keys to eliminate lower retention was proposed by:*
   a. Moyers
   b. Alex Lundstrom
   c. Raleigh Williams
   d. Nance   **(Ans: c)**

7. *Wrap around retainer is:*
   a. An extended version of spring aligner
   b. Used in periodontally weak dentition
   c. The labial and lingual surfaces of all teeth embedded in a strip of acrylic
   d. All of the above   **(Ans: d)**

8. *Band and spur retainer is used for:*
   a. Stabilizing the derotated tooth
   b. Stabilizing the midline diastema correction
   c. Stabilizing crossbite correction
   d. None of the above   **(Ans: a)**

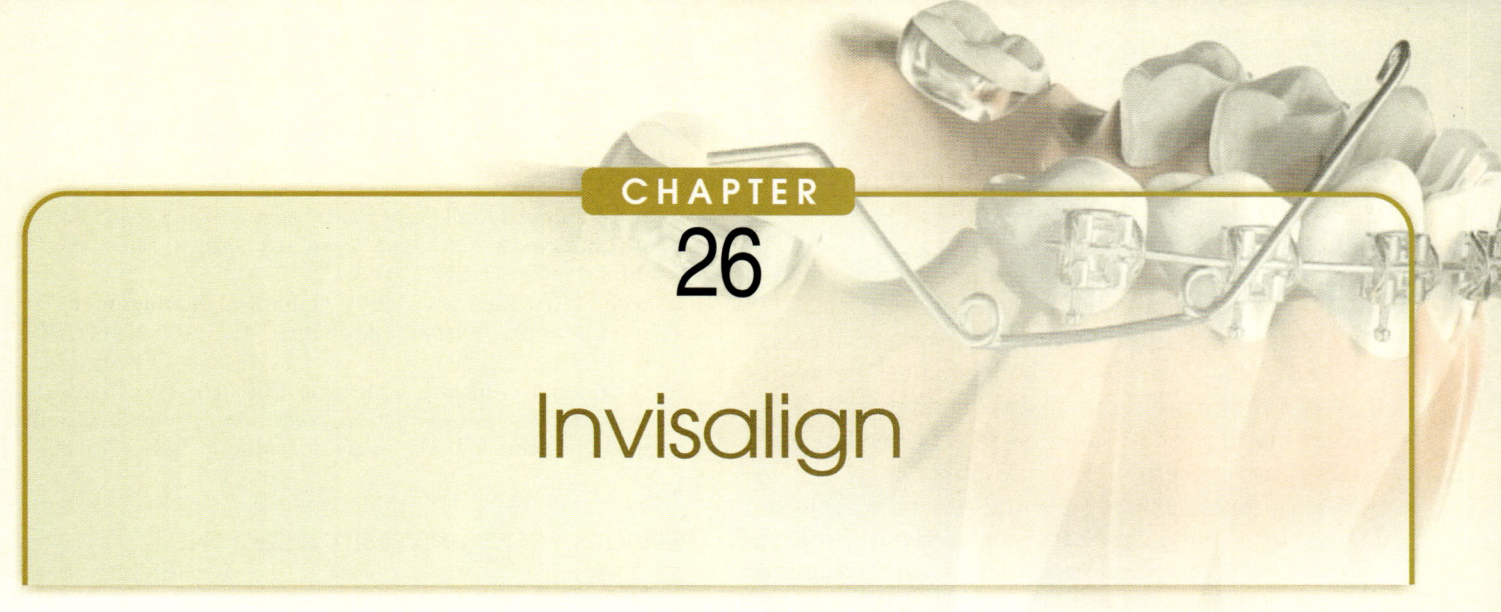

Invisalign

Invisalign is manufactured by Align Technology, a multinational medical-device company headquartered in San Jose, California. The company was founded in 1997 by Zia Chishti. Chishti conceived of the basic design of invisalign while an adult orthodontics patient. During his treatment with a retainer intended to complete his treatment, he posited a series of such devices could affect a large final placement in a series of small movements. He partnered with Kelsey Wirth to seek developers.

Invisalign takes a modern approach to straightening teeth, using a custom-made series of aligners created. These aligner trays are made of smooth, comfortable and virtually invisible plastic that is worn over the teeth. Wearing the aligners will gradually and gently shift the teeth into place, based on the exact movements the dentist or orthodontist plans out. There are no metal brackets to attach and no wires to tighten. You just pop in a new set of aligners approximately every two weeks, until your treatment is complete. You will achieve a great smile with little interference in your daily life. The best part about the whole process is that most people woold not even know you are straightening your teeth.

They are also indicated for patients who have experienced a relapse after fixed orthodontic treatment.

Clear-aligner treatment involves an orthodontist or dentist taking a mold of the patient's teeth, which is used to create a digital tooth scan. The computerized model suggests stages between the current and desired teeth positions, and aligners are created for each stage.

Each aligner is worn for 20 hours a day for two weeks. These slowly move the teeth into the position agreed between the orthodonist/dentist and the patient. The average treatment time is 13.5 months.

Clear aligners, also known as clear-aligner treatment, are orthodontic devices that are used incremental transparent aligners to adjust teeth as an alternative to dental braces. They are sold under the brand names Clear Correct and Invisalign.

A 2014 systematic review concluded that there is insufficient evidence to determine the effectiveness of these therapies. Opinion is that they are effective for moderate crowding of the front teeth, but are less effective than conventional braces for several other issues. In particular, they are indicated for "mild to moderate crowding (1–6 mm) and mild to moderate spacing (1–6 mm)".

Clear aligners are likely useful for moderate front-teeth crowding. In those with teeth that are too far forward or backward, or rotated in the socket, the aligners are likely not as effective as conventional braces. More cases of relapse of the anterior teeth have been found with Invisalign compared with conventional braces. Clear aligners are more noticeable than lingual braces, but are probably more comfortable. They can be removed, which makes cleaning of the teeth easier and they are faster for the dentist to apply.

Application

- Treatment begins with taking X-ray, photographs, a bite registration, and polyvinyl siloxane impressions of the person's teeth and gums.

- The dentist/orthodontist completes a written evaluation that includes diagnosis and treatment plan.
- Dental impressions are scanned in order to create a digital 3D representation of the teeth.
- Technicians move the teeth to the desired location with the program treat, which creates the stages between the current and desired teeth positions.
- Anywhere from 6 to 48 aligners may be needed. Each aligner moves teeth 0.25 to 0.33 mm.
- A computer graphic representation of the projected teeth movements, created in the software program ClinCheck, is provided to the doctor and patient for approval or modification before aligners are manufactured.
- The aligners are modeled using CAD-CAM (computer-aided-design and computer-aided-manufacturing) software and manufactured using a rapid prototyping technique called stereolithography.
- The molds for the aligners are built in layers using a photosensitive liquid resin that cures into a hard plastic when exposed to a laser.
- The aligners are made from an elastic thermoplastic material that applies pressure to the teeth to move into the aligner's position.
- Patients that need a tooth rotated or pulled down may have a small, tooth-colored composite attachment bonded onto certain teeth.
- More attachments can make the aligners less aesthetically pleasing.
- Reproximation, (also called interproximal reduction or IPR and colloquially, filing or drilling), is sometimes used at the contacts between teeth to allow for a better fit.

Each aligner is intended to be worn 20 hours a day for two weeks. On average, the treatment process takes 13.5 months. Treatment time varies based on the complexity of the planned teeth movements. The aligner is removed for brushing, flossing and eating. Once the treatment period has concluded, the patient is advised to continue wearing a retainer at night for the foreseeable future.

When the Invisalign system was first developed, many of the aligner manufacturing processes were carried out by hand, and computer technicians had to modify each tooth in the computerized model individually.

BIBLIOGRAPHY

1. Jean Philippe Houle, Luis Piedade, et al. The Predictability of Transverse Changes with invisalign. The Angle Orthodontist 2016;87(1):19–24.
2. Rooybeth Khosravi, Bobby Cohanim. Management of overbite with invisalign appliance. Ajo 2017; 151(4):691–699,e2.
3. Thorsten Grunheid, Charlene Loh. How accurate is invisalign in non-extraction cases? Are predicted tooth positions achieved. The angle orthodontist 2017;87(6):809–815.

PREVIOUS YEAR'S UNIVERSITY QUESTIONS

MCQs

1. *Who introduced the Invisalign?*
   a. EH Angle
   b. Cruz
   c. Align technology
   d. None of the above **(Ans: c)**

2. *In which year Align technologies introduced invisalign?*
   a. 1990
   b. 1999
   c. 1980
   d. 1993 **(Ans: b)**

3. *A typical Invisalign treatment requires:*
   a. 20–30 aligners
   b. 50–80 aligners
   c. 90–110 aligners
   d. 120–130 aligners **(Ans: a)**

4. *Benefits of Invisalign are:*
   a. Easier cleaning
   b. Invisible thus no unwanted attention to your mouth
   c. No brackets
   d. All of the above **(Ans: d)**

5. *Invisalign is:*
   a. Fixed
   b. Semi-fixed
   c. Removable
   d. Semi-removable **(Ans: c)**

6. *Models for Invisalign are made by the process called:*
   a. Steriography
   b. Stereolithiography
   c. Sterography
   d. Steroanginography **(Ans: b)**

Lab Procedures in Orthodontics

27.1 STUDY MODEL PREPARATION

Chapter Outline

- Parts of study model
- Steps in preparation of study models

ORTHODONTIC STUDY MODELS

Orthoontic study models are essential diagnostic records which are accurate plaster reproductions of the teeth and their supporing soft tissues and which help to study the occlusion and the dentition from all the three dimensions.

Parts of a Study Model (Fig. 27.1)

Orthodontic study model consists of two parts:
1. Anatamic portion
2. Artistic portion

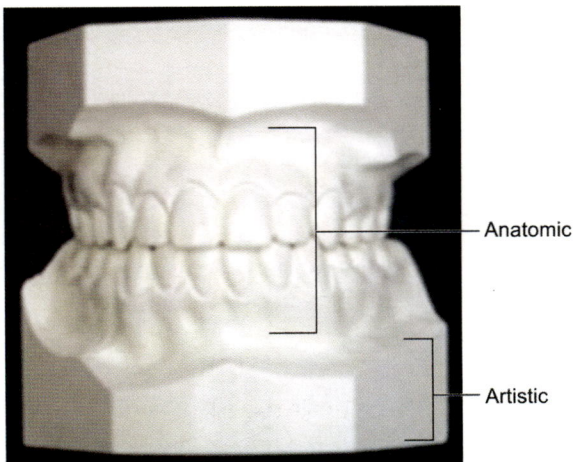

Fig. 27.1: Parts of a study model

1. *Anatomic portion:* It is the actual replica of the dental arch and surrounding tissues. This part is usually made of dental stone. It should not be disturbed while trimming.

2. *Artistic portion:* It is the base portion, which supports the anatamic portion. The artistic portion is usually made of dental plaster.

Ratio of portion of orthodontic study model: The ratio of the anatomic portion to artistic portion is 3:1, e.g. three parts of anatomic portion and one part of artistic portion.

Steps in Preparation of Study Models

The following are the sequential steps involved in fabrication of the study models:
- Step I: Impression making
- Step II: Disinfection of the impression
- Step III: Casting the impression
- Step IV: Basing and trimming of the cast
- Step V: Finishing and polishing

It is advised to soak models in water for 5 minutes before starting to trim to make trimming easier. The anatomical portion of model should not be immersed.

The following are the steps involved in trimming of the study models:

Step 1 (Fig. 27.2)

- The base of the mandibular cast should be parallel to the occlusal plane.
- The lower model is inverted over a T shaped piece of rubber and marking is circumscribed all around the base of the model using a marker mounded on a vertical stand.
- Once the marking is made, the base of the cast is trimmed up to the marking.

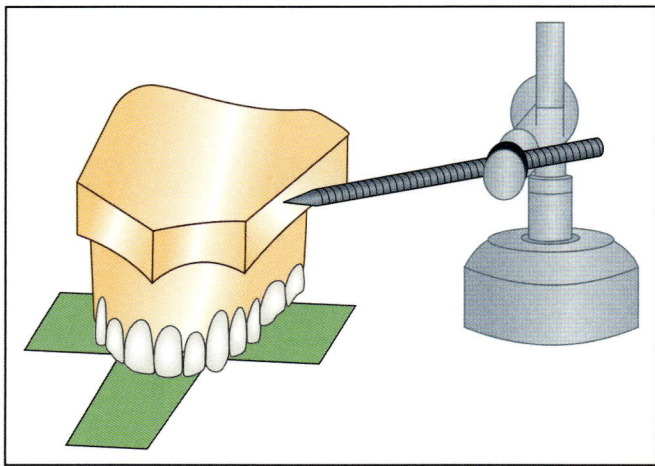

Fig. 27.2: Step 1

Step 2 (Fig. 27.3)

- Back of the mandibular cast is trimmed so that it is perpendicular to the base and a line drawn between two central incisors.
- While trimming the back of the cast, 5 mm of the plaster base should be left distal to the most posterior teeth.

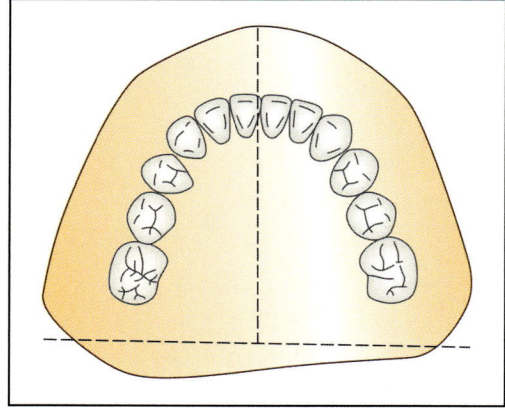

Fig. 27.3: Step 2

Step 3 (Fig. 27.4)

Occlude the upper and lower models together and trim the maxillary back surface, so that the maxillary back is in flush with the mandibular back.

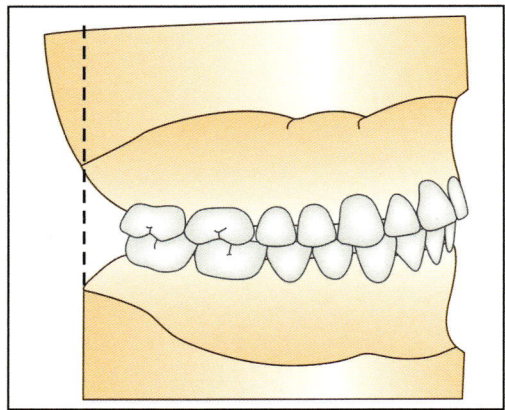

Fig. 27.4: Step 3

Step 4 (Fig. 27.5)

- The upper and lower models are occluded together and are placed on their backs on the model to the trimmer.
- The base of the maxillary cast is trimmed so that it is parallel to the base of the lower model.

After the step, the bases of maxillary and mandibular cast are parallel to each other and to the occlusal plane, and the backs of both the upper and lower casts should be perpendicular to their bases. Occlusal models should have a sharp 90° angle between their base and back.

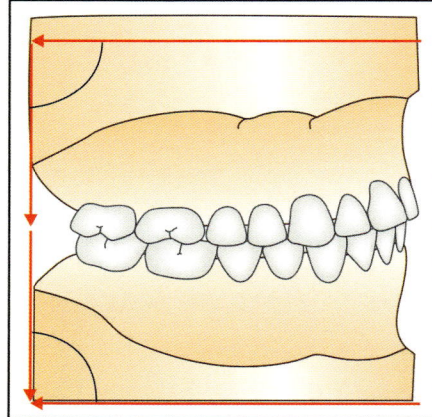

Fig. 27.5: Step 4

Step 5 (Fig. 27.6)

- The buccal cuts are made on the mandibular cast 5–6 mm away from the buccal surface of the posterior teeth.
- The buccal cuts are made 60° to the back of the model.
- The anterior segment of the lower arch is trimmed into a curve that follows the curvature of the lower anterior teeth.
- The anterior curve should be 5–6 mm away from the labial surface of the anterior teeth.

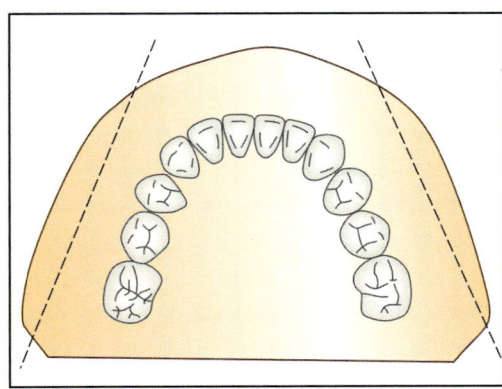

Fig. 27.6: Step 5

Step 6 (Fig. 27.7)

The anterior segment of the lower arch is trimmed into a curve that follows the curvature of the lower anterior teeth.

The anterior curve should be 5–6 mm away from the labial surface of the anterior teeth.

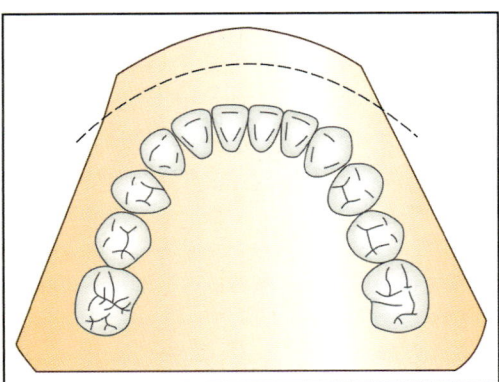

Fig. 27.7: Step 6

Step 7 (Fig. 27.8)

- The posterior cuts of the mandibular model are trimmed at approximately 115° to the back of the model.
- The linear measurement of the posterior cuts should be 13–15 mm.

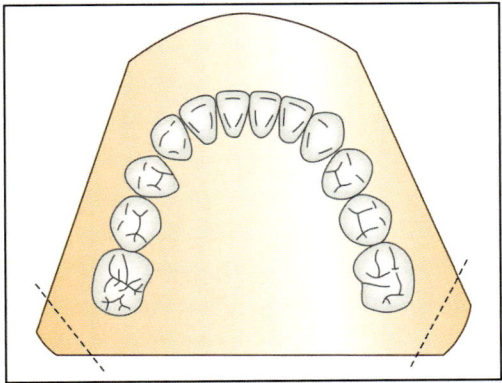

Fig. 27.8: Step 7

Step 8 (Fig. 27.9)

- The buccal cuts are made on the maxillary cast 5 mm away from the buccal surface of the most posterior teeth.
- The buccal cuts should be 65° to the back of the maxillary cast.

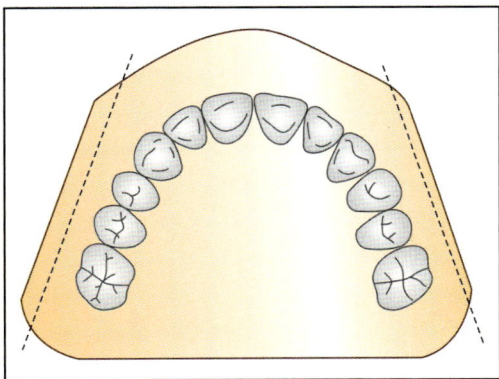

Fig. 27.9: Step 8

Step 9 (Fig. 27.10)

- The anterior cuts are made on the maxillary cast.
- The cuts on either side should be equal length and should lie 5–6 mm ahead of the labial surface of the anterior teeth.
- The anterior cuts on either side should meet at the midline of the cast and should extend till the midline of the canine.
- The anterior cuts are made 30° to the back of the cast.

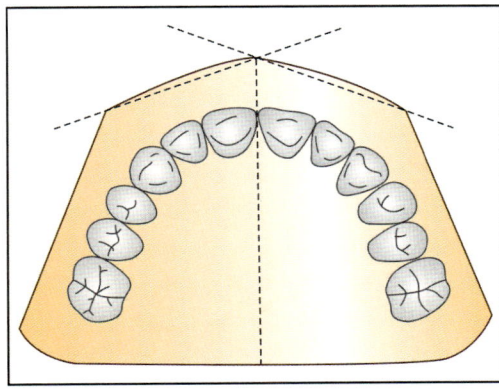

Fig. 27.10: Step 9

Step 10 (Fig. 27.11)

- The posterior cuts of the maxillary cut are made in such a way that they are in flush with the posterior cuts of the mandibular cast.
- This is done by occluding the models and trimming the maxillary posterior cuts till they are in line with the mandibular posterior cuts.

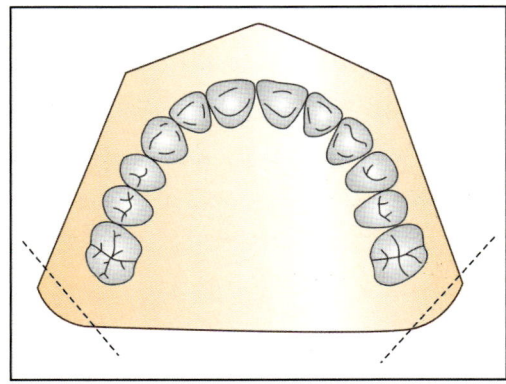

Fig. 27.11: Step 10

Bibliography

1. Proffit WR, Fields HW, Jr. Saver DM. Contemporary orthodontics, Fourth edition. st Louis Mosby. Inc. 2007;167–233.
2. Ellis PE, Benson PE. Does articulaling study casts make a difference to treatment planning? J. Orthod. 2003;30:45–49.

PREVIOUS YEAR'S UNIVERSITY QUESTIONS

Short Questions

1. Parts of a study model
2. Discuss the different steps in preparation of study models

27.2 WELDING AND SOLDERING

Chapter Outline

- Definitions
- Types of welding

- Application of welding in orthodontics
- Application of soldering in orthodontics

DEFINITIONS

Welding is the joining of two or more metal pieces directly under pressure without introduction of an intermediary or a filler material

Soldering is the joining of two or more metal pieces directly under pressure with introduction of an intermediary or a filler material called solder.

TYPES OF WELDING

Following are three types of welding:
1. Cold welding
2. Hot welding
3. Spot welding

Cold Welding

Cold welding is a process of plastically deforming a metal (usually at room temperature) accompanied by strain hardening, e.g. gold foil filling.

Hot Welding

Hot welding uses the heat of sufficient intensity to melt the metals being joined.

Spot Welding (Fig. 27.12)

Spot welding involves both heat and pressure, these two are the basic principles involved in the process of spot welding, e.g. joining of orthodontic components.

Principles of Spot Welding

Following are the two principles involved in the process of spot welding:
- Heat
- Pressure
  - Electric current (A/C) is made to pass through a step down transformer to obtain a low voltage of high amperage current that is conducted through two copper electrodes on either side of the metal being joined.
  - Resistance offered by stainless steel to the current of high amperage generates very high temperature at the electrodes.

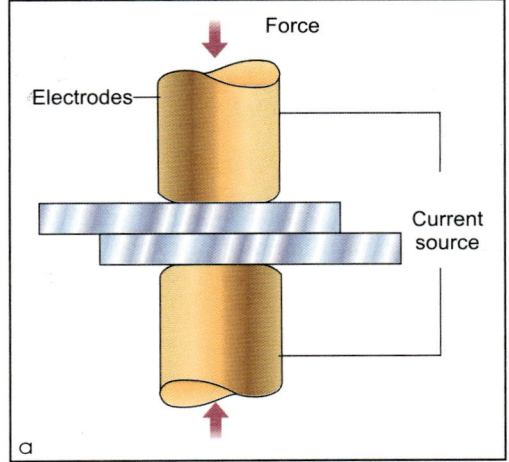

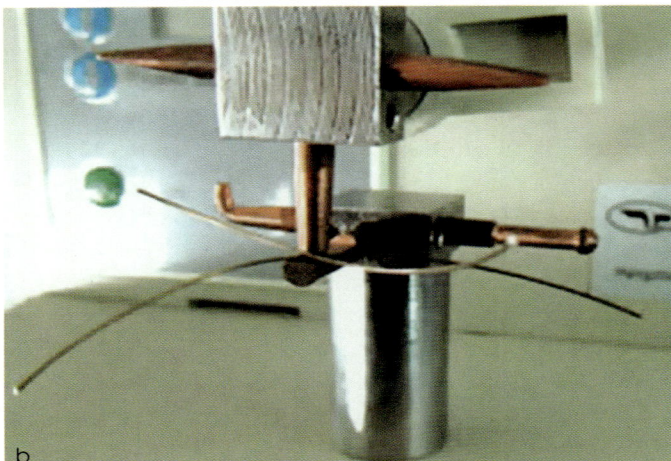

Fig. 27.12a and b: Parts of spot welder

  - Thus, the area of metal under the electrodes becomes plastic.
- The copper electrodes simultaneously apply pressure on the metals and, therefore, squeeze the metals into each other.

Copper electrodes: The copper electrodes in a welding unit serve the following purposes:
- Transmit current to the metals to be joined so as to cause a rapid increase in temperature.
- The electrodes help in conducting the heat produced away from the area so as to preserve the properties of stainless steel around the weld spot.

- The two electrodes also help in holding together the two metals to be joined.
- The electrodes are designed to apply pressure on the metals being joined. As soon as the temperature increases, the pressure exerted by the electrodes helps in squeezing the metal into each other.

Duration of current: It includes:

- It is very important that this passage of current at the weld spot of very short duration, i.e. not more than 1/10th of a second.
- In case, the current is passed for a longer duration of time, it results in weld decay due to the precipitation of carbides from the metal.

Procedure of Spot Welding

- *Selection of proper electrodes:* Select the proper electrodes for the thickness or shape of the material to be welded (Fig. 27.12a and b).
- *For welding, thin materials:* A broad electrode should be used.
- *For welding thick materials:* A narrow electrode should be used.
- *Cleansing the electrodes:* The electrodes of the welder are cleaned so as to remove any carbide precipitates.
- *Surface of electrodes:* Surface of electrodes must be smooth, flat and perpendicular to its long axis.
- *The metals being joined:* The metals being joined are placed between the electrodes.
- *Switch is turned on:* The electrode pressure can be maintained for a few seconds to help to obtain a good joint.
- Force is applied before, during and after the application of current to prevent arching at the work piece.
- In spot welding, fusion of faying surfaces of a lap joint is achieved at one location by opposing electrodes.
- When electrodes are together, they should be in total contact. If not, they should be filed until total contact is achieved. Sparking and localized over welding will result, if interface contact is not uniform.

APPLICATION OF WELDING IN ORTHODONTICS

1. Joining of metal strips during bonding.
2. Fixing attachments, such as brackets and molar tubes to the bands.
3. Attaching springs to a rigid bow wire or to bands

Advantages of Spot Welding

- Spot welding quick and easy

- No need to any flux or filler material.
- Multiple sheets are joined together at same time.
- No dangerous open flame
- Save production costs.
  Circuit diagram of spot welding machine is shown in Fig. 27.13.

Spot Welder (Fig. 27.14)

Orthodontic spot welders employ the electrode technique and are used instead of soldering in cases where the heating cycle must be very short, in order to prevent changes in the physical properties of the components being joined.

Bracket Welding with Mesh

Originally, the strands within the mesh backing were wlded to each other and to the back of the bracket. Spot welding appears to cause damage to the mesh base where the mesh is completely obliterated by the spot welding, causing the wire to fracture and leaving sharp areas exposed. Spot-weld damage not only decreases the nominal area available for retention but also produce an area of stress concentration which can initiate the fracture of the adhesive at the adhesive base interface. Inadequate spot-welding may lead to separation of the bracket from the base.

Laser Welding (Fig. 27.15a to c)

- Laser welding in an argon gas atmosphere is done to join the titanium components. Advantage using this method is that the metal is subjected to vary minimal heat influence and hence the welded joint will be composed of same pure titanium as the substrate components. Laser welding units are now available.
- The laser used is ususlly a pulsed high power neodymium laser with a very high power density.

Advantages of Laser Welding

- Lower heat generation.
- No oxide formation because of the inert argon atmosphere.
- Joint made of the same pure titanium as the components, thus reduces the risk of galvanic corrosion.

APPLICATION OF SOLDERING IN ORTHODONTICS

- Fusion of brackets and buccal tubes onto the bands in fixed orthodontic appliances
- Fixed rapid maxillary appliances
- Banded canine-to-canine retainers

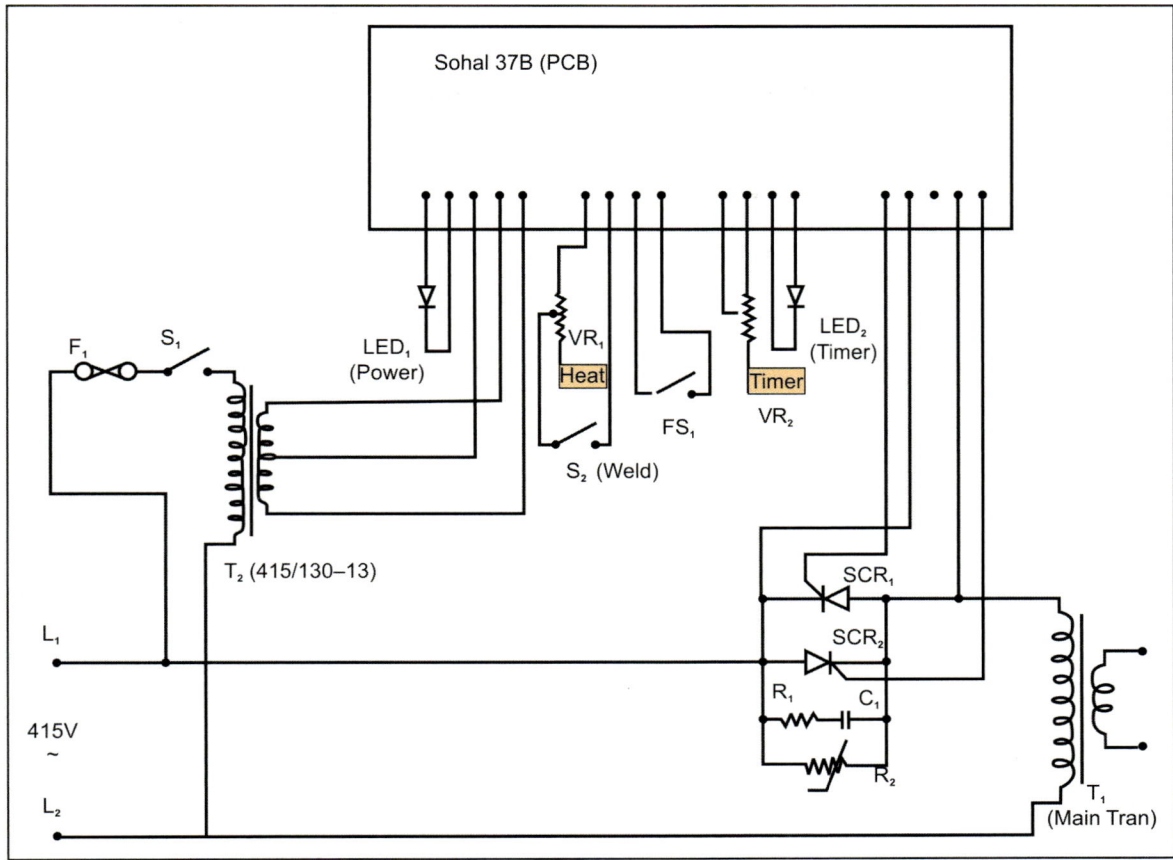

Fig. 27.13: Circuit diagram

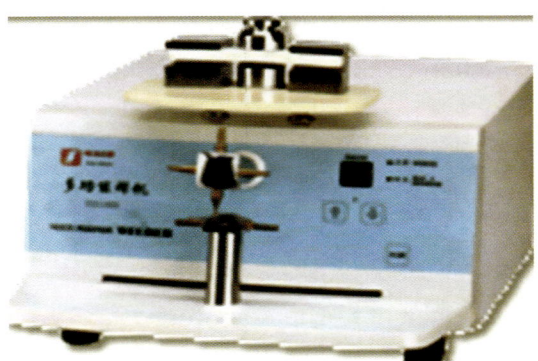

Fig. 27.14: Spot welder

- Band and spur retainers
- Habit-breaking appliances—band and loop space maintainers

Techniques for Soldering

Depending on the degree of precision to which the components are to be joined.
- Free hand soldering
- Jig soldering
- Investment soldering

Free hand soldering: Orthodontic torch can be placed on a bench so that both hands can be used to hold the parts in position (Fig. 27.16a). The process involves soldering two metallic parts together after adequate stabilization, without the use of investments to precisely hold the parts (Fig. 27.16b).

Soldering Procedure

- Ideally silver solders are used—alloy of silver, copper, zinc to which in and indium are added to lower the fusion temperature and improve solderability.
- Soldering temperature
- Technical considerations:
  a. Needle like not luminous gas air flame is used.
  b. Thinner the diameter of the flame, less the metal surrounding the joint is annealed.
  c. The work is held 3 mm beyond the tip of the blue cone in the reducing zone of the flame.
  d. Soldering should be observed in shadow against a black background so the temperature can be judged by the color of the work. The color should not exceed dull red.

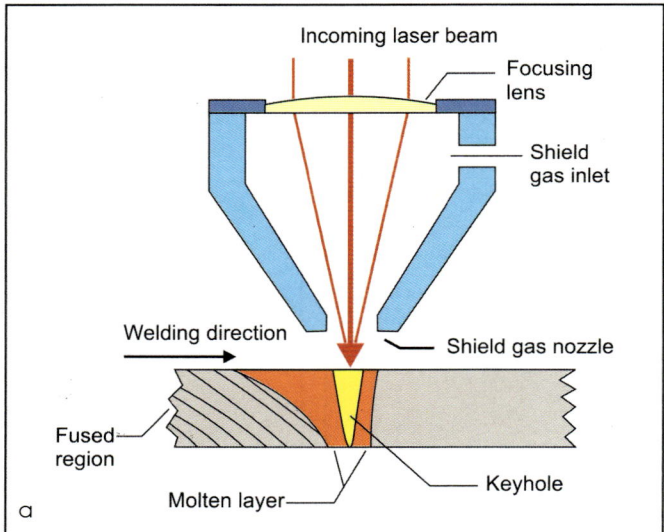

Laser welding article

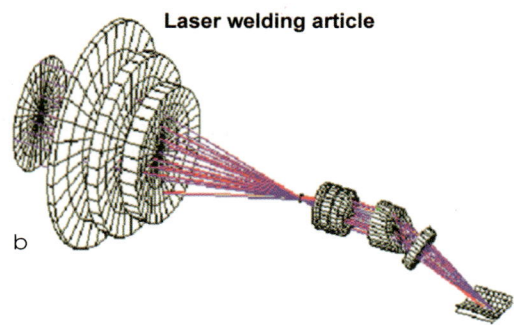

b

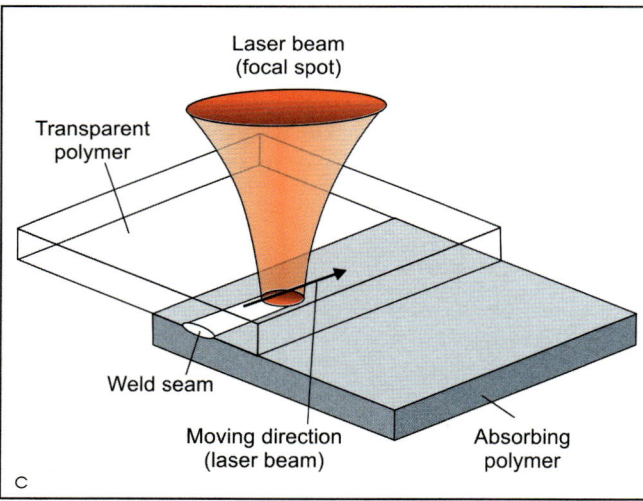

Fig. 27.15a to c: Laser welding

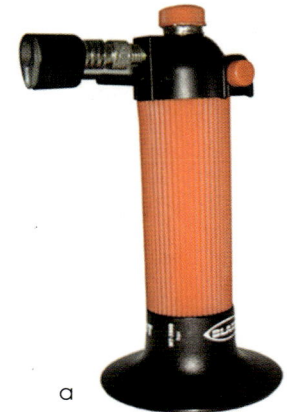

a

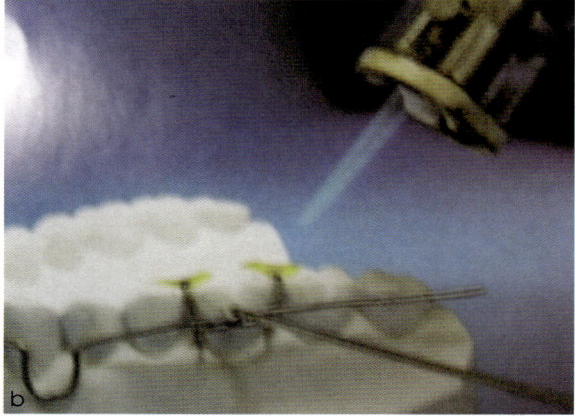

b

Fig. 27.16: (a) Torch, (b) Free hand soldering

the flux also dissolves the impurities, prevents the oxidation of the metals. Fluxes used commonly are:

- Borax—55%
- Boric acid—35%
- Silica—10%

Ideal Requirement of a Dental Solder

1. It should melt at low temperature.
2. It should be wet and flow freely.
3. Its color should match that of metal being joined.
4. It should be resistance to tarnish and corrosion.
5. It should resist pitting during heating.

When do you apply solder?

- First, flux bubbles as the excess water is driven off.
- Then, it dries becoming hard, white and crusty.
- Finally, as it gets even hotter, it melts into a molten, glistening film. This indicates that the metals are hot enough for the solder to follow toward them, if held in close proximity.

e. If possible, the parts should be tag-welded to hold the parts together.

f. *Fluxes:* Flux is Latin word meaning 'flow'. The flux aid in the removal of the oxide layer so as to increase the flow of the molten solder. In addition,

Technical Procedure

- Cleaning and preparing the surface to joined
- Assembling the parts to be joined
- Application of the flux to the parts to be joined
- Controlling the flame temperature
- Controlling the time to ensure adequate flow

  Note:
  - Zone of flame
  - The reducing zone is to be used

Investment Soldering (Fig. 27.17)

It is used when the area of contact between the metallic parts being joined is large, and whenever precision is needed in joining the metals. This procedure involves the embedding of the metallic parts in investment leaving a gap of about 0.13 mm between the metals.

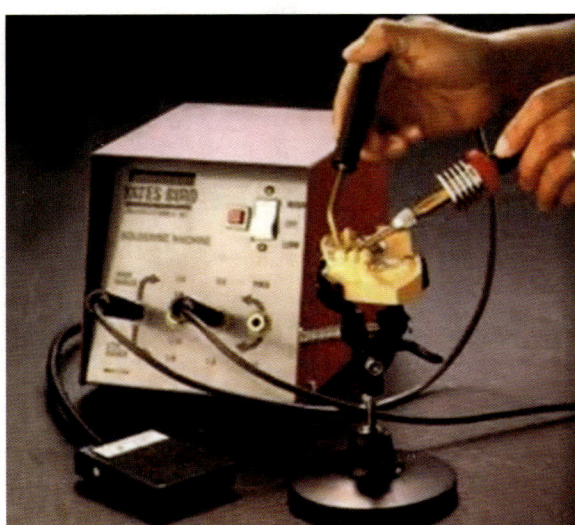

Fig. 27.17: Investment soldering

Failures in Soldering

- Overheating of the solder can lead to pitted joint of low strength
- Failure due to clean the parts to be joined
- Failure due to improper fluxing and flow of solder
- Corrosion
- Porosities, brittleness due to impurities causes failure in soldering

Bibliography

1. White Kent. Braying versus soldering TM Technologies, Tools and method for better Metal working. Archived from original on 23, June 2017, Retrieved 2 May 2018.
2. Aggarwal A, Singh H. Optimization of Maching Techniques—A Retrospective and Literature Review- Sadhana 2005;30(6):699–711.
3. Thorsten Grunheid, Charlene Loh. How accurate is invisalign in non-extraction cases? Are predicted tooth positions achieved. The angle orthodontist 2017;87(6):809–815.

PREVIOUS YEAR'S UNIVERSITY QUESTIONS

Short Questions

1. Technique of soldering procedures
2. Laser welding
3. Procedure of spot welding
4. Types of welding
5. Principles of spot welding

27.3 ORTHODONTIC INSTRUMENTS AND ORTHODONTIC MATERIAL

Chapter Outline

- Instruments used for placement of separators
- Banding instruments
- Bracket positioning instruments
- Wire forming pliers
- Utility and specialty pliers

- Wire cutting instruments
- Bracket debonding pliers
- Debanding plier
- 3D modular orthodontic instruments
- Sterilization

Instruments used for Placement of Separators

Separator placing plier is used to place the elastic ring separator in the interproximal area between the tooth to be banded and the two adjacent teeth on either side of it.

Other separators such as brass wire and Kesling metallic ring separators are placed using bird plier/light wire plier. The dumb-bell separator can be placed simply by pushing with fingers into the interdental area.

Banding Instruments

- Band cutting scissors—straight or curved
- Band contouring pliers is used to contour band
- Band pinchable pliers
- The contoured band material is placed around the tooth to be banded and it is pinched near the lingual side of the tooth using band pinchable pliers.
- Mershoon band pusher: Once the band is fabricated, Mershoon band pusher is used to push the band into its final position around the tooth to be banded.
- Band seater is used to seat and adapt the band around the tooth.
- Band-crimping plier is used to modify the band according to the contour of tooth.

Bracket Positioning Instruments

a. *Boon's gauge:* It is used to measure the bracket positioning heights of teeth and helps in proper positioning of the brackets. It has four measurements namely 3.5 mm, 4 mm, 4.5 mm and 5 mm to guide the brackets positioning on different teeth (Fig. 27.18).

b. *Bracket positioning height gauge:* It also serves the same purpose as Boon's gauge. It has certain advantage over Boon's gauge because of its rectangular design. It also helps in adjusting bracket into its final position (Figs 27.19 and 27.20).

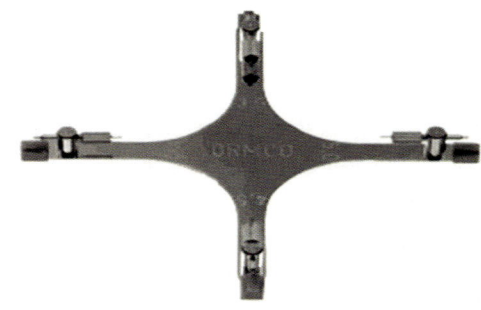

Fig. 27.18: Bracket placement marker/measuring gauge

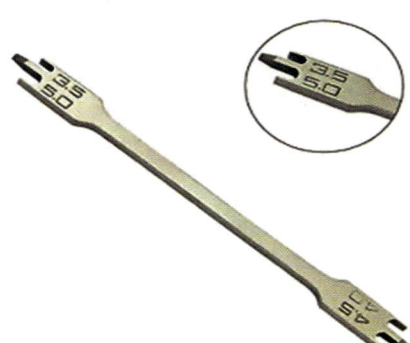

Fig. 27.19: Bracket positioning gauge

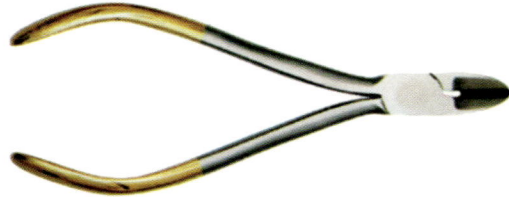

Fig. 27.20: Hard cutter plier

c. *Direct bonding bracket holder:* It is used for holding, carrying and placing the bracket on the surface of the tooth at the desired position (Fig. 27.21).

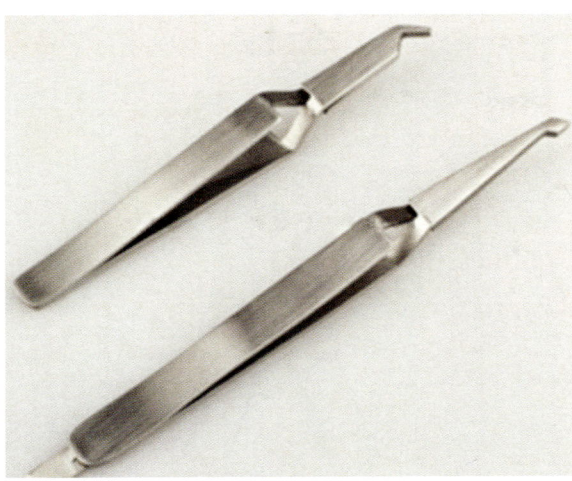

Fig. 27.21: Bracket tweezer

Wire Forming Pliers

a. *Light wire plier (bird beak plier):* It is used for adjusting and activating the 3D appliance. It can also be used for adjusting the 0,025 inch extenders on all 3D appliance.

b. *Clasp bending pliers:* Arrow clasp forming plier is used to bend arrow clasps so that the arrow head can engage the retentive for undercut. It is used for wire up to 0.7 mm/.028 inch (Fig. 27.22).

c. *Arrow clasp former:* It is used for hard wires up to 0.7 mm/0.028 inch. They form the clasp of the shape as shown in Fig. 27.23.

d. *De Le Rosa plier:* It is used in fabrication of archwire and helps to accentuate the curvature of the archwire.

e. *Loop forming plier:* It is used to form various components of removable and fixed appliances such as bows, springs, and canine retractors.

f. *Nance loop forming plier:* The working end of Nance loop forming pliers has four distinct step formations which help in forming loops of varying sizes.

g. *Tweed loop forming plier:* It is an excellent plier for making precise, consistent types of omega loops in round and rectangular wires.

Utility and Specialty Pliers

a. ***Three prong pliers:*** The working end of this instrument is used for the activation of Quad helix appliance which is often used for arch expansion.

b. ***Mathew pliers:*** There are a number of Mathews hemostats which are mainly used for tying ligature wire and fastening the elastic modules while securing the archwires in the bracket slot.

   – *Narrow tips Mathew hemostat:* It is ideal for placing the elastic modules although it can also be used for tying ligatures

   – *Standard tips Mathew:* It has slightly heavier construction with large tips. It is used for placing elastic modules and tying ligatures.

   – *Narrow tips Mathew (hollow form):* The working end has a 0.20 inch groove at both the tips. Advantage

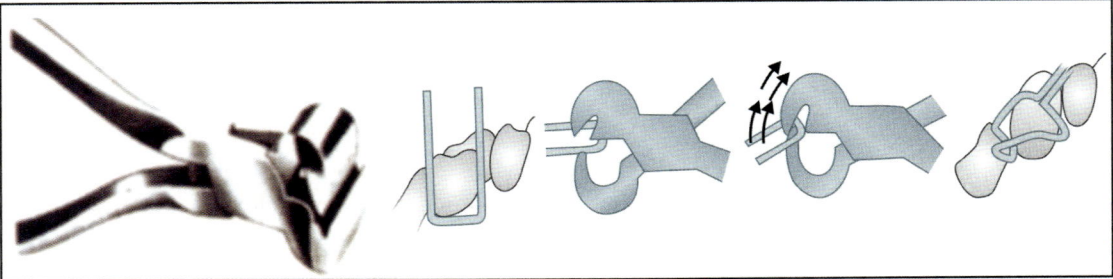

Fig. 27.22: Arrow clasp bending plier

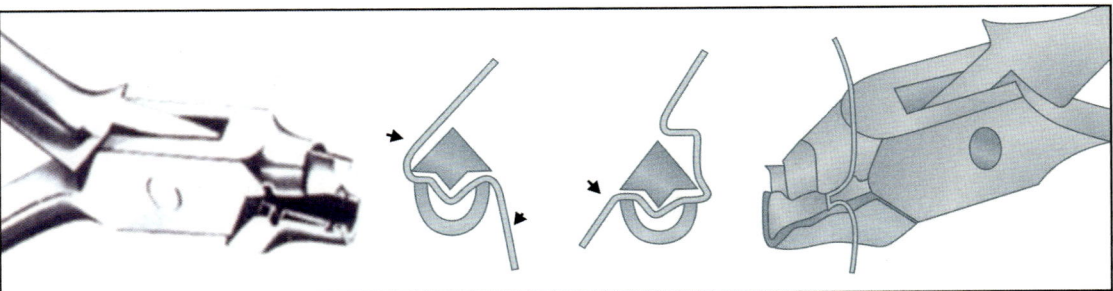

Fig. 27.23: Arrow clasp former

of the grooved tip feature of this plier is that it allows firm and positive grip of elastic module without crushing the bracket during the procedure of placement modules.

– *Crile needle holder:* It has a long handle and fine tips. It is also used for the holding and placing of elastic modules.

– *Hook tip Mathew:* The working end has a small hook at its tip which helps in securing elastic modules firmly. The hook also prevents slipping of modules out of the tip during the procedure.

– *Carbide inserted Mathew:* It has carbide cross-cut serrations on its working end which increases the longevity of this instrument. This is used for tying metal ligatures.

c. **Weingart plier** (Fig. 27.24): It is used for holding, carrying and placing the archwires in the bracket slots. There are various designs of Weingart pliers such as:

• *Standard tip Weingart plier:* It has fully serrated cross-cut beaks and a convenient working angle to avoid injury to the soft tissue during archwire placement.

• *Standard size Weingart plier:* It has non-inserted tips and is used to carry in the archwire.

• *Heavily tips Weingart plier:* This type has stubby inserted tips and is used to carry heavy arch wire.

Wire Cutting Instruments

• *Distal end cutter* (Fig. 27.25): It is used to cut the excess archwire distal to the molar band. They are provided with safety hold mechanism. Due to this design of the plier, the distal piece of wire after it is cut is held between the beaks of the cutter and thus prevents soft tissue injury and accidental swallowing. There are two designs namely:

– Micro distal end cutter with safety hold.
– Distal end cutter with safety hold.

• *Pin and ligature cutter:* It is used to cut the terminal ends of lock pins in Begg's technique and excessive

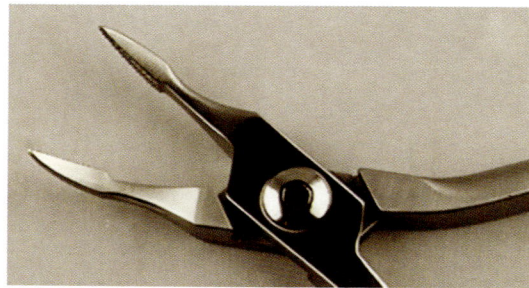

Fig. 27.24: Weingart plier

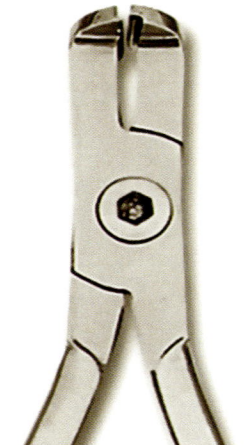

Fig. 27.25: Distal end cutter

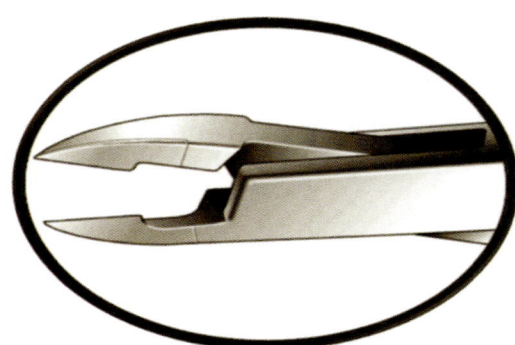

Fig. 27.26: Pin and ligature cutter

ends of ligature wire. 45° angled cutting tips for easy cutting of ligatures especially in the posterior areas and the lingual technique (Fig. 27.26)

Bracket Debonding Pliers

• Anterior debonding plier
• Posterior debonding plier (Fig. 27.27)

Angulated bracket remover—wide: It has an extra width of 6 mm and is angulated to increase accessibility in the posterior region.

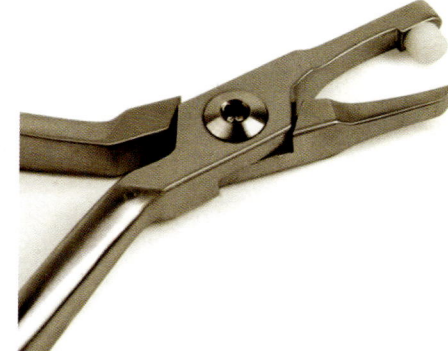

Fig. 27.27: Posterior band remover

Debanding Plier

During debanding procedure, the anterior and posterior band removers are used to remove the bands from anterior and posterior banded teeth, respectively.

3D Modular Orthodontic Instruments

a. *Howe plier:* It is used for carrying all the 3D appliances to the arch such as 3D lingual arch, 3D Wilson distalizing arch and 3D quad helix appliance. It is also used for rotating, tipping and torquing of these 3D appliances.

b. *Light wire plier (bird beak plier):* It is used for adjusting and activating the 3D appliance. It can also be used for adjusting the 0.025 inch extenders on all 3D appliances.

c. *Belzer wire cutter:* It is used to crimp omega stop and tandem yoke onto arch. It can also be used for cutting excess wire from appliances.

d. *Lingual arch forming plier:* It is used for holding the appliances with precision-seated post during fabrication. It can also be used for rotation and torquing of 3D quad helix.

e. *Jaw pliers:* It is used for:
   - Tightening wire formed 3D posts for any loose fit.
   - Adjusting quad helix appliance.
   - Adjusting 3D activators:
     1. Band director: It is used for seating of 3D posts in 3D lingual tubes
     2. Band scaler/pusher: It is used for removing 3D appliance from 3D lingual tubes.
     3. Angle wire bending plier: It is used for adjusting and activating 3D appliance.
     4. Modular Omega plier: It is used for adjusting the expansion or contraction of the omega loop on the 3D appliance.

Young universal plier: It is used for fabricating many of the wire components such as bows, clasps springs and wire components of myofunctional appliance. It is ideal for labial bows using different size loops.

Adam's plier: It was developed by Philip C Adam. It is used for fabricating Adam's clasp and all its modification. Adam's clasp bending plier is special plier for easy forming of Adam's clasps in one step. It is used for wires up to the diameter of 0.7 mm.

Three-prong plier: It has three beaks. The wire is placed between the three beaks which are perpendicular to the long axis of the plier beaks.

Optical plier: It has one round beak and one beak that is concave. The round beak fits into the concave opposite beak of the plier.

Turrets: It is used to provide an arch form to the main archwire in the edge-wise and preadjusted appliances. It is available with and without the torque options. The straight length of the archwire is simply wound in the turret to provide the desired curvature (Fig. 27.28).

Hard cutter plier: It has hard metal tips or tungsten carbide tips. This is heavier and larger than the pin and ligature cutter. This is used to cut all wires up to 0.020" round (Fig. 27.20)

Heavy wire cutter: It is also called heavy gauge side cutters. It is capable of cutting wires of up to 1.3 mm diameter. These are generally non-sterilizable and are used mainly in the lab.

Sterilization

Do's

- Always use distilled water or surgical milk for precleaning.
- The pliers should be kept separately especially when they are in an ultrasonic cleaner.

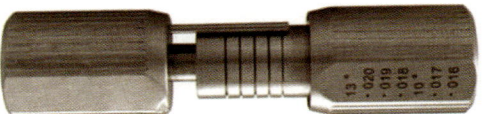

Fig. 27.28: Turrets

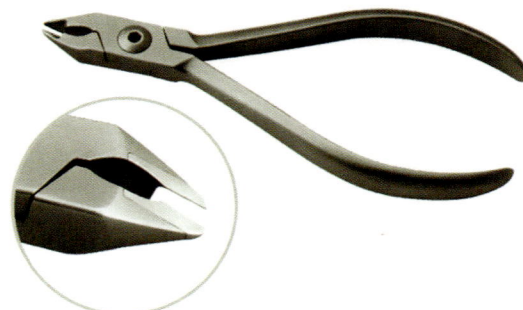

Fig. 27.29: Ceramic bracket removing plier

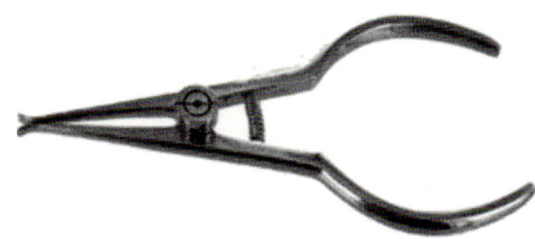

Fig. 27.30: Ligature tying plier

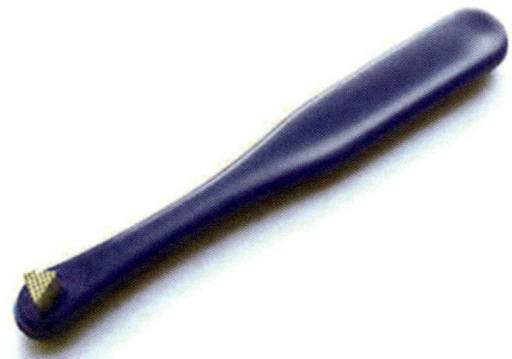

Fig. 27.31: Molar band seater

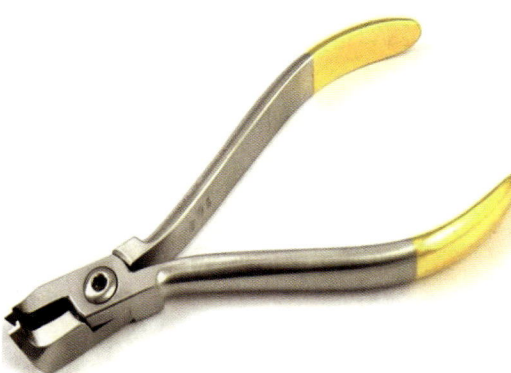

Fig. 27.32: Distal end TC cutter

- Check the wire sizes of plier cutting and bending specifications.
- Clean pliers first with Y 10 surgical milk or distilled water solution.

Don'ts

- One should never use soap and water to clean pliers. Distilled water cab is used in ultrasonic cleaner.
- Glutaraldehyde can also damage pliers. Do not put them in any glutaraldehyde solution.
- Do not brush pliers as hard brush might scratch pliers.
- Avoid excessive sterilization as it might damage the plier polish.

Bibliography

1. Adams CP. The modified arrowhead clasp-some further considerations. Dent Record 1953;73:333.
2. Graber TM, Neumann B. Removable orthodontic appliances philadelphia: WB Saunders 1984.
3. Prof H WR. Contemporary orthodontics St Louis. CV Mosby, 1986.

PREVIOUS YEAR'S UNIVERSITY QUESTIONS

Short Questions

1. What are the banding instruments?
2. Bracket positioning instruments
3. Wire cutting instruments

Photography in Orthodontics

Chapter Outline

- Introduction
- Camera
- Lens
- Aperture
- Film
- Exposure

- Flash and lighting
- Focusing
- Clinical techniques
- Intraoral photographs
- Digital photography

INTRODUCTION

The word photograph comes from the Greek words 'Phos' and 'Graphien'.

- Phos—light
- Graphien—to draw

Photograph is a picture drawn with light.

A digital camera is an important as any other equipment in a dental clinic up-to-date with technological advances. The utilization of photography is fundamental and images may be used for several purposes including registration records, pre- and post-treatment evaluation, collection of clinical cases for didactic-pedagogic use, publication of scientific articles, legal protection, improvement of professional experience, a tool for professional advertising and marketing.

However, similar to any other dental equipment, the clinician must know the photographic resources and have technical and operational expertise to improve the performance and outcomes also for the beginners.

The digital technology has revolutionized and is well established in the clinical dental photography. Images from digital cameras are available in seconds and can be displayed on computer screen in minutes, which is advantageous compared to the long time and higher costs required for the processing of conventional photographs. Image editing software allows multiple actions such as rotation, enhancement, lighting, cropping and even more sophisticated changes as desired.

In digital systems, image capture is performed by an electronic device called charge-coupled device (CCD), in which the thinner the dimensions of the CCD, the greater will be the amount of details in the image. The CCD is used instead of conventional films and has the function to convert light into electrical energy. It consists of a grid of electrodes and a silicon layer comprising a chip, i.e. the sensors are in charge of capturing the image. It is related to the digital camera as the microprocessor is related to the computer constituting the heart and mind of this system.

Conversion of the image known as one pixel, which is the basic unit of image detail, is derived from the abbreviation of picture element. Pixel is a single point that forms the image, corresponding also to the grain on the conversion paper images. The greater number of pixels, the higher the image resolution or its fidelity, in which all photographs are the same size (3.7 × 5.42 cm) but have different resolutions in pixels. If they are printed in this size, the quality of the first two would be similar and progressively worsened in the other two.

Why Photography in Orthodontics?

Radiography depicts that which cannot be seen with the naked eye; photography documents that can be seen.

Unreliable memories: Within a matter of months, patients and parents tend to forget how severe the original malocclusion was. Having slides available at every visit reminds both the orthodontist and the patient of the original situation, against which all improvements can be judged.

Medicolegal requirements: It is critical to have clinical photographs that indicate any pre-existing pathology or trauma to the teeth.

Close-up photographs are strongly advised for any marked decalcification or enamel fractures that are evident from the outset.

Teaching needs: Slides are probably the most important teaching aids in orthodontics. If cases are to be used in lectures, posters, papers, and presentations, a high standard of clinical photography is required.

Treatment evaluations: A quick scan of sequential slides with patients and parents during treatment will save lengthy explanations of biomechanics or tooth movements.

CAMERA

The camera is basically a box, with small aperture or opening where the lens is attached at one end and the film at the other. The inside of the camera must be completely dark so that the rays of light reach the film only through the aperture.

Principle

The camera works in much the same way as your eye (Fig. 28.1). The lens in the eye focuses the image onto the nerve cells in the retina and this image is sent to the brain by the optic nerve. To keep the image sharp even when the distance varies, the lens has to be moved either farther or closer to the film. This is called 'focussing' (Fig. 28.2).

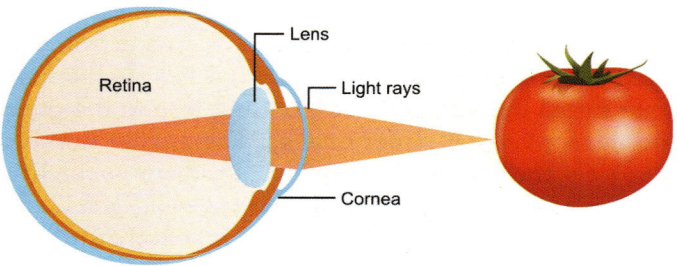

Fig. 28.1: Working nature of camera like eye

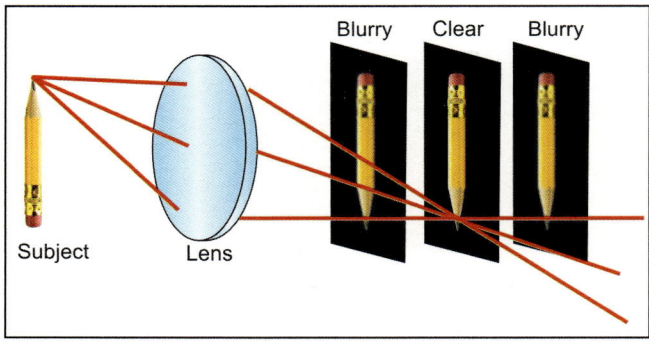

Fig. 28.2: Focusing

The diaphragm of the camera is a variable aperture which controls the amount of light allowed onto the film, much in the same way that the iris of the human eye contracts in bright sunlight but opens when the room is dark.

The light reflects from a subject, enters the camera through the lens, which focuses the rays of light into an image on the film. Light rays from the top of the subject form the lower part of the image and those from the bottom form the upper part. Thus the image on the film is upside down (Fig. 28.3).

Types of Cameras

- Single lens reflex (SLR) (Fig. 28.4a–f)
- Twin lens reflex (TLR) (Fig. 28.5a-d)
- Instant picture/polaroid
- Point and shoot
- Special cameras
- Panoramic
- Under water
- Stereoscopic
- Subminiature (spy)

LENS

Lens is a piece of transparent material that has at least one curved surface. The lens is the heart of the camera, the component that turns the three-dimensional world outside the camera into a two-dimensional image on the film inside (Fig. 28.6).

Its job is to take the beams of light bouncing off of an object and redirect them so they come together to form a real image—an image that looks just like the scene in front of the lens. The best way to understand the behavior of light through a curved lens is to relate it to a prism. A prism is thicker at one end, and light passing through it is bent (refracted) toward the thickest portion (Fig. 28.7).

A lens can be thought of as two rounded prisms joined together. Light passing through the lens is

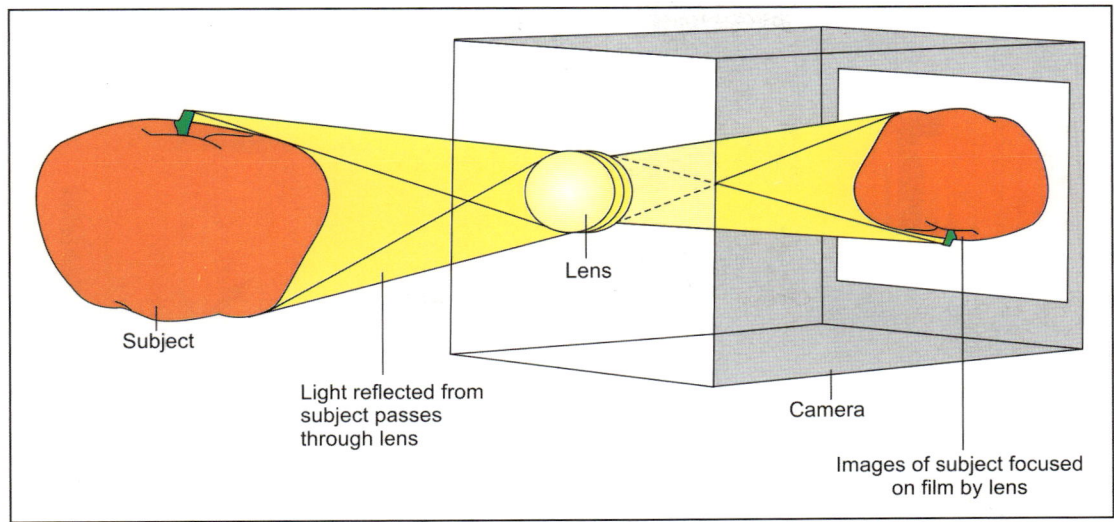

Fig. 28.3: Single lens reflex

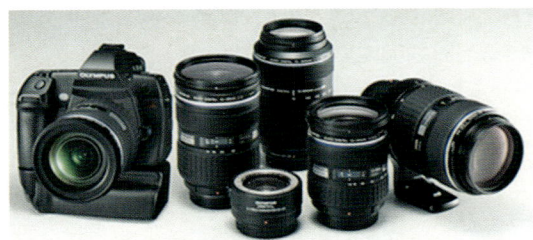

Fig. 28.4a: Single lens reflex

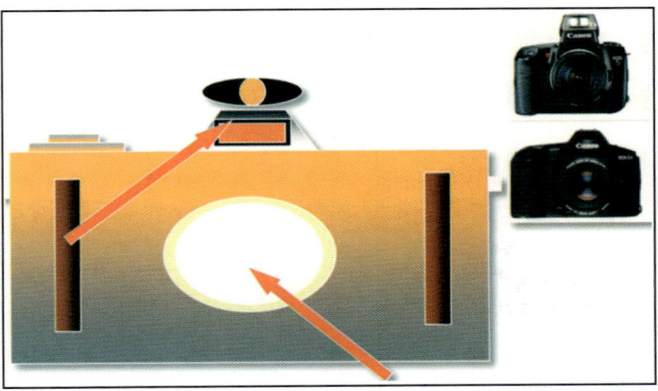

Fig. 28.4c: Single lens reflex

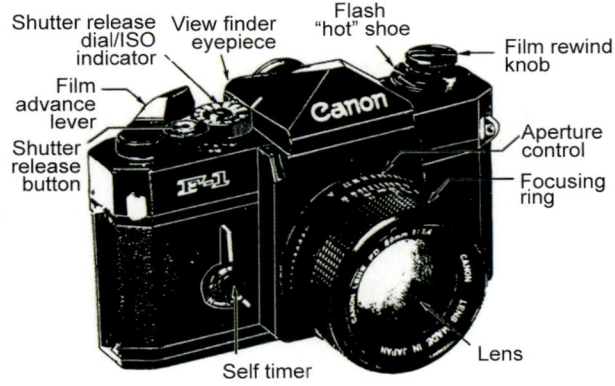

Fig. 28.4b: Parts of a 35 mm SLR camera

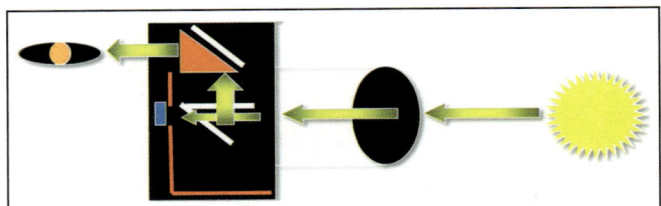

Fig. 28.4d: Single lens reflex

always bent toward the thickest part of the prisms (Fig. 28.8).

A lens produces its focusing effect because light travels more slowly in the lens than in the surrounding air. Therefore, refraction (an abrupt bending of a light beam) occurs both where the beam enters the lens and

where it emerges from the lens into the air (Fig. 28.9).

Because of the curvature of the lens surfaces, different rays of an incident light beam are refracted through different angles. Thus an entire beam of parallel rays can be caused to converge on a single point. This point is called the focal point, or principal focus, of the lens (Fig. 28.10). A long-focus lens forms a larger image of a distant object, while a short-focus lens forms a small image (Fig. 28.11).

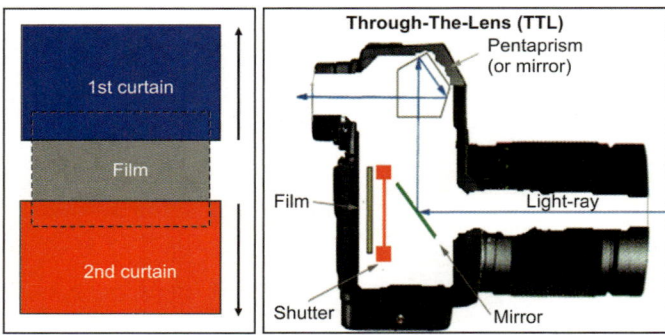

Fig. 28.4e: Single lens reflex

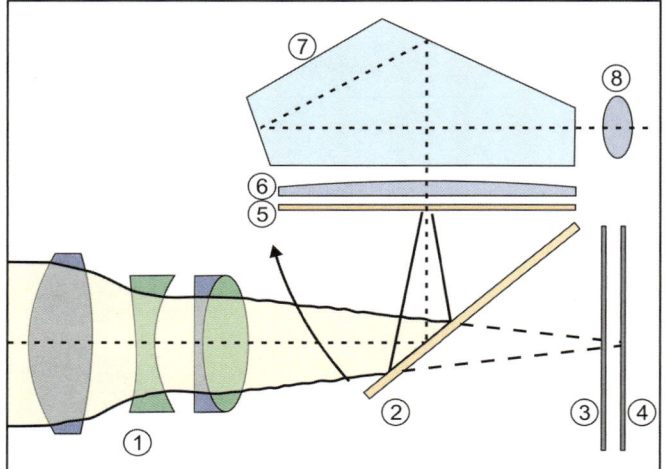

Fig. 28.4f: Cross section view of SLR system.

Note:
1. Front mount lens (four element tessar design)
2. Reflex mirror at 45° angle
3. Focal plane shutter
4. Film or sensor
5. Fousing screen
6. Condenser lens
7. Optical glass pentaprism (or pentamirror)
8. Eyepiece (can have diopter correction ability)

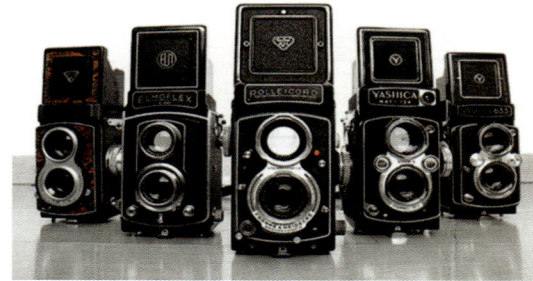

Fig. 28.5a: Twin lens reflex

Refraction of the rays of light reflected from or emitted by an object causes the rays to form a visual image of the object.

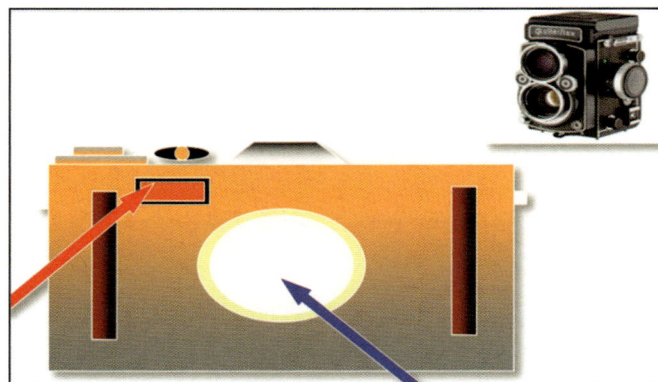

Fig. 28.5b: Twin lens reflex

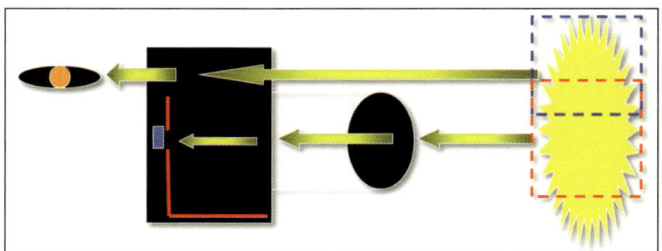

Fig. 28.5c: Twin lens reflex

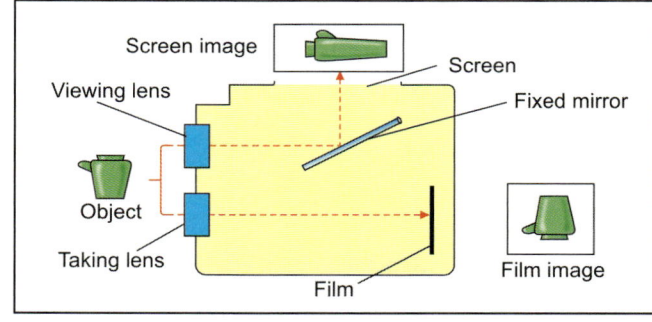

Fig. 28.5d: The fixed mirror deflects light rays coming through the viewing lens to a top screen, which shows the image upright but laterally reversed. Light from the object also goes through the taking lens, which is mounted on a common panel with the viewing lens, and is projected on the film

This image may be either:
- Real—photographable or visible on a screen or
- Virtual—visible only upon looking into the lens, as in a microscope.

The focal length of a lens is the distance from the center of the lens to the point at which the image of a distant object is formed (Fig. 28.12).

A long-focus lens forms a larger image of a distant object, while a short-focus lens forms a small image. The closer that you move an object to the lens, the larger it will appear on the film or photograph.

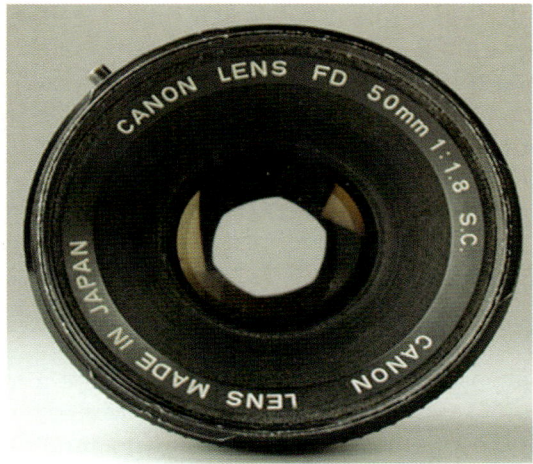

Fig. 28.6: Lens

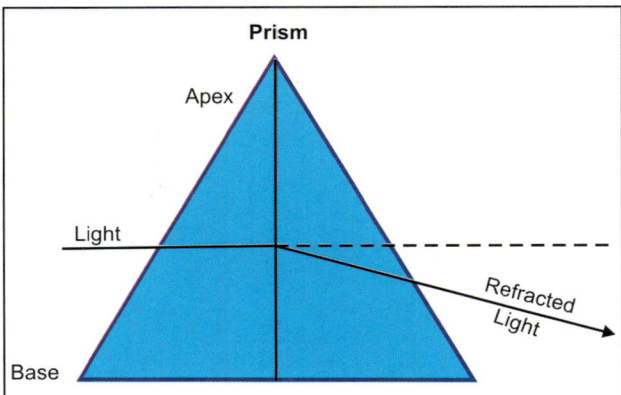

Fig. 28.7: Prism

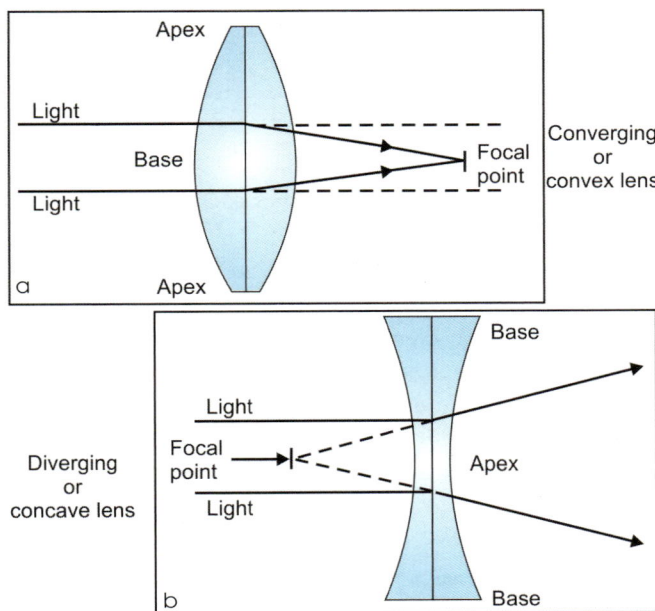

Fig. 28.8: (a) Converging or convex lens; (b) Diverging or concave lens

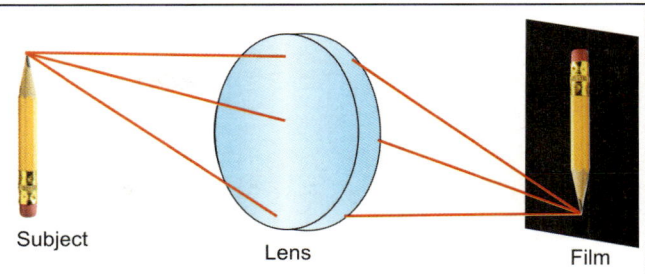

Fig. 28.9: Retraction

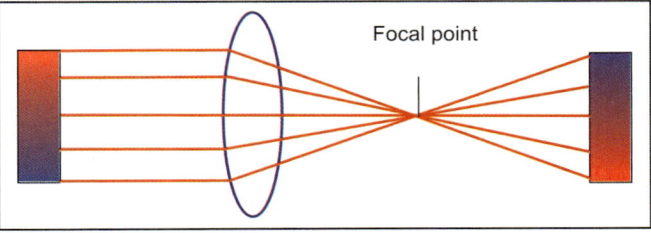

Fig. 28.10: Focal point

The image may be much larger or smaller than the object, depending on:
- The distance between the lens and the object, and
- The focal length of the lens.

There is a limit to how close you can move an object in order to enlarge an image size. If you move too close to an object, with a lens which is not suited to that distance, then the image will get distorted.

This is one of the most important concepts in dental photography, with regard to lenses.

Types of Lens

- Fisheye lens
- Wide angle lens
- Telephoto lens
- Zoom lens
- Macro lens

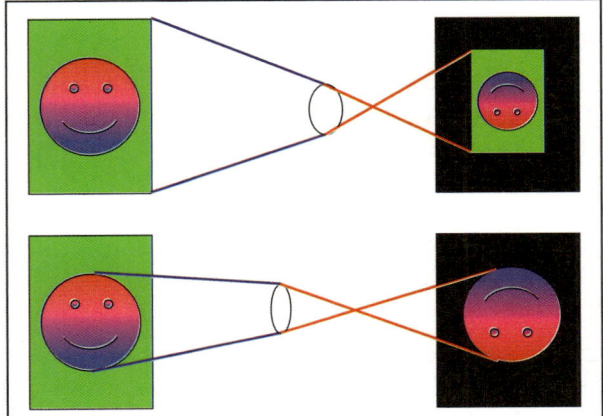

Fig. 28.11: Long and short focus larger ans small in eye respectively

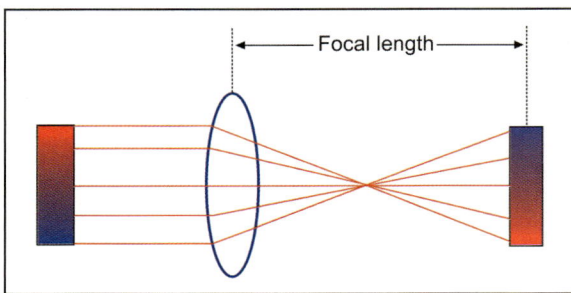

Fig. 28.12: Focal length

Fisheye Lens

- The fisheye is an ultrawide-angled lens.
- Typically, it will have a focal length of between 6 mm and 16 mm.
- For shooting interiors or other confined spaces, where an extreme angle of view is needed.

Wide Angle Lens

- Includes focal lengths ranging from around 15 mm to 35 mm
- Particularly, well suited to landscapes and architectural photography

Normal or standard:
- 50 mm lens
- Suitable for all general photography
- Usually are the cheapest available for cameras

Telephoto Lens

Short telephoto lenses range from 85 to 250 mm. Long telephoto lenses range from around 300 to 1000 mm, and beyond. Both these groups have multitude of uses including landscape photography, sports photography and wildlife photography. In addition, a short telephoto lens is considered ideal by many photographers for portrait photography.

Zoom Lenses

It is designed to have variable focal length from 24 to 80 mm, or 80 to 200 mm, etc. These are very handy pieces of equipment for, in one lens, you get two or three normal lenses. It is expensive, but when you consider that they take the place of two or three lenses these are quite economical.

Macro Lens

Macro lenses offer a steep less range of magnifications and shooting distances. They make good portrait lenses. Macro-photography is a term that covers the photography of subjects on a life size scale (1:1) or larger

than life size perhaps up to ten times (1:10). Dental photography is 100–105 mm macro lens. Some zooms can be set at a macro-setting, although the image magnification is not as great. In addition, because of the variable focal ability, it is almost impossible to make zoom lenses as sharp as a fixed focal length macro lens. Depending on the preference of the photographer and the situation, a wide variety of choices can be exercised in order to get the required effect from the lens.

Shutter Speed

The purpose of the shutter is to protect the film from light until the chosen moment. Simply to put, the shutter speed is the length of the exposure time. Shutters have speeds ranging from ½ sec to 1/8000 sec (Fig. 28.13).
- Fast shutter speed (1/2000 sec, 1/4000 sec)—the shutter is open only for a brief moment.
- Slower shutter speed (1/30 sec, ½ sec)—the opposite; the exposure is made for longer.

Each speed will allow half as much of light strike the film as the preceding one, e.g. 1/30 will allow twice as much light as 1/60 would.

A shutter speed shown as '2000' means 1/2000—meaning very fast. Usually, in dental photography, we have standard situations which are static. Therefore, the shutter speeds are also standard, viz. 1/60. The fraction indicator of 1/60 is left out to 'simplify' things.

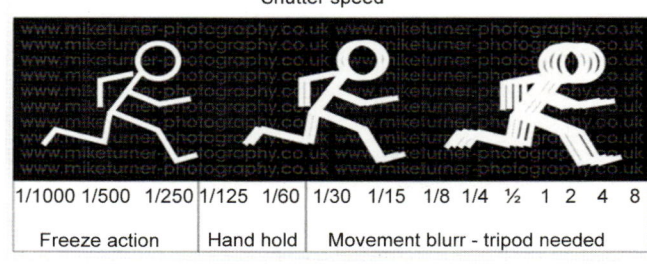

Fig. 28.13: Shutter speed

APERTURE (Fig. 28.14)

The aperture is an opening through which the light passes from the subject to the film. The aperture size is a measure of the size of that opening. It controls the amount of light that is allowed to pass through the lens, and eventually strike the film.

The aperture does this either by opening or closing, and allowing more or less light to pass through. The various sizes of the aperture are called 'f' stops or 'f' numbers.
- The f-stops start from 1.4 and go up to 32.
- Easy calculation: 1.4, 2, 2.8, 4, 5.6, 8, 11, 16, 22, 32 (Figs 28.15 and 28.16).

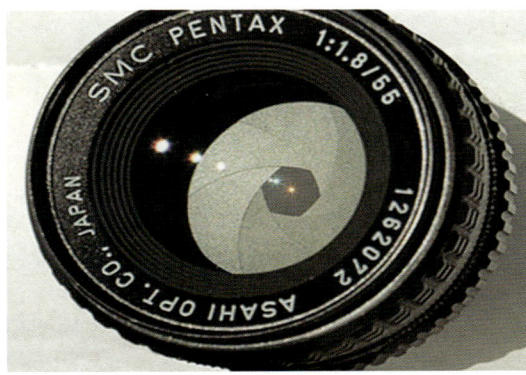

Fig. 28.14: Aperture

Some lenses have a rotating ring on the lens barrel called the aperture selection ring. Other cameras have an electronic dial to control this setting.

These numbers refer to the size of the lens aperture, but not the diameter of the aperture. The f number is the number by which the focal length of the lens must be divided to yield the diameter of the aperture, e.g.

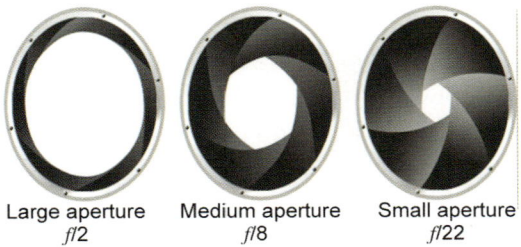

| Large aperture | Medium aperture | Small aperture |
| *f*/2 | *f*/8 | *f*/22 |

Fig. 28.15: Various size of apertures

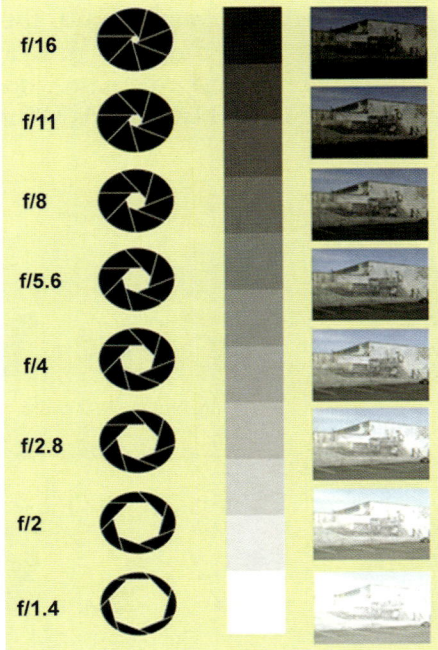

f/16
f/11
f/8
f/5.6
f/4
f/2.8
f/2
f/1.4

Fig. 28.16: Various size of apertures F' stops

- In a 50 mm lens, the lens is set to f/2 aperture.
- Therefore, the diameter of the aperture must be 50/2, i.e. 25 mm.
- Similarly, in a 100 mm lens, an aperture setting of f/2 means a diameter of 100/2, i.e. 50 mm.

Caution

A 50 mm lens set at f/8 will allow exactly the same amount of light that is allowed to pass through as does a 200 mm lens set at f/8.

This can be explained on the basis of the Inverse Square Law. The intensity of light is inversely proportional to the square of the distance that it travels. The 200 mm is longer than the 50 mm lens. Therefore, the light has to travel further to reach the film. Thus, on the 200 mm lens, the opening has to be bigger, at f/8, to allow the same amount of light as a 50 mm lens set at f/8. Remember in this case too, the higher the number the lesser the amount of light that is allowed to pass through.

FILM

Types (Fig. 28.17)

- Black and white
- Color
- Color reversal (for slides)
- Also, instant film (polaroid)

Speed

- Film speed is the amount of time required for the film to react to light.
- The photographic film is similar to the radiographic film in this respect.
- The photographic film is also composed of light-sensitive grains (silver halide particles), which when exposed, produce an image of the subject.
- Thus, the larger the grains, the more sensitive it is to light. This is called a fast film.

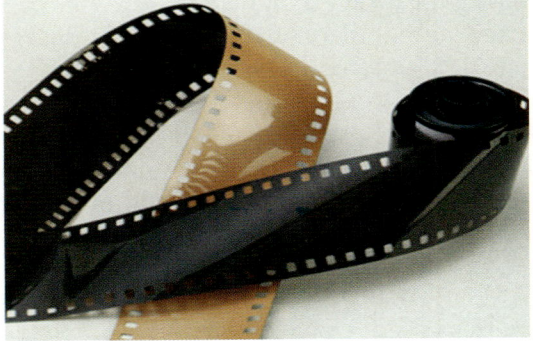

Fig. 28.17: Film

- A slower film would have smaller crystals that are less sensitive to light.
- However, smaller grains, i.e. slower films always would produce sharper images vis-à-vis faster films with larger grains.
- Previously, film speed was either denoted with an ASA (American Standards Association) number or a DIN (Deutsche Industrie Norm) number.
- Now film speed ratings have been standardized and are indicated by an ISO (International Standards Organization) number.
- The film speeds available range from ISO 25 to ISO 3200.
- ISO 25 being the slowest and ISO 3200 being the fastest.
- Slow (25–64) films are used for stationary objects in a well-illuminated scene or when fine detail is essential.
- A fast film (400–3200) is used for scenes that have dim light or involve fast action.
- A medium (100–300) speed film is suitable for average conditions of light and movement.
- In this case too, as you move from one film number to the next, you would require twice as much light to get the same exposure.
- For example when you move from ISO 50 to ISO 100, you need half as much light for the ISO 100 to get the same photograph.
- For dental photography, the ideal film would be ISO 100 that provides adequate sharpness and detail.
- Light would not be a constraint in these situations as the conditions are static and well illuminated with a flash.

Exposure

- Exposure is the total amount of light reaching the film in the camera.
- If too much light enters the camera, the film will be over exposed and the picture will be too bright.
- If there is insufficient light, the film will be under exposed and will result in a dark uninteresting picture.

If too much light enters the camera, the film will be over exposed and the picture will be too bright. If there is insufficient light, the film will be under exposed and will result in a dark uninteresting picture (Fig. 28.18).

The three factors that affect the exposure are:
1. Aperture setting (smaller number)
2. Shutter speed (smaller number)
3. Film speed (larger number)

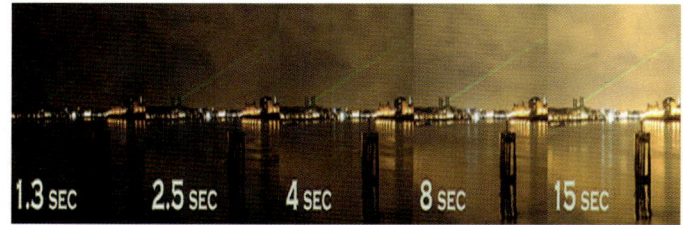

Fig . 28.18: Variation in light exposure affects picture

To obtain the correct image for your object, you must combine the three so that the correct quantity of light strikes the film. Usually speaking, the shutter speeds and the aperture are variable, but the speed of the film is not.

Depth of Field (Fig. 28.19)

- A photographic term, which defines what, is in focus within your shot, both in front of, and behind your point of focus.
- In other words, it is the zone of the 'in-focus' elements in front and behind.
- The area within the depth of field appears sharp, while the areas in front of and beyond the depth of field appear blurry.

Factors Affecting DOF

1. Aperture size
2. Focal length of the lens
3. Distance of the subject from the camera

It should be noted that the depth of field does not extend equally in front of, and behind, the point of focus. As a general rule, the DOF produced by a particular lens will extend approximately one-third in front the point of focus, and two-thirds behind.

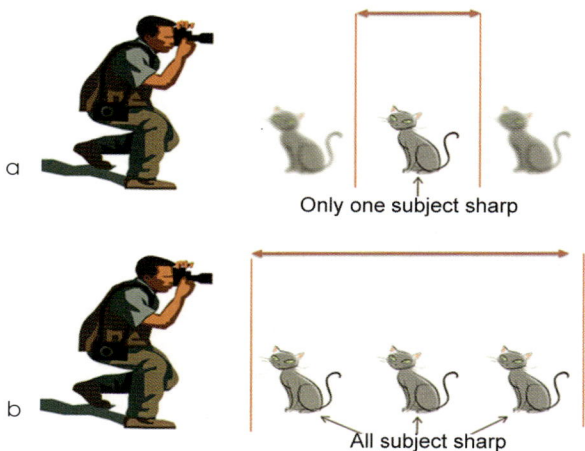

Only one subject sharp

All subject sharp

Fig. 28.19: (a) Shallow depth of field; (b) Large depth of field

FLASH AND LIGHTING

The two most important sources of light are:
- Natural
- Artificial/flash

Using different combinations of the two can enable the photographer to obtain a wide variety of results, often with dramatic effects.

In dental photography, the flash gun is always employed, irrespective of the type, i.e. I/O or E/O photography.

Types of Flash

- Ring flash (Fig. 28. 20)
- Built in flash (Fig. 28. 21)
- Dedicated point flash (Fig. 28. 22)

Important Characteristics

- Flash guide number—indicates how powerful the flash is.
- A GN of 40 is adequate for dental photography when using an ISO 100 film.
- Recycle time: 5–10 secs

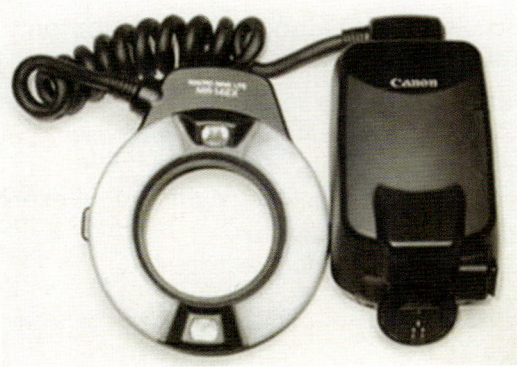

Fig. 28.20: Ring flash

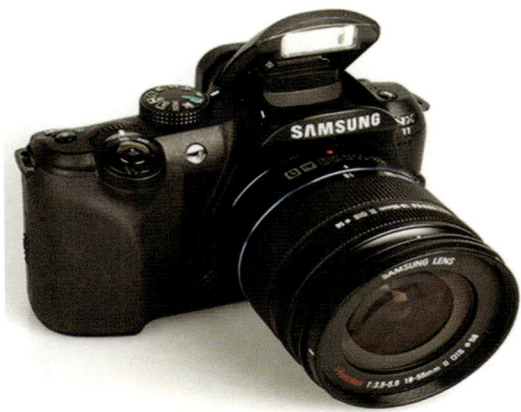

Fig. 28.21: Built in flash

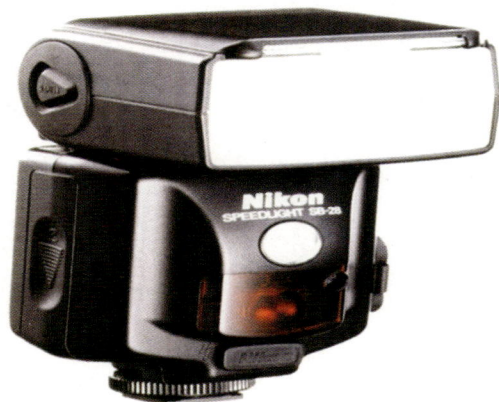

Fig. 28.22: Dedicated point flash

Synchronization

- The duration of the electronic flash is very short, often less than 1/1000 second, and it goes off instantaneously.
- Hence, flashes can be used at shutter speeds slow enough for the whole film to be exposed simultaneously.
- This is where flash synchronization comes into the picture.
- If your shutter is adjusted to higher speeds as prescribed by the manufacturer, you may end up with partially lit photographs.
- The shutter speed that is synchronized with the flash is often marked in red or has this sign marked next to it
- This shutter speed should be the one selected for dental photography.

Red-Eye

Where do the red eyes come from? The red color comes from light that reflects off of the retinas in our eyes—what you see is the red color from the blood vessels nourishing the eye (Fig. 28.23).

Eliminating Red-Eye

Many cameras have a 'red-eye reduction' feature. In these cameras, the flash goes off twice—once right before the picture is taken, and then again to actually take the picture. The first flash causes people's pupils to contract, reducing 'red eye' significantly. Another trick is to turn on all the lights in the room, which also contracts the pupil. Red-eye normally occurs when the angle of the light, striking the subject and being reflected off the camera is 2.5° or less. Thus, if possible, move the flash away from the camera. You can also try bouncing the flash off the ceiling, if that is an option

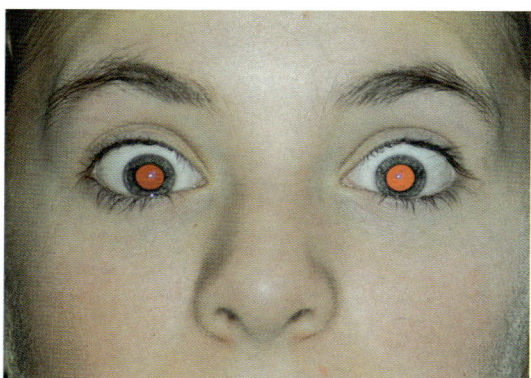

Fig. 28.23: Red-eye

Table 28.1: Uses of extraoral photographs

a. Evaluation of craniofacial relationships and proportion before and after treatment
b. Assessment of soft tissue profile
c. Proportional facial analysis and/or photographic analysis of Schwarz
d. Important for conducting the total space analysis
e. Monitoring of treatment progress (if standardized)
f. Invaluable for longitudinal study of treatment and post-treatment follow-up
g. Detection and recording muscle imbalances
h. Detecting and recording facial asymmetry
i. Identifying patients.

and have the subject look slightly away from the camera.

CLINICAL TECHNIQUES

Extraoral photographs are considered essential records and should be taken before starting treatment and after completion of treatment. The information provided by these photographs is invaluable and this is one record that the patient can really relate to. American Board of Orthodontics had laid down guidelines for these photographs (Table 28.1).

It is recommended that at least three extraoral photographs be taken for all patients. These include (Fig. 28. 24):

- Frontal facial with lips relaxed
- Facial profile with lips relaxed
- Three quarter view, smiling or
- Frontal facial smiling.

For facial deformity cases or cases likely to undergo orthognathic correction, it is recommended that all the four photographs mentioned above should be complemented.

FRONTAL FACIAL

According to Profit

- Frontal view with lips relaxed
- Frontal view with lips together
- Profile view with lips relaxed
- Profile view with lips together
- Smile (angular or frontal)

American Board of Orthodontic Requirements for Extraoral Photographs (ABO)

- Quality prints either in black and white or color.
- Head oriented accurately in all 3 planes of space and in F-H plane.
- 1 lateral view—facing to the right, serious expression, lips closed lightly.
- 1 anterior view—serious expression
- Background free of distractions.

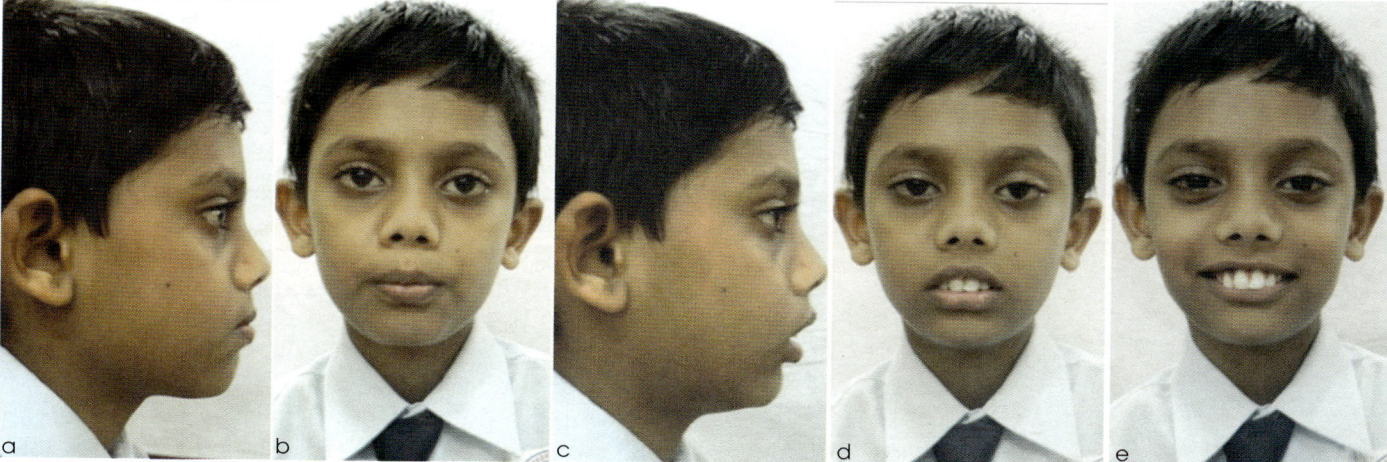

Fig. 28.24: (a) Profile view with lips together; (b) Frontal view with lips together; (c) Profile view with lips relaxed; (d) Frontal profile with lips relaxed; (e) Frontal facial smiling

- Optional—one frontal view, serious expression
- 1 lateral view, 1 anterior view (optional)—with lips apart
- 1 anterior view—smiling.
- Quality lighting with no shadows.
- Ears exposed for purpose of orientation.
- Eyes opened, looking straight; glasses removed.

Intraoral Photographs

They are helpful in explaining and motivating the patient. They are also used to monitor treatment progress and results. They are also useful in medicolegal cases involving the texture and color of teeth (Table 28.2).

The American Board of Orthodontics, guidelines are practically universally followed (Table 28.3).

Sandler, Murray (JO 2002)

- 9 pre-treatment and 9 post-treatment photos are absolute necessary.
- Photographic details at each wire change and at any other important stage is the gold standard.
- 36 per patient allow full photographic documentation of the average case.

Frontal View

A. Outer canthus to superior attachment of the ear (C-SA line);
B. Interpupillary line
C. Encompassing area (crown to collar bone).

Table 28.2: Uses of intraoral photographs

a. Record the structure and color of enamel
b. Patient motivation
c. Assessing and recording health or disease of the teeth and soft tissue structures
d. Monitoring of treatment progress
e. Study of relationships before immediately following and several years after treatment to improve treatment planning

Table 28.3: The American Board of Orthodontics, guidelines for intraoral photographs (Fig. 28.25)

a. Quality standardized intraoral color prints
b. Photographs should be oriented accurately in all three planes of the space
c. One intraoral photograph in maximum intercuspation
d. Two lateral views—right and left
e. Optional—two occlusal views-maxillary and mandibular
f. Free of distractions—retractors, labels, etc.
g. Quality lightening revealing anatomical contours and free of shadows.
h. Tongue should be retracted posteriorly
i. Free of saliva and /or bubbles
j. Clean dentition

Jonathan Sandler, Vincent Kokich (AJODO 2009): Assessed the quality of photographs taken by orthodontists to see whether those taken by orthodontic auxiliaries and professional photographers are of comparable quality.

- Most of the photos taken by the 3 groups of photographers are judged to be good or acceptable.

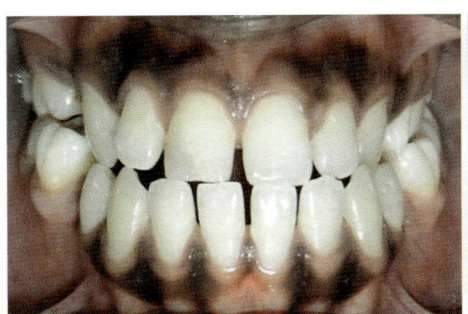 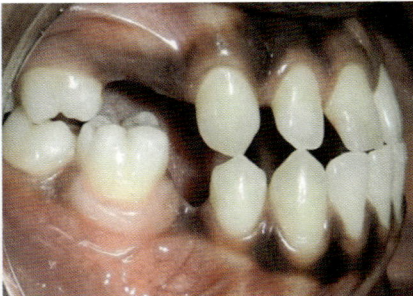 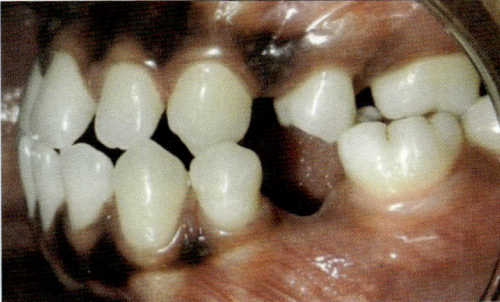

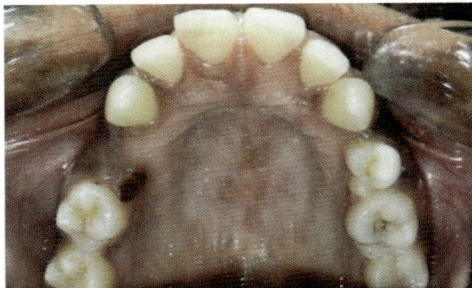 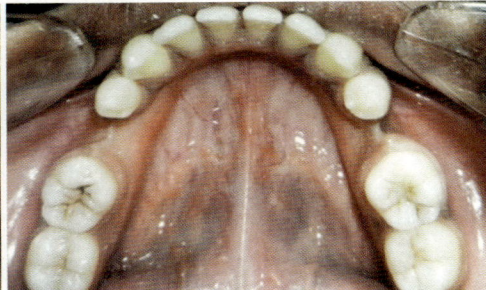

Fig. 28.25: Intraoral photographs

- The results for extraoral photographs showed no statistically significant differences between the 3 groups for good and acceptable images.
- The results for intraoral photographs showed that the orthodontists produced significantly more good-quality intraoral photographs.

Clinical Tips

- The direction of pull of the retractors is always side ways and slightly forward away from the gingival tissues. This maximizes the field of view and minimizes patient discomfort.
- Wetting the retractors just before insertion eases the process of positioning them properly with minimum patient discomfort.
- When taking occlusal mirror shots, slightly warming the mirror in warm water prior to insertion helps prevent fogging of the mirrors which would prevent a clear image.
- During occlusal mirror shots, instruct the patient to open wide just prior to pressing the camera button. This helps in obtaining the maximum mouth opening at the right moment and minimizes the patient's fatigue during the procedure.
- It is recommended that all photographic records be taken before impression taking, to eliminate the possibility of impression material being stuck between the teeth or the face during photographic record-taking.
- Clean the target site of debris, excess saliva and air bubbles before taking photograph.
- Target area should be moist but not desiccated.
- Isolate the target site (include only what is necessary in photograph).
- Use retractors as appropriate to afford an unrestricted view of the target area (Fig. 28.26)
- Use a high quality mouth mirror as appropriate to view the target area.
- Control fogging by dipping mirror into hot water the drying it with a soft tissue.
- Alternatively, use a light stream of air from the air syringe to keep the mirror from fogging.
- Keep the patient's nose out of a palatal view of maxillary incisors.
- Keep finger tips, mirror edges and retractors out of the picture.
- Include reference measuring device (as for biopsies)

Ideal Head Position and Perspective for a Frontal View

Useful four types are (Fig. 28.27):
- *Frontal at rest:* If lip incompetence present, lip should be in repose and mandible in rest position.

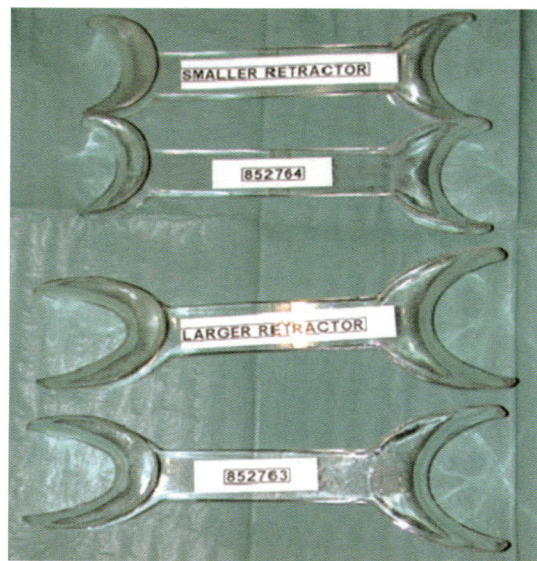

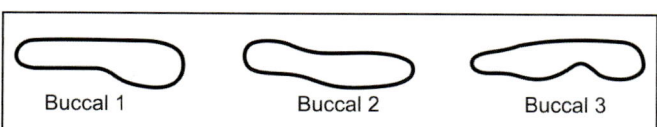

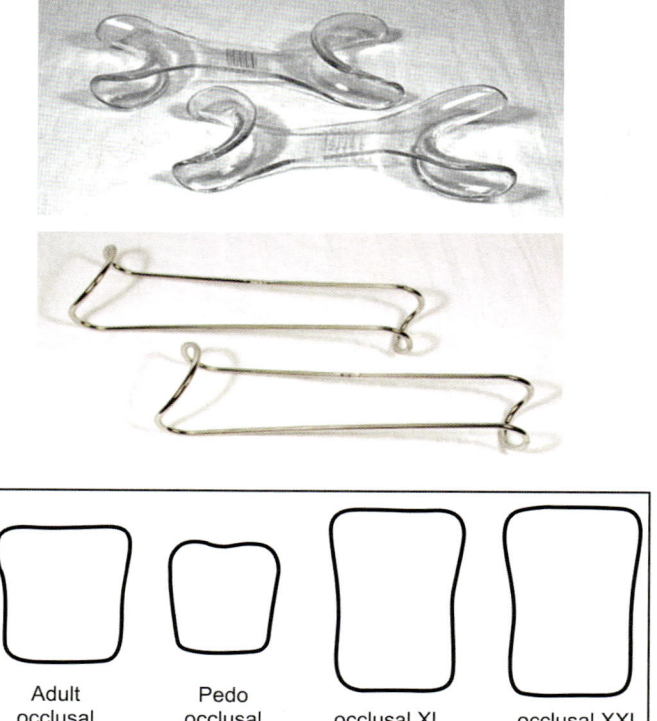

Fig. 28.26: Large and small retractors

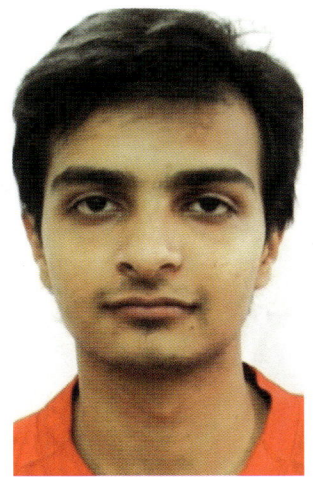

Fig. 28. 27: Frontal at rest

- *Frontal view with teeth in maximum intercuspation:* With lips closed even if this strains the patient gives clear documentation of lip strain and esthetic effect. Lip together picture recommended in patient with lip incompetence.
- *Frontal dynamic (smile):* Demonstrates amount of lip exposure display and any excessive gingival display.
- *Close up image of posed smile:* Recommended as standard photo for careful analysis of smile relationship.

Lateral/Profile View

Outer canthus to superior attachment of ear (A) and encompassing area of crown to collar bone (C) (Fig. 28.28).

Two useful profile images are:
- Profile at rest: Lip relaxed (Fig. 28.29)
- Profile smile: For angulations of maxillary incisors, important esthetic factors.

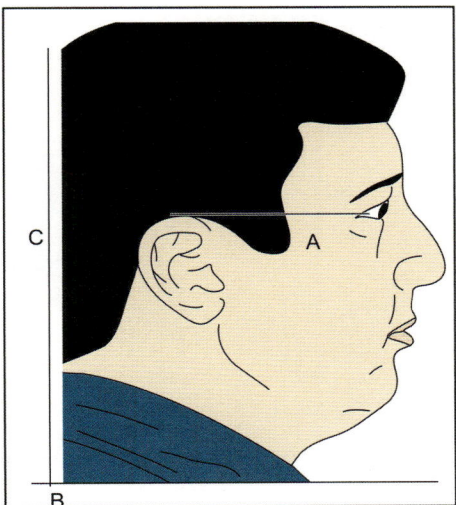

Fig. 28. 28: Profile view

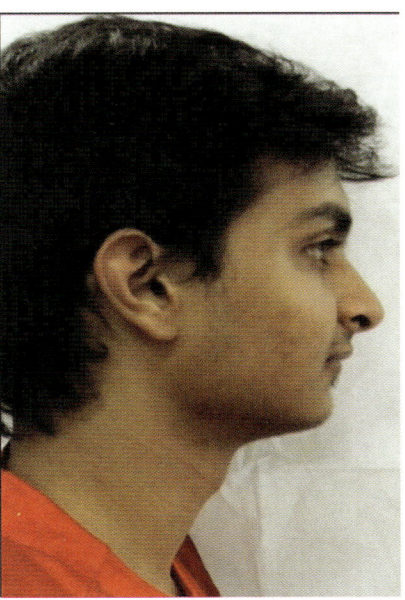

Fig. 28.29: Profile at rest

The success of an orthodontic treatment is frequently related to the improvement gained in the patient's facial appearance, which includes the soft tissue profile. Cephalometric measurement of the face in terms of esthetics can be difficult and misleading due to the variability of the intracranial reference lines. Extra-cranial references are more accurate, but can be time-consuming to apply.

- *NM Bass (JO 2003):* To overcome the problems of bony landmarks in cephalograms—proposed the *esthetic horizontal reference line*, which is related to the esthetic or photographic position of the facial profile, familiar to all orthodontists.
- The variability of this reference line has been shown to be considerably less than other methods of orientating the facial profile, with a method error of only 1.36°.

The analysis permits straight forward assessment of the orthodontically important lower facial third and the location of the dentition in the face to be determined in an individualistic way, taking the soft tissues into consideration. Spurious and misleading bony landmarks are avoided by the use of the esthetic horizontal line—an easily reproducible datum line with a low method error. Esthetic changes in the profile can subsequently be accurately assessed for treatment monitoring, using progress radiographs (Fig. 28.30)

- *Xingzhong Zhang, Mark G Hans (AJODO 2007)* compared craniofacial measurements from cephalometric radiographs with analogous measurements from standardized facial photographs using 326 subjects.

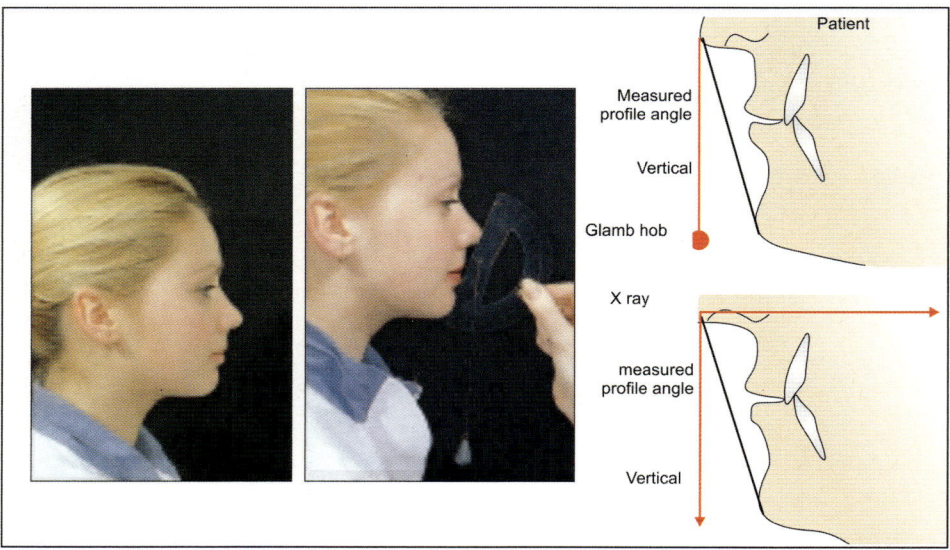

Fig. 28.30: Esthetic horizontal reference line depicting esthetic

- Three angular, 3 linear, total face heights, and lower face height cephalometric measurements were compared with 4 angular and 4 linear measurements from standardized photographs.
- Both linear and angular measurements useful for characterizing facial morphology can be reliably measured from facial photographs.
- However, the correlations between analogous photographic and cephalometric measures suggest that these modalities measure different aspects of facial morphology and cannot be used interchangeably.
- Cephalometrics remains the method of choice for clinical patient care, and photographs might be better for large-scale epidemiologic studies, especially when there is a need for a low-cost, non-invasive method that can be used in diverse clinical and field settings.

Oblique View (Fig. 28.31)

- Make sure that about half of opposite upper lid eyelashes show all or far side pupil should not show.
- *Oblique view-2:* Another oblique view, showing about half of subject's pupil, most of her upper lashes, and none of her lower lashes (Fig. 28.32)
- *Oblique view smile:* The final extraoral photograph to be taken, this shot conveys the patient as in 'social interaction', and can give valuable informtion about the smile esthetics changes pre- and post-treatment (Fig. 28.33)
- *Oblique at rest:* Useful for examination of the midface for deformity and nasal deformity. Also reveals the characteristics like chin neck area, prominence of gonial angle, length and definition of border of mandible. Also focus on lip fullness, vermillion display, and facial asymmetry.

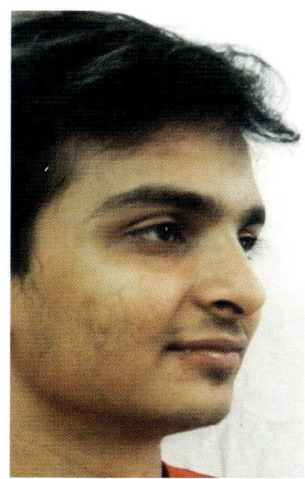

Fig. 28.31: Oblique view

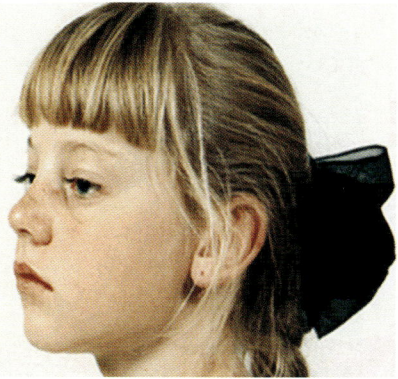

Fig. 28.32: Oblique view 2

- *Oblique on smile:* To observe the anteroposterior cant of occlusion. The occlusal plane is consonant with the curvature of the lower lip on smile (smile arc).

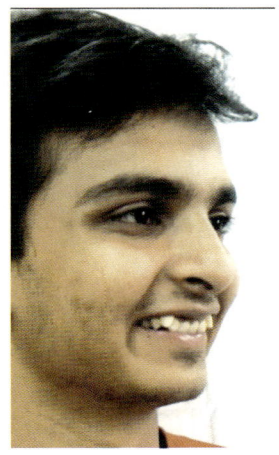

Fig. 28.33: Oblique view smile

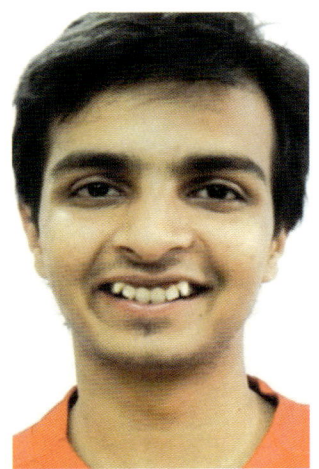

Fig. 28.34: Smile

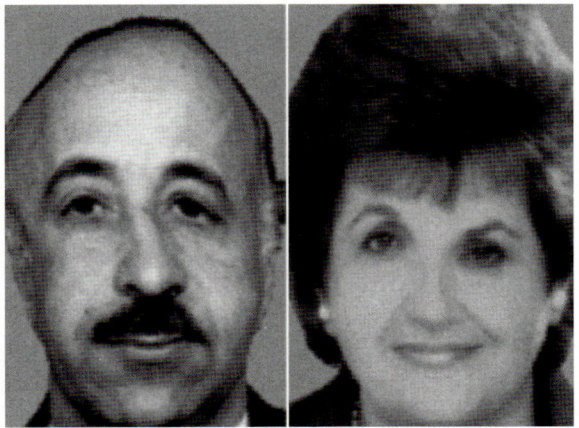

Fig. 28.35: Distorted views

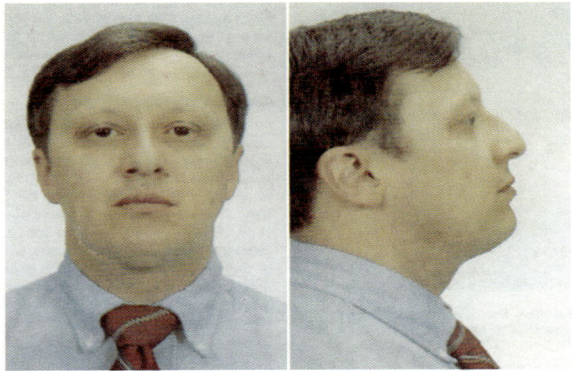

Fig. 28.36: Patient should always look straight-up

- B, centric occlusion;
- C, extreme protrusive position.

Note
- Chin and neck should show, preferably up to the clavicles.
- Use Frankfort horizontal line to be sure that head is level.

Hairstyle can distract Facial Analysis

Hair should be pulled back, in a ponytail, if necessary. This allows for auricular analysis and for relationship between tragus and infraorbital rim to be evaluated. Same applies to hair down over forehead (Fig. 28.45).

Frontal intraoral photograph: Positioning camera at 12 O'clock position parallel to occlusal plane gives proper exposure to field without shadows.

Lateral intraoral photograph: Position camera perpendicular to occlusal plane while flash should be facing anteriorly to eliminate shadows.

Maxillary occlusal intraoral photograph: Position camera again at 12 O'clock position and at 45° angulation from photographic mirror.

- *Smile:* As broad grin as possible with the teeth showing. Otherwise it is similar to frontal view (Figs 28.34, and 28.42–28.44).

Backward tilt of head: Distorted view caused by backward tilt of head. The chin appears prominent, particularly in the lateral view (Figs 28.35–28.37).

Lateral head rotation: The view is not symmetrical. The distance from outer canthus to hairline is not equal on both sides (Figs 28.38 and 28.39).

Viewpoint distortion caused by a 35 mm wide-angle lens (Fig. 28.40). Distorted view caused by incorrect camera position:

A. Camera too high
B. Camera too low.

Three mandibular positions as shown in lateral views (Fig. 28.41). Differences between each of the positions are easily discerned:

- A, Centric relation;

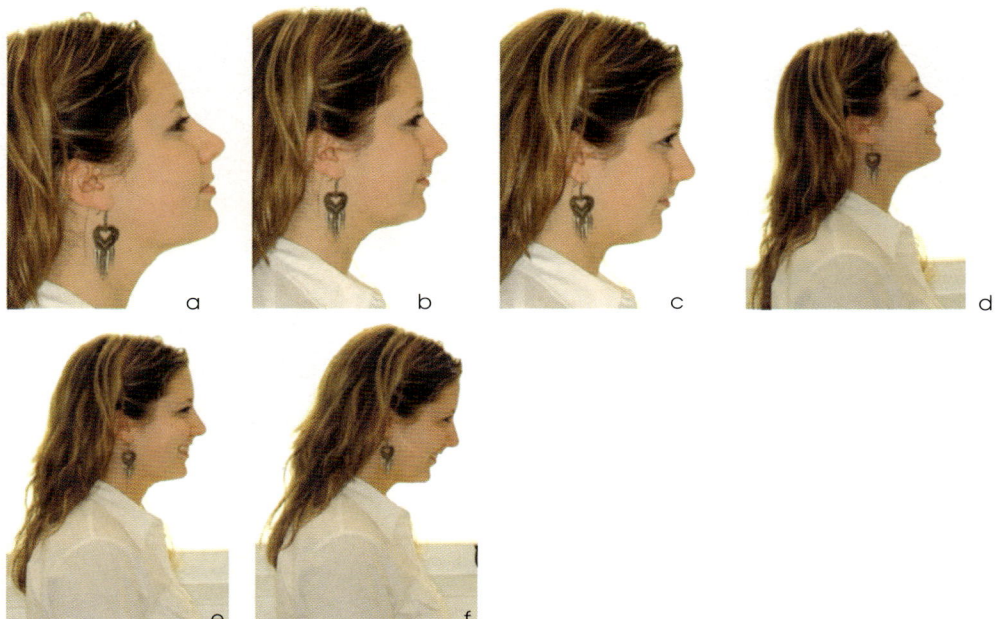

Fig. 28.37: (a) Class III, (b) Class I. (c) Class II. (d-f) Differing skeletal pattern purely due to patient positioning errors

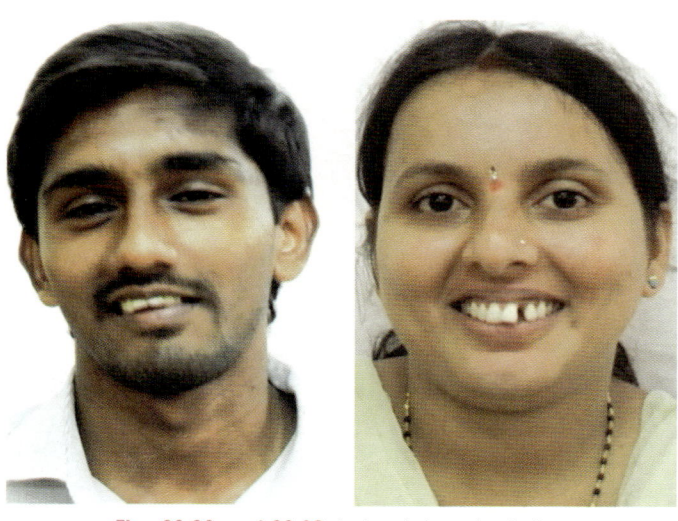

Figs 28.38 and 28.39: Laterals head rotation

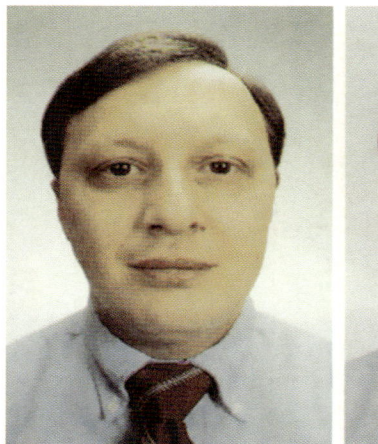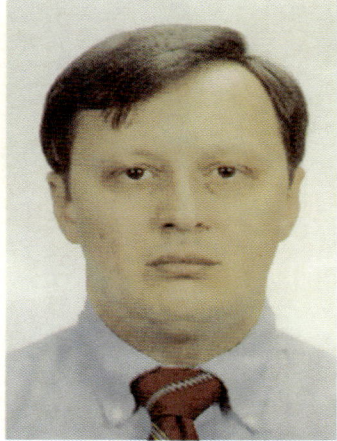

Fig. 28.40: Viewpoint distortion caused by a 35 mm wide-angle lens

Mandibular occlusal intraoral photograph: Position camera at 6 O'clock position and at 45° angulation from photographic mirror

- Clean the target site of debris, excess saliva and air bubbles before taking photograph.
- Target area should be moist but not desiccated.
- Isolate the target site (include only what is necessary in photograph)
- Use retractors as appropriate to afford an unrestricted view of the target area
- Use a high-quality mouth mirror as appropriate to view the target area.

- Control fogging by dipping mirror into hot water then drying it with a soft tissue.
- Alternatively, use a light stream of air from the air syringe to keep the mirror from fogging.
- Keep the patient's nose out of a palatal view of maxillary incisors.
- Keep fingertips, mirror edges, and retractors out of the picture.
- Include reference measuring device (as for biopsies)
- Camera settings remain the same:
  - f/22
  - 1/60 sec

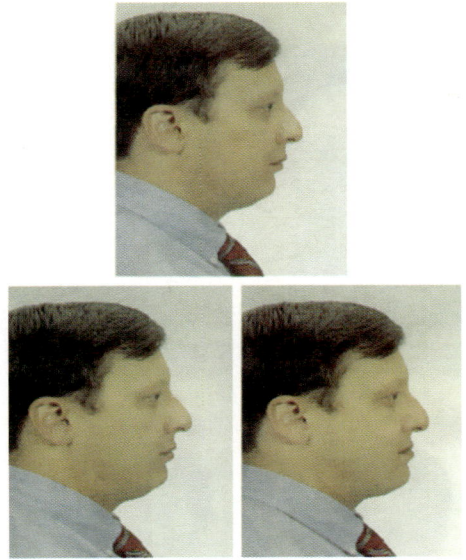

Fig. 28.41: Three mandibular positions as shown in lateral views

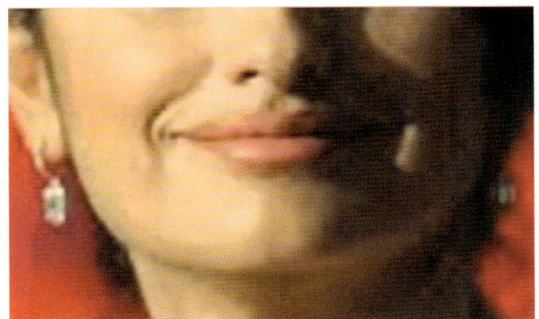

Fig. 28.42: Lips together smile

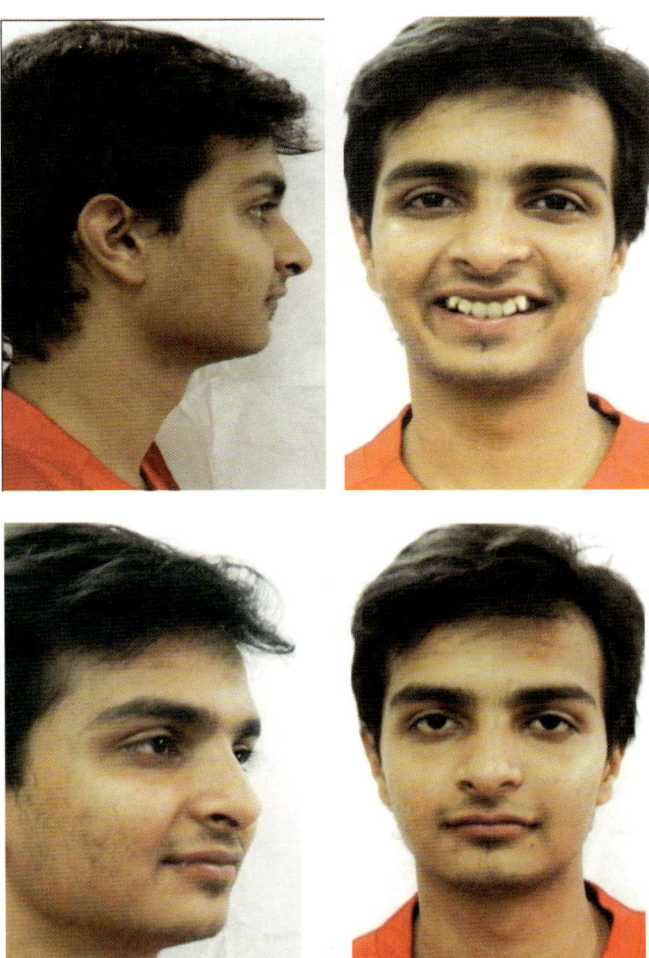

Fig. 28.44: All views equal

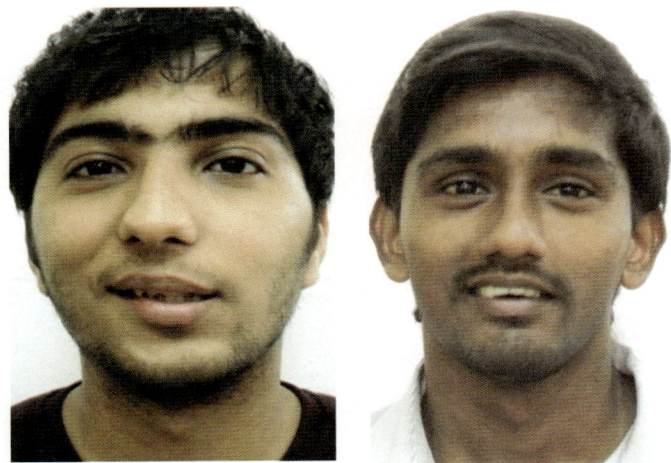

Fig. 28.43: Smile

Casts and Articulators (Fig. 28.46)

- Background used can be black or a pastel shade.
- The backdrop should be 'seamless', i.e. without any creases or folds.

- The background chosen could be a cloth or paper, with the latter being the more preferred one.
- If possible, this should not have any texture at all and not much reflection.
- f/16 or f/11 with 1/60 sec and a flash should be used.
- Shadows may be eliminated with a side mounted flash unit or a half-on ring flash.
- Names, OP nos., etc. imprinted on the sides make record keeping easy.

Radiographs (Fig. 28.47)

To take X-ray photos, the following clinical tips should be followed.

- Do NOT use the flash (Fig. 28.47)
- Use an illuminated background, like a medical X-ray view box.
- Mask the radiograph about an inch on all sides to exclude the light around the sides.
- f/5.6 or f/8 is sufficient.

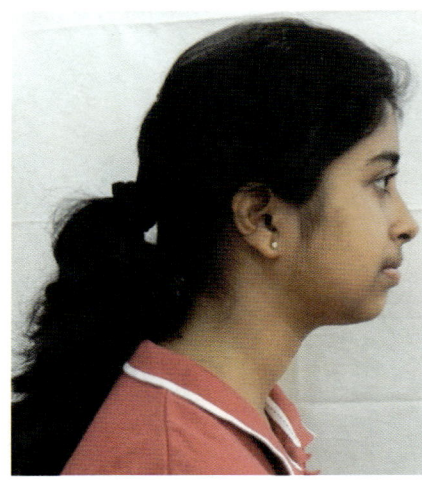
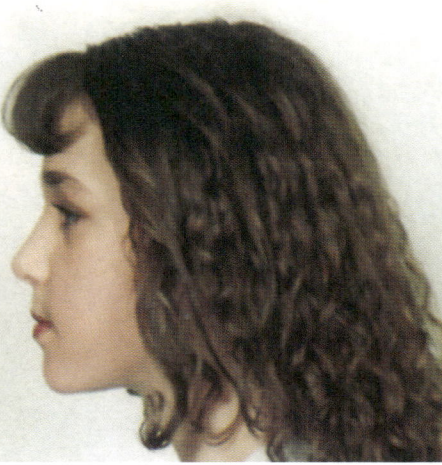
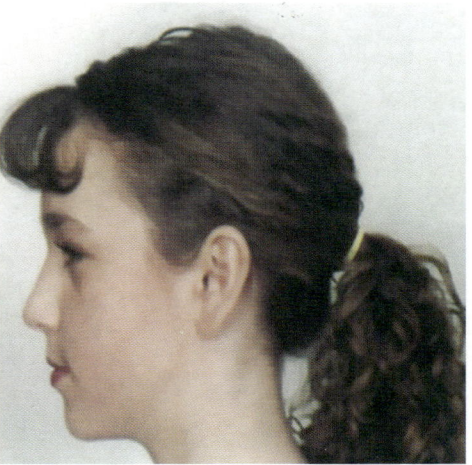

Fig. 28.45: Hair style distract facial analysis

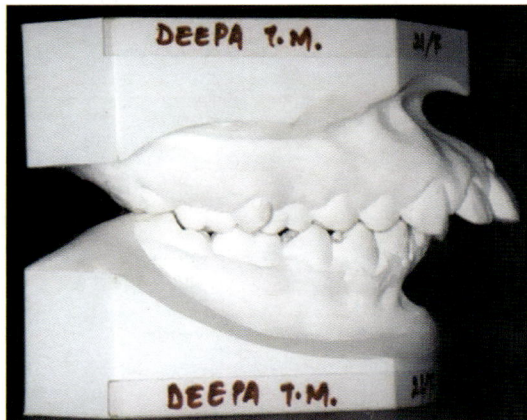

Fig. 28.46: Articulation

DIGITAL PHOTOGRAPHY

The images can be displayed on a screen immediately after they are recorded. It can store thousands of images on a single small memory device and delete images to free storage space. The majority including most compact cameras can record moving video with sound as well as still photographs. Some can crop and stitch pictures and performs other elementary image editing. Some have GPS receiver built in and can produce geotagged photographs.

The first recorded attempt at building a digital camera was in 1975 by Steven Sasson, an engineer at Eastman Kodak. The new solid CCD image sensor chips were developed by Fairchild Semiconductor in 1973. The camera weighed 8 pounds (3.6 kg), recorded black and white images to a cassette tape, had a resolution of 0.01 megapixels (10,000 pixels), and took 23 seconds to capture its first image in Dec 1975. Digital photography has been generally available since 1981. In 1991, Autotrader were the first mass market publication to move completely to digital recording of images.

With digital imaging, it is now possible with a reasonable investment, to digitally acquire, archive and easily retrieve clinical images of our patients. Special diagnostic software allows the orthodontist to customize the presentation of text, graphics and photographs.

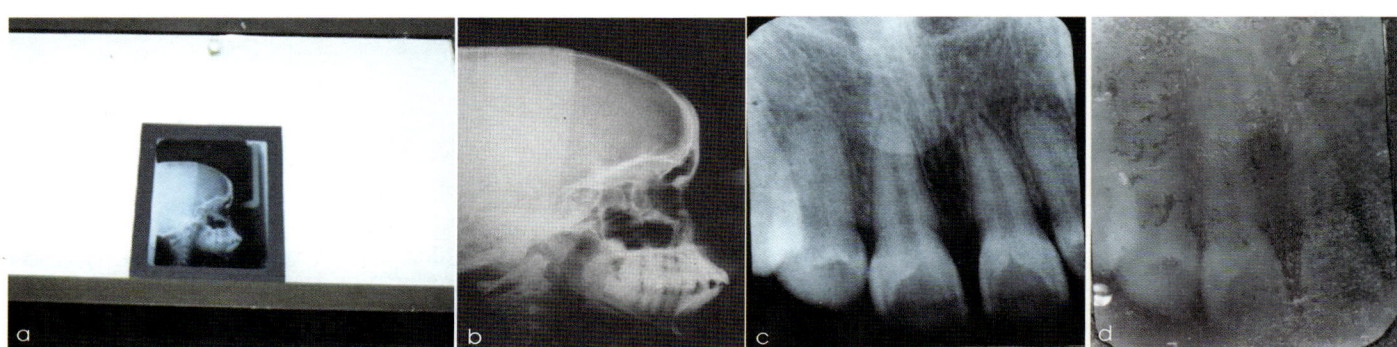

Fig. 28.47: (a and b) Photos using radiogrphs; (c) Without flash; (d) With flash

Computerized Digital Photography

The term 'Computerized photography' actually describes the blending of video and digital photography along with the processing of those images. It can be divided into three principal functions like input, processing and output.

The input procedure is the most technique-sensitive and has a dramatic impact on the image quality. Digital images used in orthodontics are input from one of three sources;

1. Video signal
2. Digital camera
3. Scanner

Images from a video camera are usually output as an analog signal which is coverted to a digital image by a digitizer or frame grabber built into the computer.

A digital camera captures the image directly from the CCD sensor and requires no analog-to-digital conversion. The digital images are stored in the camera on small electronic 'flash cards' or on a miniature hard disk drive. They can then be downloaded to a computer.

Digital Images

Digital images are made up of picture elements (pixels) comprising red, green and blue light each set at a level between 0 and 255. Varying the level of each of the three colors results in the gamut of 16.7 million colors. Numerical values for each of these colors are stored on the charged couple device (CCD). The number of pixels combined with the degree of compression determines the quality of the final output.

The quality of the digital image depends on a number of factors:

1. Camera optics
2. Lighting
3. Pickup device (the CCD sensor in the camera)
4. Analog signal quality (composite, S-video or component)
5. Digitizer resolution

Digital cameras can be divided into two main groups (Figs 28.48 to 28.50):

1. Compact digital cameras
2. Professional cameras with digital interface. A professional reflex camera meets all the requirements for clinical orthodontic photography.

File Format and Software Compression

Once an image has been acquired by the CCD, it is stored in the camera's memory as a file. Image files can be of different formats and more important, can be

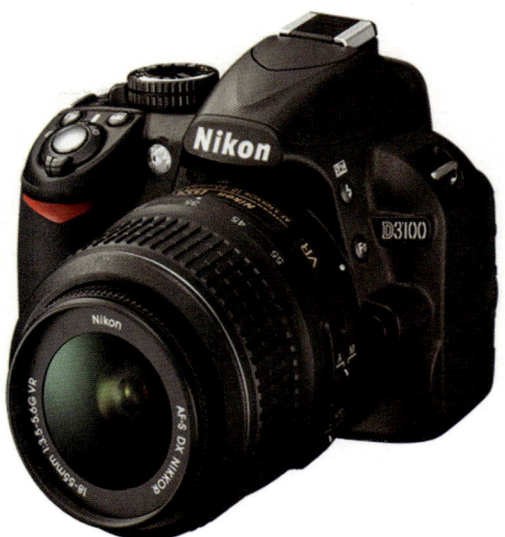

Fig. 28.48: Nikon D3100 SLR

Key Features

Type of camera	Single-lens reflex digital camera
Effective pixels	14.2 million
Image sensor	Nikon DX format (23.1 × 15.4 mm) CMOS sensor
Image size (pixels)	4,608 x 3,072 (L) 3,456 x 2,3404 (M) 2,304 x 1,536 (S)
Sensitivity	ISO 100 to 3200 in steps of 1 EV plus HI-1 (ISO 6400) and HI-2 (ISO 12800)

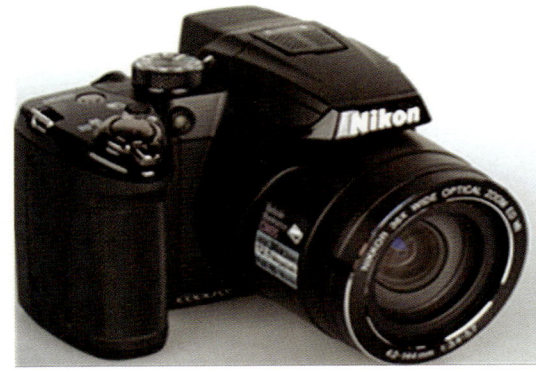

Fig. 28.49: Nikon Coolpix P500 Digital SLR Camera

Key Features

- 36× zoom lens (35 mm equivalent: 22.5–810 mm)
- 12.1 Mp CMOS image sensor
- 7× anti-blur
- 3in 921,000 dot, tiltable LCD monitor
- Full (1080p) HD movie recording with stereo sound
- HDMI connector for output to an HDTV.
- Side zoom control
- Exposure modes (P/S/A/M)
- Easy Panorama 360°/180°
- High-speed continuous shooting (8fps) at full 12.1 megapixel resolution

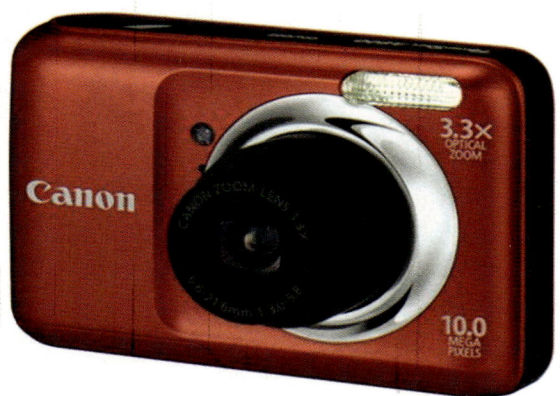

Fig. 28.50: Canon poweshot A800 digital camera: 10 megapixel, 3.3x optical zoom, 2.5" LCD screen

compressed. Compresssion increases the number of images that can be stored in memory; but it also causes a decay of the image quality; the higher the compression, the greater the decay.

Number of images stored in memory: There are two types of image storage:
1. Built-in (internal) memory
2. Removable memory

Four types of removable memory:
1. Solid State Floppy Disk Card (SSFDC) or 'Smart card'
2. Miniature card
3. Compact flash card
4. 3.5" floppy disk

SSFDCs can store only as much as 8 MB of data, while miniature cards store as much as 24 MB.

Compact flash card: It can be found in sizes from 2 MB to more than 100 MB. The amount of space taken by one image depends on its resolution and on the file compression. An uncompressed image with a resolution of 1280 × 1024 takes up 3.75 MB, while an 800 × 600 image can be compressed to only 100 KB.

There are two different ways to transfer the images from the camera to the computer:
1. *Cable connection:* Most digital cameras can be connected to a PC through a serial or parallel port. This kind of connection is extremely slow, and serial transfer is slower than parallel.
2. Transfer from removable memory through a computer drive.

Morphing: An image (as done by orthodontic software) for patient education, growth prediction and treatment prediction is a regular and accepted practice.

Conventional vs Digital Photography
Traditional Orthodontic Photography

Advantages
- Superior image quality
- Relatively inexpensive hardware (camera, optics, lighting)
- Mature, stable hardware
- Availability of technical assistance

Disadvantages
- Long processing time
- Delay in viewing
- Frequent need for retakes
- Ongoing film and processing expenses
- Physical storage requirements
- Possibility of lost or misplaced photographs
- Expense, time, and degradation of quality involved in duplication
- Difficulty of remote transmission

Disadvantages of Digital Photography
- Cameras prices are still high but they are decreasing in prices everyday.
- Digital image can be retouched and would not be useful for medicolegal requirements as the traditional negative.
- Since digital quality and technology are advancing, actual digital cameras will be absolutes in a few years.

Advantages of Digital photography
- A digital camera captures the image directly from the CCD sensor and requires no analog-to-digital conversion.
- The digital images are stored in the camera on small electronic 'flash cards' or on a miniature hard disk drive. They can then be downloaded to a computer.
- Ability to view the image as soon as it has been taken both in the camera screen or in the PC, allowing the doctor or operator to rectify it, repeat it or show it to the patients in order to motivate them.
- The absence of film, slides or processing cost is very well welcome for everybody.
- The ability to store records electronically is useful since after a number of years working, the space needed to store a large number of pictures records is significant.
- Image copies can be made automatically and easily with no economic cost.
- Digital photos are suited for immediate data transmission automatically everywhere to a colleague with the advantage of keeping original ones.

- There is not dust, scratch or damage of slides with time, even though it is necessary to make security copies very often.
- Digital records allow complete more confidentiality as the number of people involved in the processing and storage procedure is reduced.
- Digital records are easily and automatically introduced in main lectures, oral communications or PC presentations for teaching purposes.
- Any competent assistant can be trained to take digital photos.

To Conclude

The ability to produce high-quality photographs is an important clinical skill that has applications across all aspects of dentistry. Photography is not necessarily covered in sufficient detail in undergraduate training. Its inclusion could be rewarding. The technology in photography is changing rapidly, with new products reaching the market constantly. Therefore, a photography system needs to be selected with this in mind.

BIBLIOGRAPHY

1. Coimbra O, Lomheim C. Digital imaging and orthodontics. Am J Orthod 1999;115:103–105.
2. Doldo T, Fiorelli G, Patanè B. A comparison of three digital cameras for intraoral photography. J Clin Orthod 1999;33: 588–593.
3. Fiorelli G, Pupilli E, Patanè B. Digital photography in the orthodontic practice. J Clin Orthod 1998;32:651–656.
4. Mah J, Ritto K. The Cutting Edge. Imaging in Orthodontics: Present and Future. JCO 2002;36(11):619–625.
5. Maheshwari A, Kumar M. Understanding Pixel of Camera and Its Implication. JIDA 2010; 4(12): 524–525.
6. Pirttiniemi. Mastering digital dental photograph. EJO 2006; 28:624–30.
7. Sandler PJ, Murray A. Digital photography in orthodontics. J Orthod 2001;28:197–201.
8. Sandler PJ, Murray AM, Bearn D. Digital records in orthodontics. Dent Update 2002;29:18–24.
9. Sandler PJ, Murray AM. Recent developments in clinical photography. British Journal of Orthodontics 1999;26:269–274.
10. Scholz RP. Orthodontic technolocity. Am J Orthod 2001; 119:325–326.
11. Quintero JC, Trosien A, Hatcher D, Kapila S. Craniofacial imaging in orthodontics. Historical perspective, current status, and future developments. Angle Orthod 1999; 69:491–506.

PREVIOUS YEAR'S UNIVERSITY QUESTIONS

Short Questions

1. Digital photography in orthodontics—Discuss
2. American Board of Orthodontic requirements for extra- and intra-oral photography

Computers in Orthodontics

Chapter Outline

- Use of computer application in orthodontics
- Total digital radiography
- Digital Cephalometrics
- Videocephalometry
- Digital photography

Computers are especially useful as diagnostic aids due to their capability for storing large amount of data, objective approach and ability to perform complex calculation relatively easily in a short span of time. It is practically used in all the facets of any dental practice today. Computers have become especially useful to orthodontist as given in Table 29.1.

Types of Computers

- Super computers
- Mainframe computers
- Mini computers
- Desktop computers
- Notebooks/laptop computers
- Palmtop/tablet computers

USE OF COMPUTER APPLICATION IN ORTHODONTICS
(Table 29.2)

- Digital photography
- Digital radiography
- Digital cephalometrics
- Video cephalometric
- 3-D imaging
- Digital study models

Digital Image (Table 29.3)

A digital image is a matrix of square pieces or picture elements referred to as pixels that are displayed upon

Table 29.1: Clinical/graphic application

Conventional	Computerized
• Case sheet	• Data sheet
• Impression and diagnostic casts	• 3D photography
• Radiographs	• RVG, digital radiography
• Manual tracing	• Digitized tracing
• Cephalometric analysis	• Advanced software like Nemoceph, AudaxCeph,
• Diagnostic set-up	• VTO/VTP
• Treatment preformed system	• Treatment customized
• Mid-term evaluation	• Continuous monitoring

a flat panel display or a CRT and constitute the image space. The image space on a monitor is made up of pixels arranged in a series of horizontal lines called **'raster lines'**.

The significance of the pixels and their accumulation is seen in the resolution of an image. The pixels are arranged in a matrix .512 × .512. Matrix contains 262, 144 pixels. If a large number of pixels are used to represent an image, their discrete nature becomes less apparent.

A digital image is stored in a matrix of rows and columns of pixels values known as a bitmap image. Resolution basically refers to the density of pixels in a bitmapped image. Pixels/inch or pixels/mm, i.e. the spatial resolution of an image increases as the number

Table 29.2: Uses of computers in dental practice

Administrative applications

- Patient case records
- Recall appointments
- Patient scheduling
- Accounts
- Patient correspondence
- Billing
- Inventory lists
- Prescription formats
- Post-treatment instructions
- Insurance claims
- Referral information

Clinical applications

- Patient photographs—analysis and storage
- Patient radiographs—analysis and storage
- Interspecialty referral and opinion
- Patient motivation
- Appliance design using CAD CAMs
- Growth predictions
- Visual treatment objectives
- Generation of pre- and post-treatment photographs
- Patient interaction and information on the internet

Miscellaneous applications

- Survey information/epidemiological data
- Presentations
- Continuing dental/medical education
- Literature reviews
- Entertainment

of pixels increase. A digital image when enlarged exhibits graininess-pixelization. The value of each pixel is stored in one or more "bits" of data.

Sample Depth

Number of bits used to represent each pixel, i.e. each pixel has a digital value that represents the intensity of the information recorded for its detection. Information in computers is stored as 1's and 0's basically in a binary state. Each pixel of n bite/pixel is capable of 2n different colors and intensities.

In a 6 bit image, each pixel has 64 different values and in a 8 bit image each pixel has 256 different intensities or colors.

Grayscale images, such as a radiograph, need to possess 8 bits of data/pixel to be perceived as a continuous tonal range. Presently 12 bits (4096 shades of gray) is considered optimal.

Color images are usually represented by 24 bits of data/pixel (16.7 million possible color), i.e. 8 bits of data of each in RGB. Therefore, in each RG and B channel, 256 colors exist. If the colors chosen from the palette match the tones of image, image quality can be remarkably good.

Image Archiving/Storage

The storage of cephalometric radiographs and/or other radiographs is expensive and this cost could be reduced by image archiving. Such archiving of radiographs could prove extremely useful in long-term growth studies or treatment analysis studies utilizing radiographs. The problem of image storage increases with an increase in the number of pixels or sample depth.

However, an aid in the storage and transmission of images is the system of image compression. It is possible to compress data with no significant loss of image quality at compression ratios of up to 3:1. This is termed lossless compression.

For greater compression, some loss of information would occur but clinically acceptable pictures would be obtained at compression ratios up to 20:1—long compression.

Joint photographic experts group (JPEG) is the most commonly used compression method where 95% of storage space reduction is achieved. The JPEG works on 8 × 8 blocks of pixels and creates artifacts at the corner of blocks as data is encoded.

Table 29.3: Advantages and disadvantages of digital imaging

Advantages	Disadvantages
- Elimination of darkroom and automatic processing equipment	- Initial cost
- No chemical procesing waste	- Image quality
- Elimination of radiographic film	- Sensors can be bulky for patients
- Instant viewing of images	- Need a computer and/or network
- Less radiation dose to the patient	- Lack of a hard copy without additional equipment
- Low per image cost	- Panoramic and cephalometric units are more expensive than similar film units
- Ability to manipulate the images	- Acceptance by third party carriers is variable
- Images can be sent via E-mail	- Integration of radiographic software into practice
- Remote access to images outside the office	

Image Display

A normal monitor exhibits 625 lines. To be able to optimally view images 2048 lines are considered necessary.

TOTAL DIGITAL RADIOGRAPHY

The concept of total digital radiography is today a reality, i.e. an entire radiology department would utilize solely digital imaging facilities. Here there is a central storage and retrieval system which would facilitate the distribution of images to many locations within the hospital.

The immense volume of data, which is considered difficult to manage (12.81 terabytes/year) could be viewed at various locations—'multimodality viewing'. This would permit the display of not just the patients history, but also conventional radiographs, CT scans, photographs and other information. Patient's history and all other information integrated with radiographs would definitely be more informative to any clinician irrespective of his/her field of specialization.

Advantages and disadvantages of digital radiography are seen in Table 29.4.

Teleradiology

Transmission of radiographs to various sites via telephone lines/satellite link. This is dependent upon the:

- System used
- Size of the pixel matrix
- Time reuired

It is being done, but requires higher configuration systems and relatively lesser picture size (pixel mass).

Various Methods of Digital Radiography

Three methods are available for acquiring digital grayscale images of radiographs:

- Phosphor plate technique
- Direct receptor technique
- Transparancy scanner technique

Photo Stimulable Phosphor Plates

Step 1: Conventional X-ray tube end is used to expose the plate.

Step 2: Activating its phosphor coating and formation of a latent image.

Step 3: Sensitivity of the plate causes decrease of X-ray exposure by about 90%.

Step 4: The plate is passed over a laser scanner.

Step 5: The laser scanner stimulates the phosphor coating to emit visible light proportional to the X-ray exposure.

Step 6: The light is detected and converted to a gray-scale intensities creating a digital image which is tranferred to a computer and saved on a local or network storage.

Step 7: The latent image is then removed by placing the plate over a bright light for a few minutes; plates are reusable and can be used for several thousand exposures.

The image is obtained at 12 bits/pixel but can be down sampled to 8 bits/pixel.

Direct Receptors

These use a photosensitive sensor such as a:

- Charged couple device
- Complementary metal oxide semiconductor (CMOS)

Table 29.4: Advantages and disadvantages of digital radiography	
Advantages	*Disadvantages*
• Easy to operate	• Requires adequate infection control protocols
• Requires minimal training	• Initial cost of system and cost for replacement equipment
• Eliminates processing chemicals and equipment	• Discomfort of sensors due to bulkiness and interference of cord
• Hard copies can be printed	• Must have appropriate lighting for interpretation
• Allows for communication with third party via internet	• Technical difficulties with equipment
• Easily viewed on any computer monitor	• Concern with rapidly advancing technology and compatibility in the future
• Can reduce radiation exposure	• Ease of retakes, "Preferred" image density and smaller dimensions of direct digital sensors can result in higher levels of radiation exposure
• Viewing of the image is immediate	
• Long-term cost of equipment can work out to less when compared to film processing chemicals, purchasing film and maintenance	

Conventional X-ray tube is used to expose the sensor and activate thousands of tiny light-sensitive fields.

As with the phosphor plate method, exposure decreases by about 90%.

The phosphor plate systems require two steps— exposure and scanning; direct receptors display images immediately on the monitor.

Intraoral sensors are suitable for periapical and bitewing radiography. A small and large sensor for cephalometry is also available.

Flatbed Transparency Scanner

- Many orthodontists contemplating digital cephalometry find this method to be simplest and least expensive method of digital image acquisition.
- A conventional X-ray film is placed on the scanners flat transparent surface and is scanned by a light source.
- The transmitted light is detected by a CCD and is converted into grayscale intensities.
- A new class of flatbed scanners that can obtain images at 12 bits/pixel and a resolution of 600 pixels/ inch are now available.
- However, the images obtained by this method require a lot of memory space.
- 3D digital models using laser technology: A new laser scan based approach called e-models was developed to improve the accuracy and efficiency of orthodontic diagnosis, treatment planning and bracket placement.

Automatic Identification of Landmarks (Table 29.5)

The cephalometric radiograph is scanned into the computer. The computer automatically loads the landmarks and performs the analysis. This overcomes the errors usually encountered in the manual identification of landmarks.

The procedure of computerized automatic identification has the potential to increase accuracy, and improve our ability to correctly diagnose orthodontic problems. Also the very use of computerization might make the application of alternative methods of form

Table 29.5: The various manual errrors in the analysis of cephalograms

A. Reproducibility errors
B. Variation in image acquisition
C. Landmark identification
    i. Interobserver variation
    ii. Intraobserver variation
D. Measurement errors

description, other than lines and analysis possible. Techniues such as FEM, allometric models, Mesh diagram, etc. have the potential of becoming more clinically applicable.

The common approach to identify landmarks have a similar approach in that
- Image pixels in the regions of high intensity gradient or edges are identified.
- These edges are assumed to be object boundaries.
- Landmarks are then found in relation to these labeled boundaries.

This approach involves four steps:
- Remove noise
- Label pixels according to their engines
- Count pixels and label edge
- Find landmark band on position or relationship to labeled edgs.

DIGITAL CEPHALOMETRICS

Cephalograms are two-dimensional representation of 3D anatomy. Our ability to derive meaningful information from head films depends on the reliability with which the anatomic relations can be evaluated.

Fortunately, orthodontists around the world have agreed on a reasonably high level of standardization in the methods used to acquire a cephalogram. The head position and orientation, source object distance and radiographic enlargement have been standardized to a degree that permits a common descriptive language of dentofacial morphology and the development of consistent methods of anthropometric landmark identification.

The information inherent in the large data collections that cephalometric studies ential is of fundamental importance to orthodontic diagnosis and understanding craniofacial changes due to growth or orthodontic therapy.

The analysis and acquiring of cephalometric data can be streamlined and made more efficiently by using a new approach or a new analytic tool. This technology must be able to store, score, retrieve and analyze vast collections of imformation.

This new approach has two important features. First it applies powerful mathematical technology to describe and analyze morphologic structures and secondly, this can be analyzed by the computer.

In the past two decades, we have witnessed the development of number of systems for the computer-aided encoding of data from lateral cephalograms for use in craniofacial research and clinical treatment planning (Fig. 29.1).

Comparison between Manual and Computerized Prediction

The cephalometric application workflow is as follows:

Digitization

Digitization is the form by which analog information is converted to digital form. The methods involved can be either direct or indirect.

During digitization, X-Y coordinates of cephalometric landmarks are recorded and stored in data set. This data set is the starting point for the formulation of various computer generated VTOs and STOs.

Direct Computer Digitization

A digitizing tablet or digitizer is used for this purpose.

Digitizers may be opaque, transparent digitizers can be backlit, allowing direct digitization of cephalogrmas without any intermediate acetate tracing.

Resolution and Accuracy

Resolution is the smallest distance that can be resolved by the digitizer in the order of 1000 lines/inch.

Accuracy is the precision with which a digitizer can record reported movements over various regions on its surface. It should be in the order of ±0.25 mm for cephalometric application.

The anatomical points are entered using on electronic pen or instrument. The digitizing tablet is made up of a fine electric grid that includes registration points as fine as 0.009 mm apart. This electronic instrument emits an electronic signal either on command or continuously.

Various varieties of instruments are available for this purpose. The two most commonly used are:
1. Electronic pen
2. Crosshair cursor

Electronic pen: An electronic pen is activated to emit a signal when the tip of the pen is pressed against the film or a button on the pen is pressed. Electronic signals are emitted directly from the pen to the grid completing the circuit.

Crosshair cursor: This potentiometer consists of two wires arranged in a crosshair pattern which are embedded into a glass window. The electronic registration signal is emitted from the junction of the wires. The operator presses a button to activate the potentiometer.

The crosshair cursor is less popular now because:
1. The digitizer is bulky and not very easy to use.
2. Glow from the glass in which the wires are embedded prevents optimum mapping of the various landmarks.

Indirect Digitization

For indirect digitization, a video camera or mapper captures an image of the cephalometric radiograph and stores it in the computer. The video camera must be calibrated with the cephalometric film being plowed into the computer. The digital radiography is another method of data input into the computer.

The image is then displayed on a monitor and the landmarks are identified using a mouse. The only disadvantage of this method is that the digitizing

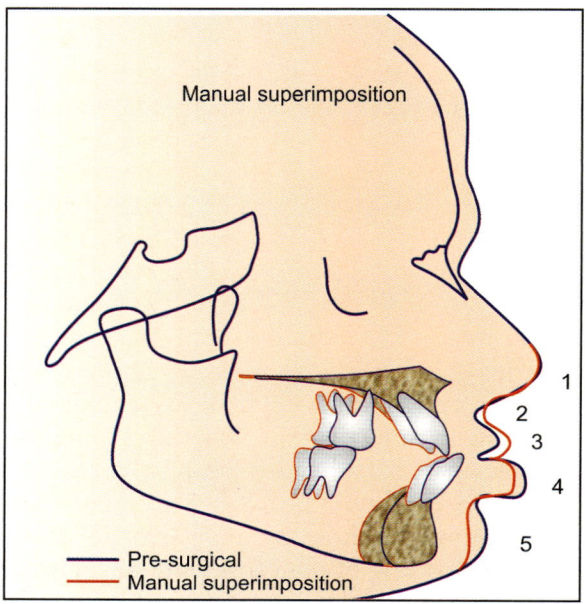

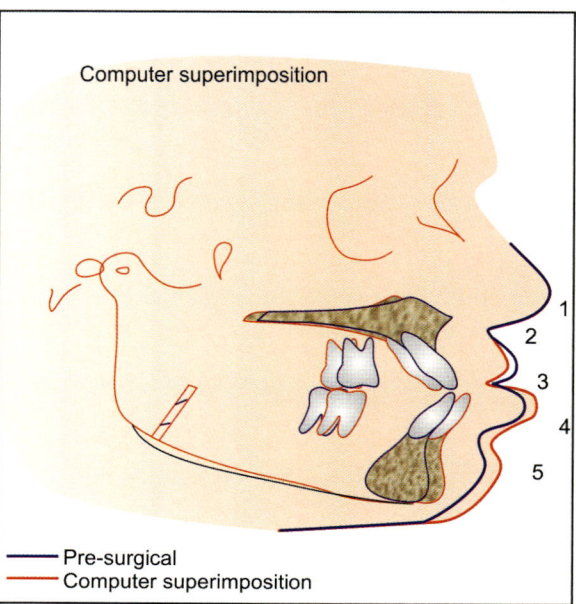

Fig. 29.1: Comparison between manual and computerized prediction

resolution obtained is lessar than that obtained with a digitizer.

Mode of Digitization

- Point mode
- Stream mode

Point mode: The user sequentially locates landmarks in a predetermined order recording one coordinate pair for each landmark. It basically involves the direct location of individual landmarks.

A visual representation of a cephalogram is generated by connecting discretely located points due to their proximity and sequence, making a visual representation of a cephalogram possible.

Stream mode: Here the operator traces a cephalogram using the digitizing device and the tracing thus obtained in the form of a stream of points controlled ny a programmable option. The points are recorded as a specific number of coordinate points per second or after the cursor has moved a certain distance.

The points were joined from audible contour and this analogy is easily accepted by the computer.

Advantages and Disadvantages

Point mode digitization is more time consuming but more accurate.

Stream mode digitization is less accurate due to the manner in which the data is acquired.

The location of hard and soft tissue landmarks must be provided to the predictive software. Point mode reliably provides location of the landmarks whereas the stream mode does not.

A coordinate pair may not be transmitted as the cursor passes over a landmark such as the subnasale. Thus, the accuracy of landmark location suffers here.

Also, to locate a point and determine a change in its position over time it is helpful to know the precise position of the landmarks relative to its origin. The accuracy of such information can be obtained only by way of point digitization.

Direct Digitization

Computer softwares that allow direct digitization of cephalometric radiographs are currently available. These software programs perform various orthodontic and surgical movemets based upon parameters entered by the user into the program.

'Dentofacial planner' program has a digitization regimen for the lateral cephalogram consisting of 68 landmarks of which 43 are soft tissue landmarks and remainder are hard tissue landmarks.

'Quick ceph' another commercially available program uses a 28-landmark regimen with all points representing hard tissue landmarks.

Both programs can perform a variety of functions with the digital cephalometric radiograph including:

- Cephalometric analysis
- Superimposition (Fig. 29.1)
- Growth estimation
- Orthodontic treatment planning
- Surgical prediction

The hard tissue positions as predicted in the expected surgical procedure are fed into the program and the expected soft tissue cahnges are then calculated. The soft tissue profile prediction is made possible by the application of ratios of soft tissue and hard tissue changes to the surgical movements that are within the program.

These ratios are based upon retrospective studies of stability and soft tissue changes.

Cephalometric Analysis and Treatment Planning

The various tasks that make up cephalometrics can be broadly divided into static and dynamic function.

Static function: Information derived from the radiograph contours on a cuurent film or collection of films.

Dynamic function: Dynamic functions include elements of cephalometric representation that are transformed or manipulated such as growth prediction.

Orthodontic/Surgical Text Planning

Static Cephalometric Function

Cephalometric applications use the digitized coordinates for a sequence of landmarks for the anatomic structures they represent. Vector mathematics is used to compute a variety of commonly used cephalometric movements, the angle between 2 lines and the perpendicular from a point to a line, etc.

Movements derived from a patient's digital cephalogram are reported in comparison to a data of age and sex specific values.

To accommodate cephalometric enlargement, the coordinates of all digital landmarks are scaled by a factor that reduces the dimension of the overall representation to a corrected size. Digitized cranial base or reginally stable landmarks are used for imposition of digitized landmarks. Incorporating magnitudes and dimension of change. Analyses can be conducted for all superimposed coordinate sets.

The basic problem with using software programs for superimposition is that unlike in manual superimposition where stable landmarks are superimposed on one another or the best fit contours are matched in cephalometric computer applications, superimpositions are done using landmarks already stored in their data sets, this can potentially result in errors due to poor landmark location.

Dynamic Cephalometric Function

The concept of cephalometric prediction rapidly for planning combined surgical and orthodontic treatment is well established. These are basically growth and treatment visualization systems.

Treatment decisions are entered into the system and immediately evaluated. Landmarks sufficient to render an adequate distribution of the structures involved must be digitized.

Cephalometric growth forecasting is still a region of some controversy. However, it is well documented that it is possible to estimate growth to a certain degree using cephalometry.

The rickets growth prediction methodology is widely used and is easily implemented in various softwares. It applies increments of growth to a series of landmarks along reference lines determined by the subjects exisitng anatomy. These can be refined by the use of growth increments senstitve to the subject's skeletal age.

Cephalometric applications allow the user to manipulate the position and inclination of skeletal and dental structures to create orthodontic and surgical treatment plans. Software 'Handles' are available that allow the manipulation of the position and orientation of a specific structure.

The profile changes in an individual in response to manipulation can be visualized and algorithms exist that can predict the patients soft tissue profile following such alterations. Soft tissue profile changes are a combination of a number of factors (growth + orthopedic changes + orthodontics).

Profile changes in an adult are relatively easier to evaluate, especially if the only manipulation is surgical in nature. Hence, it is easier to study the effects of surgery or orthodontic treatment in adults rather than growing individuals especially upon soft tissue profile.

Studies have shown that software predictive models to be at least as effective as manual prediction.

Advantages of using computers for cephalometry include:
1. Speed—1 minute for digitization
2. Luxury of exploring many treatment options simultaneously and weighing the results vs variables.
   - Extraction vs nonextraction.
   - Surgery vs pure orthodontic approach.

3. Can share the information with colleagues/referral sources.
4. Collabrate with the surgeon on treatment plan.
5. The laborious measurement of angles and distances by the manual use of a protractor is eliminated as measurements are made virtually instantaneously by the computer.
6. All the various cephalometric data can be converted to digital data and any number of analyses can be performed.
7. Data bases can be created for various ethnic communities. Gender/sex, even in private practices.
8. Speeds up the process of constructing a visaul treatment objective (VTO).

VIDEOCEPHALOMETRY

Prior to the advent of the present graphic capabilities of the computer video imaging technique, the profile that predicted the result of orthognathic surgery was communicated via profile tracings and verbal descriptions. Photo modification, as it was called, involved the sectioning of photographs using a pen-like device and the lines were then rearranged to provide visualization of treatment results.

Profile Video Image Modification

The evolution of relatively inexpensive and accessible computer technology has made it possible to incorporate graphics into the plannning and communication phases of orthodontic treatment. Computer assisted 'cut and paste' movements are used to modify the image in an effort to describe the anticipates profile or facial result from dental or surgical movements.

The need for video cephalometry stems from the fact that unlike for plastic surgery when just the soft tissue result of a particular procedure is required, in orthodontics a knowledge of the effect of the treatment upon the underlying skeletal and soft tissue structures too is essential. The computer results required, because of the manipulation of both the hard and soft tissues dictates the need for the superimposition of the cephalometric radiograph over the face (Table 29.6).

Quantified Profile Modification through Extrapolation

As the development of imaging software progressed, an effort was made to quantify the movements produced on a computer screen to allow for planning to correlate the required changes to the facial changes for correction of malocclusion.

The company 'Orthographic' was the first to introduce treatment visualization using video images.

Table 29.6: Common clinical errors in video imaging

- If facial images and cephalograms are not taken simultaneously, it may result in significant differences in head position and image magnification discrepencies
- A minor alteration of either cephalogram or video image is at times required to obtain best fit between the alteration, this in turn raises questions regarding the validity of the video-cephalometric study
- Errors in head position during image capture might have a deleterious effect upon perception planning of profile
- The video image and cephalometry both might show a different soft tissue position
- Differences exist in soft tissue response in differently gathered subjects and corrections might have to be built in the softwares used for such alterations
- Distortion of image might orginate from the use of a particular camera
- Distortion could be due to distortion on the computer monitor (this can be avoided or at least minimized by using flat screen monitors)

A video image was made and the software in the computer was capable of measuring the image in real life size.

A lead rod was stuch to the image and since the size of the markes was known, the computer software could then be calibrated to the size of the rod based on its size on the computer image.

Photocephalometry

Photocephalometry consisted of taking radiograph and photographs from a similar distance. The photograph negative could then be enlarged and accurately superimposed onto the photograph to visualize profile changes due to orthognathic surgical procedures.

Techniques of Image Superimposition upon Cephalogram

There are four basic ways in which a cephalometric image can be superimposed over a video image of the patient.

1. Digitization of the cephalogram then sizing the profile video image to the cephalogram.
2. Digitized followed by sizing of the cephalogram to an existing video image.
3. Gathering a video image of the cephalogram and matching it to an existing video image, with the cephalogram being digitized on screen.
4. Simultaneous cephalometric and video image gathering. To acieve consistently matching profiles it is recommended that the video camera be exactly correlated to the cephalometric source. Yet, since this

is not possible always, certain errors are bound to get incorporated in the process.

The two ways that are most frequently used for the correlation of the video and the cephalometric images are:

Direct digitization: Two or more points digitized and the distance between them is noted and these act as a reference for all other points on the video image.

Indirect digitization: A grid is placed on the radiograph/image and the digitization in the computer is done on a preset grid that matches the grid on the image.

DIGITAL PHOTOGRAPHY

Digital photography has revolutionized the way photographs are now taken and stored. The technology available to us now allows all but the most demanding of photographic application to be executed with consummate ease. Orthodontic photographic needs through essential, are basic and easily accomplished using digital cameras.

The procedure involved is practically the same as conventional photography, except that it stores images in digital form on a storage media. Also, it provides many advantages over conventional photography. The most important being that it is simple to tranfer and manipulate such data (Table 29.7).

Pixels and Resolution

800 × 600 and 1800 × 1600 pixels are believed to be adequate for orthodontic purpose.

Input Devices

The big difference between traditonal film camera and digital camera is that unlike traditonal cameras that capture the image on film, here there is a solid state device called an image sensor.

Exposure

When shutter release is pressed a metering cell measures the amount of light coming through the lens and accordingly sets the aperture and shutter speeds for the correct exposure when the shutter opens briefly.

Each pixel on the image sensor records the brightness of light that falls on it as an electric charge. The more light that hits a pixel the higher the charge, i.e.

- Lights from brightly lit areas—high charges
- Light from shadows—low charges

Pixels only capture brightness and not color! Colors are recorded on the image sensor as red, green or blue. Each pixel on the sensor has a filter so that it can record

Table 29.7: Advantages of digital photography over-conventional photography

- Versatility—incredibly easy to:
  - Alter photographs
  - Store and distribute
  - E-mail: Post on website
- Less chance of poor shots due to the back screen
- Saves money in the long run
  - No rolls
  - Development
- Instant knowledge regarding the appearance of pictures
- Pictures can be identified before printing
- Eco-friendly
- No waiting for film to be processed
- Sound and video possible

only that light that forms through the filter and other colors are blocked. Only that particular colors brightness can be evaluated. But when a color other than that of the three types of pixels is transmitted onto the sensor a process known as interpolation is used to calculate the third color.

By combining the color registered with the color directly, detected by the pixel the actual color can be arrived at. All these calculations are performed by a microprocessor.

Types of image sensors frequently used:
- Charged couple device (CCD)
- Complementary metal oxide semiconductor (CMOS)

Both these image sensors capture light on a grid of small pixels on their surfaces. How they process the image is what it differentiates them from each other. A charge couple device (CCD) gets its name from the way the charges on its pixels are read after exposure. After exposure, the charges are transferrred onto a plane on the register called the read out register, then to an amplifier, and then onto an analog to digital converter. Once the row has been read out, and registered its charges on the read out row are deleted.

The charges on each row are compiled onto one above so that when one moves down the one above can move down to the read out register.

Complementary metal oxide semiconductor (CMOS) is a technology used to make millions of chips for computer processors and memory. With CMOS, the costs are greatly reduced. CMOS has processing circuits on the same unit. Here the only problem is the noise associated with pictures.

Image Resolution

The optical resolution of a camera or scanner is an absolute number because the image sensor pixels are photo elements, i.e. physical devices that can be counted.

Interpolated resolution is the enhancement of a picture by adding software pixels. This is not acceptable because it is just a make believe enhancement and a burden on the memory, yet it is frequently used to enhance photograph quality.

Imgae Storage Format

The size of an image file is huge when compared to other file fromats. With increased resolution the requirement of memory also increases.

Image storage can be done in two forms depending upon their attachment to the digital cameras. The storage facility may be removable and fixed.

Older cameras have fixed storage, that limits the number of photos that can be taken. All the present day cameras have some form of removable storage enabling the photographer to take any number of photos as he wishes and is limited only by the amount of media he possesses.

Advantages of Removable Storage

i. Erasable and reusable
ii. Usually removable
iii. Easy transfer to computer

Removable Storage Devices

- Flash cards
- Smart media
- Floppy drive
- Micro drive

Photography Software

i. Download software
ii. Photo-editing device
iii. Album software
iv. Photo-printing software

The softwares basically allow for the manipulation of the digital photographs for various purposes. They permit the required detail to get highlighted and depending upon the function required for the image can be stored or printed. They are extremely important for patient motivation as the pretreatment photographs can be modified to show approximate or expected post-treatment changes.

Three-Dimensional Imaging

Even though we tend to visualize and plan treatment using two-dimensional aids such as cephalogram and facial photographs the current paradigm shift in orthodontics and the keen interest in esthetics has resulted in an interest in three-dimensional visualization and diagnosis to plan treatment for what is a three-dimensional structure.

Craniofacial Imaging and Animation with the Laser Scanner

This is significant technology breakthrough in facial 3D image reconstruction. Vivid 700 was the first commercially visible laser scanner introduced by Minolta. A Class II laser is used to scan the face. Facial photographs are taken using a CCD camera, that is present adjacent to the scanning outlet. A beam splitter facilitates the capture of the laser scan simultaneously with color texture map.

Laser scanners record the distortion of lasers when passed over a face and infer their distortion to provide a surface map. Color/texture map is recorded simultaneously using a digital camera and this is superimposed over the surface map to obtain a composite image.

The problem with laser scanning is an inability to scan transparent, bright white and black objects.

Digital Study Models

Now computerized softwares are commercially available which are capable of scanning study models and storing the scanned data as three-dimensional images. The scanned data is caliberated to the actual size of the study models. Either the impression can be scanned or the plaster cast can be scanned using a laser scanner. If impressions are scanned, then there is no need of making the plaster cast.

Advantages of Digital Study Models

- Image/data can be stored without damage for a long time.
- Data can be easily transformed from one place to another within seconds.

- Minimal storage is required.
- No need of plaster models.
- Virtual setup can be done.
- Laboratory storage space and cost is eliminated.
- The 3D data can be printed to make physical models in a variety of materials such as plaster, wax, synthetic materials with the use of 3D printers.

Disadvantages of Digital Models

- Increased cost
- Backup is needed as digital model can be lost/deleted.

BIBLIOGRAPHY

1. Adams GL, Gansky SA, Miller AJ, et al. Comparison between traditional two-dimensional cephalometry and a three-dimensional approach. Am J Orthod 2002;122(1):117–20.
2. Harrell WE Jr, Hatcher DC, Bolt RL. In search of anatomical truth: three-dimentional modeling and the future of orthodontics. Am J Orthod 2003;122(3):325–30.
3. Hutchinson I, et al. Digital cameras and orthodontics: An overview. Dent Update 1999;26:144–9.
4. Mozzo P, et al. A new volumetric CT machine for dental imaging based on the cone-beam techniue: preliminary results. Eur Radil 1998;8:1558–64.

PREVIOUS YEAR'S UNIVERSITY QUESTIONS

Short Questions

1. Uses of computer application in orthodontics
2. Uses of computer application in dental practice
3. Advantages and disadvantages of digital imaging
4. Advantages and disadvantages of digital radiography
5. Photocephalometry
6. Advantages of digital photography over conventional photography
7. Digital photography
8. Digital study models

Adult Orthodontics

Chapter Outline

- Introduction
- Indications for orthodontic treatment in adults
- Contraindications for orthodontic treatment in adults
- Biomechanical considerations when treating adult patients
- Types of treatment in adults

INTRODUCTION

At one time, orthodontic treatment was limited to the adolescent age group. But today, with the development of newer techniques and better understanding of the biologic basis of tooth movement, the age up to which orthodontic treatment is considered possible has increased considerably. Today more and more adult patients are visiting orthodontic clinics for attaining treatment. The reason is of increased awareness about dental health that motivates the patients to visit dentists and/or orthodontists (Table 30.1).

Since orthodontic treatment is easily available and acceptable to the patients, the general dentists are also recommending orthodontic intervention more frequently than ever before. The prevalence of periodontal problems and their established association with malaligned teeth has also helped advocate the case for orthodontics.

For all practical purposes, an adult is defined as a person who has to grow. Biologically, this happens at around 18 years of age. For orthodontic purposes, it is better to classify adult patients as:

Group I: 18 to 25 years of age

Group II: 26 to 35 years of age

Group III: 36 years and older

The first group patients are generally treated as other adolescent patients. They may exhibit heightened

Table 30.1: Reasons why adults seek orthodontic treatment
- Did not want orthodontic treatment as children.
- Parents or they themselves did not know about orthodontics as children.
- Orthodontist was not available in the vicinity.
- Dentist did not advise orthodontic treatment when younger.
- Parents could not afford orthodontic treatment.
- Incomplete or relapsed orthodontic treatment as children.
- Gum (periodontal) problems because of the malocclusion present.
- Concerned about appearance.
- Can afford orthodontic treatment now.
- Malocclusions like spacing/crowding becoming more prominent with age.
- Advised by prosthodontist, prior to fixed replacement of teeth.
- Advised by periodontist, to prevent further deterioration of periodontal condition.
- TMJ problems arising due to the malocclusion.
- Overall heightened concern about dental health.

concerns for esthetics, but otherwise are periodontally healthy. The second group exhibits more periodontal and restorative problems. Whereas, the third group will invariably present prosthodontic complications and may lack a full complement of teeth.

INDICATIONS FOR ORTHODONTIC TREATMENT IN ADULTS

- Why take orthodontic treatment in adults?

- Is it only to improve the esthetic demands of the patient or just because we have better techniques today?
- Indications for orthodontic treatment can be broadly classified into four categories:
  - Prosthodontic
  - Periodontal
  - Temporomandibular joint (TMJ)
  - Esthetic

Prosthodontic Indications for Orthodontic Treatment of Adults

Prosthodontists are advocating fixed prosthesis in more and more patients. Certain criteria need to be fulfilled before teeth can be used as abutments, these relate to parallelism of abutment teeth, redistribution and redirection of occlusal and incisal forces, improvement of crown/root ratio, etc.

Orthodontic appliances can upright teeth that have tilted into extraction spaces. They are even more frequently used to acieve parallelism of abutment teeth. They are also used to distribute teeth more favorably both inter- and intra-arch. Teeth that have supraerupted and prevent the placement of prosthesis in the opposing arch can be intruded. Orthodontic appliances can act as space regainers, and can help achieve regain lost space into which prosthesis may be placed.

Periodontal Indications for Orthodontic Treatment in Adults

Crowding of teeth: It is a proven fact that crowding of teeth leads to accumulation of plaque. If not removed can cause subsequent periodontal breakdown. Crowded teeth are difficult to clean as the bristles of the routinely used toothbrushes cannot reach the embrasures. Once these teeth become well aligned, oral hygiene procedures can be carried out more easily and efficiently.

Spacing between teeth is not only unsightly but also provides an ideal location for food lodging. This can lead to the formation of periodontal pockets and associated loss of bone. Spacing in the anterior segment is often associated with periodontal breakdown following pregnancy in middle-aged women. An orthodontist can close these gaps and help to maintain the results.

Temporomandibular Joint Dysfunction

The term is a symptom and encompasses a varied number of underlying causes. It can often be the result of over-closure, caused due to an early loss of posterior teeth or/and decrease in the lower facial height. Orthodontist can elevate symptoms and use of splints can be beneficial before any prosthetic rehabilitation.

Esthetics

This remains and will remain the most important motivation for a patient to seek orthodontic treatment. An incisor drifting anteriorly, or a crossbite which was acceptable for 30 years suddenly becomes unsightly as the malocclusion starts worsening following a generalized loss of periodontal health.

CONTRAINDICATIONS FOR ORTHODONTIC TREATMENT IN ADULTS

The buzz word is—'doesn't over do it.' Yes, science has progressed, but the bottom line remains that do not try it if you think it is not possible. The situation may arise because of four main reasons:

1. *Medical:* The patient is medically compromised to an extent that bone formation itself is likely to be compromised. Especially in diseases like diabetes mellitus, the healing capacity of the tissues is much below normal and treatment should be avoided.
2. Periodontal condition of the patient is poor, with multiple mobile teeth. Patients who do not maintain good oral hygiene are poor candidates for orthodontic treatment irrespective of the age of the patient (Fig. 30.1).
3. Skeletal malocclusions, which require surgical intervention, also might not be undertaken because of the extent of medical and for physical condition of the patient.
4. Motivation of the patient is essential. Do not start treatment, if at the time of evaluation itself it is felt that the patient is skeptical of the procedure being advocated. It is advised not to proceed with the treatment unless the patient is found to be determined to see the therapy through to completion.

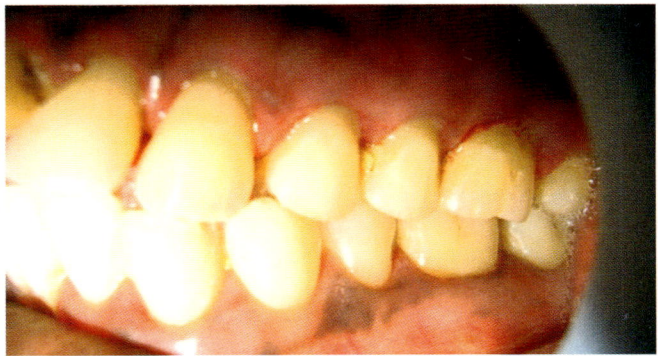

Fig. 30.1: Poor periodontal condition unsuitable for orthodontic treatment

Difference between Adolescents and Adults

Both adolescents and adults, if cooperative, can be treated equally well orthodontically. The two differences which can paly havoc with any orthodontic appliance therapy are growth and the degree of periodontal breakdown. Growth is a factor that can be ignored for allpractical purposes in adults. In a way, this makes it easier for the clinician as he is expected to undertake only dental changes, which are usually simpler to achieve as compared to growth modification procedures. Periodontal disease, which is rarely seen in growing children, becomes a major factor when planning orthodontic treatment for adults. The degree of periodontal beakdown and the resultant bone loss around teeth might determine and at times even dictate the course of treatment for adults.

Generally, adult patients are better motivated and will stanby their commitments on oral hygiene and appliance maitainance. Adults definitely take longer to get used to the appliance, but they appreciate results better and hence, it is a more satisfying experience treating adult patients (Table 30.2).

BIOMECHANICAL CONSIDERATIONS WHEN TREATING ADULT PATIENTS

Orthodontic appliance should always be chosen depending upon the malocclusion and in the case of adults—the patient's expectations. Expectations can be with regard to the esthetics of the appliance or the results desired. The capability of the orthodontist to treat cases with different appliances also plays a major role here.

The most esthetic appliance is the lingual appliance but labially placed esthetic brackets might be more commonly used. This is because a few orthodontists are trained in the lingual technique. Also, a lingual orthodontic treatment will be much more expensive as compared to treatment with any other appliance.

The traditional adolescent treatment objectives are toned down without necessarily compromising treatment results to incorporate minimal dental manipulation appropriate for the individual case. In other words, move only those teeth that are essential to achieve acceptable results. At times, space may be created by proclining teeth or extracting a single tooth or single arch extractions are more commonly done, rather than the routine all first premolar extraction. The scope for segmental treatment is increased in adult patients.

With advancing age, certain changes take place in the oral tissues which have a bearing on orthodontic tooth movement. Some such changes are seen in all adult patients treated, these are as follows.

Changes in the Tooth Structure

Occlusal Facets

Occlusal facets are more common in adults as compared to adolescent. These might cause resistance to tooth movement, as the teeth tend to interdigitate better and more perfectly.

Dental Caries

Adults are most susceptible to recurrent dental caries, and these might increase the chances of the tooth being root canal treated. Root canal treated teeth might show more root resorption as compared to normal healthy teeth.

Table 30.2: Differences between adolescent and adult patients		
Characteristic	Adolescent patient	Adult patient
Growth potential	Growth modification may be possible	No growth possible. Correction limited tot tooth movement
TMJ adaptability	Adaptable	Frequently shows signs of TMJ dysfunction
Periodontal problems	Rarely show signs of periodontal disease	Periodontal problems are frequently encountered
General health	Rarely a consideration	Might be of major concern, especially if surgery is planned
Appliance esthetics	Rarely of concern	Of major concern to the patient
Retention planning	Usually short- term and with removable appliances	Long term and actually fixed
Appliance tolerance the	Will usually tolerate and get used to all orthodontic appliances soon	More time is required to get accustomed to appliance
Speech	Adjust quickly	Adjustment takes time and effort
Motivation and cooperation	Ranges from poor to excellent	Usually good

Restorative Failures

As the patient's age progresses, so do the chances of him/her having dental restorations.

Restoration with:
- Improper contours leading to the loss of proper contacts.
- Proximal overhangs—causing formation of periodontal pockets.
- Deficient occlusal carving may cause loss of occlusal carving may cause loss of occlusal contacts, decreasing the chewing capability of the patient.
- Teeth restored with ceramic crowns or laminates may also pose problems while bonding of orthodontic attachments.

Changes in the 'U' (peridontium)

As the age advances, the periodontium is weakened and its reparative capacity is reduced.

Adults exhibit higher susceptibility to periodontal bone loss as compared to adolescent. Decrease in the alveolar bone height of teeth tends to decrease periodontal support.

Forces have to be accordingly decreased to move such compromised teeth. Also, this causes a change in the center of resistance which shifts more apically. Hence not only the magnitude of the force has to be decreased but bracket placement might have to be altered. The further away the point of application of force from the center of resistance, the more the chances for the tooth to tip. Tipping movement is the easiest to achieve.

The adult bone is denser and less vascular. Also, as age progresses, the overall rates at which cells are produced decreases. And this in turn might lead to decrease in the rate at which adult teeth move and stabilize. The more slowly the bone forms the longer and more critical the retentive phase becomes.

Missing Teeth

Premature Loss

Premature loss of teeth might cause:
- If replaced in time, presence of removable or fixed prosthesis in the patient's mouth, or
- If not replaced within a reasonable period of time:
  - Supraeruption of the tooth in the opposing arch
  - Tipping of the tooth distal to the extraction site. This often leads to narrowing of the bone at the site of extraction—moving a tooth into such a site

is usually difficult and might lead to loss of attachment and mobility

Temporomandibular Joint

The temporomandibular joint is one thing that is often not considered   important while treating adolescent. This is mainly because they exhibit high degree of adaptability and rarely any symptoms of TMJ dysfunction. It is exactly the opposite with adults and the joint should be evaluated not only while diagnosing the case but also monitoring during and after treatment.

TYPES OF TREATMENT IN ADULTS

Adults present with multiple problems and these need not be only classified as simple malocclusions. Orthodontic treatment needs to take into consideration the periodontal and/or prosthodontic rehabilitation of the patient, depending upon the intensity of malocclusion and the amount of orthodontic correction required.

Proffit classified adult orthodontic procedures as:
- Adjunctive orthodontic treatment
- Comprehensive orthodontic treatment
- Surgical orthodontic treatment

Adjunctive Orthodontic Treatment

These are procedures which are done as precursors or in conjunction with other dental procedures. These are generally done to facilitate further prosthodontic or periodontal rehabilitation of the patient. These are the most commonly undertaken procedures in the patients who fall in the Group II and III age groups.

The goals of adjunctive orthodontic treatment include:
- Parallelism and/or deterioration of abutment teeth
- Elimination of crowding
- Elimination of anterior spacing, which might be causing frequent food lodgement or esthetic problems.
- Establishing a more favorable distribution of teeth.
  a. Inter-arch
  b. Intra-arch—to facilitate prosthetic rehabilitation
- Establishing a more favorable crown-to-root ratio and/or intrusion of specific teeth.

Adjunctive Treatment Procedures

- Uprighting of molars
- Forced eruption
- Alignment of anterior teeth
- Positioning tooth for implants
- Crossbite correction
- Diastema closure

Uprighting of Molars

- Many adults will have loss of posterior tooth usually first permanent molars.
- When a first molar is lost, the adjacent teeth drift, tip and rotate.
- The gingival tissue gets folded and there is formation of periodontal pocket, and poor interproximal contact.
- Uprighting molars eliminate the periodontal problems, create space for pontic or close the space if there is negligible residual space.

Appliance Used

- Partial fixed appliances with uprighting springs.
- Prosthesis should be given within 6 weeks after completion of uprighting (as a guideline)

Reasons for Alignment of Anterior Teeth

- To facilitate placement of normally contoured crowns and pontics.
- To improve access and to facilitate proper placement of restorations.
- To repositioning the roots.
- To facilitate proper placement of implants.

Positioning Tooth for Implants

In some cases, implants are placed for replacement of teeth.

- The teeth have to properly position for efficient placement of implants.
- Implants for prosthesis are placed after the cessation of vertical growth.
- In boys, it will be about early 20s and in girls, 15–17 yrs.

Crossbite Correction

Crossbite in adults can be corrected using:

- Removable appliances
- Fixed appliances
- Removable appliances are indicated when the correction requires only tipping movements.
- Fixed appliance: If vertical control is critical and if bodily movement is required, then arch appliances are utilized.

Diastema Closure

- For better esthetics, partial closure of the incisor space and redistribution of the space is done.
- And followed by composite build-up.

Comprehensive Orthodontic Treatment

Comprehensive treatment is similar to treatment undertaken in adolescent. It involves full fledged treatment with or without extraction of teeth. The orthodontic appliance is usually the bonded kind and esthetic brackets are frequently used (Fig. 30.2).

The treatment objectives of comprehensive orthodontic treatment for adults are the same as for adolescent, namely:

- Dentofacial esthetics
- Stomatognathic function
- Stability

According to Proffit, comprehensive orthodontic treatment would last for duration of more than 6 months. Generally, fixed appliance therapy may last from 1–1½ years. Comprehensive treatment may or may not be combined with surgical orthognathic treatment.

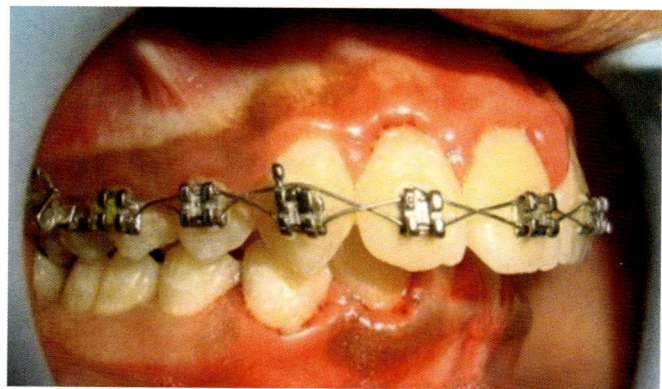

Fig. 30.2: Comprehensive orthodontic treatment in adult patients

Surgical Orthodontic Treatment

A team approach like:

a. *Presurgical orthodontics leveling of arches individually:* It helps in achieving a proper alignment.

b. *Orthognathic surgery proper:* The surgical procedures are sed to establish a proper skeletal relationship. This involves the planned skeletal fracturing of individual skeletal bones—maxilla, mandible and their repositioning with the help of bone plates or wiring as required. Jaw discrepancies in all three planes of space can be corrected.

c. *Post-surgical orthodontics:* It helps to achieve proper interdigitations and final positions of teeth for balance, stability and esthetics.

Bibliography

1. Gustke CJ. Treatment of periodontitis in the diabetic patient. A critical review. J Clin Periodontal 1999;26:133–7.
2. Nattrass C, Sandy JR. Adult orthodontics—a review. Br J Orthod 1995; 22:331–7.

PREVIOUS YEAR'S UNIVERSITY QUESTIONS

MCQs

1. *Generally duration of adjunctive treatment is:*
   a. 8–12 months
   b. More than 12 months
   c. 6 months or more
   d. More than 24 months   **(Ans: c)**

2. *Comprehensive orthodontic treatment patient is usually carried out in:*
   a. 6–7 years
   b. 7–9 years
   c. Young adults
   d. Older individual   **(Ans: c)**

3. *Generally, the duration of comprehensive orthodontic treatment is:*
   a. 8–2 months
   b. 8–16 months
   c. 7–24 months
   d. 4–6 months   **(Ans: b)**

4. *Comprehensive orthodontic treatment refers:*
   a. Orthodontic treatment requires less time
   b. Complete treatment to achieve the best balance between dental and facial esthetics ideal occlusal relationships and dentoalveolar stability
   c. Both a and b
   d. None of the above   **(Ans: b)**

5. *Following are examples of adjunctive orthodontic treatment in adults, except:*
   a. Opening for insertion of single tooth implant
   b. Elimination of interproximal black space
   c. Full fledged orthodontic treatment with or without extraction
   d. None of the above   **(Ans: c)**

6. *The following is a prosthodontic indication of adjunctive orthodontic treatment in adults:*
   a. Paralleling the abutment teeth
   b. Space opening for insertion of single tooth implant
   c. Uprighting of tilted teeth and regaining of space prior to prosthetic replacement of missing teeth
   d. All of the above   **(Ans: d)**

7. *Orthodontist may have to alter the position of bracket placement while treating an adult patient due to:*
   a. Loss of alveolar bone height that shifts the center of resistance of the tooth more apically
   b. Position of bracket placement need not be altered in adults
   c. Loss of alveolar bone height that shifts the center of resistance of the tooth more coronally
   d. Both a and b   **(Ans: d)**

8. *While treating adult orthodontic patients with multiple missing teeth anchorage can be gained by:*
   a. Teeth
   b. Ridge
   c. Mini-implants
   d. All of the above   **(Ans: c)**

Index

3d modular orthodontic instruments 433
4-4 bonded retainer 414
10 measurement analyses 190

Aanchorage 158
Abnormal
    eruptive path 92
    labial frenum 92
    pressure habits 88
    swallowing habit 216
According to Profit 444
Ackerman and Proffit classification 18
Acrylic components 263
Activator 267
Active
    finger sucking habit after 4 years 212
    vertical corrector by Eugene Dellinger
      (1986) 391
Adaptive swallowing behavior 216
Address and occupation 96
Adjunctive orthodontic treatment 469
Advantages of
    Angle's system 13
    digital photography 454
    Katz's classification 18
    laser 378
    screw over spring 246
    spot welding 426
Age 96
Age determination using growth chart 131
Airway obstruction-treatment 360
Alveolar process 51
American Board of Orthodontic (ABO) 444
American cleft palate association's
    classification (1962) 355
Amniotic lesion 87
Anatomy of hand-wrist 131
ANB angle 110
Anchor units 294
Anchorage
    for the herbst aappliance 292
    loss 159
    planning 162
Andresen and Haupl concept 267
Andrew's six keys (1970) 14
Angle of
    convexity 116
    mandible 49
Angle's class
    I malocclusion 8
    II malocclusion 8
    III malocclusion 11

Angle's classification 7, 320
Angulation of inclined plane 259
Ankylosis 92
Anomalies
    in tooth number 88
    of tooth shape 90
    of tooth size 90
Antegonial notch 50
Anterior
    and posterior expansion 248
    inclined bite plane 242
    open bite 324, 336
Aperture 440
Apical base method 408
Appliance therapy 214
Application of 419
    3d imaging to modern orthodontic 403
    laser in orthodontics 378
    soldering in orthodontics 426
    welding in orthodontics 426
Applied anatomy 252
Aramentarium 125
Arch perimeter analysis 122
Argon laser 377
Articular angle 117
Ashley Howe's analysis 122
Assessment of
    anteroposterior jaw relationship 98
    facial asymmetry 97
    vertical skeletal relationship 99
Asymmetrical mandibular prognathism 188
Attributes 223
Australian wires (AJ wilcock wires) 282
Automatic identification of landmarks 459
Autonomous fixed appliance (Darendilier
    and Joho (1992) 391

Ballard's classification 14
Band and
    bar type 169
    loop 168
    spur retainer 414
Banded
    canine-to-canine retainer 414
    tooth- and tissue-borne appliances 253
Banding instruments 430
Bands 281
Base plates 243
Basic
    chin cup appliance design 305
    principles of distraction osteogenesis 194
    tennets of growth: pattern, variability
      and timing 33
    theorems of retention 409

Bauru Yardstick for BCLP 356
Begg appliance or light force technique or
    differential force technique 286
Begg's retainer 411
Behavior learning theory-Palermo (1956) 206
Benefits
    of orthodontic treatment 2
    of the early treatment approach 333
    to patients 333
    to practitioners 334
Benjamin's theory (1962) 206
Bennett's classification of malocclusion 16
Beta angle 117
Biochemical control of tooth movement 151
Biologic
    concept of magnetic force and
      histologic changes 388
    control of tooth movement 146
Biology of tooth movement 146
Biomechanical considerations 304
    when treating adult patients 468
Biomechanics of vertical pull headgear 305
Bionator 270
    types 270
Bite planes 241
    registration 273
Bitewing radiograph 395
Bjork, Grave and Brown method 135
Bjork-Jarabak analysis 117
Blood flow theory/fluid dynamic theory 150
Body of mandible 49
Bolton's analysis 123
Bondable brackets 285
Bonded
    retainer with multistranded wire 413
    retainers 412
    RME 254
Bone
    adaptation 408
    bending piezoelectric theory 149
    implant interaction 374
Bows 225
Bracket
    debonding pliers 432
    positioning instruments 430
    welding with mesh 426
Brackets 282, 284
Branches of orthodontics 2
British standard institute classification
    (incisor classification) 16
Bruxism 219
Buccal
    bar 170
    tubes 281

Buccally displaced maxillary canines and incisors 182
Buccinator mechanism 70
Bulb prosthesis 369
Butler's field theory 84

Calculation of dai scores 26
Camera 436
Canine
    classification 16
    impaction 180
Canines 309
Carey's analysis 122
Caries control 166
Case history 96
    and clinical examination 95
Casts and articulators 451
Causative factors 212
Causes for anterior crossbite 317
Causes of relapse 408
Caution 441
Cell division 77
Cemented type of inclined plane 259
Center of
    resistance 141
    rotation 142
Cephalic and facial examination 97
Cephalocaudal gradient of growth 33
Cephalogram 108
Cephalometric
    analysis 108
    analysis and treatment planning 461
    findings of bimaxillary protrusion 113
    findings of class III malocclusion 113
    for orthognathic surgery 190
    landmarks 109
    landmarks and planes 109
    radiograph 397
Cephalostat 108
Ceramic brackets 285
Cervical
    headgear 301
    vertebrae as indicators of skeletal maturity 135
Changes in the 'U' 469
    mandibular arch 64
    maxillary arch 64
    tooth structure 468
Characteristics of lines of forces 387
Chief complaint 96
Chin 51
Chin cup appliance 304
Choice of teeth for extraction 309
Chronological age 130
Cinefluororadiography 404
Circumferential supracrestal fibrotomy (CSF) 185
Clasp 228
Class III malocclusion 102
Classification based on abnormal skeletal pattern 321

Classification of
    appliances 223
    class II malocclusion 320
    cleft lip and cleft palate 353
    distraction device 195
    FR 262
    functional appliances 257
    implants for orthodontic anchorage 372
    occlusion 66
    open bite 335
    oral habits 204
    retainers 410
    space maintainers 167
    thumb sucking 209
    treatment modalities with DO 195
Clinical
    and radiographic signs of impaction 181
    features of lip habits 219
    frankfort mandibular plane angle (FMA) 99
    implications of genetics in orthodontics 81
    significance of growth spurts 35
    techniques 444
Clip-on retainer or spring realigner 411
Closing diastemas 391
CO$_2$ 377
Coffin spring 249
Cold welding 425
Common indications for placement of implants 372
Comparison between manual and computerized prediction 460
Complex (skeletal) deep bite 345
Componenets of
    class II malocclusion 319
    fixed appliance 276
    FR 263
    FRD 296
    removable appliance 224
Comprehensive orthodontic treatment 470
Computerized digital photography 453
Concept of viscoelastic property 267
Concepts of growth 33
Contraindications for
    orthodontic treatment in adults 467
    space maintainers 166
Control of biofilms during orthodontic treatment 385
Controlled and uncontrolled tipping 143
Conventional vs digital photography 454
Coronoid process 51
Correction of
    anterior crossbite 317
    mandibular abnormalities 191
    maxillary abnormalities 192
Corrective orthodontics 3
Cortical anchorage 160
Couple 142

Cranial
    base 41
    vault 40
Craniofacial imaging and animation with the laser scanner 465
Cranium
    development of the skull 40
    occipital or parietal anchorage 160
Criteria for a good retainer 410
Crossbite 341
Cross-sectional studies 32
Crowding 324, 349
Crown and loop 171
    appliance 168
    with rest 171
Cytotoxicity 389

Davis and Ritchie classification (1922) 353
Debanding plier 433
Deciduous dentition stage 58
Deep bite 344
Definition
    and introduction 68
    of growth and development 28
    of habits 204
    of thumb sucking 209
Deglutition (swallowing) 71
Degree of
    root resorption and root resorption index 155
    severity of root resorption 155
Delayed eruption of permanent teeth 92
Demerits 19
Dens evaginatus 92
Dental
    aesthetic index (DAI) 25
    age 131
    caries 92
    changes 268
    deep bite 344
    factors 327
    health component 23
    history 96
    parameters 116
    problems 334, 361
Dentoalveolar
    distraction vs periodontal distraction 154
    open bite 335
Dentofacial changes associated with prolonged sucking habit 216
Depth of field 442
Dermatoglyphics and skeletal malocclusion 105
Design and construction 272
Determination of
    anterior ratio 124
    overall ratio 124
Developing anterior crossbite 318
Development of
    habit 205

removable appliances 224
thyroid 40
tongue 40
Developmental spacing 58
Dewey's modification for Angle's classification 13
Diagnostic
database 196
feature for midline diastema 347
Dietary problems (nutritional deficiency) 88
Difference between adolescents and adults 468
Different
extraction procedure 310
methods of correction 347
methods of gaining space 307
methods to accelerate tooth movement 153
types of tooth movement 143
ways of expansion 246
Digit sucking 211
Digital
cephalometrics 459
image 456
images 453
photography 452, 463
radiography 401
study model 128, 465
substraction radiography 405
Digitization 460
Dilaceration 92
Dimensional changes in the dental arches 64
Diode laser 377
Direct
bonding technique 288
digitization 461
Disadvantages of digital photography 454
Distal jet/the lingual distalizer system 313
Distal shoe space maintainer 169
Distraction osteogenesis 193
Down's analysis 115
Drawback of
Angle's classification 13
Pont's analysis 123
the analysis 125
Duration of treatment 259
Dynamic cephalometric function 462

Edard's technique 186
Edgewise brackets 285
Effect
of drugs/medications on tooth movement 152
of rapid maxillary expansion 255
on interarch relationship 216
Elastics
and elastomerics 277
in removable appliance 243
Embryological background 357
Energy product 387

Environment 87
Equilibrium theory 70
Erbium laser 377
Eric Johnson and Brent Larsson (1993) 206
Essential diagnostic aids 95
Essix 171
Esthetic
component 23
problems 361
wires 283
Esthetics 467
Etiologic classification 18
Etiological factors of
angle class III malocclusion 327
class II malocclusion 319
Etiology of
bruxism 219
canine impaction 181
cleft lip and palate 356
crowding 350
deep bite 345
midline diastema 347
open bite 338
tongue thrusting 207
Evaluation of facial proportions 99
Evaluation of the relationship between rest position and habitual occlusion in the vertical plane 102
transverse plane 102
Exercise for tongue 178
Exercises for the lips 177
Expansion appliance 245
Experimental approach 31
Extraction of
first molars 310
second permanent molar 310
second premolars 309
third molar 310
Extraoral
anchorage 160
examination 97
radiograph 396
Extrusion of fractured teeth 391

Facial
divergence 98
esthetic analysis 189
profile 97
Factors
affecting growth and maturation 30
to be considered for space maintenance 166
Failure to eliminate the original cause 408
Failures in soldering 429
Family history 96
Features
and effects of deep overbite 346
of open bite 335
Feeding
appliance 362
problems 358

Fiber-reinforced polymeric wires 284
File format and software compression 453
Film 441
First
classification 257
premolars 309
transition period 60
Fishman's skeletal maturity indicators 134
Fixed
anterior bite planes 242
appliances 276
functional appliances 292
lingual mandibular growth modificator-a new appliance for class II correction 296
retainers-types 412
space maintainer 167
Flash and lighting 443
Fluoride application 308
Fogh Andersen (1942) 354
Force 141
module 294
Forces according to their duration 144
Forsus fatigue resistant device 296
Fourth classification 257
FR III appliance 266
FR V appliance 266
Frankel philosophy 261
Frenectomy 186
FR-I appliance 263
FR-IV appliance 266
Frontal
facial 444
view 445
Functional
analysis 101
development 70
orthopaedic magnetic appliances (FOMA) (vardimon) 390

General
examination 97
factors 87
Genetic
code within the DNA molecule 76
disorders 81
disorders and inheritance 80
factors 30
influences on tooth size, number, morphology 84
Genetics and malocclusions 84
Gerber space regainer 177
Glass fiber-reinforced composite resin (GFRCR) as a space maintainer 170
Goals of early orthodontic treatment 332
Gonial angle 118
Goslon Yardstick for UCLP 355
Graber's classification 87
Grades of AJ wilcock wires 283
Gradings 23

Greulich and Pyle method 133
Groper fixed anterior bridge 171
Growth 28
    at sutures 53
    at tissue level 29
    fields 36
    hormones and growth factors 30
    modification 381
    rotation 37
    sites 36
    spurts 35
    theories 44
Gum pad stage 58

Hairstyle can distract facial analysis 449
Hand-wrist radiograph 400
    predictable 129
Handicapping labiolingual deviation
    index (HLD index) 24
Hard magnets-resistant to
    demagnetization 386
Hawley's appliance 410
    with split acrylic dumb-bell spring 177
Hazards, indications and contra-
    indications 255
Headgear 300
Hearing problem 360
Herbst appliance 292
Hereditability and functional component
    of occlusion 84
High pull headgear 306
Historical perspective 174
Holography 379
Hot welding 425
Huckaba radiographic analysis 126
Human chromosomes 73

Icon scoring method 24
Ideal
    occlusion 65
    requirement of a dental solder 428
    requirements 129
    requirements of space maintainer 167
Illness 30
Image
    archiving/storage 457
    display 458
    resolution 464
    storage format 464
Impact of nanotechnology on dental
    implants 384
Implant
    material 373
    sizes 374
Importance of
    first permanent molars 7
    genetics 81
Important characteristics 443
Improper restoration 92
Incisor
    impaction 183
    relationship 60

Incline plane 258
Incomplete and complete deep bite 345
Index of complexity outcome and need
    (ICON) 24
Index of orthodontic treatment needs
    (IOTN) 23
Indications
    for orthodontic treatment in adults 466
    for placement of implants 373
    of hand and wrist X-rays 129
    of space maintainers 166
Indirect
    bonding 290
    digitization 460
Input devices 463
Installation of FRD 296
Instructions to prevent relapse 259
Instruments used for placement of
    separators 430
Interceptive orthodontics 2
Interincisal angle 112
Intermaxillary anchorage 162
International confederation for plastic and
    reconstructive surgery classification
    (1968) 355
Interpretation of growth data 33
Intertransitional period 62
Interventions for accelerating orthodontic
    tooth movement 153
Intramaxillary anchorage 161
Intraoral
    anchorage 160
    photographs 445
    priapical radiograph 395
    radiographs 395
Investment soldering 429

Jasper Jumper appliance 294

Kansal's retainer 412
Katz's classification 18
Kernahan's striped 'y' classification 354
Kesling
    diagnostic setup 126
    tooth positioner 411
Korkhaus analysis 123

Large maxillomandibular advancement
    possible 195
Laser
    Doppler flowmetry 381
    holography 404
    safety 380
    tissue interaction 376
    welding 426
Lashal classification 355
Lateral/profile view 447
Lens 436
Ligature wires 282
Limitations of cephalometry 108
Limitations 311

Limited or short-term retention 407
Linder harth index 123
Line of direction of force 305
Lingual
    arch space maintainer 168
    arch with stops 168
    attachments 280
    brackets 286
    technique 287
    tuberosity 51
Lip
    bumper 313
    habits 218
    print and skeletal malocclusion 104
Lischer's classification 13
Local factors 88
Lock pins 282
Lokar distalizer 312
Longitudinal studies 32

Magnetic
    activator device 392
    brackets 390
    force systems in orthodontics 389
    induction 387
    moment 387
    properties relevant 387
    resonance imaging 401
    retainer 391
    substances 386
    twin blocks 390
Magnets 313
    with fixed appliances (abraham
        blechman, 1985) 389
Maintaining lower incisor position during
    late mandibular growth 414
Management during mixed dentition 322
Management of
    class I malocclusion 317
    class II division 2 malocclusion 323
    class II malocclusion 319, 321
    class II malocclusion in adults 323
    class III malocclusion 327
    cleft lip and palate 362
    deep bite 273
    functional disturbances 322
    palatally displaced canines 181
    skeletal anterior crossbite 318
Mandible at birth 47
Mandibular
    condyle 50
    distraction devices 196
    foramen 50
    incisors 309
    incisor school 408
    plane 110
Mastication 70
Maturation assessment by Hagg and
    Taranger 134
Maturity indicators 129

Maxilla 42
Maxillary
    central incisors 309
    deficiency 328
    lateral incisors 309
    second molar extraction in maxillary
        first molar distalization 311
    sinus 53
    tuberosity 53
Measurement
    and interpretation 115
    approach 30
    of malocclusion 22
Mechanics of tooth movement 141
Mechanism of bone growth 36
Medical history 96
Meiosis 77
Memory screw 252
Mental age 130
Merits 19
Metal brackets 284
Methods of
    classification of malocclusion 4
    placement 372
    studying physical growth 30
    studying role of genes 82
    tongue examination 103
Methods to assess skeletal maturity 132
Midline diastema 346
Millard's classification (1977) 354
Minor surgical procedure 180
Missing teeth 469
Mitosis 77
Mixed dentition
    analysis 125
    period 60, 318
Mixed/semilongitudinal studies 33
Mode of action 261
Model analysis 122
Modes of collection of growth data 32
Modifications of oral screen 261
Modified
    bonded space regainer 176
    ribbon arch brackets in Begg
        technique 285
Molar distalization 311, 390
    in lower arch 311
Molar uprighting simple technique
        (MUST) 315
Moment 142
    to force ratio 142
Mouth breathing 103
    habit 217
Moyer's classification 320
Moyer's mixed dentition analysis 126
Muscle exercises 177
Muscular anchorage 161
    forces 408
Musculature school 408
Myofunctional treatment 55

Nance holding arch 168
Nanocoatings in archwires 384
Nanoparticle delivery from elastomeric
        ligature 385
Nanoparticle in orthodontic adhesive 384
Nanotechnology
    for craniofacial bone and cartilage
        tissue engineering 383
    in orthodontics 384
Nasal cavity 53
Natal
    and neonatal teeth 57
    factors 320
Nd:YAG laser 377
Need for
    classification 4
    orthodontic treatment 2
Neodymium-iron-boron magnets 388
Neural age 130
Neurotropic process in orofacial growth 54
New molar distalizers 314
Newton's first law 141
Nickel titanium expander 250
Non-radiographic 125
Normal development of maxillary
        canine 180
Numerical disorders 81
Nutrition 30

Objectives of this analysis 114
Oblique view 448
Obturator 368
Occlusal
    bar 170
    interdigitation 66
    pad 171
    plane angle 111
    radiograph 396
    splint 220
Occlusion 65
    school 408
Occlusogram 127, 405
One-phase early orthodontic treatment 332
Open
    and closed coil springs 280
    bite 334
    coil space regainer 177
OPG 396
Oral
    drive theory 206
    gratification theory 206
Orbit 53
Origin of mandible 41
Original design 273
Orthodontic
    instruments and orthodontic
        material 430
    study models 421
    surgical text planning 461
    treatment 184
    treatment protocol 200

Orthodontics during distraction and
        consolidation phase 200
Orthognathic surgery 187
Orthopedic
    appliances 299
    changes in class III malocclusion 302
Ossification of the mandible 41
Osteotomy procedures 191
Other
    characteristic features of magnets 387
    diagnostic aids 104
    theories related to craniofacial
        growth 46
Over correction 200

Palatal remodeling and increase in
        maxillary height 54
Palate 42
Parental counseling 166
Parts of
    a study model 421
    face mask 302
    implant 374
Pattern 33
Patterns of genetic transmission 82
Peck and Peck classification 20
Peer assessment rating 24
Pendulum appliance 311
Periodontal
    indications for orthodontic treatment in
        adults 467
    ligament traction 408
Periods of growth and dental
        development (Hellman) 57
Permanent dentition 318
Pharyngeal
    arches 39
    pouches 39
Phases of
    early orthodontic treatment 332
    growth 29
    tooth movement 151
Philosophy of
    bionator 270
    chin cup therapy 305
Photocephalometry 403, 463
Physiological and biochemical age 130
Pitch, roll and yaw in systematic
        description 20
Pixels and resolution 463
Planes and lines 109
Plastic brackets 284
Polynorborgen 284
Pont's analysis 122
Position and eruption 84
Possible mechanism for formation of
        isolated cleft palate 357
Possible stages of orthodontic treatment
        timing 334
Post-distraction orthodontics 201

Posterior
  bites plane 242
  crossbite 325, 327
  open bite 341
Postnatal
  cranial base 43
  factor 320
  growth of craniofacial complex 43
  growth of mandible 47
  growth of nasomaxillary complex 52
  growth of the cranial vault 43
  history 97
  influences 87
Postural habit 219
Powell's aesthetic triangle 101
Power scope 298
Predisposing metabolic climate and
    disease 87
Preformed posterior space maintainer 169
Premature loss of deciduous teeth 90
Prenatal
  factors 319
  growth of craniofacial region 38
  history 96
Pressure tension theory 147
Presurgical orthodontics 190
Preventive
  measures undertaken 166
  orthodontics 2
Primary
  atypical swallowing behavior 217
  translation/displacement 52
Principle of laser 375
Principles of retention 407
Problems with anterior bite planes 241
Profile video image modification 462
Prolonged retention of deciduous 91
Propellant unilateral magnetic appliance
    (PUMA) 390
Properties of magnets 386
Prosthodontic indications for orthodontic
    treatment of adults 467
Protein synthesis 76
Proximal reduction 308
Pseudo class III 328
Psychoanalytic theory 206
Psychological problems 361
Psychological stress 30

Quad helix appliance 249
Quantified profile modification through
    extrapolation 462
Quantifying the classification 18

Radiographic assessment of canine
    position 181
Radiographs 451
Raleigh Williams' six keys to eliminate
    lower retention 416
Ramus 48
Rapid maxillary expansion (RME)
    appliances 252

Rare earth magnets and impaction 390
Reactivation of twin block 274
Recent advances 127, 155
  in diagnosis 118
  of FFD 296
Reciprocal anchorage 160
Recycling 393
Red-eye 443
Relapse due to growth related changes 408
Reliability of simon norms 16
Removable
  functional appliances 257
  functional regulator (FR) 261
  of soft tissue and bony barrier to enable
    eruption of teeth 186
  orthodontic appliances 223
  space maintainers 167
Replication of nucleic acid 76
Requirements
  of DNA 75
  of orthodontic index 23
  to do model analysis 121
Respiration 72
Respiratory tract infections 359
Rest position 102
Retainers 410
Retention
  class II 415
  class III 415
Reverse pull headgear 302
Ribbon arch brackets 285
Risk factors for root resorption 156
Risk factors of root resorption after
    orthodontic treatment 155
Role of
  growth pattern on treatment
    decisions 55
  occlusion 409
  orthodontist in cleft lip and palate 366
  radiography in orthodontics 394
  third molars 409
Root resorption 155

Saddle angle 117
Safety valve mechanism 65
Sagittal
  appliance 248
  type crossbite (anterior crossbite) 341
Salient features 19
Salzman's classification 86
Samarium-cobalt magnets 388
Sample depth 457
Scammon's growth curve 34
Schools of retention 408
Season and circadian rhythm 30
Second
  classification 257
  transitional period 60
Secondary translation 52
Secular trends 30

Separators 276
Serial extraction 173
Severity ratings of AP system 19
Sex 96
Sexual/pubertal age 130
Shape memory polymers in
    orthodontics 385
Short notes 55, 393, 406
Shutter speed 440
Side effects 302
Significance of anthropoid spaces 60
Simon's classification 16
Simple anchorage 159
Singer's method of assessment 133
Single gene disorders 81
Sites of placement 372
Skeletal
  age 131
  changes 268
  class III 328
  factors 327
  malocclusion 16
  maturity indicators 129
Slow expansion appliance 246
Slow type 246
Smart brackets with nanomechanical
    sensors 385
Smile 103
SNB angle 110
Soft tissue analysis 112
Soldering procedure 427
Space
  maintainers 166
  maintenance 165
  regainers 175
  regaining 175
Speech 72
  problem 360
  prosthesis 368
Speed 441
Spot
  welder 426
  welding 425
Springs 236, 286
Stability of class III malocclusion 330
Stage I: use of presurgical orthopedics 362
Stage II: treatment of CLCP in deciduous
    dentition 365
Stage III: treatment of CLCP in mixed
    dentition 366
Stage IV: treatment of CLCP in permanent
    dentition 366
Stages of
  development used by Bjork and
    Helm 252
  twin block 273
Stationary anchorage 159
Steiner's analysis 110
Steps in
  fabrication 262

fabrication of oral screen 261
  preparation of study models 421
Sterilization 433
Straight
  pull headgear 305
  wire technique 288
Strategies of class II division 1
    malocclusion 321
Structural disorders 82
Structure of nucleic acid 74
Study model and model analysis 121
Study model preparation 421
Submucous cleft 367
Superimposition 118
Supplemental diagnostic aids 96
Surface bone remodeling 53
Surgical
  assisted rapid palatal expansion 193
  orthodontic treatment 470
  orthodontics 3
Synchronization 443
Syndromic cleft 356
Synonyms 267, 307

Tanaka and Johnston 126
Technical procedure 429
Techniques 286
  for soldering 427
Teeth mineralization as skeletal maturity
    indicator 137
Teflon-coated wires 284
Teleradiology 458
Temporary anchorage device (TAD) 163
Temporomandibular joint
    dysfunction 467
Tests to diagnose the mode of
    respiration 217
Theorem 1–7 409
Theorem 8–10 410
Theories of
  cleft lip and palate 357
  tooth movement 146
Third classification 257
Three-dimensional imaging 464
Thumb/finger sucking habit 209
Timing of distalization 311
Timing of growth 35
Tip-edge
  brackets 285
  technique 287

Tipping 143
To conclude 455
Tomography 401
Tongue thrusting habit 206
Tooth-borne appliances 253
Total digital radiography 458
Tracing
  of the polygon 117
  supplies and equipment 109
  technique 109
  the gene in family pedigree studies 82
Trajectories of mandible 69
Transition twin block 274
Transpalatal
  arch (Goshgarian arch) 169
  with omega loop 169
Transverse
  expansion 247
  type crossbite (posterior crossbite) 342
Treatment
  during adulthood 329
  for deep bite 325
  modalities in growing and non-
    growing patients 346
  of adolescent child 329
  of class II malocclusion 321
  of midline diastema 348
  of preadolescent child 329
  of tongue thrust habit 208
  plan for class III malocclusion 329
Trident of habit factors 88, 212
Trimming 271
  the activator for vertical control 269
Tweed's
  analysis 113
  classification of anchorage
    preparation 162
  growth trends 114
Twelve keys to stability of lower incisors 417
Twin
  block appliance 272
  studies 82
Two-phase treatment 333
Two-stage interalveolar corticotomy 183
Types of
  activator 268
  cameras 436
  computers 456
  crowding 349

expansion screw 246
flash 443
growth 29
growth data 32
index 22
laser 377
lens 439
magnetic materials 388
retention 407
root resorption 155
space maintainers 167
treatment in adults 469
welding 425

Unfavorable sequelae of malocclusion 2
Uprighting 144
  of molars 315
Use of computer application in
    orthodontics 456
Uses 121
  and limitations of cephalometry 108
  of cephalometry 108
  of diagnostic setup 126
  of orthodontic implants 373
Utility and specialty pliers 431

Vacuum-formed (Essix) retainer 412
Variability 33
Variations of Angle's classes 12
Various
  methods of digital radiography 458
  problems 357
Veau's classification (1931) 354
Vestibular screen 260
Videocephalometry 462
Viscoelastic activity 268
Visual treatment objective (VTO) 258

W-arch appliance 249
Weldable brackets 285
Welding and soldering 425
Wilson 3d lingual arch 171
Wire
  cutting instruments 432
  forming pliers 431
Wits appraisal 115
Wolff's law of transformation of bone 68
Wrap around retainer 411

Xeroradiography 400

Zygoma 54